# Food and Nutrition: A Human Health Perspective

# Food and Nutrition: A Human Health Perspective

Editor: Zoey Watson

MURPHY & MOORE
www.murphy-moorepublishing.com

**Murphy & Moore Publishing,**
1 Rockefeller Plaza,
New York City, NY 10020, USA

Visit us on the World Wide Web at:
www.murphy-moorepublishing.com



ISBN: 978-1-63987-228-2 (Hardback)



**Cataloging-in-Publication Data**

Food and nutrition : a human health perspective / edited by Zoey Watson.
p. cm.
Includes bibliographical references and index.
ISBN 978-1-63987-228-2
1. Food. 2. Nutrition. 3. Health. I. Watson, Zoey.

RA601 .F66 2022

641.3--dc23

# Table of Contents

# Preface

Nutrition refers to the physiological and biochemical process for the utilization of food by living organisms to support life. Food nutrients, such as carbohydrates, proteins, minerals, vitamins, fats, fiber and water help organisms to grow, survive and reproduce. When the essential nutrients are not made available through diet in the right proportion, deficiency diseases may occur such as anemia, scurvy, blindness, stillbirth, preterm birth, etc. High consumption of certain nutrients can also lead to conditions such as metabolic syndrome, obesity, diabetes, and cardiovascular diseases, among others. This book is a compilation of chapters that discuss the most vital concepts and emerging trends in the field of food and nutrition. Different approaches, evaluations, methodologies and advanced studies on nutrition and human diet have been included herein. This book is a collective contribution of a renowned group of international experts.

The researches compiled throughout the book are authentic and of high quality, combining several disciplines and from very diverse regions from around the world. Drawing on the contributions of many researchers from diverse countries, the book's objective is to provide the readers with the latest achievements in the area of research. This book will surely be a source of knowledge to all interested and researching the field.

In the end, I would like to express my deep sense of gratitude to all the authors for meeting the set deadlines in completing and submitting their research chapters. I would also like to thank the publisher for the support offered to us throughout the course of the book. Finally, I extend my sincere thanks to my family for being a constant source of inspiration and encouragement.

**Editor**

# 1

# Inhibitory effects of quail egg on mast cells degranulation by suppressing PAR2-mediated MAPK and NF-kB activation

Priscilia Lianto[1,2], Fredrick O. Ogutu[3], Yani Zhang[2], Feng He[2] and Huilian Che[1,2*]

[1]Beijing Advanced Innovation Center for Food Nutrition and Human Health, College of Food Science and Nutritional Engineering, China Agricultural University, Beijing, 100083, P.R. China; [2]College of Food Science and Nutritional Engineering, China Agricultural University, Beijing, 100083, P.R. China; and [3]Food Technology Division of Kenya Industrial Research and Development Institute, South C – Popo Rd., Off Mombasa Rd., PO Box 30650-00100, Nairobi, Kenya

*Abstract*

***Background:*** Quail egg (QE) has been reported to possess an anti-allergic and anti-inflammatory activity. We have demonstrated that whole QE was able to attenuate the allergic symptoms in food allergy–induced EoE murine model, but whether QE albumen or QE yolk plays a more important role still remains unclear.
***Objective:*** In this current study, we investigated the suppressive role of QE in mast cell degranulation and cytokine production of the effect phase response.
***Method:*** A passive cutaneous anaphylaxis (PCA) mouse model was used to confirm the anti-allergic effect of QE. Besides, HMC-1 cell model was used to study its suppressive role in more detail. In this *in vitro* study, we divided QE into three groups: whole QE, QE albumen, and QE yolk. The effect of QE treatment on mast cell degranulation and intracellular calcium influx was investigated. Moreover, the effect of QE allergy– related mediators, genes, and proteins were also assessed by ELISA, RT-PCR, and western blotting.
***Results and discussion:*** Our data showed that the extent of mast cell degranulation–mediated ear vascular permeability in IgE-mediated PCA mice treated with whole QE (17 mg/kg) was decreased significantly up to 43.31 ± 0.42% reduction. HMC-1 cell–based immunological assay *in vitro* indicated that QE, particularly its albumen, acted as a 'mast cell stabilizer'. Under the concentration of 70 μg/mL, QE albumen effectively suppressed the releases of β-hexosaminidase, histamine, and tryptase, as well as Th2 and pro-inflammatory cytokine production; reached 30 up to 50% reduction. Besides, QE albumen was also able to significantly modulate the upregulation of IL-10 up to 58.30 ± 5.9%. Interestingly, our data indicated that QE yolk still had a significant inhibitory effect on modulating Th2 cytokines in its highest concentration (100 μg/mL), while QE albumen showed no inhibitory effect. Western blot analysis showed QE albumen effectively down-regulated the expressions of calcium-related protein (TRPC1, Orai1, STIM1, PLC-γ and IP3R), facilitated the reduction of PAR-2 and induced the reduction of phosphorylation of JNK, IKKα, p50 and p65 protein expressions.
***Conclusion:*** As confirmed by PCA and HMC-1 cell-based immunology assay, QE albumen and QE yolk may work together through exerting anti-allergy activity and can be used as a potential anti-allergic nutrient in the future.

Keywords: *quail egg; mast cells; anti-allergic; PAR-2; degranulation; activation*

Pervasiveness of allergic diseases such as atopic dermatitis, asthma, food allergy, hives, and hay fever is a serious health issue. These diseases are classified into type I hypersensitivity caused by release of the granule-stored mediators such as histamine, proteases, lipid mediators, and cytokines from mast cells (1). In addition, mast-cell mediators apparently through the protease-activated receptor (PAR)-2 may likewise contribute to the development of unending and allergic inflammation by supporting the inflow of inflammatory cells, such as eosinophils, macrophages, lymphocytes and basophils, prompting tissue inflammation (2). Thus far, there are no treatments accessible to cure allergic diseases entirely. However, a few pharmaceuticals as well as mast cell stabilizers (disodium cromoglycate, sodium hydroxypropylcromate, ketotifen, etc.), anti-histamine drugs (diphenhydramine, chlorpheniramine maleate, terfenadine, etc.), and immune suppressors (adrenal cortical hormones, dexamethasone, hydrocortisone, etc.) are essentially utilized to help relieve unfavorable allergic symptoms and reduce the distress of anaphylaxis through stabilizing mast cells for treating allergic disease. When mast cells are stabilized, they are not readily triggered by stimulatory factors, such as allergens, to engage in steps leading to the discharge of preformed pharmacologic mediators and the new synthesis of inflammatory lipid mediators and cytokines (3). However, these medications not only have side effects but also do not counteract symptom reoccurring. Therefore, natural anti-allergic ingredients would be a suitable option for anti-allergic strategy.

Previous studies suggest that quail egg (QE) is different from other bird eggs. This distinction particularly originates from its egg albumen, which is richer in proteins that have anti-allergic and anti-inflammatory effects (4–6). A patent on the role of QE in controlling the immune cell function, particularly eosinophils and neutrophils, in the treatment of hypersensitivity, was issued in 2015 by the United States (patent number: US2015/0057232A1) (7), giving strong establishments of the unique role of QE. A number of clinical studies have also indicated the therapeutic effect of QE as allergic asthmatic (8) and rhinitis treatments (9). More recently, our study has also shown the therapeutic potential of QE in in attenuating the symptoms of murine model food allergy induced Eosinophilic esophagitis like disease (10). However, the suppressive role by which QE inhibits mast cell degranulation and allergic type I responses is not well defined.

In this study, we investigated the suppressive effect of QE on modulating mast cell activation–mediated immediate allergic response. Herein, we used PCA and HMC-1 *in vivo* and *in vivo* mast cell model experiments to describe suppressive effects of QE on modulating mast cell degranulation–mediated immediate allergy hypersensitivity.

## Materials and methods

### *Chemicals*

The chemicals were obtained from the following suppliers: monoclonal anti-Dinitrophenyl antibody produced in mouse (anti-DNP IgE, D8406), dinitrophenol-human serum albumin (DNP-HSA), Compound 48/80 (C48/80, C2313), water-soluble tetrazolium-8 (WST-8, 96992), 4-nitrophenyl N-acetyl-b-D-glucosaminide (N9376), Evans blue (E2129), and Fluo-3AM (39294) (Sigma–Aldrich Corp., USA); TransCript One-Step gDNA Removal and cDNA Synthesis SuperMix (AT311) and TransStrart Top Green qPCR SuperMix (AQ131) (TransGen Biotech, China); Commercial human ELISA kits (eBioscience, Inc., San Diego, CA); BCA Protein Assay Kit (CW0014S, CW-Biotech, Beijing China). Anti-β-actin antibody (ab36861), anti-Transient Receptor Potential Channel 1 (TRPC-1) antibody (ab192031), anti-Calcium Release Activated Calcium Channel Protein 1 (Orai1) antibody (ab83751), anti-Stromal Interaction Molecule 1(STIM1) antibody (ab59342), anti-*Phospholipase C-gamma* (PLC-γ) antibody (ab37384), anti- and Inositol 1, 4,5-Trisphosphate Receptor (IP3R) antibody (ab38557), anti-Extracellular Signal-Regulated Kinase (ERK1/2) antibody (ab30258), anti-p38 antibody (ab30359), anti c-Jun N-Terminal Kinase (JNK1/2) antibody (ab303154) (Abcam, UK); anti-IkappaBalpha (IKK-α) antibody (397700), anti-Nuclear Factor Kappa B (NF-kB) p50 antibody (14-6732-81), anti NF-kB p65 antibody (14-6731-63), (eBioscience, Inc., San Diego, CA). All other reagents used in this study were of analytical grade.

### *Sample preparation*

Normal, commercially available, fresh QE (*Coturnix* sp.) were obtained from a local egg market. QE were divided into three groups: whole QE (egg albumen and yolk), QE albumen (albumen separated from egg yolk), and QE yolk (yolk separated from egg albumen). Each of the groups was mixed using mixer (Joyoung Co Ltd.), freeze-dried and powdered using vacuum freezer (Alpha 1-2 LD plus, Martin Christ, Germany), and then packed and stored at −20°C.

### *Animals and management*

Female BALB/c mice aged 7–8 weeks were purchased from Weitong Lihua Experimental Animal Technology Co., Ltd. (Beijing, China; No: SCXK(Jing)2016-0001) and acclimatized to their new housing for a week before beginning experimental protocols. Animal experiments employed age-, gender-, and genetic-strain-matched controls to account for any variations in data sets compared across experiments. Mice were bred and housed under specific pathogen-free (SPF) conditions in the animal laboratory of College of Food Science and Nutritional Engineering, China Agricultural University (Beijing, China). Experimental mice rooms were maintained at a temperature of 23 ± 3°C, relative humidity of 40–70%, light/dark cycle of 12 h, and air exchanges at 15 times/hour. Experimental mice were provided with *ad libitum* access to fresh filtered water and standard rodent diet (moisture, ash, crude protein, fat, crude fiber, calcium, and phosphorus) produced by Ke Ao Xie Li Feed Co., Ltd. (Beijing, China). It met Chinese Standard GB14924.3-2010 feeding condition requirement, and the limit of detection for aflatoxin was below 20 μg/kg. All experiments were performed under the China Agricultural University Animal Experimental Welfare and Ethical Inspection Committee approved protocols and in accordance with its guidelines. All efforts were made to minimize the suffering of experimental animals.

### *Establishment of IgE-mediated PCA model in BALB/c mice*

The PCA assay was carried out following procedure previously described by Knoops et al. (11). Basically, one ear of the animal is injected with anti-DNP-IgE, and the other is left alone. Thus, 1 h post-dosing animals are challenged with a tail vein injection of DNP-HSA diluted in Evan's blue dye. Signs of blue reaction and swelling from the site of IgE-sensitized ear represent mast cell degranulation. One hour after the last injection, mice are euthanized and ear punch biopsies from both ears are harvested to quantify Evan's blue content in the ear tissue using spectrophotometric techniques for measuring dye extravasation into the tissue. The PCA assay in this study was performed according to the schedule set-forth in this study protocol with slight modifications.

Ten female BALB/c mice (4 weeks old, weighing 18–22 g) were divided into two groups ($n$ = 5). All tested mice received an intradermal injection of 0.5 μg of anti-DNP IgE in 30 μL of saline in the right ear. A week prior to sensitization, BALB/c mice were given 17 mg/kg·bw of daily oral egg treatments. The amount for oral administration was followed by the recommended dietary intake of QE by Integrative Therapeutics (integrativepro.com/allqlear • 800.931.1709) which is 84 mg/day for humans (12). For the dose conversion of QE dietary treatment, we followed a Simple Practice Guide for Dose Conversion between Animals and Human by using the average weight of human body in China, which is around 60 kg (13). The formula of calculation is:

$$\text{Human equivalent dose}\left(\text{mg}/\text{kg}\right) = \text{mouse equivalent dose}\left(\text{mg}/\text{kg}\right) \times \frac{\text{dosage conversion factors for mouse}}{\text{dosage conversion factors for human}}$$

$$\frac{84\,\text{mg}}{60\,\text{kg}} = \text{mouse equivalent dose}\left(\text{mg}/\text{kg}\right) \times \frac{3}{37}$$

Therefore, in this experiment, the dose of QE was 17 mg/kg weight body/animal. During the experiment period, QE-treated BALB/c mice were also given concurrently continuous access to QE by feeding water containing 17 mg/L QE. On day 8, each mouse was injected intraperitoneally with 200 μL of DNP-HSA and Evans blue solution (100 μg DNP-HSA and 2% Evans blue in 0.9% NaCl). After challenge, Evans blue extravasation in the right ear was captured by a Canon Electro Optical System (EOS) camera (Canon, Inc., Japan) as a qualitative analysis of vascular permeability. The mice were sacrificed 40 min after treatment with DNP-HSA, and right ears were collected. The ear dye color was extracted by incubating ear with formamide at 64°C for 12 h. The absorbance of the dye was determined at 620 nm using the Thermo Scientific Varioskan Flash (Thermo, USA) to quantitatively assess the vascular permeability.

*HMC-1-cells-based immunological assay*

The human mast cell line (HMC-1) obtained from national platform of experimental cell resources (Beijing, China) was cultured in RPMI 1640 medium supplemented with 10% fetal bovine serum (FBS) and $1\times10^5$ U/L penicillin/streptomycin at 37°C in a humidified 5% $CO_2$ incubator. Thus, this study using HMC-1 mast cell line conducted mast cell viability and degranulation experiment assays.

Cell numbers of HMC-1 after QE pre-treatments were examined using WST-8 assay kit according to manufacturer's instructions. WST-8 is reduced by dehydrogenases in cells to give an orange-colored product (formazan), which is soluble in the tissue culture medium. The amount of the formazan dye generated by dehydrogenases in cells is directly proportional to the number of living cells (14). In brief, $1\times10^4$ HMC-1 cells/mL medium were pre-incubated with various concentrations of 0, 50, 100, 500, and 1000 μg/mL of QE groups. After incubation for 30 min, 10 μL of WST-8 was added for incubating for another 30 min at 37°C. Finally, supernatants were transferred into another 96-well plate for measurement at 450 nm with a Thermo Scientific Varioskan Flash plate reader (Thermo, USA).

The HMC-1 cell–based immunological assay was carried out following procedure previously described by Hohman & Dreskin with some modification (15). Firstly, the cells were pre-incubated with QE group treatments with various concentrations (0, 50, 70, 100 μg/mL) for 30 min. Afterward, the cells were stimulated with 100 μg/mL C48/80 for 45 min at 37°C. After stimulation with C48/80 for 1 h, cell solution was centrifuged at 1,500 rpm for 5 min, 30 μL of supernatant was collected and transferred to a 96-well plate and incubated with 50 μL of p-Nitrophenyl-N-Acetyl-β-D-Glucosaminide (1.3 mg/mL in 0.1 M citric acid buffer, pH 4.5) for 1 h at 37°C. The reaction was terminated by adding 200 μL stop solution (0.1 M $Na_2CO_3$/$NaHCO_3$, pH 10.0). Each well absorbance was measured at 405 nm using a Thermo Scientific Varioskan Flash microtiter plate reader (Thermo, USA). The total release of β-hexosaminidase was determined in HMC-1 cells without egg treatments and the spontaneous release of HMC-1 cells was evaluated by adding 50 μL of medium only instead of C48/80 to each well. Aliquots of the cell lysate or culture supernatant were sonicated in 130 μL of the modified medium containing 0.1% Triton X-100 at 37°C for 45 min. The release of β-hexosaminidase activity was measured using 4-nitrophenyl 2-acetamido-2-deoxy-β-D-glucopyranoside (PNAG) as described previously by Kuehn et al. (16). The formula of the release of β-hexosaminidase calculation is:

$$\beta\text{-hexosaminidase release}\left(100\%\right) = \frac{Absorbance_{supernatant} - Absorbance_{blank\ of\ supernatant}}{Absorbance_{total\ release} - Absorbance_{cell\ lysate}} \times 100\%$$

*Measurement of allergic mediators and cytokines*

The HMC-1-based immunological assay on detecting histamine and tryptase release levels was performed similar to the β-hexosaminidase release detection assay, while for the detection of Th2 cytokines (IL-4, IL-5, IL-10 and IL-13) and pro-inflammatory cytokines (IL-6, IL-8, and TNF-α), this study conducted a slight modification of cell stimulation time. After QE-pretreated HMC-1 cells were stimulated with C48/80 for either 1 h or 8 h, cell solution was centrifuged at 1,500 rpm for 5 min. Culture supernatants of cells were collected and stored in −80°C prior to mediator and cytokine level analysis. All these allergic mediators and cytokines were determined using ELISA kit according to the manufacturer's instructions (eBioscience, Inc., San Diego, CA).

In brief, each mediator standard was set and 50 μL standard diluent was added to standard well. 10 μL testing sample was added to testing sample well, and then was followed by addition of 40 μL sample diluent. Blank wells were not added anything. 100 μL of horseradish peroxidase-conjugated streptavidin (HRP labelled avidin working fluid) was added to each well, covered with an adhesive strip, and incubated at 37°C for 60 min. Each well was aspirated and washed five times with phosphate-buffered saline (pH 7.4) containing 0.1% Tween-20 (PBST washing dilution). 50 μL chromogen solution A and 50 μL chromogen solution B were added, gently mixed, and incubated at 37°C for 15 min with no light condition. In the end, 50 μL terminate solution (100 μL of 2 N sulfuric acid) was added to each well, gently mixed, and then within 5 min, the absorbance value of each hole was measured at 450 nm wavelength using a microplate reader Thermo Scientific Varioskan Flash (Thermo, USA). The detection limits of allergic mediators and cytokines were as follows: histamine (0.1 ng/mL), tryptase (1.0 ng/mL), IL-5 (0.1 pg/mL), IL-4, IL-6, IL-10, IL-13, (1.0 pg/mL), TNF-α (1.7 pg/mL), and IL-8 ECP (2.0 pg/mL).

*Measurement of intracellular calcium ($Ca^{2+}$) concentration*

Intracellular calcium influx was measured according to the previous method described by Huber et al. (17). Cells were seeded into a 96-well black opaque cell culture plate. After pre-incubation with or without QE treatments, cells were incubated with 5 μM of Fluo-3AM for 30 min at 37°C in the dark condition. Following a 30s baseline recording, cells were challenged for another 300s with 100 μg/mL of C48/80. The fluorescence intensity (FI) was recorded using the Thermo Scientific Varioskan Flash microtiter plate reader (Thermo, USA) with excitation wavelength at 488 nm and emission wavelength at 525 nm. The formula of $[Ca^{2+}]_i$ calculation is:

$$[Ca^{2+}]_I \text{ (nm)} = K_d[(F-F_{min})/(F_{max}-F)]$$

where $F_{min}$ is the background fluorescence with 5 mM EGTA and $F_{max}$ is the maximum fluorescence with 0.1% Triton X-100 instead of C48/80. The effective dissociation constant (Kd) of Fluo-3 and $Ca^{2+}$ is 400 nM.

*RT-PCR analysis*

QE-pretreated HMC-1 cells were stimulated with C48/80 for 6 h. Total RNA was extracted using Trizol reagent and cDNA was transcribed using the TransScript One-Step gDNA Removal and cDNA Synthesis SuperMix. RT-PCR was conducted using the TransStart Top Green qPCR SuperMix for PAR-2 and β-actin. PCR for HMC-1 was performed with primers as follows:

5'-TTTCTCTCGGTGCGTCCAG-3' (sense) and
5'-GTTCCTTGGATGGTGCCACT-3' (anti-sense) for PAR2;
5'-CTCGCCTTTGCCGATCC-3' (sense) and 5'-GGG GTACTTCAGGGTGAGGA -3' (anti-sense) for β-actin.

Quantitative real-time PCR conducted under the thermal cycling conditions involved denaturation step at 95°C for 1 min, followed by 40 cycles at 94°C for 30s, 60°C for 30s, 72°C for 30s, and the final melting curve program with raping rate 0.5°C/0.05 sec from 55°C to 95°C. Using β-actin as the internal control gene, the relative quantitative level of mRNA was calculated by $2^{-\Delta\Delta Ct}$ method $C_t$ is the threshold cycle and ΔCt was calculated from test $C_t$-β actin $C_t$.

*Western blotting*

Western blotting was performed according to the previous method described by Mahmood & Yang (18). For the detection of calcium channel–related protein expression, QE-pretreated HMC-1 cells were stimulated with C48/80 for 1 h, while for the detection of mitogen-activated protein kinases (MAPK) and nuclear factor-kappaB (NF-kB) cell signaling pathway–related protein expression, cells were stimulated for 6 h. After stimulation, HMC-1 cell samples were lysed with lysis buffer containing protease inhibitors, and centrifuged at 4°C and 12,000 g for 15 min. The supernatants were collected and the protein concentration of the supernatant was determined using a BCA Protein Assay Kit. The total cell lysates (50–70 μg of total protein) from different samples were subjected to 10% SDS-PAGE, transferred to nitrocellulose membranes blocked in TBST solution containing 5% BSA for 1 h at room temperature. After blocking with 5% BSA in TBST solution, the membrane was, respectively, incubated overnight at 4°C with primary antibodies against β-actin, TRPC1, Orai1, STIM1, PLC-γ, and IP3R, ERK1/2, JNK1/2, NF-kB p50, and p65, (1:1000), or IKK-α (1:400). After washing six times with TBST, the membranes were next probed with HRP-conjugated secondary antibody and incubated for 1 h at room temperature. Protein bands were visualized with enhanced chemiluminescence reagent and exposed to an X-ray film (Sage creation Mnin Chemi II, China).

*Statistical analysis*

Statistical analysis was determined by one-way analysis of variance (ANOVA) using GraphPad Prism 5.01 (GraphPad Software, Inc., USA). All data are presented as the mean values ± standard error of the mean (*SEM*) with three times experimental replicates and statistical significance was set at $p < 0.05$.

## Results

*The effect of QE on mast cell activation in IgE-mediated PCA response mice model*

Type I allergic hypersensitivity is characterized by the abundant activation of mast cells, inducing immediate allergic reactions (19). In order to investigate the role of QE in type I allergic hypersensitivity, the anti-allergic activity of QE *in vivo* was evaluated using IgE-mediated PCA mice. As shown in Fig. 1a, the IgE-mediated PCA was successfully induced by the sequential injections of IgE and DNP-HSA within 40 min after injection. This PCA response was in parallel with vastly occurring capillary dilatation and the increase of ear vascular permeability, by which manifestation was visibly shown by the leakage of Evans blue dye into the ears, indicating the occurrence of mast cell degranulation at site of IgE-sensitized mice ears. When QE was orally administered to IgE-mediated PCA mice, the extent of mast cell degranulation–mediated ear vascular permeability was lessened, as indicated by the intensity of blue color of the ear and Evans blue extraction of the ears. The absorbance of the dye showed that the PCA reaction was significantly suppressed by oral administration as compared to control group (1.27 ± 0.12 vs 0.72 ± 0.09; $p < 0.05$; Fig. 1b).

From the PCA experiment, we might identify the effect of oral QE treatment in inhibiting mast cell degranulation–regulated mice vascular permeability symptom in IgE-mediated PCA mice. The suppressive effect of 17 mg/kg of QE was similar to our previous study using food allergy–induced EoE murine model (10). In order to elucidate the detail suppressive role of how QE modulates mast cell activation, we conducted further experiment using HMC-1 cell line. We divided QE into three groups: whole egg, egg albumen, and egg yolk in order to investigate which parts of QE could act as anti-allergic and inflammatory agents.

*The effect of QE on HMC-1 mast cell activation*

In most cases of using therapeutic compound treatment, it can influence the viability of treated cells (14). We first examined the cytotoxic effect of QE on HMC-1 cells using the WST-8 assay. HMC-1 cells were treated for 30 min at final QE group concentrations of 10, 50, 100, 500, and 1000 μg/mL. The results showed that the viabilities of cells treated with different QE groups were not affected within the treated concentration range, except for cells

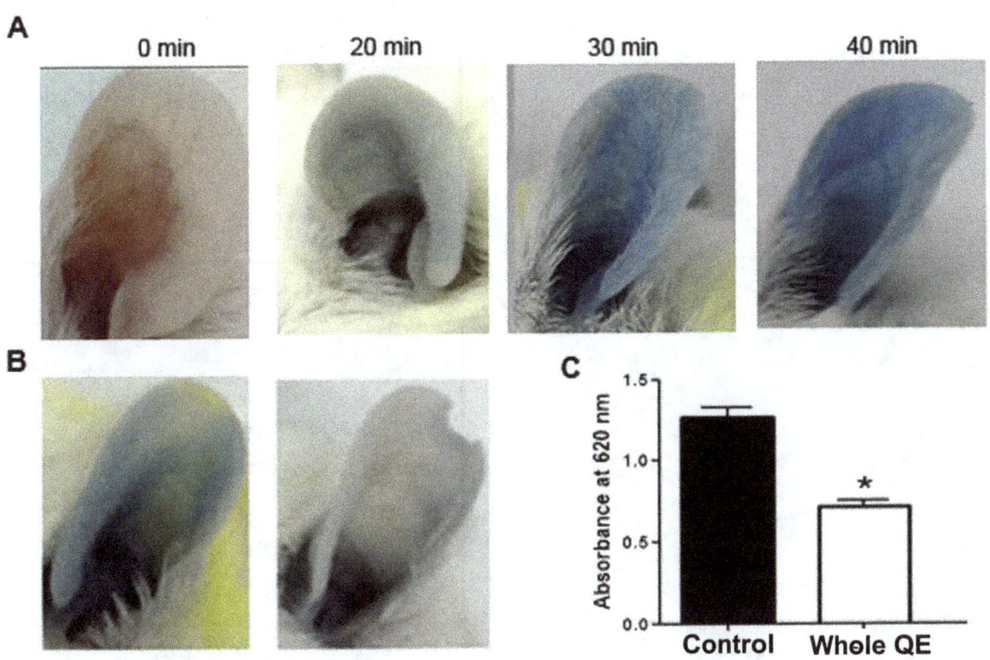


*Fig. 1.* The effects of QE treatment on the vascular permeability and mast cell stabilization *in vivo.* (a) The change of ear color after 40 min DNP-HSA stimulation. (b) Qualitative and (c) quantitative detection of the vascular permeability after Evan's Blue Dye/DNP-HSA stimulation. Results are expressed as mean ± SEM. *$p < 0.05$ as compared to the control group.

treated with QE yolk, as shown in Fig. 2a. In addition, we found no significant difference between cells treated with either whole or albumen QE groups and control group ($p > 0.05$). However, we found significant reduction of cells treated with QE yolk at concentrations ranging from 500 to 1000 μg/ mL, which reduced almost 40% from original numbers of cells (1.40 ± 0.05 vs 0.82 ± 0.07; $p < 0.05$). Therefore, we used QE concentrations ranging from 10 to 100 μg/ mL for all subsequent experiments.

Degranulation is an important sign of mast cell activation. In order to carry out a more comprehensive examination of degranulation levels, we investigated not only the level of β-hexosaminidase release but also the levels of histamine and tryptase release which are valid biomarkers for mast cell degranulation (14). The effect of various QE treatments on degranulation of HMC-1 cells was examined. HMC-1 cells were treated with various QE treatments, and degranulation was induced by C48/80. As expected, the release of β-hexosaminidase was significantly increased over the incubation time with C48/80 as shown in Fig. 2b.

Accordingly, C48/80 challenged HMC-1 cells were incubated for 1 h to determine the effect of QE on β-hexosaminidase release. QE suppressed the release of β-hexosaminidase in a dose-dependent manner (Fig. 2b). On the contrary, histamine and tryptase were also robustly released following the C48/80 stimulation (Fig. 2c-d). In line with β-hexosaminidase, QE treatments indicated similar inhibition effect on modulating histamine and tryptase release from HMC-1 cells (Fig. 2c-d). QE suppressed the β-hexosaminidase, histamine, and tryptase released *in vitro* with HMC-1 in a dose-dependent manner, which showed significant effect in the range concentrations of 50–100 μg/mL ($p < 0.05$), reached 30 up to 50% degranulation reduction. Data also indicated that the degranulation suppression of QE albumen was stronger than QE yolk ($p < 0.05$). This reduction difference could be shown by the comparison degranulation reduction levels for β-hexosaminidase, histamine, and tryptase between QE albumen and yolk groups, wherein reductions, under 100 μg/mL QE concentrations, reached 47.03 ± 1.23% vs 29.15 ± 1.96%; 72.41 ± 0.08% vs 30.04 ± 0.42%; and 50.43 ± 1.92% vs 34.99 ± 1.83%, respectively. In addition, cells treated with the highest concentration of QE yolk (100 μg/mL) showed a recovery level of mediator releases wherein reductions were lower than cells treated with 70 μg/mL of QE yolk (β-hexosaminidase: 44.67 ± 1.53; histamine: 5.91 ± 0.15; tryptase: 1109.52 ± 5.52). These results suggest that QE suppressive effect on modulating mast cell degranulation is likely derived from QE albumen.

### *The effect of QE on HMC-1-released Th2 cytokines*

Mast cells have a vital role as crucial effector and controlling cells in the initiation of the allergic immune response by regulating Th2 lymphocyte differentiation and thus

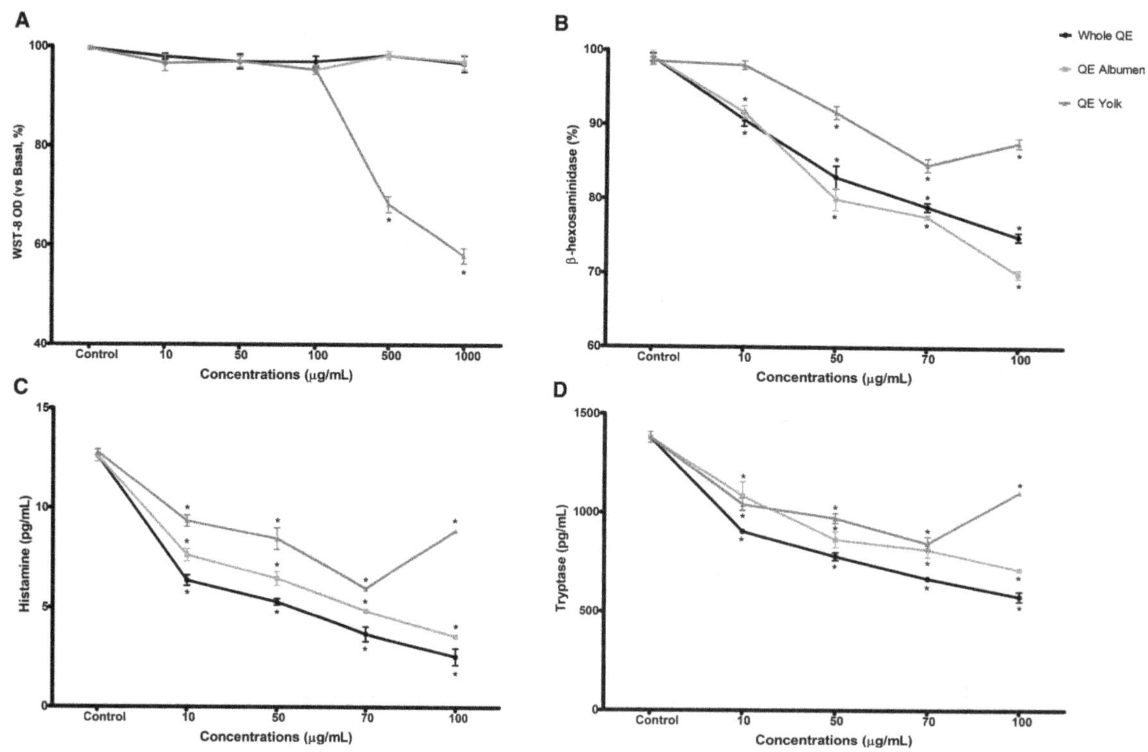


*Fig. 2.* The effects of QE treatments on HMC-1 mast cell stabilization *in vitro.* (a) Cell viability and cell degranulation–mediated mediator release. (b) β-hexosaminidase, (c) histamine, and (d) tryptase levels. Results are expressed as mean ± SEM. *$p < 0.05$ as compared to control group.

prompting the generation of Th2-associated cytokines (20). We, therefore, investigated the effect of QE on Th2-cytokines (IL-4, IL-5, and IL-13). As shown in Fig. 3a-c, the inhibitory effects of different QE treatments on modulating Th2 cytokines (IL-4, IL-5, and IL-13) showed similar results. As compared to control group, all QE treatments showed inhibitory effects on modulating these Th2 cytokine levels in a reverse dose-dependent manner. The higher the concentrations of QE, the weaker the inhibition effects on modulating Th2 cytokines ($p < 0.05$).

As compared to control group, the significant inhibitory effects of whole QE and QE albumen on modulating IL-4 (whole QE: 31.77 ± 2.53; QE albumen: 30.93 ± 2.47 vs C group: 36.68 ± 2.29) and IL-13 (whole QE: 28.67 ± 2.21; QE albumen: 29.52 ± vs C group: 33.68 ± 0.64) cytokine levels were only up to 50 μg/mL concentration, while the significant inhibitory effects of whole QE and QE albumen on modulating IL-5 cytokine level were up to 70 μg/mL concentration (whole QE: 54.14 ± 3.82; QE albumen: 55.41 ± 3.67 vs C group: 62.50 ± 1.80). Yet, under the highest concentration of QE treatment (100 μg/mL), we found no significant IL-4 (whole QE: 37.78 ± 1.79; QE albumen: 36.21 ± 1.68 vs C group: 36.68 ± 2.29), IL-5 (whole QE: 59.39 ± 3.85; Q albumen: 60.04 ± 3.05 vs C group: 62.50 ± 1.80), and IL-13 (whole QE: 34.58 ± 1.28; QE albumen: 36.38 ± 1.90% vs C group: 33.68 ± 0.64) level differences. In contrast, as compared to control group, QE yolk, up to 100 μg/mL concentration, still showed significant inhibitory effects on the releases of IL-4 (30.09 ± 4.70 vs 36.68 ± 2.29) and IL-5 (46.59 ± 1.01 vs 62.50 ± 1.80) but not in the release of IL-13 (29.84 ± 0.22 vs 33.68 ± 0.64; $p < 0.05$). All of these results indicated that QE yolk was likely the most effective regulator in modulating the release of Th2-associated cytokines.

Mast cell-derived IL-10 restricts leukocyte infiltration, inflammation, tissue damage associated with innate response and thereby preventing damage to the organ (21). As shown by Fig. 3d, all QE treatments showed a similar effect on upregulating IL-10 level of HMC-1 cells in dose-dependent manner. As compared to control group (127.52 ± 4.17), data indicated that treated cells under the highest concentration of whole QE, QE albumen, and QE yolk (100 μg/mL) demonstrated a marked upregulated IL-10 level, reaching up to 315.51 ± 5.86, 305.84 ± 8.81, and 247.56 ± 3.92, respectively ($p < 0.05$). However, QE yolk showed the weakest upregulation effect on modulating the level of IL-10 release, which was almost 20% lower than whole QE or QE albumen IL-10 upregulated levels ($p < 0.05$). This finding indicated that QE albumen was more effective in upregulating the release of IL-10 rather than QE yolk.

*The effect of QE on HMC-1-released pro-inflammatory cytokines*

Mast cell activation also results in the vast release of pro-inflammatory mediators (22), leading to the exacerbation

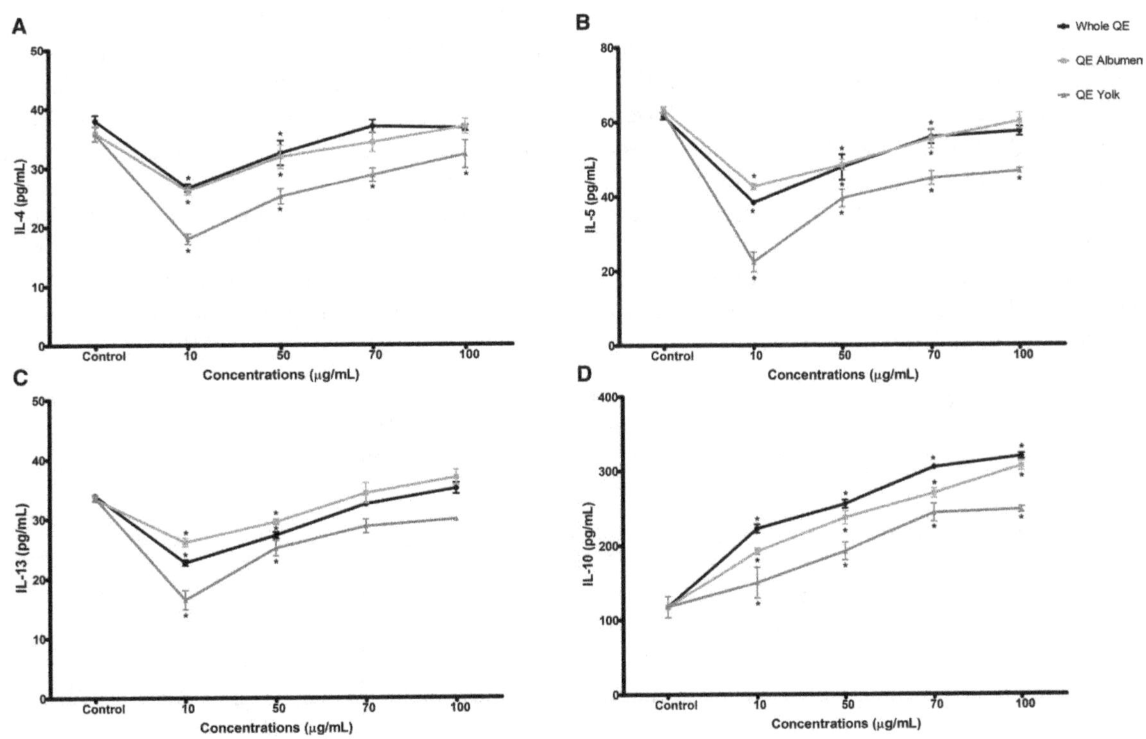


*Fig. 3.* The effect of QE treatments on HMC-1 released Th2 cytokines. (a) IL-4, (b) IL-5, (c) IL-13, and (d)IL-10. Results are expressed as mean ± SEM. *$p < 0.05$ as compared to the control group.

of allergic response. *Therefore,* we also investigated whether various QE treatments were able to modulate the release of pro-inflammatory cytokines. Hence, we measured the levels of IL-6, IL-8, and TNF-α release from HMC-1, as shown in Fig. 4.

As compared to the control group, QE albumen and QE yolk showed similar significant inhibitory effect on the release of IL-6 in a reverse dose-dependent manner, in the highest concentration of treatment (100 μg/mL), and was able to reach the highest value of IL-6 cytokine release (QE albumen: 301.49 ± 11.45; QE yolk: 282.32 ± 6.12 vs C group: 399.22 ± 17.95; Fig. 4a, $p < 0.05$). In addition, whole QE which conversely showed significant inhibitory effect on the release of IL-6 in a dose-dependent manner, in the highest concentration of treatment (100 μg/mL), was able to reach the lowest value of IL-6 cytokine release (Whole QE: 238.00 ± 11.56 vs C group: 399.22 ± 17.95; Fig. 4a, $p < 0.05$).

Meanwhile, for the release of IL-8 cytokine, all QE treatments showed significant inhibition effect on modulating IL-8 cytokine level in a reverse dose-dependent manner. As compared to control group, cells treated with the highest concentration of whole QE and QE albumen (100 μg/mL) were able to reach the IL-8 level of control group (whole QE: 82.24 ± 3.40; QE albumen: 77.12 ± 2.97 vs C group: 83.86 ± 0.75, Fig. 4b, $p > 0.05$). In contrast, even QE yolk inhibition effect also showed a reverse dose-dependent manner, but the highest concentration of QE yolk still showed significant inhibitory effect on modulating IL-8 level (64.22 ± 2.32 vs 83.86 ± 0.75, Fig. 4b, $p < 0.05$). The highest concentration of QE yolk (100 μg/mL) was only able to lower the release of IL-8 cytokine level up to 23.42 ± 2.11%, whereas the lowest concentration of QE yolk (10 μg/mL) was able to lower the release of IL-8 up to 52.47 ± 3.78% (Fig. 4b, $p < 0.05$), suggesting the higher the concentration of QE yolk, the weaker the inhibition effect on the release of IL-8 level.

In contrast to the other two pro-inflammatory cytokine release patterns, all QE treatments showed a significant inhibitory effect on modulating the release of TNF-α in a dose-dependent manner (Fig. 4c, $p < 0.05$). The highest concentration of QE treatments (100 μg/mL) was able to suppress the release of TNF-α to reach 209.31 ± 4.25; 238.77 ± 2.89; 294.3 ± 3.72 for whole QE, QE albumen, and QE yolk, respectively, as compared to the control group (428.29 ± 13.47). This suppression effect of whole QE, QE albumen, and QE yolk on the release of TNF-α caused a marked reduction up to 51.13 ± 2.17%; 44.25 ± 2.58%; 31.28 ± 2.85%, respectively. Not similar with the IL-6 and IL-8 cytokine modulating trend observed in this study, the inhibition effect of QE albumen on modulating TNF-α was stronger than QE yolk (Fig. 4c, $p < 0.05$). Overall, we concluded that each of the QE treatments likely through differently regulating cell signaling pathways brought different results in modulating pro-inflammatory cytokines.

As most of the cases we found in this study indicated that 70 μg/mL of QE treatments were effective to modulate the inhibition response of HMC-1 cells; therefore, we used this range of concentration of QE treatments for further experiments.

*The effect of QE on the influx of intracellular ion calcium ($Ca^{2+}$) of HMC-1 cells*

As reported, the degranulation of mast cells depends on intracellular calcium ion $[Ca^{2+}]_i$ release from the endoplasmic reticulum (ER) and calcium release–activated calcium-mediated $Ca^{2+}$ influxes (23). We further investigated the effect of QE treatments on $Ca^{2+}$ influx. Fluo-3AM, a fluorescent $Ca^{2+}$ indicator, was used to determine the $[Ca^{2+}]_i$. As shown in Fig. 5a, $[Ca^{2+}]$i in the control cells rapidly increased after stimulation with C48/80. Elevation of $[Ca^{2+}]$i in the cells treated with whole QE and albumen QE was significantly suppressed until it reached level 183.31 ± 1.92 and 180.15 ± 0.62, as compared to control group wherein $[Ca^{2+}]$i influx level was still high during 120s up to reaching 279.99 ± 0.82 ($p < 0.05$), and kept its gradual progression. In addition, QE yolk also showed suppressive effects on $[Ca^{2+}]_i$ even though its suppressive effect was weaker than other QE treatments, by which it

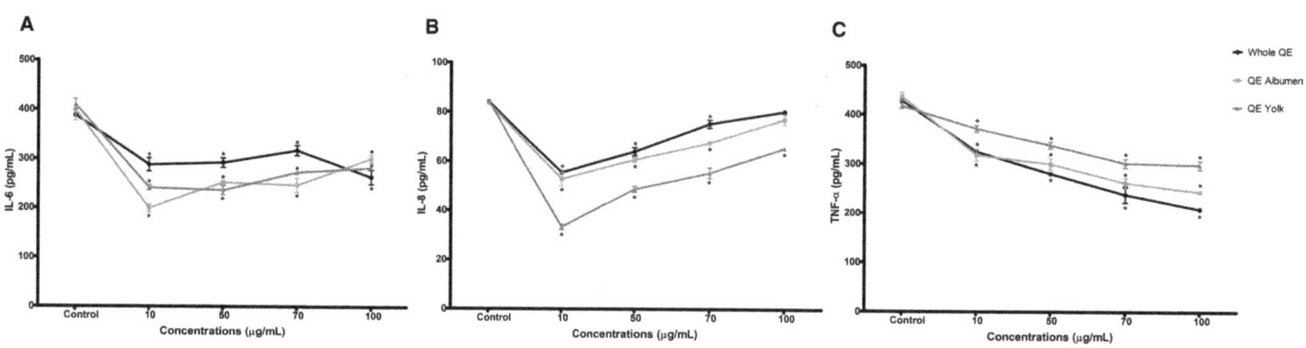


*Fig. 4.* The effect of QE treatments on HMC-1 released pro-inflammatory cytokines. (a) IL-6, (b) IL-8, and (c) TNF-α. Results are expressed as mean ± SEM. *$p < 0.05$ as compared to the control group.

reached only 219.18 ± 0.54 ($p < 0.05$). These results indicated that QE, particularly its albumin, was effective in inhibiting the elevation of C48/80-stimulated $Ca^{2+}$ influx.

We further investigated the expression of $Ca^{2+}$ influx–related proteins (TRPC1, Orai1, STIM1, *PLC-γ*, and IP3R). Based upon western blotting results, the expression levels of TRPC1, Orai1, PLCγ, and IP3R were significantly decreased by whole QE and QE albumen ($p < 0.05$, Fig. 5b-g), resulting in almost 45–75% fold reduction in protein expression. In addition, even though the inhibition effects of QE on these protein expressions were not as strong as QE albumen ($p < 0.05$), which resulted only in 20–40% fold reduction in protein expression, QE yolk also showed significant inhibition effects on the expression of TRPC1, Orai1, and IP3R, as compared to control group ($p < 0.05$; Fig. 5c-d;g). However, QE yolk showed no modulation effect on regulating STIM-1 and PLCγ protein expressions ($p > 0.05$; Fig. 5e-f). We then confirmed that QE, particularly its albumin, had a more significant effect on the depletion of ER calcium store, as compared to QE yolk, by stabilizing mast cells through significantly suppressing the $Ca^{2+}$ influx due to the lower expression of calcium channel proteins (TRPC1, Orai1, STIM1, PLC-γ, and IP3R).

### *The effect of QE on the PAR-2-mediated MAPK and NF-kB cell signaling pathways of HMC-1 cells*

It has been reported that QE plays an important role in the treatment of allergy disease by acting as a PAR-2 inhibitor which is able to enhance mast cell stabilization (6). In addition, our recent study has also indicated the significant PAR-2 activation in peanut allergy–induced EoE-like disease murine model and oral QE treatment was able to diminish the elevation of PAR-2 expression. Then, in this experiment, the effect of QE treatments on expression of PAR2 was examined by RT-PCR. Indeed, we found a similar trend with our previous study. As shown in Fig. 6a, PAR-2 expression was significantly elevated in the HMC-1 control group and whole QE and QE albumen treatments were able to significantly inhibit PAR-2 expression ($p < 0.05$), while QE yolk inhibition was weaker as compared to other QE treatments ($p < 0.05$).

Because the activation of MAPK and NF-κB is critically required for the transcriptional regulation of PAR-2-mediated allergic response (24), we further investigated whether the inhibition of allergic responses by QE are mediated through the MAPK and nuclear translocation of NF-κB pathway in C48/80-stimulated HMC-1 by western blot analysis. As shown in Fig. 6b-e, C48/80 markedly stimulated the phosphorylation of ERK 1/2, JNK 1/2, and p38 MAPK as well as IKKα, nuclear translocations of p50 and p65 subunit of NF-κB in HMC-1 (Fig. 6f-i). QE pretreatment, particularly QE albumen, significantly suppressed the C48/80-induced activation of JNK MAPK ($p < 0.05$, Fig. 6e), resulting in 47.10 ± 1.39% fold protein reduction, but did not affect the phosphorylation of ERK or p38 ($p > 0.05$; Fig. 6c-d), and QE yolk did not show any inhibition effect ($p > 0.05$; Fig. 6b-e). Furthermore, IKKα,

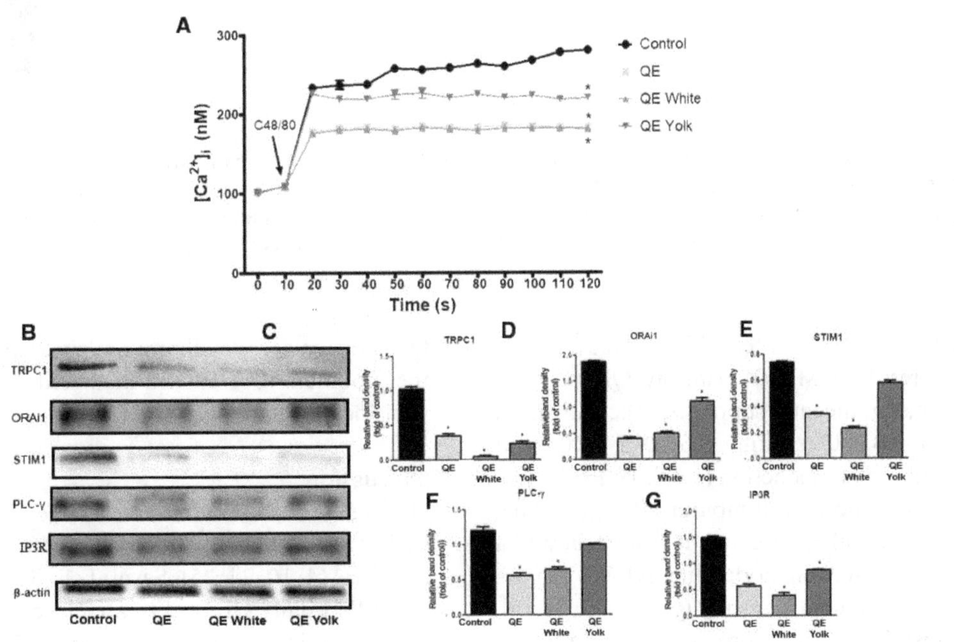


*Fig. 5.* The Effect of QE on the influx of intracellular ion calcium ($Ca^{2+}$) of HMC-1 cells. (a) Intracellular $Ca^{2+}$ influx concentration. (b) Western blotting of calcium protein expression. Fold activation data analysis: (c) TRPC1, (d) ORAi1, (e) STIM1, (f) PLCγ, and (g) IP3R. Results are expressed as mean ± SEM. *$p < 0.05$ as compared to control group.

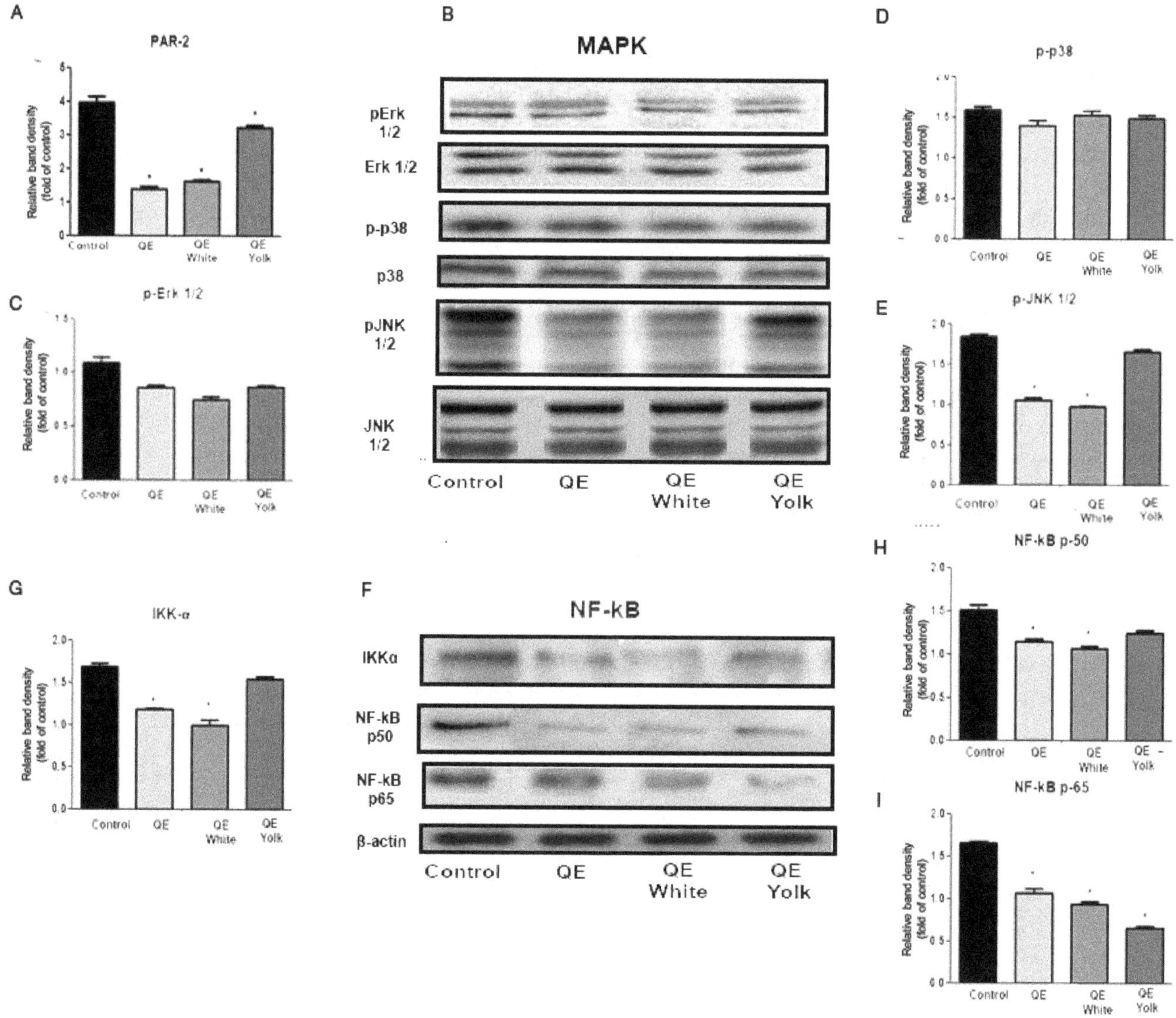


*Fig. 6.* The effect of QE on the PAR-2-mediated MAPK and NF-kB cell signaling pathways of HMC-1 cells. (a) mRNA fold induction of PAR-2. (b) Western blotting of MAPK signaling. MAPK fold activation data analysis: (c) pERK1/2, (d) p-p38 and (e) p-JNK1/2. (f) Western blotting of NF-kB signaling. NF-kB fold activation data analysis: (g) IKK-α, (h) NF-kB p50, and (i) NF-kB p65. Results are expressed as mean ± SEM. *$p < 0.05$ as compared to the control group.

NF-kB p50, and p65 were also affected by C48/80 (Fig. 6f-i). Similar to the result of MAPK pathway, QE, particularly QE albumen, significantly suppressed the activation of IKK-α and NF-kB p50, resulting in 54.29 ± 1.21% and 16.67 ± 1.14% fold protein reduction ($p < 0.05$; Fig. 6g-h), while QE yolk did not show any inhibition effect ($p > 0.05$; Fig. 6g-h). Surprisingly, all QE treatment groups showed a significant inhibition effect on modulating NF-kB p65 activation as compared to control group ($p < 0.05$; Fig. 6i), resulting in almost 40–60% fold protein reduction where QE yolk appeared as the most effective treatment among the others which resulted in 58.83 ± 1.15% fold protein reduction ($p < 0.05$; Fig. 6i). All the results indicated that QE, particularly its albumin, played an important role in the modulation of PAR-2-mediated MAPK and NF-kB translocation signaling pathways.

## Discussion

QE has been shown to have diverse biological activities, such as anti-allergic, anti-inflammatory, and anti-cancer activities (4–10, 24, 25). Several clinical studies have indicated that daily QE oral treatment could attenuate allergic asthmatic and rhinitis symptoms (5, 8, 9). In addition, our recent study found that QE was able to modulate the inflammatory response of food allergy–induced EoE-like disease by modulating PAR-2 transduction pathway in peanut-sensitized mice (10). Even though we have reported that QE inhibited the activation of PAR-2 in EoE murine model which represented delayed allergic response, the suppressive effect of QE on modulating mast cell degranulation in immediate allergic response is not yet well defined. So far, *in vitro* studies have just reported the role of QE on modulating the activation of basophils, neutrophils, and eosinophils. Therefore, to verify this, we firstly confirm the role of QE as 'mast cell stabilizer' *in vivo* using a IgE-mediated immediate allergic response in PCA mice model by which the report in accordance to this appears to be minimal. Then, we used HMC-1 mast cell lines to study the suppressive effect of QE on mast cell degranulation.

As summarized in Fig. 7, this present study found that QE possessed an anti-allergic activity through suppressing mast cell activation. It has been well-established that allergic mediator releases, like histamine, tryptase, Th2, and pro-inflammatory related cytokines, are closely associated with various allergic and inflammatory diseases. Thus, the inhibition of allergic mediators' generation by mast cells is an important therapeutic strategy in the context of allergic-inflammatory disease. In this present finding, we observed that QE albumen played the most effective role as compared to QE yolk in modulating mast cell degranulation by suppressing the release of β-hexosaminidase, histamine, and tryptase, as well as pro-inflammatory cytokines (IL-6, IL-8, and TNF-α) and upregulating the release of IL-10 in a dose-dependent manner, by which data showed that the lowest concentration QE albumen (10 μg/mL) already had significant inhibitory effect on modulating these mediators. In addition, even though QE yolk also showed significant therapeutic effect to modulate these mediators, these modulation effects were not as strong as QE albumen, by which its significant inhibition effects started in

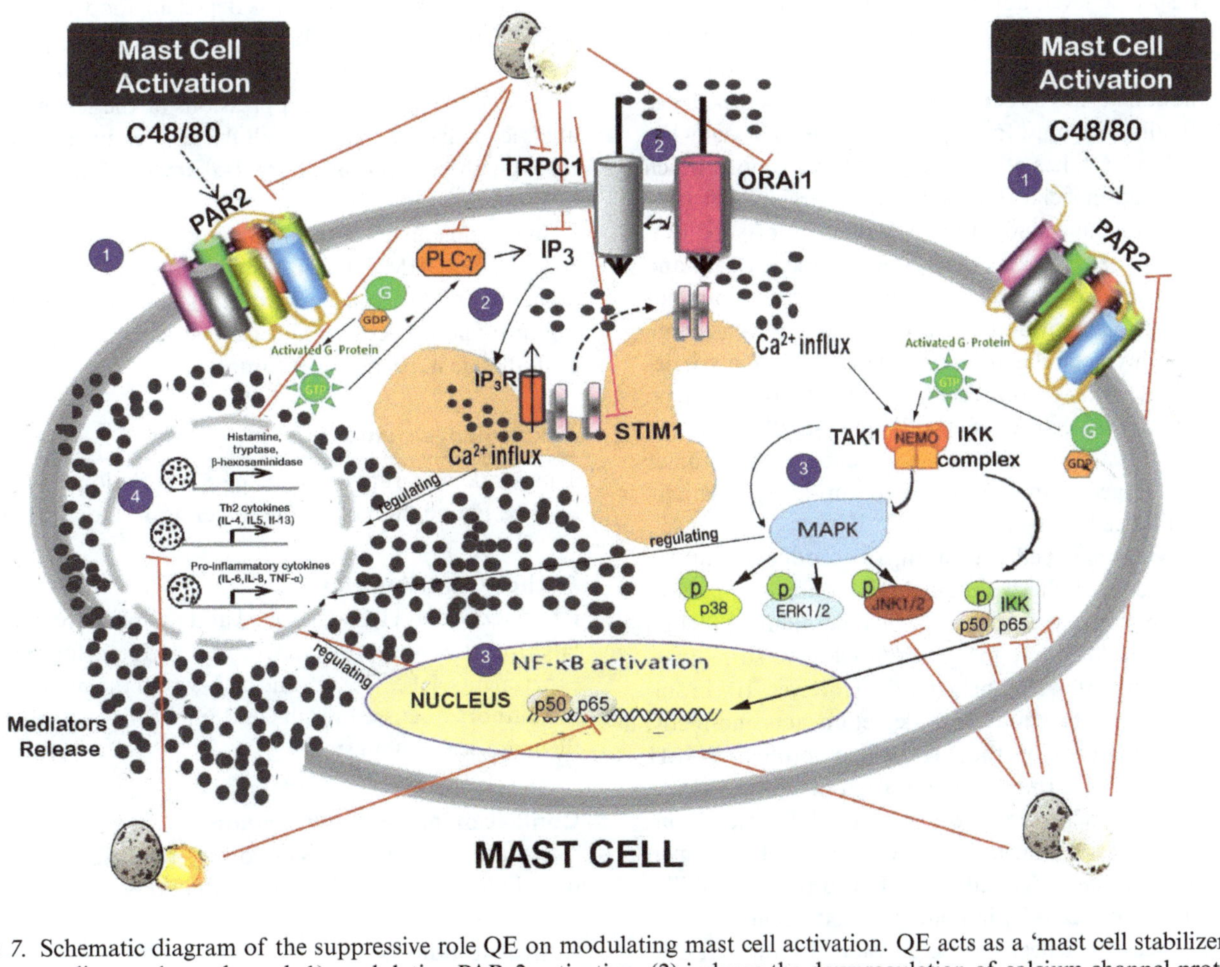


*Fig. 7.* Schematic diagram of the suppressive role QE on modulating mast cell activation. QE acts as a 'mast cell stabilizer' to reduce mediator release through 1) modulating PAR-2 activation; (2) induces the downregulation of calcium channel proteins (TRPC1, Orai1, STIM1, PLC-γ, and IP3R); (3) leads to the reduction of phosphorylation JNK, NF-kBp50, and p65, as well as IKK-α contributed in MAPK and NF-kB signaling pathways related to mast cell degranulation stimulated by antigen; and thus (4) promotes the decrease level of secretion mediators (β-hexosaminidase, histamine, tryptase) including Th2 (IL-4, IL-5, and IL-13) and pro-inflammatory related cytokines (IL-6, IL-8, and TNF-α) release.

concentration of 50 μg/mL. Interestingly, although QE albumen in lower concentration also showed significant inhibitory effects on mast cells released Th2 (IL-4, IL-5, IL-13) and pro-inflammatory cytokines (IL-6, IL-8), QE yolk showed a greater significant inhibition effect as compared to QE albumen on modulating those allergic related cytokines, even though its inhibition effect was also in a reverse dose-dependent manner.

The augmentation of Th2 cytokines in a higher concentration of QE was not surprising as it is largely known that QE itself contained many described egg allergens which also may act on immune pathway regulation to provide benefit in the occurrence of allergy reactions. Besides, the effective effect of QE yolk on modulating Th2 cytokines likely due to its high nutrient contents which likely also play an important role as anti-allergic agents (26). In contrast, study using chicken egg albumen to treat trimellitic anhydride (TMA) induced allergy murine model supported our finding. This study reported that TMA-sensitized mice treated with chicken egg albumen did not show any increase of IgE specific level, but the consumption of chicken egg albumen by TMA-treated mice could not modulate mice Th2 immune responses (27). However, it is still difficult to take the conclusion by comparing the effect of chicken egg and QE albumen only. Even though a proteomic study has reported that QE has other special protein fractions which may play a beneficial role as an anti-allergic agent (28), another proteomic study using egg albumen of six different bird species (chicken, duck, goose, turkey, quail, and pigeon) discovered that the content of QE albumin major protein allergens (ovalbumin, ovomucoid, ovotransferrin, lysozyme) were similar to other bird egg albumin species (29). Therefore, we considered no modulation effect on Th2 cytokines in cells treated with high QE albumen concentrations was likely due to the presence of these major protein allergens. However, detailed anti-allergic activity of QE still needs to be elucidated.

Following mast cell activation, the production of $IP_3$ allows calcium influx through both non-calcium selective canonical transient receptor channel family (TRPC) channels, and/or the highly calcium selective store-operated calcium entry channels (Orai). However, $IP_3$ in initiating internal calcium store depletion acts indirectly, which is identified by the ER resident protein STIM1 (30, 31), that in turn causes activation of Orai channels (32–34). The increased level of intracellular $Ca^{2+}$ concentration was significantly reduced after QE albumen treatment, which suggested that QE also plays a stabilizing role on mast cells by inhibiting the extracellular Ca2+ influx process. The decreased expression of Orai1, STIM1 and TRPC1 in protein levels indicate that GA might suppress the Ca2+-dependent degranulation due to the lower expression of these calcium channel proteins. Besides, the downregulation of IP3R protein expression in mast cell treated with QE albumen indicated that QE also has an effect on the depletion of ER $Ca^{2+}$ store. A marked upregulation of the calcium channel proteins activation provokes the activation of PAR-2. Its activation, through coupling with G proteins, induces a variety of signaling cascades including PLCγ activation, which thus evokes $[Ca^{2+}]_i$ rise and then triggers both MAPK and NF-kB signaling pathways in mast cells, leading to the release of mediators. In this study, we also found that QE albumen effectively suppressed the activation of PLC-γ in protein level. Next, we also found that QE also significantly suppressed the phosphorylation of JNK, p50, p65, as well as IKKα which represented MAPK and NF-kB signaling pathways, respectively. In addition, even though QE yolk's role in modulating mediators release is not as strong as QE albumen, QE yolk shows a significant effect on modulating NF-kB downstream signaling pathway through effectively modulating the phosphorylation of p65. This finding is in line with our previous study which shows that QE can block the activation of PAR-2 through inhibiting the phosphorylation of NF-kB p65 in food allergy–induced EoE mice model. Taken together with our previous results (10), the anti-allergic inflammatory activity of QE appears to be due to the suppressions of the secretions of allergic mediators and intracellular $Ca^{2+}$ influx generation through the inhibition of PAR-2 downstream signaling transduction pathway.

In conclusion, as confirmed by passive cutaneous anaphylaxis and HMC-1 cell-based immunology assay, QE albumen and QE yolk may work together through exerting anti-allergy activity and can be used as a potential anti-allergic nutrient in the future.

## Acknowledgements

This work was supported in part by National Natural Science Foundation of China under grant No. 81573158.

## Author Contributions

P.L., F.O.O. and H.C. conceived and designed the project. H.C. oversaw the project. P.L. and H.F. performed the experiments. P.L., F.O.O., and Y.Z. wrote the manuscript. All authors discussed results and implications and edited the manuscript at all stages.

## Conflict of interest and funding

The authors have not received any funding or benefits from industry or elsewhere to conduct this study.

## Ethical standards

All procedures performed in this article involving animals were in strict accordance with the China Agricultural University Animal Experimental Welfare and Ethical Inspection Committee approved protocols and in accordance with ethical standard guidelines of China Agricultural University. The manuscript does not contain clinical studies or patient data.

## References


1. Theoharides TC, Kalogeromitros D. The critical role of mast cells in allergy and inflammation. Ann N Y Acad Sci 2006; 1088: 78–99.
2. Minai-Fleminger MY, Schaffer FL. Mast cells and eosinophils: the two key effector cells in allergic inflammation. Inflamm Res 2009; 58(10). 631–8.
3. Cook EB, Stahl JL, Barney NP, Graziano FM. Mechanisms of antihistamines and mast cell stabilizers in ocular allergic inflammation. Curr Drug Targets Inflamm Allergy 2002; 1(2): 167–80.
4. Feeney RE, Means GE, Bigler JC. Inhibition of human trypsin, plasmin, and thrombin by naturally occurring inhibitors of proteolytic enzymes. J Biol Chem 1969; 244(8): 1957–60.
5. Bruttman G. 'Ovix' Quail egg homogenate: a clinical evaluation. La Medicina Biologica 1995; 2: 25–9.
6. Vergnaud S, Bruttmann G. Effetto inibitorio dell'ovomucoide di uovo di quaglia gaipponese sull'attivita. La Medicina Biologica 2007; 2: 5–13.
7. Melsens P, Waterloo BE, Jean L, Saint-Junien FR. Anti-inflammatory composition for modulating the cell response of neutrophils and eosinophils. United States Patent, US2015/0057232. 2015.
8. Truffier JC. Approche therapeutique de la maladie allergique par ingestion d'oeufs de caille. La Clinique 1978; 22: 2–4.
9. Benichou AC, Armanet M, Bussiere A, Chevreau N, Cardot JM, Tetard J. A proprietary blend of quail egg for the attenuation ofnasal provocation with a standardized allergenic challenge: a randomized, double-blind, placebo-controlled study. Food Sci Nutr 2014; 2(6): 655–63.
10. Knoops L, Louahed J, van Snick J, Renauld JC. IL-9 promotes but is not necessary for sytemic anaphylaxis. J Immunol 2005; 175(1): 335–41.
11. Integrative Therapeutics. ALLQLEAR™ Fast-acting seasonal support Therapeutics Integrative http://data.integrativepro.com/product-literature/info/allqlear-info-sheet.pdf (cited: 12.06.2016).
12. FDA. Guidance for industry-estimating the maximum safe starting dose in initial clinical trials for therapeutics in adult healthy volunteers. Department of Health and Human Services, Food and Drug Administration; 2005. Available from: https://www.fda.gov/downloads/Drugs/GuidanceComplianceRegulatoryInformation/Guidances/UCM078932.pdf.
13. Tominaga H, Ishiyama M, Ohseto F, Sasamoto K, Hamamoto T, Suzuki K, et al. A water-soluble tetrazolium salt useful for colorimetric cell viability assay. Anal Comm 1999; 36(2): 47–50.
14. Hohman RJ, Dreskin SC. Measuring degranulation of mast cells. Curr Protocols Immunol 2001; 26(7): 1–7.
15. Kuehn HS, Radinger M, Gilfillan AM. Measuring mast cell mediator release. Curr Protocols Immunol 2010;7:38.
16. Huber M, Helgason MP, Scheid V, Duronio R, Humphries RK, Krystal G. Targeted disruption of SHIP leads to steel factor-induced degranulation of mast cells. Eur Mol Biol Organ J 1998; 17(24): 7311–9.
17. Mahmood T, Yang PC. Western Blot: technique, theory, and trouble shooting. N Am J Med Sci 2012; 4(9): 429–34.
18. Schroeder JT. Basophils: emerging roles in the pathogenesis of allergic disease. Immunol Rev 2011; 242(1): 144–60.
19. Masuda A, Yoshikai Y, Aiba K, Matsuguchi T. Th2 cytokine production from mast cells is directly induced by lipopolysaccharide and distincly regulated by c-Jun N-Terminal Kinase and p38 pathways. J Immunol 2002; 169(7): 3801–10.
20. Grimbaldeston ME, Nake S, Kalesnikoff J, Tsai M, Galli SJ. Mast cell-derived interleukin 10 limits skin pathology in contact dermatitis and chronic irradiation with ultraviolet B. Nat Immunol 2007; 8(10): 1095–104.
21. Theoharides TC. Mast cells and inflammation. Biochimica et Biophysica Acta 2012; 1822(1): 21–33.
22. Vig M, Kinet JP. Calcium signaling in immune cells. Nat Immunol 2009; 10(1): 21–7.
23. Jacquet A. The role of innate immunity activation in house dust mite allergy. Trends Mol Med 2011; 17(10): 604–11.
24. Liu WH, Means GE, Feeney ER. The inhibitory properties of avian ovoinhibitors against proteolytic enzymes. Biochimica et Biophysica Acta 1971; 229(1): 176–85.
25. Bogard WC, Kato I, Laskowski M. A Ser162/Gly162 polymorphism in Japanese quail ovomucoid. J Biol Chem 1980; 255(14): 6569–74.
26. Tolik D, Polawska E, Charuta A, Nowaczewski S, Cooper R. Characteristics of egg parts, chemical composition and nutritive value of Japanese quail eggs-a review. Folia Biologica (Krakow) 2014; 62(4): 287–92.
27. Park GH, Jeon SJ, Ryu JR, Choi MS, Han SH, Yang SI, et al. Essential role of mitogen-activated protein kinase pathways in protease activated receptor 2-mediated nitric-oxide production from rat primary astrocytes. Nitric Oxide 2009; 21(2): 110–9.
28. Hu S, Qiu N, Liu Y, Zhao H, Gao D, Song R, et al. Identification and comparative proteomic study of quail and duck egg white protein using 2-dimensional gel electrophoresis and matrix -assisted laser desorption/ionization time-of-flight tandem mass spectrometry analysis. Poultry Sci 2016; 95(5): 1137–44.
29. Sun C, Liu J, Li W, Xu G, Yang N. Divergent proteome patterns of egg albumen from domestic chicken, duck, goose, turkey, quail, and pigeon. Proteomics 2017; 17(17–18); 1–12.
30. Liou J, Kim M, Heo W, Jones J, Myers JW, Ferrell JE, et al. STIM is a $Ca^{2+}$ sensor essential for $Ca^{2+}$ store depletion triggered $Ca^{2+}$ influx. Curr Biol 2005; 15(13): 1235–41.
31. Yuan JP, Zeng W, Dorwart MR, Choi Y J, Worley P F, Muallem S. SOAR and the polybasic STIM1 domains gate and regulate Orai channels. Nat Cell Biol 2009; 11(3); 337–43.
32. Liao Y, Erxleben C, Yildirim E, Abramowitz J, Armstrong DL, Birnbaumer L. Orai proteins interact with TRPC channels and confer responsiveness to store depletion. Proc Natl Acad Sci U S A 2007; 104(11): 4682–7.
33. Prakriya M. The molecular physiology of CRAC channels. Immunol Rev 2009; 231(1): 88–98.
34. Vig M, Peinelt C, Beck A, Koomoa DL, Rabah D, Koblan Huberson M, et al. CRACM1 is a plasma membrane protein essential for store operated $Ca^{2+}$ entry. Science 2006; 312(5777): 1220–3.



***Huilian Che**

Beijing Advanced Innovation Center for Food Nutrition and Human Health,
Beijing, China,
College of Food Science and Nutritional Engineering,
China Agricultural University,
Beijing, 100083, P.R. China
Email: chehuilian@cau.edu.cn

2

# Hypolipidemic activities of partially deacetylated α-chitin nanofibers/nanowhiskers in mice

Wenbo Ye[1], Liang Liu[1], Juan Yu[1], Shilin Liu[2], Qiang Yong[1] and Yimin Fan[1,*]

[1]Jiangsu Co-Innovation Center of Efficient Processing and Utilization of Forest Resources, Jiangsu Key Lab of Biomass-Based Green Fuel and Chemicals, College of Chemical Engineering, Nanjing Forestry University, Nanjing, China;
[2]College of Food Science and Technology, Huazhong Agricultural University, Wuhan, China

*Abstract*

Partially deacetylated α-chitin nanofibers/nanowhiskers mixtures (DEChNs) were prepared by 35% sodium hydroxide (NaOH) treatment followed by disintegration in water at pH 3–4. The aim of this study was to investigate the hypolipidemic effects of DEChNs at different dosage levels in male Kunming mice. The male mice were randomly separated into five groups, that is, a normal diet group, a high-fat diet group, and three DEChN groups that were treated with different doses of DEChN dispersions (L: low dose, M: medium dose, H: high dose). Primarily, the DEChNs significantly decreased body weight (BW) gain and adipose tissue weight (ATW) gain of mice. Meanwhile, the decreasing extent of weight ratios between ATW and BW was dependent on the dose of DEChNs. Moreover, the DEChNs prevented an increase in plasma lipids (cholesterol and triacylglycerol) in mice when they were fed a high-fat diet. Histopathological examination of hepatocytes revealed that the DEChNs were effective in decreasing the accumulation of lipids in the liver and preventing the development of a fatty liver. The results suggested that the DEChNs reduced the absorption of dietary fat and cholesterol *in vivo* and could effectively reduce hypercholesterolemia in mice.

Keywords: *chitin; nanofibers/nanowhiskers; hypolipidemic effects; cholesterol*

Hyperlipidemia is a major cause of coronary atherosclerosis and subsequent related cardiovascular disease, which has always been related to obesity to some extent (1). In recent years, most studies have examined how to decrease plasma lipid concentrations and the absorption of fat in the intestinal tract to reduce diet-related chronic disease (2). The conventional therapeutic modalities for hyperlipidemia are lipid-lowering drugs such as atorvastatin, lovastatin and fibrates (3). These synthetic drugs are available and effective but may cause adverse effects at the same time (4). Therefore, the antihyperlipidemic activity of many biologically active components from natural materials, such as polysaccharides and dietary fiber, has been explored. Polysaccharides, such as *Ulva pertusa*, *Ulva lactuca*, chitosan, and chitosan derivatives, are novel potential hyperlipidemic agents (3). Other dietary fibers, such as pectin and psyllium, also exhibit potent hypolipidemic effects (5).

Studies have shown that chitosan has a beneficial lowering effect on plasma cholesterol, which may play an important role in the prevention and treatment of cardiovascular disease (6, 7). Some previous research work has revealed the hypolipidemic mechanism of chitosan hypolipidemic activity of low molecular weight chitosan was better than high molecular weight chitosan (8, 9). The positively charged amino groups of chitosan may have the ability to bind negatively charged molecules, such as lipids and bile acids, and subsequently be excreted in the feces (10). The adsorption of chitosan to oil droplets affects the digestibility of oil. Access to the oil by digestive enzymes is decreased, thereby decreasing oil digestion.

Chitosan is a derivative of chitin. Chitosan is a cationic polysaccharide produced by the deacetylation of chitin under alkaline conditions, normally with a degree of deacetylation (DDA) greater than 0.7. Chitosan is, consequently, a copolymer of N-acetyl-D-glucosamine and D-glucosamine, which is similar to chitin structurally (11). Chitin, the source of chitosan, is the second most abundant renewable natural polysaccharide after cellulose. Chitin is the main component of the exoskeleton of arthropods, such as crabs, prawns, and shrimp, as well as the cuticles of insects and the cell walls of certain fungi, coexisting with various types of proteins and certain minerals (12). Isolated chitin is composed of β-(1-4)-linked 2-acetamido-2-deoxy-β-D-glucose units and a small amount of D-glucosamine. Because a large amount of crab and shrimp shell–derived chitins is discarded every year, utilizing chitin as a functional material or commodity is highly beneficial (13). In addition to converting chitin to its highly deacetylated derivative, chitosan, which may be used in a variety of applications, chitin itself has the potential to be converted into individual nanofibers through some downsizing processes.

One of the methods, partial deacetylation with 30–35 wt% NaOH treatment followed by disintegration in water at a pH of 3–4, was used to prepare partially deacetylated α-chitin nanofiber/nanowhisker mixtures (DEChNs) from α-chitins. The as-prepared DEChNs had DDA values of 0.25–0.35 and a high density of cationic charged C2-amino groups on the surface (14). The DEChNs had lower DDA values (0.25–0.35) than chitosan (normally >0.70) and did not dissolve at a molecular level but dispersed at a nanofibril level, maintaining high crystallinity (14). Our previous studies showed that partially deacetylated α-chitin can be converted to nanofiber/nanowhisker mixtures by mechanical pretreatment under acidic conditions (15). The DEChNs have been studied as nanostructured materials for further applications, such as gels and films (16). Other research work has been conducted to study the biochemical properties of DEChNs. Kazuo Azuma et al. evaluated the effects of oral administration of surface-deacetylated chitin nanofibers, chitosan, and cellulose nanofibers on hypercholesterolemia in rats and indicated that chitin nanofibers suppressed an increase in serum total cholesterol (TC), chylomicron, very-low-density lipoprotein (VLDL), and phospholipid (PL) levels while increasing alanine transaminase levels, vacuolar degeneration, and accumulation of lipid droplets in liver tissue (17). Recently, Anraku et al. proposed that surface-deacetylated chitin nanofibers are more effective in decreasing renal injury and oxidative stress than deacetylated chitin powder in 5/6 nephrectomized rats (18). The result of this study suggested that ingestion of chitin nanofibers, not chitin powder, resulted in significantly reduced levels of pro-oxidants, such as uremic toxins, in the gastrointestinal tract, thereby inhibiting the subsequent development of oxidative stress in the systemic circulation. All of these studies stated the potential of chitin in the biotechnology field, emphasizing the importance of nanofibrillation of chitin. However, research has rarely reported the mechanism and the effects of chitin nanofibers/nanowhiskers on hypolipidemic function. Although the DEChNs and chitosan have similar macromolecular structures, DEChNs are characterized by nanofibril morphology, lower amino groups, and higher crystallinity. Thus, it is worth further examination of the relationship between the biochemical properties of DEChNs and their hypolipidemic effects.

In the present study, the hypolipidemic effects of the DEChN dispersions were investigated in male Kunming mice at different dosage levels. The effects of the DEChNs on the weight of the body, organ tissue, and adipose tissue were examined in this study. Serum blood chemistry analysis and histopathological examination of the liver were also performed.

## Materials and methods

### *Materials*

The α-chitin was purified from swimming crab (*Portunus trituberculatus*) shells collected from Nantong, a seaside city in Jiangsu Province, China, as follows (11). Discarded crab shells were soaked in 1 M HCl for 12 h to remove the mineral salts. The sample was then washed thoroughly with distilled water, followed by treatment with 1 M NaOH for 12 h to remove the proteins. These two steps were repeated three times. The obtained residual solid was decolored by immersing it in 0.5% (w/w) $NaClO_2$, and the pH was adjusted to 5 using acetic acid. The suspension was heated for 2 h at 70°C. The purified α-chitin solid residues were obtained by filtration, rinsed with distilled water, and stored at 4°C for further use. TC, triacylglycerol (TG), high-density lipoprotein cholesterol (HDL-C), and low density lipoprotein cholesterol (LDL-C) kits were purchased from Nanjing Jiancheng Bioengineering Institute, Nanjing, China. All other reagents and solvents were of analytical grade.

### *Preparation of deacetylated α-chitin nanofiber/nanowhisker mixtures*

The α-chitin (1 g) was suspended in 35% (w/w) NaOH solution (25 mL) at 90°C for 4 h with continuous stirring. The final partially deacetylated chitin product with a DDA of 0.29 was collected and thoroughly washed with deionized water until a neutral pH was obtained and then stored at 4°C (14). The DDA of the original and partially deacetylated chitins were determined by the electrical conductivity titration method (19). In this case, a dried sample (0.1 g) was added to water (60 mL), and a small amount of 0.5 M NaOH was used to adjust the pH to 9. The slurry was stirred for 30 min for adequate distribution. Afterward, 0.1 M HCl was added to adjust the pH to 2.5–3.0, and a 0.05 M NaOH solution was added at a rate of 0.1 mL/min to adjust the pH to 11 using a pH-stat titration system. The conductivity and pH curves obtained reflect the amount of C2-amino groups in the chitins.

The partially deacetylated chitin was suspended in deionized water at a concentration of 0.1% (w/v), and the pH of the suspension was adjusted from the original pH of 6–7 to 3–4 by adding acetic acid with constant stirring. Next, this suspension was homogenized and treated with ultrasonication, the DEChNs were obtained after centrifugation, and the dispersions were successfully prepared (16).

*Animals and diets*

Kunming mice (males, Specific pathogen free (SPF), 18–20 g) were used as the experimental animals. The mice were procured from the Animal Center for Disease Prevention and Control in Hubei Province, China. All animal protocols were approved by the institutional animal care and use hospital of Huazhong Agricultural University (Wuhan, China). The animal study was performed under strict adherence to the international rules for animal experiments and the internationally accepted ethical principles for laboratory animal use and care. The mice were housed in cages in a controlled environment (25 ± 2°C, 50–70% relative humidity, 12±1 h light–dark cycle). There were five mice in each cage, and these mice were allowed free access to food and water for 5 days. Then, the mice were randomly divided into five groups as follows (10 mice per group). The normal fat control group (blank group, $n = 10$) received a normal fat diet and saline solution. The normal fat diet consisted of 40% corn starch, 22% wheat, 20% soybean, 7% peptone (fish), 4% casein, 4.2% mineral mixture, 0.8% amino acid, 0.3% vitamin mixture, 0.2% choline chloride, and 1.5% fat. The high-fat control group (control group, $n = 10$) received a high-fat diet and dilute acetic acid solution. Finally, there were three DEChN groups, namely, the L-DEChN ($n = 10$), M-DEChN ($n = 10$), and H-DEChN groups ($n = 10$), which received a high-fat diet and low, medium, or high doses of DEChN dispersions, respectively, dispersed in dilute acetic acid at a pH of 3–4. The high-fat diet consisted of 10% lard, 10% egg yolk powder, 2% cholesterol, 0.5% sodium deoxycholate, and 77.5% normal fat diet.

*Experimental design*

All mice were fed under experimental conditions for 21 days. The male mice were randomly separated into five groups: a normal diet group, a high-fat diet group, and three DEChN groups that had been treated with different doses of DEChN dispersions (low, medium, and high). During the experimental period, the method described by Qi et al. (20) was employed in this study. The mice were allowed free access to food and water for 5 days to acclimate to the animal facility and were weighed and randomly divided into five groups as described above. Each day the body weights (BW) were recorded, and in the DEChN groups, the mice were intragastrically administered DEChN dispersions at dosages of 18.75 mg/kg·bw·d (L-DEChN group), 37.5 mg/kg·bw·d (M-DEChN group), and 75 mg/kg·bw·d (H-DEChN group). Correspondingly, each day the mice in the blank group were given saline solution, and the mice in the control group were given dilute acetic acid solution. At the end of the third week, mice fasted for 18 h prior to blood withdrawal. Necropsies were performed on all mice after blood withdrawal, and organ and adipose tissues were collected and measured.

*Collection of blood and bioassay*

All blood samples for the bioassay were obtained by retro-orbital blood collection from mice that fasted overnight (18 h). Blood samples were centrifuged at 3,000 g for 10 min to separate the serum for lipid profile estimation and stored at –4°C. The serum TC, TG, HDL-C, and LDL-C concentrations were measured by an enzymatic colorimetric method using commercially available kits. Meanwhile, liver, kidney, and spleen samples were also collected and weighed.

*Statistical analysis*

Statistical analyses were performed using Student's $t$-test and compared to the control group (21). The data are presented as the mean ± standard deviation; $p < 0.05$ was considered a statistically significant difference.

## Results and discussion

*Characterizations of deacetylated α-chitin nanofiber/nanowhisker mixtures*

The atomic force microscopy image of the DEChNs is shown in Fig. 1a. Complete individualization of DEChNs was achieved by partial deacetylation and the following downsizing process. The as-prepared individual DEChNs had widths that ranged consistently between 10 and 30 nm and lengths that ranged between 150 and 500 nm. The DDA of the DEChNs was 0.29.

Photographs of the DEChNs in water at pH 1.5–6 are shown in Fig. 1b. The DEChNs were well dispersed in water at pH 1.5–4.5; however, at pH 6.0 there was severe turbidity with white flocculent particles, indicating that DEChNs flocculate in water at higher pH values. The well dispersion of DEChNs at pH 1.5–4.5 was in accordance with its high zeta-potential (+30–70 mV), which indicated the high cationic surface charges of DEChNs. Thus, the addition of acetic acid cationized the C2-amino groups on the DEChNs, promoting the fibrillation of the DEChNs into nanofibrils by electrostatic repulsion and stable dispersion in water. However, DEChNs lost a certain amount of positive charge when the zeta-potential decreased to +24.1 mV at pH 6.0 and therefore became flocculent and precipitated.

While pH is normally neutral in most parts of the body, it is acidic in the gastric environment. The changes in the zeta-potential and dispersion-flocculation that occurred in relation to the pH value of the DEChNs reflect

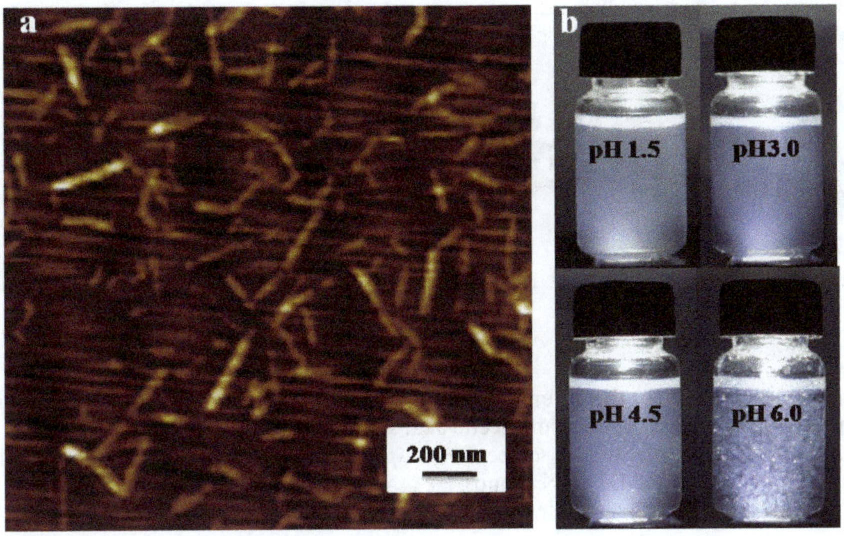


*Fig. 1.* Characterizations of partially deacetylated α-chitin nanofibers: (a) atomic force microscopy observation of partially deacetylated α-chitin nanofiber/nanowhisker mixtures (DEChNs) prepared from α-chitin; (b) photographs of dispersions of DEChNs in water at pH 1.5–6.

the potential of DEChNs to bind molecules such as lipids, cholesterol, and bile acid in the stomach at pH < 4.5 (acidic gastric juice) and to flocculate with the binding molecules at a higher pH in the intestine for excretion outside of the body.

### *Body and tissue weight of mice*

The BW and BW gain of experimental mice are shown in Fig. 2a and b, respectively. The DEChN dispersions were divided into the following three dosage groups: L-DEChNs, M-DEChNs, and H-DEChNs, in which the mice were fed dosages of 18.75, 37.5, and 75 mg/kg·bw·d of DEChN dispersions, respectively. The mice were fed the DEChNs along with a high-fat diet to estimate their effect on the resulting weight change of the mice. As a control, because the DEChNs were dispersed under acidic conditions mediated by acetic acid, the dilute acetic acid solution was given to the mice along with the high-fat diet.

As shown in Fig. 2a and b, the mice fed the high-fat diet plus the dilute acetic acid solution (control group) showed decreases in BW during the experimental period, compared with those mice fed the normal-fat diet plus a saline solution (blank group). This indicates that the dilute acetic acid could reduce the weight gain of the mice even though they were fed the high-fat diet. Until Day 14, there were some differences in the BW of mice fed the L-DEChNs and mice in the control group. However, after 14 days, the BW of these two groups showed little difference. The results suggested that the L-DEChN (18.75 mg/kg·bw·d) dispersion dosage slightly mitigated increases in the BW of mice fed a high-fat diet after the initial 2 weeks, when mice had acclimated to the feeds. Compared with the control group and the L-DEChN group, there was significantly less BW gain in mice that had been fed the M-DEChN and H-DEChN doses. Especially for the mice that received H-DEChNs along with a high-fat diet, a minimal increase in the BW was observed.

Overall, the BW of the mice obviously changed; both acetic acid and DEChNs were able to prevent the weight gain of mice, even those fed a high-fat diet, and the degree of prevention was correlated with the dosage of DEChNs.

Necropsies were performed on the experimental mice after 21 days. The tissue weights (TW) of the mice (including liver weight, kidney weight, and spleen weight) are shown in Table 1. As shown in Table 1, compared with the control group, the TW of the mice fed DEChN dispersions were significant lower along with a lower overall BW. The results suggest that DEChNs reduced both the BW and TW gain of mice. In contrast, the ratios of liver, spleen, and kidney weights to BW (TW/BW) showed no significant differences among all groups.

### *Adipose tissue and serum lipids*

The adipose tissues (including renal, epididymal, and mesenteric adipose tissue) of experimental mice were collected and measured. The adipose tissue weight (ATW) and the ATW/BW ratios are shown in Table 2. Compared with the mice fed the normal-fat diet plus a saline solution (blank group), the mice fed the high-fat diet plus a dilute acetic acid solution (control group) showed an increase in ATW at the end of the experimental period. This indicates that feeding the mice a high-fat diet resulted in a high accumulation of lipids.

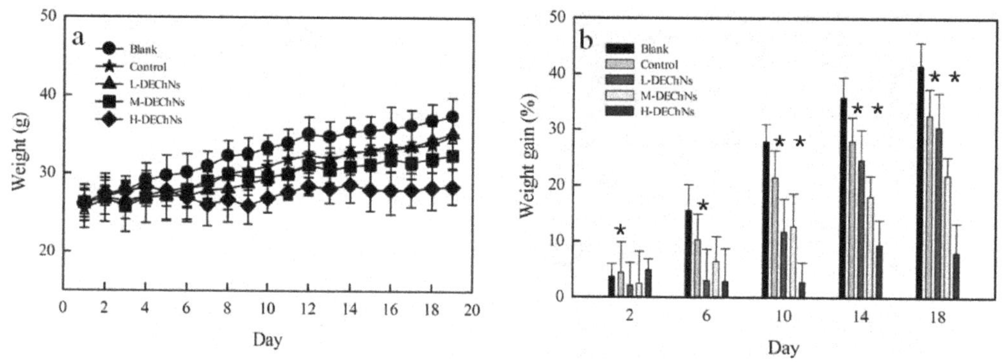


*Fig. 2.* (a) Changes in body weight and (b) the difference in body weight gain in the blank group (fed a normal diet and saline solution), control group (fed a high-fat diet and dilute acetic acid solution), and L-, M-, and H-DEChN groups (fed a high-fat diet and low, medium, and high doses of DEChN dispersions). $^{*}p < 0.05$ control group compared with the DEChN groups. $^{**}p < 0.01$ control group compared with the DEChN groups.

*Table 1.* Body and tissue weights of mice

| Groups | Blank[a] | Control[b] | L-DEChNs[c] | M-DEChNs[d] | H-DEChNs[e] |
|---|---|---|---|---|---|
| BW (g) | 33.63 ± 2.87 | 34.19 ± 1.89 | 31.88 ± 3.02* | 30.36 ± 3.26** | 26.58 ± 2.08** |
| Liver weight (g) | 1.92 ± 0.18 | 1.87 ± 0.30 | 1.67 ± 0.15* | 1.64 ± 0.14* | 1.46 ± 0.04** |
| Liver weight/BW (%) | 5.70 ± 0.30 | 5.48 ± 0.55 | 5.23 ± 0.31 | 5.40 ± 0.34 | 5.51 ± 0.21 |
| Spleen weight (g) | 0.116 ± 0.035* | 0.139 ± 0.016 | 0.133 ± 0.022 | 0.1195 ± 0.03 | 0.113 ± 0.046 |
| Spleen weight/BW (%) | 0.34 ± 0.08* | 0.41 ± 0.04 | 0.42 ± 0.08* | 0.39 ± 0.05* | 0.43 ± 0.06 |
| Kidney weight (g) | 0.672 ± 0.124 | 0.681 ± 0.09 | 0.637 ± 0.067 | 0.571 ± 0.131* | 0.497 ± 0.024* |
| Kidney weight/BW (%) | 1.996 ± 0.345 | 1.99 ± 0.14 | 1.999 ± 0.141 | 1.88 ± 0.33 | 1.87 ± 0.16 |

BW, body weight[a]

Blank group (fed normal diet and saline solution); [b]control group (fed high-fat diet and dilute acetic acid solution); [c,d,e]L-, M-, H-DEChN groups (fed high-fat diet and low, medium, high dose, respectively, of DEChN dispersions). Data are presented as mean ± standard error. $^{*}p < 0.05$ compared with the control group; $^{**}p < 0.01$ compared with the control group.

Compared with the control group, a decrease in the weights of the renal, epididymal, and mesenteric adipose tissues were observed in the H-DEChN and L-DEChN groups. The H-DEChN group showed a greater decrease than the L-DEChN group. The weights of the renal ATW of mice in the L-DEChN group and the H-DEChN group were 0.235 ± 0.068 and 0.146 ± 0.041 g, respectively, compared with 0.418 ± 0.148 g in the control group and 0.234 ± 0.116 g in the blank group. The weights of the epididymal adipose tissue of mice in the L-DEChN and H-DEChN groups were 0.621 ± 0.16 and 0.412 ± 0.098 g, respectively, compared with 0.819 ± 0.238 g in the control group and 0.695 ± 0.107 g in the blank group. The weights of the mesenteric adipose tissue of mice in the L-DEChN and H-DEChN groups were 0.476 ± 0.187 and 0.471 ± 0.097 g, respectively, compared with 0.728 ± 0.085 g in the control group and 0.616 ± 0.17 g in the blank group. The weights of the renal, epididymal, and mesenteric adipose tissues of mice in the M-DEChN group were 0.268 ± 0.075, 0.700 ± 0.159, and 0.594 ± 0.115 g, respectively. There was an obvious decrease in the weights of the collected adipose tissue compared with the control group, while there was no significant difference in the renal, epididymal, and mesenteric ATW/BW ratios of the M-DEChN group and the blank group. The results indicated that DEChNs could interfere with the absorption of dietary fat and cholesterol *in vivo*. This finding was likely a result of the unique ability of chitin to bind lipids and bile acids. The H-DEChN group (75 mg/kg·bw·d DEChNs) was more effective than the L-DEChN group (18.75 mg/kg·bw·d DEChNs) or the M-DEChN group (37.5 mg/kg·bw·d DEChNs) in decreasing the accumulation of lipids in tissue and preventing the development of obese mice.

The serum lipid concentrations of mice were measured, including TC, TG, HDL-C, and LDL-C. The results are shown in Table 3. After 21 days of experimental diets, the serum TC concentration of the mice fed the high-fat diet was higher than that of the mice fed a normal-fat diet. However, the serum TC and HDL-C concentrations of

*Table 2.* Adipose tissue weight of mice

| Groups | Blank[a] | Control[b] | L-DEChNs[c] | M-DEChNs[d] | H-DEChNs[e] |
|---|---|---|---|---|---|
| Renal ATW (g) | 0.234 ± 0.116* | 0.418 ± 0.148 | 0.235 ± 0.068* | 0.268 ± 0.075* | 0.146 ± 0.041** |
| Renal ATW/BW (%) | 0.69 ± 0.30** | 1.21 ± 0.37 | 0.72 ± 0.21* | 0.88 ± 0.19* | 0.54 ± 0.11** |
| Epididymal ATW (g) | 0.695 ± 0.107 | 0.819 ± 0.238 | 0.621 ± 0.16 | 0.700 ± 0.159 | 0.412 ± 0.098* |
| Epididymal ATW/BW (%) | 2.06 ± 0.27 | 2.38 ± 0.72 | 1.95 ± 0.47 | 2.20 ± 0.22 | 1.54 ± 0.23* |
| Mesenteric ATW (g) | 0.616 ± 0.17 | 0.728 ± 0.085 | 0.476 ± 0.187 | 0.594 ± 0.115* | 0.471 ± 0.097* |
| Mesenteric ATW/BW (%) | 1.83 ± 0.35* | 2.13 ± 0.61 | 1.48 ± 0.40* | 1.96 ± 0.38* | 1.75 ± 0.31 |

ATW, adipose tissue weight; BW, body weight[a]

Blank group (fed a normal diet and saline solution); [b]control group (fed a high-fat diet and dilute acetic acid solution); [c,d,e]L-, M-, H-DEChN groups (fed a high-fat diet and low, medium, high doses, respectively, of DEChNs dispersions). Data are presented as mean ± standard error. *$p < 0.05$ compared with the control group; **$p < 0.01$ compared with the control group.

*Table 3.* Serum lipid levels of mice

| Groups | Blank[a] | Control[b] | L-DEChNs[c] | M-DEChNs[d] | H-DEChNs[e] |
|---|---|---|---|---|---|
| TC (mmol/L) | 3.562 ± 0.786 | 3.910 ± 0.596 | 3.321 ± 0.589* | 3.801 ± 0.883* | 3.429 ± 0.507* |
| TG (mmol/L) | 1.389 ± 0.430 | 1.247 ± 0.559 | 1.385 ± 0.514 | 1.311 ± 0.660 | 0.709 ± 0.234 |
| HDL (mmol/L) | 1.665 ± 0.406 | 1.658 ± 0.830 | 0.842 ± 0.346** | 0.702 ± 0.176** | 0.678 ± 0.263* |
| HDL/TC | 0.468 ± 0.225 | 0.424 ± 0.133 | 0.253 ± 0.134 | 0.185 ± 0.084** | 0.198 ± 0.124 |
| LDL (mmol/L) | 0.614 ± 0.198 | 0.697 ± 0.210 | 0.812 ± 0.271 | 0.849 ± 0.313 | 0.728 ± 0.166 |

TC, total cholesterol; TG, triacylglycerol; HDL-C, high density lipoprotein cholesterol; LDL-C, low density lipoprotein cholesterol[a]

Blank group (fed a normal diet and saline solution); [b]control group (fed a high-fat diet and dilute acetic acid solution); [c,d,e]L-, M-, H-DEChN groups (fed a high-fat diet and low, medium, high doses of DEChN dispersions, respectively). Data are presented as mean ± standard error. *$p < 0.05$ compared with the control group; **$p < 0.01$ compared with the control group.

the mice in the H-DEChN group were lower than those of mice in the control group; the value of high density lipoprotein cholesterol (HDL-C) 1.658 mmol/L in the control group decreased to 0.678 mmol/L in the H-DEChN group, which is approximately a 2.44-fold decrease, indicating that while feeding the mice a high-fat diet normally resulted in a higher accumulation of lipids in the blood, DEChNs can suppress hyperlipidemia in mice that are fed high-fat diets.

#### *Liver histological examination*

The livers from the mice were subjected to histopathological examination, and the results are shown in Fig. 3. At the end of the experiment, the livers of the mice from the control group had become swollen, oily, and orange. By comparison, the livers from the blank and DEChN groups were normal and dull red in color. As shown in Fig. 3, there were no evident fat vacuoles in the cytoplasm from the blank group, while hepatocytes from mice in the control group had accumulated a large number of fat vacuoles. The results indicated that feeding the mice a high-fat diet resulted in a higher accumulation of lipids in the livers of mice, thereby leading to a severe fatty liver. Histopathological examination of hepatocytes from mice in the DEChN groups revealed that livers had a small number of droplet accumulation compared with those in the control group. In addition, there was no evidence of fat vacuoles in the cytoplasm among the DEChN groups and the livers of the DEChN groups appeared normal, that is, similar to the blank group. These results suggested that a small dosage of DEChN dispersions was effective in decreasing the accumulation of lipids in the liver, thus preventing the development of a fatty liver. The histopathological examination of the liver was consistent with the data collected for BW gain, ATW gain, and serum lipid levels, thereby proving that DEChNs possesses effective hypolipidemic activity.

#### *Optimum dosage of deacetylated α-chitin nanofiber/nanowhisker mixtures*

Azuma et al. recently proposed that an oral administration of surface-deacetylated chitin nanofibers (SDCNFs) decreased the diet-induced increase in serum TC, chylomicron, very-low-density lipoprotein, phospholipid levels, and suppressed vacuolar degeneration and accumulation of lipid droplets in liver tissue (17). They also suggested that administration of SDCNFs did not affect BW change or organ weights. However, our study showed that DEChNs significantly reduced the BW and ATW gains in mice when fed a high-fat diet. The difference may be attributed to the dosage of DEChN dispersions. In the present study, the dosage was under precise control and the DEChNs were intragastrically administered.

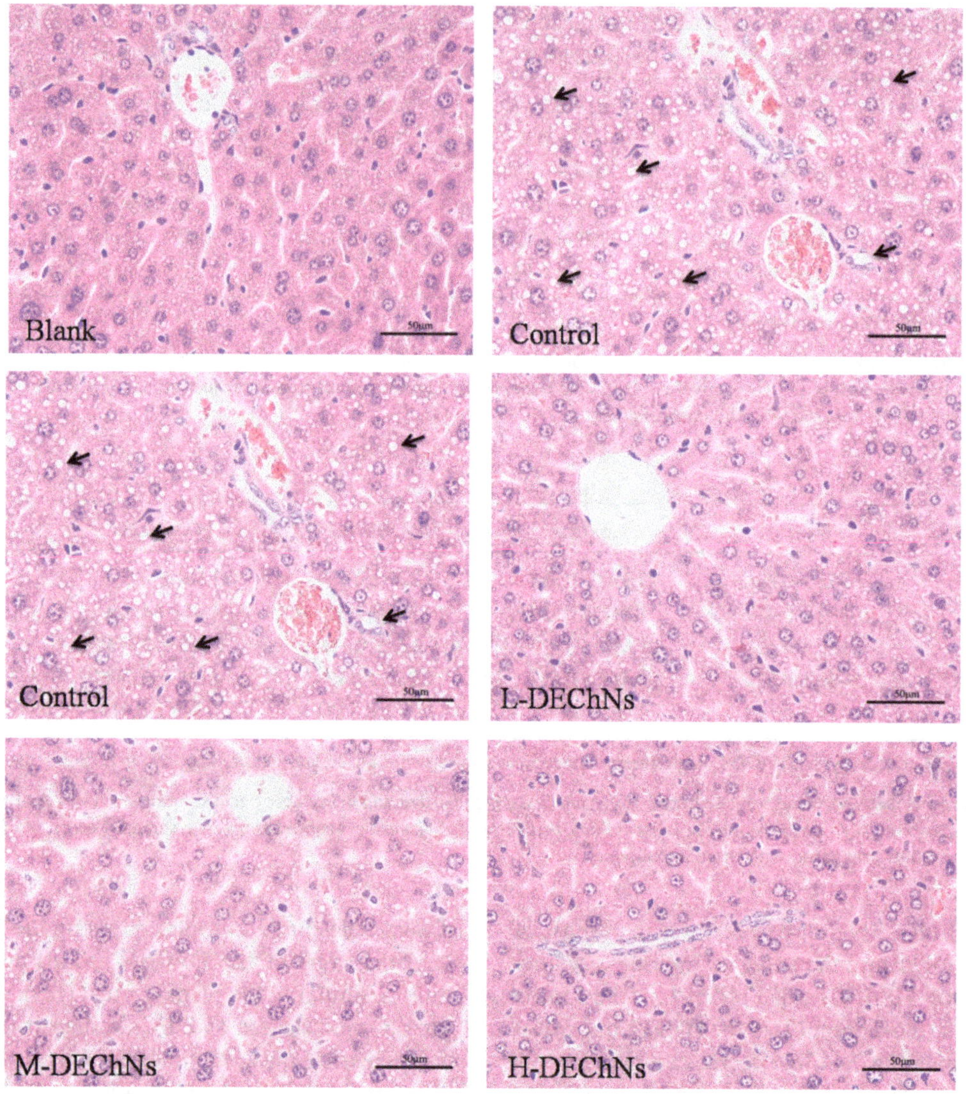


*Fig. 3.* Histological examination of liver tissues from mice in the blank group (fed a normal diet and saline solution), control group (fed a high-fat diet and dilute acetic acid solution), and the L-, M-, H-DEChN groups (fed a high-fat diet and low, medium, high doses of DEChN dispersions, respectively). The arrows point out the fat vacuole in the cytoplasm.

The present study suggests that the BW and ATW gains of the mice in the DEChN groups were significantly lower than those of the control group and changed dramatically in the H-DEChN group. On the contrary, the changes of the weight ratio between tissue and body were observed to be slight. For the H-DEChN group, the suppression of BW gain and the reduction of adipose tissue accumulation were the most obvious. The drastic changes may indicate that mice fed excessive DEChNs exhibited a pathological growth state. Therefore, in consideration of the efficacy of ATW loss and ensuring healthy growth of mice as mentioned above, a dosage of 37.5 mg/kg·bw·d DEChNs (the M-DEChN dose), in the medium dosage range, was recommended and proposed in the present study.

At the recommended optimum dosage, DEChNs can facilitate weight loss and reduce accumulation of fat in diet-induced obese mice and significantly reduce the rise of liver lipid levels in mice when fed a high-fat diet. Meantime, at this dosage, the DEChNs reduced the plasma lipid levels, the serum TC, and TG concentration as well. These values were lower than those of mice fed the high-fat diet and dilute acetic acid solution, indicating that DEChNs can effectively prevent hypercholesterolemia when consuming a high-fat diet. The most probable explanation for this is the binding of lipids to the DEChNs, thereby reducing the absorption of dietary fat and cholesterol *in vivo*.

Chitosan, with an average molecular weight of 650 kDa or greater, was approved by the Ministry of Health, Labour and Welfare (Japan) in 1997 as a specific healthy functional food, and the approved oral dosage of chitosan was 0.5–3 g per day in humans (22). In particular, doses between 2 and 5 g/kg were used to evaluate the hypolipidemic effects of chitosan. In this study, the best dosage of DEChNs for optimal hypolipidemic effects was 37.5 mg/kg·bw·d, which is much lower than the recommended dosage of chitosan. Thus, we conclude that the hypolipidemic effects of DEChNs are more efficient than those of chitosan.

#### *Possible hypolipidemic mechanism of deacetylated α-chitin nanofiber/nanowhisker mixtures*

According to previous reports, chitosan, a derivative of chitin, can reduce BW and ATW gains in mice that are fed high-fat diets (22). The hypolipidemic mechanism of chitosan was investigated in male Sprague-Dawley rats and the results suggested that chitosan reduced the absorption of dietary fat and cholesterol *in vivo*, thereby effectively reducing the occurrence of hypercholesterolemia in rats (23). There have been many studies that have attempted to explain the mechanisms of chitosan in inhibiting hyperlipidemia. A classical perspective, which is widely accepted, is that chitosan binds lipids in the gastrointestinal tract, which are then excreted in the feces (23, 24). DEChNs have a similar molecular structure to chitosan but can be identified by their nanofibrillar morphology, lower amino groups, and increased crystallinity. However, there have not been many research studies that have examined the use of DEChNs in supporting the hypolipidemic activities of mice, as well as the underlying mechanisms of how the DEChNs inhibit hyperlipidemia.

Our zeta-potential detection revealed that even though the DEChNs possess lower amino groups (DDA values approximately 0.25–0.35) than chitosan (DDA values normally >0.70), they still possess high cationic surface charges under acidic conditions. That is to say, chitin, as well as chitosan, may have the unique ability to bind lipids and bile acids. Moreover, the nanofibrillar morphology and high crystallinity might be the other advantages. In detail, the C2-amino groups on the surface of the DEChNs were cationized in gastric juice (pH 1–2), which gave the DEChNs a high zeta-potential of +30–70 mV in the stomach. Positively charging the DEChNs allowed for the attraction and accumulation of anions, such as large amounts of lipids, cholesterol, and bile acid, to the DEChNs via electrostatic attraction. It is noteworthy to mention that the DEChNs do not dissolve at a molecular level but disperse at a nanofibril level in the stomach. Therefore, the DEChNs adsorb to the surface of an oil droplet, decreasing its accessibility to digestive enzymes, thereby decreasing its digestion. Moreover, the DEChNs could act as an emulsifier, affecting the emulsification and adsorption of lipids because DEChNs and oil could contribute to a large accumulation through hydrophobic interaction and nano-effects. Therefore, the binding of lipids and the emulsification could be the main cause for the hypolipidemic action of DEChNs. When the protonated DEChNs enter the intestine (pH 7–7.5), they lose the positive charge then flocculate and precipitate along with the lipids, cholesterol, and bile acid. Thereafter, these precipitates are trapped in the intestine and eventually excreted.

## Conclusions

The present study examined the following effects of DEChNs: 1) reducing accumulation of adipose tissues, 2) preventing increases in plasma in mice that are fed a long-term high-fat diet, and 3) guarding against the symptoms of hypercholesterolemia and fatty liver in mice. Further studies are needed to examine the pharmacokinetics and biodegradability of DEChNs. Finally, the TC and lipid levels of the liver, serum, and liver enzymes and receptors regulating the lipid metabolism were not examined in this study. Therefore, these areas also need further examination.

## Acknowledgments

This research was financially supported by the National Key R&D Program of China (2016YFD0600803), the National Natural Science Foundation of China (No. 31100426), the Doctorate Fellowship Foundation of Nanjing Forestry University, and the Priority Academic Program Development of Jiangsu Higher Education Institutions (PAPD). Thanks to Professor Jiuliang Zhang from Huazhong Agricultural University for his guidance and assistance.

## Conflict of interest and funding

The authors have not received any funding or benefits from industry or elsewhere to conduct this study.

## References

1. Prasad K, Kalra J. Oxygen free radicals and hypercholesterolemic atherosclerosis: effect of vitamin E[J]. Am Heart J 1993; 125(4): 958–973.
2. Zhang HL, Tao Y, Guo J, Hu YM, and Su ZQ. Hypolipidemic effects of chitosan nanoparticles in hyperlipidemia rats induced by high fat diet[J]. Int Immunopharmacol 2011; 11(4): 457–461.
3. Liu X, Sun Z, Zhang M, Meng X, Xia X, Yuan W, et al. Antioxidant and antihyperlipidemic activities of polysaccharides from sea cucumber Apostichopus japonicus[J]. Carbohydr Polymers 2012; 90(4): 1664–1670.
4. Knopp RH. Drug treatment of lipid disorders[J]. N Engl J Med 1999; 341(7): 498–511.
5. Vergara-Jimenez M, Conde K, Erickson SK, and Fernandez ML. Hypolipidemic mechanisms of pectin and psyllium in guinea pigs fed high fat–sucrose diets: alterations on hepatic cholesterol metabolism[J]. J Lipid Res 1998; 39(7): 1455–1465.
6. Anandan R, Ganesan B, Obulesu T, Mathew S, Kumar RS, Lakshmanan PT, et al. Dietary chitosan supplementation attenuates isoprenaline-induced oxidative stress in rat myocardium[J]. Int J Biol Macromol 2012; 51(5): 783–787.
7. Zhang J, Liu J, Li L, and Xia W. Dietary chitosan improves hypercholesterolemia in rats fed high-fat diets[J]. Nutr Res 2008; 28(6): 383–390.

8. Zhang J, Zhang W, Mamadouba B, and Xia W. A comparative study on hypolipidemic activities of high and low molecular weight chitosan in rats[J]. Int J Biol Macromol 2012; 51(4): 504–508.
9. Anraku M, Michihara A, Yasufuku T, Akasaki K, Tsuchiya D, Nishio H, et al. The antioxidative and antilipidemic effects of different molecular weight chitosans in metabolic syndrome model rats[J]. Biol Pharmaceut Bull 2010; 33(12): 1994–1998.
10. Baker WL, Tercius A, Anglade M, White CM, and Coleman CI. A meta-analysis evaluating the impact of chitosan on serum lipids in hypercholesterolemic patients[J]. Ann Nutr Metabol 2009; 55(4): 368–374.
11. Liu L, Lv H, Jiang J, Zheng K, Ye W, Wang Z, et al. Reinforced chitosan beads by chitin nanofibers for the immobilization of β-glucosidase[J]. RSC Adv 2015; 5(113): 93331–93336.
12. Kumar MNVR. A review of chitin and chitosan applications[J]. React Funct Polymers 2000; 46(1): 1–27.
13. Fan Y, Fukuzumi H, Saito T, and Isogai A. Comparative characterization of aqueous dispersions and cast films of different chitin nanowhiskers/nanofibers[J]. Int J Biol Macromol 2012; 50(1): 69–76.
14. Fan Y, Saito T, Isogai A. Individual chitin nano-whiskers prepared from partially deacetylated α-chitin by fibril surface cationization[J]. Carbohydr Polymers 2010; 79(4): 1046–1051.
15. Zhang Y, Jiang J, Liu L, Zheng K, Yu S, and Fan Y. Preparation, assessment, and comparison of α-chitin nano-fiber films with different surface charges[J]. Nanoscale Res Lett 2015; 10(1): 1.
16. Liu L, Wang R, Yu J, Jiang J, Zheng K, Hu L, et al. Robust self-standing chitin Nanofiber/Nanowhisker hydrogels with designed surface charges and ultralow mass content via Gas Phase Coagulation[J]. Biomacromol 2016; 17(11): 3773–3781.
17. Azuma K, Nagae T, Nagai T, Izawa H, Morimoto M, Murahata Y, et al. Effects of surface-deacetylated chitin nanofibers in an experimental model of hypercholesterolemia[J]. Int J Mol Sci 2015; 16(8): 17445–17455.
18. Anraku M, Tabuchi R, Ifuku S, Nagae T, Iohara D, Tomida H, et al. An oral absorbent, surface-deacetylated chitin nano-fiber ameliorates renal injury and oxidative stress in 5/6 nephrectomized rats[J]. Carbohydr Polymers 2017; 161: 21–25.
19. Fan Y, Saito T, Isogai A. Preparation of chitin nanofibers from squid pen β-chitin by simple mechanical treatment under acid conditions[J]. Biomacromol 2008; 9(7): 1919–1923.
20. Qi H, Huang L, Liu X, Liu D, Zhang Q, and Liu S. Antihyperlipidemic activity of high sulfate content derivative of polysaccharide extracted from Ulva pertusa (Chlorophyta)[J]. Carbohydr Polymers 2012; 87(2): 1637–1640.
21. Xu W, Zhou Q, Yin JJ, Yao Y, and Zhang JL. Anti-diabetic effects of polysaccharides from Talinum triangulare in streptozotocin (STZ)-induced type 2 diabetic male mice[J]. Int J Biol Macromol 2015; 72: 575–579.
22. Sumiyoshi M, Kimura Y. Low molecular weight chitosan inhibits obesity induced by feeding a high-fat diet long-term in mice[J]. J Pharm Pharmacol 2006; 58(2): 201–207.
23. Liu J, Zhang J, Xia W. Hypocholesterolaemic effects of different chitosan samples in vitro and in vivo[J]. Food Chem 2008; 107(1): 419–425.
24. Xia W, Liu P, Zhang J, and Chen J. Biological activities of chitosan and chitooligosaccharides[J]. Food Hydrocolloids 2011; 25(2): 170–179.

***Yimin Fan**
College of Chemical Engineering
Nanjing Forestry University
159 Longpan Road, Nanjing 210037, China
E-Mail: fanyimin@njfu.edu.cn

# 3

# Immunomodulatory activity of *Lactobacillus plantarum* KLDS1.0318 in cyclophosphamide-treated mice

Yueyue Meng, Bailiang Li, Da Jin, Meng Zhan, Jingjing Lu, and Guicheng Huo*

Key Laboratory of Dairy Science, Ministry of Education, Northeast Agricultural University, Harbin, China

*Abstract*

***Background:*** Probiotics in fermented foods have attracted considerable attention lately as treatment options for immune diseases, the incidence of which has been increasing throughout the world.
***Objective:*** The objective of the present study was to investigate the immunomodulatory activity of *Lactobacillus plantarum* (*L. plantarum*) KLDS1.0318 in cyclophosphamide-treated mice.
***Design:*** To investigate the immune-enhancing effects of *L. plantarum* KLDS1.0318, we used a immunosuppressive model. Ninety female six-week-old BALB/c mice were randomly divided into six groups: normal control (NC) group, model control (MC) group, immunosuppression plus *L. plantarum* KLDS1.0318 groups with three different doses (KLDS1.0318-L, KLDS1.0318-M, and KLDS1.0318-H), and plus levamisole hydrochloride as positive control (PC) group.
***Results and discussions:*** Results showed that the thymus and spleen indexes of the four treatment groups were significantly higher than those of the MC group (2.01±0.16) ($p < 0.05$). The capacity of lymphocyte proliferation, the activity of natural killer (NK) cell and macrophages phagocytosis were significantly increased ($p < 0.05$) in four treatment groups as compared with the MC group (0.327±0.022, 62.29±0.8, 0.087±0.008, respectively). The levels of relative immune factors (IL-2, IL-6, and IFN-γ) showed similar patterns ($p < 0.05$).
***Conclusions:*** This study suggested that orally administered *L.plantarum* KLDS1.0318 may effectively accelerate the recovery of immunosuppressive mice caused by cyclophosphamide (CTX). The immunomodulatory activity of the srtain recommended that *L. plantarum* KLDS1.0318 could be used as a powerful medicinal treatment against immunosuppression.

Keywords: *Lactobacillus plantarum KLDS1; 0318; splenocyte proliferation; NK cell activity; macrophages phagocytosis; cytokine*

Immunosuppression is a state of temporary or long-lasting immunity dysfunction that results in making the organism more sensitive to pathogens because of the impairment of the immune system (1–4). For example, the human immunodeficiency virus epidemic caused one of the most significant populations of immunocompromised hosts (5), which often brings about a low antibody level or ineffective vaccination in a vaccinated host. For the purpose of controlling viral infectious diseases and preventing secondary infection, vaccines and immunopotentiating drugs, such as levamisole at a high dose, have to be used for long-term cure, which often leads to a great deal of side effects, such as serious neurological symptoms, gastric hemorrhage, colic, anemia, and vasculitis (6–8). Accordingly, investigating and developing new and safer immunomodulating agents is one of the most effective and efficient methods for prevention and treatment of immunosuppressive diseases (9).

People have been seeking an effective means to prevent and remedy immunosuppressive diseases for years, but the progress is slow. In the meantime, the application of traditional probiotics in immunoregulation has acquired some achievements. Probiotics have complicated nutritional requirements and are found in a variety of habitats, such as human and animal mucosal membranes, material of plant origin, sewage, and fermented dairy products and spoiled food (10). They play a vital role in immunomodulation, maintaining the intestinal microbial balance, and preventing gastrointestinal infection. Previous research indicated that lactobacilli can be used for immune stimulation to increase early lines of defense against invading harmful bacteria (11).

Lactobacilli are able to promote immunity in mice, and this effect is dose and strain reliant (12, 13). As the expression profiles of cell wall proteins and content of DNA unmethylated cytidine guanine dinucleotide varied in different probiotics, different probiotic strains and dosages may bring about different immune responses (14–18). A great many studies have reported that *Lactobacillus plantarum* has immunoregulatory function: activation of Th1 immune responses (19), promotion of IgA secretion and prevention of influenza virus infection (20), enhancement of the cytokine profile against mite allergy (21), and improvement of natural killer (NK) cell activity, for instance (22).

*L. plantarum* KLDS1.0318, a newly identified probiotic, was preserved in our laboratory. Its effects on the activity of immune cells *in vitro* were previously investigated and it is considered to be possessed of a higher immunomodulatory activity (23). However, the immunoregulatory effects of *L. plantarum* KLDS1.0318 *in vivo* are not fully clear yet and neither is its immunoregulatory mechanism.

Cyclophosphamide (CTX), a classical myelotoxic agent, was used in a previous study to establish an experimental model applicable to the evaluation of immunomodulation by antibiotics in normal and immunocompromised mice (24). The aim of this experiment was to establish an immunosuppressive model by treating BALB/c mice with CTX. Using this model, the possible effects of *L. plantarum* KLDS1.0318 on the immune system of immunocompromised hosts were investigated.

## Materials and methods

### *Experimental animals*

Ninety female-specific pathogen-free BALB/c mice with a body weight of 20.0 ± 2.0 g were obtained from Beijing Vital River Laboratory Animal Technology Co., Ltd. (Beijing, China). Animals were acclimatized to laboratory conditions for 1 week before commencement of the animal experiment. They were housed in plastic cages at an ambient temperature of 23 ± 1°C, 50 ± 10% humidity, and a 12/12 h light–dark cycle, fed standard laboratory chow, and allowed water *ad libitum*. Animals used in this study were cared for in accordance with the *Guide for the Care and Use of Laboratory Animals* published by the US National Institutes of Health (NIH Publication 85-23, 1996), and all experimental procedures were approved by the Animal Care Review Committee, Northeast Agricultural University.

### *Preparation of bacterial strain*

*L. plantarum* KLDS1.0318 (preserved at Key Laboratory of Dairy Science, Ministry of Education, Northeast Agricultural University) was grown in de Man, Rogosa & Sharpe (MRS) medium (peptone 10.0 g, beef extract 10.0 g, glucose 20.0 g, yeast extract powder 5.0 g, sodium acetate 5.0 g, dipotassium hydrogen phosphate 2.0 g, triammonium citrate 2.0 g, magnesium sulfate 0.5 g, manganese sulfate 0.05 g, Tween 80 1.0 g, distilled water 1,000 mL, pH 6.5) (25) for 18 h at 37 °C. Bacteria were subcultured twice before inoculation of the batch culture at $10^7$ colony-forming units (CFUs)/mL. For the preparation of gavages, the bacteria were harvested by centrifugation (2,000 × g, 10 min), washed twice in sterile phosphate-buffered saline (PBS), and resuspended in sterile PBS. In the pre-experiment, for the assessment of approximate concentrations of viable bacteria, suitable dilutions of the culture were plated onto MRS broth at 37°C for 48 h. The concentrations of *L. plantarum* KLDS1.0318 were found to reach $5 \times 10^9$ CFU/mL. The bacterial strain was diluted in sterile PBS to produce suspensions of designated doses for oral administration.

### *Chemicals*

Roswell Park Memorial Institute (RPMI) 1640, fetal bovine serum (FBS), concanavalin A (ConA), and levamisole hydrochloride were purchased from Sigma Co. (St. Louis, MO, USA). Enzyme-linked immunosorbent assay (ELISA)–based cytokine kits were purchased from Cloud-Clone Corp. (Houston, TX, USA). CTX was purchased from Beijing Solarbio Science & Technology Co., Ltd. (Beijing, China).

### *Experimental design*

All mice were randomly divided into six groups: a normal control (NC) group, model control (MC) group, three *L. plantarum* KLDS1.0318 groups with different doses (KLDS1.0318-L, $5 \times 10^7$ CFU/mL; KLDS1.0318-M, $5 \times 10^8$ CFU/mL; KLDS1.0318-H, $5 \times 10^9$ CFU/mL, 0.2 mL/d), and levamisole hydrochloride (40 mg/kg) as a positive control (PC) group. Except the NC group, the other five groups were injected intraperitoneally with CTX 80 mg/kg/d of body weight in sterile saline for three consecutive days to induce immunosuppression. Body weight was used as a measure of immunosuppression effect (26). All treatments were conducted with 10 mL/kg body weight by oral administration once daily for 20 days. The NC group mice were injected and received an equivalent volume of sterile PBS as the immunosuppression group. An equivalent volume of sterile PBS was administered to MC group mice in the same way.

## Analysis of body weight

Animal body weight was monitored every 4 days throughout the experiment.

## Analysis of immune organ index

The mice were weighed before being sacrificed 20 days after the commencement of oral administration. The thymus and spleen were immediately excised surgically and weighed. The immune organ index was calculated according to the following formula:

$$\text{spleen or thymus indices (mg/g)} = \frac{\textit{spleen or thymus weight}\,(mg)}{\textit{body weight}\,(g)} \quad (27).$$

### *Assay of splenocyte proliferation induced by T-cell mitogen conA*

Mouse spleens were aseptically removed, placed in 0.1 M cold PBS, gently homogenized, and passed through a

200-mesh sieve to generate single-cell suspensions, as previously described (28). Erythrocytes were rapidly washed by hypoosmotic hemolysis. Next, the cells were suspended at a final density of $1 \times 10^6$ cells/mL in RPMI 1640 medium supplemented with 10% FBS. Splenocytes were placed into 96-well flat-bottomed microplates in triplicate at $2 \times 10^5$ cells/well, and then 2.5 μg/well of conA was added to the wells. The cells were then cultured at a total volume of 200 μL/well at 37°C in 5% $CO_2$. Serum-free RPMI 1640 medium was used as the control. After 48 h of incubation, 20 μL CCK-8 (Dojindo Laboratories, Kumamoto-ken, Japan) was added to each well and the plate was incubated for another 2.5 h. Finally, the absorbance at 450 nm was measured using a microplate reader (XD711, Shanghai Xunda Medical Instrument Co., Ltd., Shanghai, China).

#### *Assay of NK cell activity*

NK cell activity was determined using a CCK-8 assay kit (Dojindo Laboratories). Splenocytes were prepared as section Assay of splenocyte proliferation induced by T-cell mitogen conA. Briefly, blank control (RPMI 1640) and spleen cells ($1 \times 10^6$ cells/mL) were added at the level of 0.1 mL per well. One hundred microliters of $1 \times 10^4$ cells/mL YAC-1 cells, used as the target cells, were added into the wells as mentioned above, RPMI 1640 and spleen cells were added at 0.1 mL per well, used as the effector cells. The plates were then incubated at 37°C in 5% $CO_2$ for 20 h. Next, 20 μL of CCK-8 was added. Following another 4 h of co-culture, the optical density of each well was measured using an XD711 microplate reader (Shanghai Xunda Medical Instrument Co., Ltd.). In addition, absorbance measurements were also recorded for the target cell control, blank control, and effector cell control. The percentage of NK cell activity was determined by the following equation:

% of NK cell activity

$$= \left( 1 - \frac{\begin{array}{c} \textit{optical density value of test samples} - \\ \textit{optical density value of effector cell control} \end{array}}{\textit{optical density value of target cell control}} \right) \times 100 \quad (29)$$

#### *Determination of pinocytosis of peritoneal macrophages*

Mice were sacrificed and peritoneal cells were harvested by peritoneal lavage with 4 mL of RPMI 1640 medium supplemented with 10% heat-inactivated FBS. Three milliliters of cell-rich lavage fluid was aspirated and centrifuged at 1,500 rpm for 5 min. The pellet was resuspended at $1 \times 10^6$ cells/mL in RPMI 1640 medium and seeded in 96-well plates at 200 μL/well (30). The plates were then incubated for 3 h at 37°C in 5% $CO_2$, washed three times, and nonadherent cells were removed by aspiration. Attached cells were used as peritoneal macrophages (31). The cells were resuspended in 200 μL RPMI 1640 containing 10% FBS. After 24 h culture at 37°C under 5% $CO_2$, the culture medium was discarded and 100 μL of 0.072% neutral red was added to each well and cultured for another 0.5 h. Then, the mixed solution was discarded and each well was washed thrice with PBS buffer to remove the excess dye and was blotted dry. The cells were resuspended in 50% ethanol containing 1% glacial acetic acid (lysis solution) and maintained overnight at 4°C. Optical densities were then read at 540 nm and expressed as the phagocytosis index.

#### *Cytokine quantitation*

To measure IL-2, IL-6, and IFN-γ by ELISA, the blood of each mouse was collected from the orbital cavity under diethyl ether anesthesia. The fresh blood was kept standing for 10 min at 37°C and then for 15 min at 4°C. Serum was obtained by centrifugation at 3,000 rpm for 10 min and then stored at −40°C until use (30). Concentrations of cytokines (IL-2, IL-6, and IFN-γ) in serum were determined using ELISA assay kits (Cloud-Clone Corp.), according to the manufacturer's instructions. The results were expressed as the concentration of cytokines per milliliter of mouse serum by standard cytokines provided in the kits.

### Statistical analysis

Results were expressed as mean ± standard deviation (SD) of at least three replicates, and the data were analyzed with SPSS 20.0 software (SPSS Inc., Chicago, IL, USA). The statistical significance of data comparisons was determined using one-way analysis of variance, followed by Duncan's multiple range test. Values of $p < 0.05$ were considered to be statistically significant.

## Results

#### *Body weight*

Animal body weight of all the groups was monitored six times in total throughout the experiment. As shown in Fig. 1, there were no big differences in initial body weights on Day 2, after acclimatization in the animal house for 1 week. Subsequently, all five immunosuppressed mice groups, compared with the NC group, showed a dramatic decrease in body weight following the injection of CTX ($p < 0.05$). Compared with the MC group, the KLDS1.0318-L, KLDS1.0318-M, KLDS1.0318-H, and PC groups exhibited more body weight gain throughout the remaining experimental period.

### Immune organ index

As shown in Table 1, compared with the MC mice, the thymus indexes in the PC, KLDS1.0318-M, and KLDS1.0318-H groups were significantly improved ($p < 0.05$); however, there was no significant difference in the low dose of KLDS1.0318 ($p > 0.05$). As for spleen indexes, they were significantly increased ($p < 0.05$) in each KLDS1.0318 treatment group and PC group as compared

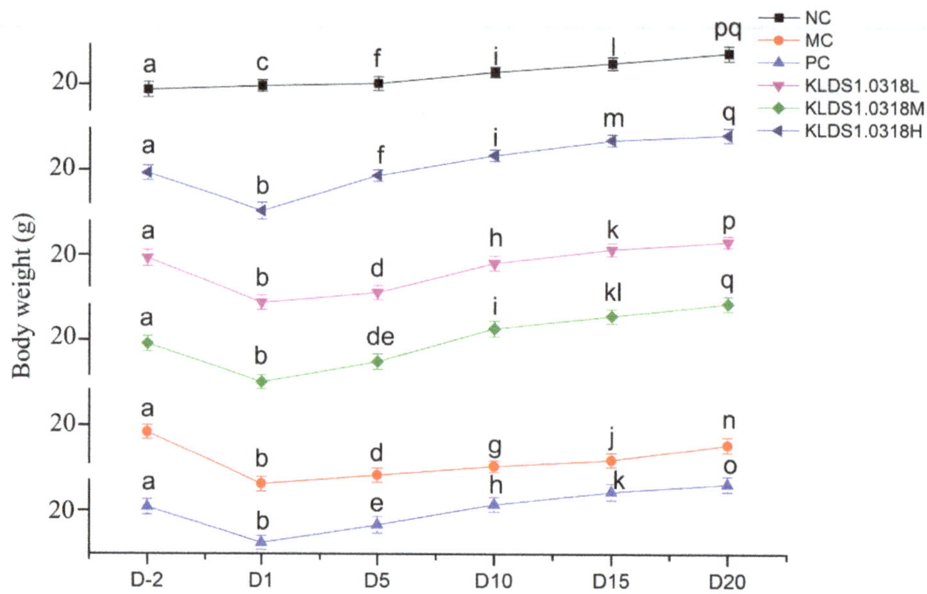


*Fig. 1.* Changes of body weight in the six groups of mice. NC, non-immunosuppression + sterilized PBS; MC, immunosuppression (IM) + sterilized PBS; PC, IM + levamisole hydrochloride (40 mg/kg); KLDS1.0318-L, IM + 5 × $10^7$ CFU/mL *Lactobacillus plantarum* KLDS1.0318; KLDS1.0318-M, IM + 5 × $10^8$ CFU/mL *L. plantarum* KLDS1.0318; KLDS1.0318-H, IM + 5 × $10^9$ CFU/mL *L. plantarum* KLDS1.0318. Data are expressed as the mean ± SD ($n$ = 15). Different letters represent significant differences between groups in the same time point ($p < 0.05$). NC, normal control; PBS, phosphate-buffered saline; MC, model control; PC, positive control; CFU, colony-forming units.

*Table 1.* Effect of *Lactobacillus plantarum* KLDS1.0318 on thymus and spleen indices in mice

| Group | Thymus index (mg/g) | Spleen index (mg/g) |
|---|---|---|
| NC | $2.67 \pm 0.22^{b}$ | $5.83 \pm 0.19^{d}$ |
| MC | $2.01 \pm 0.16^{a}$ | $4.44 \pm 0.17^{a}$ |
| PC | $2.75 \pm 0.15^{b}$ | $5.56 \pm 0.21^{cd}$ |
| KLDS1.0318-L | $2.20 \pm 0.11^{a}$ | $4.81 \pm 0.16^{b}$ |
| KLDS1.0318-M | $2.60 \pm 0.20^{b}$ | $5.24 \pm 0.19^{c}$ |
| KLDS1.0318-H | $3.15 \pm 0.17^{c}$ | $5.63 \pm 0.24^{d}$ |

NC, non-immunosuppression + sterilized PBS; MC, immunosuppression + sterilized PBS; PC, IM + levamisole hydrochloride (40 mg/kg); KLDS1.0318-L, IM + 5 × $10^7$ CFU/mL *L. plantarum* KLDS1.0318; KLDS1.0318-M, IM + 5 × $10^8$ CFU/mL *L. plantarum* KLDS1.0318; KLDS1.0318-H, IM + 5 × $10^9$ CFU/mL *L. plantarum* KLDS1.0318. Data are expressed as the mean ± SD ($n$ = 15). Significant differences ($p < 0.05$) between the groups are indicated with different letters above the data.

with those of the MC group. In addition, KLDS1.0318 treatment exhibited a stronger effect on the thymus index than that of the levamisole hydrochloride–treated mice at a dose of 5 × $10^9$ CFU/mL (0.2 mL/d) ($p < 0.05$).

### *Effect of L. plantarum KLDS1.0318 on conA–induced lymphocyte proliferation*

The effect of *L. plantarum* KLDS1.0318 on the proliferation of splenic T lymphocytes is shown in Fig. 2. The spleen lymphocyte proliferation capacity was significantly increased in the KLDS1.0318-treated groups when compared with the MC group ($p < 0.05$). Moreover, each KLDS1.0318-treated group showed a large increase in a dose-dependent manner, and the change was significant ($p < 0.05$). There was no significant difference in the NC, PC, and KLDS1.0318-H groups ($p > 0.05$). The results indicated that *L. plantarum* KLDS1.0318 could stimulate a T-lymphocyte–specific proliferative response.

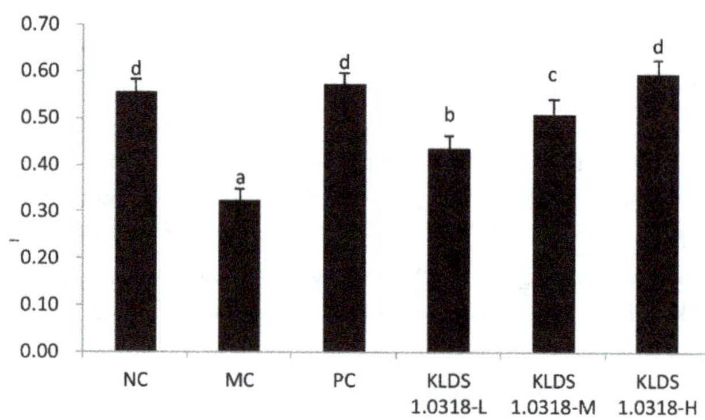


*Fig. 2.* Effect of *L. plantarum* KLDS1.0318 on lymphocyte proliferation in mice. NC, non-immunosuppression + sterilized PBS; MC, immunosuppression + sterilized PBS; PC, IM + levamisole hydrochloride (40 mg/kg); KLDS1.0318-L, IM + 5 × $10^7$. CFU/mL *L. plantarum* KLDS1.0318; KLDS1.0318-M, IM + 5 × $10^8$ CFU/mL *L. plantarum* KLDS1.0318; KLDS1.0318-H, IM + 5 × $10^9$ CFU/mL *L. plantarum* KLDS1.0318. Data are expressed as the mean ± SD ($n$ = 15). Significant differences ($p < 0.05$) between the groups are indicated with different letters above the bars.

### *Effect of L. plantarum KLDS1.0318 on NK cell activity*

As shown in Fig. 3, the results showed that KLDS1.0318 treatment significantly improved ($p < 0.05$) NK cell activity in mice (L, M, H) in a dose-dependent manner. Levamisole hydrochloride treatment also exhibited strong effects on NK cell activity in the PC group mice in comparison with the MC group ($p < 0.05$). Moreover, there was no significant difference between the NC and PC groups ($p > 0.05$). In addition, it was found that *L. plantarum* KLDS1.0318 treatment exhibited a stronger effect on NK cell activity than the PC (levamisole hydrochloride–treated mice) group at a dose of $5 \times 10^8$ and $5 \times 10^9$ CFU/mL (0.2 mL/d) ($p < 0.05$).

### *Effect of L. plantarum KLD1.0318 on phagocytic activity of macrophages*

On Day 20, after oral administration of KLDS1.0318 to CTX-treated mice, we isolated the macrophages and examined their phagocytosis activity. The pinocytosis activity of the mouse peritoneal macrophages was measured by the neutral red uptake method, which is quantitative spectrophotometric determination of neutral red in macrophages. As shown in Fig. 4, while the treatment with CTX alone (MC group) significantly reduced the phagocytosis activity of the macrophages, the treatment with KLDS1.0318 or levamisole hydrochloride significantly restored it ($p < 0.05$). The effect of KLDS1.0318 [$5 \times 10^7$ and $5 \times 10^8$ CFU/mL (0.2 mL/d)] was comparable to that of levamisole hydrochloride, and there was no significant difference between them ($p > 0.05$). However, the high dose of KLDS1.0318 exhibited a stronger effect on the phagocytic activity of macrophages than that of the PC (levamisole hydrochloride–treated mice) group ($p < 0.05$).

### *Effect of L. plantarum KLDS1.0318 on cytokine production*

To evaluate the effect of *L. plantarum* KLDS1.0318 on cytokine production, the levels of cytokines IL-2, IL-6, and IFN-γ in mouse serum were examined. As demonstrated in Table 2, compared with the other five groups, CTX injection caused significant reduction in the concentrations of cytokines (IL-2, IL-6, and IFN-γ) in the MC group ($p < 0.05$). Simultaneously, our results showed that the levels of all the cytokines in the KLDS1.0318 treatment groups (L, M, H) were significantly decreased in a dose-dependent manner when compared with those of the MC group ($p < 0.05$). Furthermore, the levels of IL-2, and IFN-γ in the KLDS1.0318 treatment indicated more significant increase ($p < 0.05$) than those of the PC group at the medium and high dose levels (M, H), while the IL-6 levels in the KLDS1.0318 treatment at the high dose group were markedly enhanced when compared with those of the PC group ($p < 0.05$).

## Discussion

As an alkylating agent, CTX has been most extensively used in chemotherapy. Along with a significant clinical effect, it can significantly damage the structure of DNA, impair immune cells, and strongly interfere with the proliferation and differentiation of T and B cells, reducing the number of normal T and B cells. Meanwhile, it reduces levels of inflammatory cytokines (32, 33), thus suppressing the cellular and humoral immune responses of

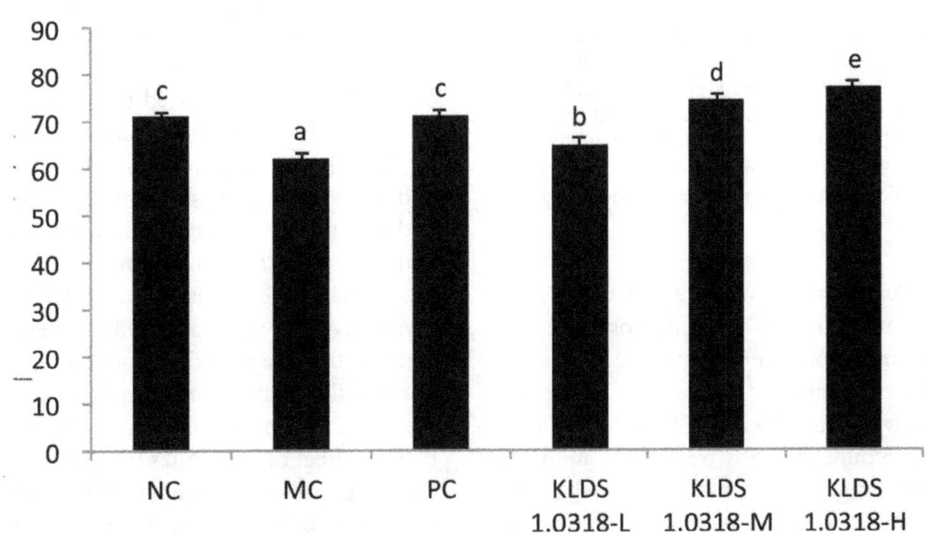


*Fig. 3.* Effect of *L. plantarum* KLDS1.0318 on NK cell activity in mice. NC, non-immunosuppression + sterilized PBS; MC, immunosuppression + sterilized PBS; PC, IM + levamisole hydrochloride (40 mg/kg); KLDS1.0318-L, IM + $5\times10^7$ CFU/mL *L. plantarum* KLDS1.0318; KLDS1.0318-M, IM + $5\times10^8$ CFU/mL *L. plantarum* KLDS1.0318; KLDS1.0318-H, IM + $5\times10^9$ CFU/mL *L. plantarum* KLDS1.0318. Data are expressed as the mean ± SD ($n = 15$). Significant differences ($p < 0.05$) between the groups are indicated with different letters above the bars.

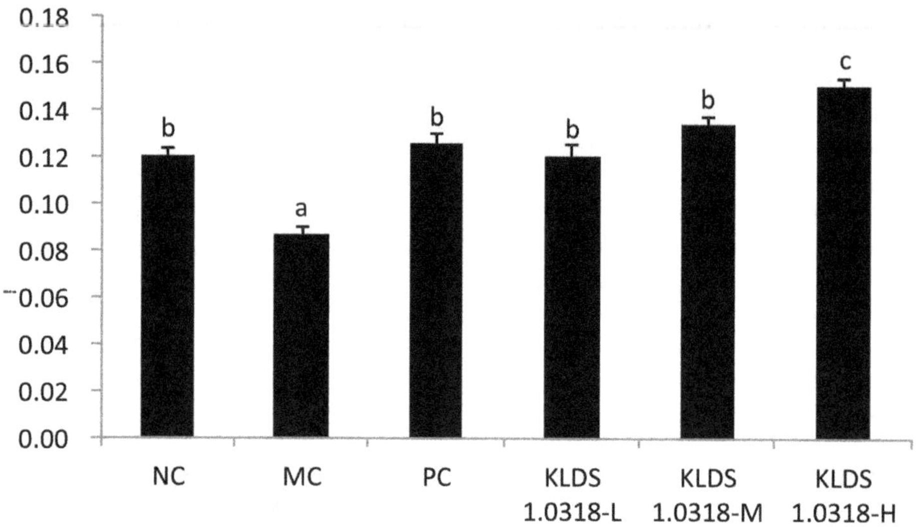


*Fig. 4.* Effect of *L. plantarum* KLDS1.0318 on phagocytic activity of macrophages in mice. NC, non-immunosuppression + sterilized PBS; MC, immunosuppression + sterilized PBS; PC, IM + levamisole hydrochloride (40 mg/kg); KLDS1.0318-L, IM + 5 × $10^7$ CFU/mL *L. plantarum* KLDS1.0318; KLDS1.0318-M, IM + 5 × $10^8$ CFU/mL *L. plantarum* KLDS1.0318; KLDS1.0318-H, IM + 5 × $10^9$ CFU/mL *L. plantarum* KLDS1.0318. Data are expressed as the mean ± SD ($n$ = 15). Significant differences ($p < 0.05$) between the groups are indicated with different letters above the bars.

*Table 2.* Effect of *L. plantarum* KLDS1.0318 on levels of cytokines in serum in mice

| Group | IL-2 (pg/mL) | IL-6 (pg/mL) | IFN-γ (pg/mL) |
|---|---|---|---|
| NC | 58.2 ± 2.7$^b$ | 33.2 ± 1.1$^c$ | 82.3 ± 3.2$^b$ |
| MC | 34.4 ± 2.5$^a$ | 15.4 ± 1.2$^a$ | 60.1 ± 2.8$^a$ |
| PC | 64.5 ± 1.3$^c$ | 31.4 ± 1.7$^c$ | 87.5 ± 3.7$^{bc}$ |
| KLDS1.0318-L | 59.3 ± 1.7$^b$ | 20.7 ± 1.6$^b$ | 92.4 ± 2.9$^c$ |
| KLDS1.0318-M | 71.7 ± 2.2$^d$ | 32.8 ± 2.1$^c$ | 102.4 ± 4.1$^d$ |
| KLDS1.0318-H | 79.6 ± 2.3$^e$ | 37.4 ± 1.9$^d$ | 123.5 ± 2.5$^e$ |

NC, non-immunosuppression + sterilized PBS; MC, immunosuppression + sterilized PBS; PC, IM + levamisole hydrochloride (40 mg/kg); KLDS1.0318-L, IM + 5 × $10^7$ CFU/mL *L. plantarum* KLDS1.0318; KLDS1.0318-M, IM + 5 × $10^8$ CFU/mL *L. plantarum* KLDS1.0318; KLDS1.0318-H, IM + 5 × $10^9$ CFU/mL *L. plantarum* KLDS1.0318. Data are expressed as the mean ± SD ($n$ = 15). Significant differences ($p < 0.05$) between the groups are indicated with different letters above the data.

the organism (9). Accordingly, mice treated with CTX were used as an animal model of an immunosuppressed state to validate the immunoenhancement of *L. plantarum* KLDS1.0318 in this experiment.

In the present study, treatment with CTX (80 mg/kg, i.p.) in mice can notably reduce the body weight and immune organ index, inhibit the proliferation of spleen cells, and lower the phagocytosis activity of the macrophages. Moreover, the levels of cytokines IL-2, IL-6, and IFN-γ were decreased by CTX. These experimental data are in accord with previous reports (26, 32, 34). The results described above expressly indicated that the immune functions of BALB/c mice were significantly repressed by CTX and suggested that the immunosuppressive model of mice was successfully established.

Lactic acid bacteria, such as *Lactobacillus acidophilus and Bifidobacterium bifidum*, have been reported to influence one or more components of humoral, cellular, or activate nonspecific immunity (35, 36). For example, it was shown that *Lactobacillus casei* and *L. acidophilus* were capable of enhancing the number of IgA-producing plasma cells *in vivo* in a dose-dependent manner. Probiotics also promoted splenocyte proliferation in response to mitogens for T and B cells in mice and increased the cytokine production of TNF-α, IL-1β, IL-6, and IFN-γ in immune cells (37). Hence, we tested the ability of lactobacillus to reinstate CTX-induced immunosuppression in mice.

The impact of *L. plantarum* KLDS1.0318 on the thymus and spleen indices was determined first, since the thymus and spleen are such important immune organs in the body and the places of growth and proliferation of immunological cells. The thymus is the immune organ in which T lymphocytes develop, proliferate, differentiate, and mature, whereas the spleen mainly contains T and B cells. Consequently, the immune organ index is usually used to reflect the growth of immune organs and evaluate the immunoregulatory effect of probiotics (38, 39). Li et al. (40) reported that some lactobacilli significantly improved the immune organ index. In the present study, our results showed that the thymus and spleen indexes in four treatment groups were obviously greater than those in the MC group at the end of the experiment. The results indicated that *L. plantarum* KLDS1.0318 could resist the influence of immunosuppression on the development of immune organs.

Lymphocyte proliferation in response to corresponding mitogens is commonly determined when evaluating the efficacy of immunomodulatory agents; thus, lymphoproliferation assays have been used to analyze the effects of probiotics on immune function (41). Ren et al. (30) tested the immunomodulatory effects of *Lactobacillus salivarius* CICC 23174 and *L. plantarum* CGMCC 1.557 and found that the splenocyte proliferation index was prominently increased by the two strains in a dose-dependent manner. To test the effect of *L. plantarum* KLDS1.0318 on the cellular immune response, we isolated the splenocytes of mice and examined their proliferation and the activity of NK cells. Our results showed that *L. plantarum* KLDS1.0318 markedly enhanced splenocyte proliferation and the activity of NK cells, suggesting that the strain could improve humoral immunity and cell-mediated immunity and correspondingly could have potential immune activity. We also examined phagocytosis of macrophages in response to *L. plantarum* KLDS1.0318, given that phagocytosis by macrophages is the primary line of defense of the immune system to defend against microbial attack. The results showed a strong increase in phagocytic activity, indicating that *L. plantarum* KLDS1.0318 played a crucial role in the initiation and modulation of nonspecific immune responses by some cytokines and reactive intermediates secreted by macrophages, which is consistent with a previous report (42).

Given that cytokines play a significant role in the development of immune response, the effect of the lactobacillus strain on the production of IL-2, IL-6, and IFN-γ was evaluated. IL-2 is a cytokine essential for the survival and proliferation of T cells. Accordingly, IL-2 secretion increased by KLDS1.0318 may stimulate T-cell proliferation and IFN-γ production, which in turn improves the immune response against cancer and pathogen-infected cells. IL-2 also induces NK cell activation, which restrains the growth and metastases of tumors (43). IL-6 secreted by Th2 cells can regulate humoral immunity (44) as one of the most essential immune and inflammatory mediators that modulate diverse cell functions, such as proliferation and differentiation of B and T cells (45). IFN-γ released by Th1 cells can effectively mediate cellular immunity (46) as one of the dominant immunoregulatory molecules that enhance potent immune responses against pathogenic bacteria and exogenous infectious agents (47). Investigation by Jang et al. (48) showed that *L. casei* HY7213 can induce the production of antitumorigenic cytokines (e.g. IL-2 and IFN-γ). In this study, the concentrations of the three cytokines in each of the KLDS1.0318 dose groups were much higher than those in the MC group. This indicated that *L. plantarum* KLDS1.0318 could highly induce the secretion of some cytokines and help maintain a balance between Th1 and Th2 type cytokines, which play an important role in host immunity.

In summary, the present study has demonstrated that *L. plantarum* KLDS1.0318 improved immunity by promoting immune organ development; enhancing lymphocyte proliferation; increasing the activity of NK cells; improving the activity of macrophage phagocytosis; and upregulating the levels of IL-2, IL-6, and IFN-γ. Consequently, these results suggest that *L. plantarum* KLDS1.0318 is an effective immunomodulating agent and may be effectively used to improve the immune function in humans.

## Acknowledgements

The present research work was financially supported by the National Key Research and Development Program of China (No. 2017YFD0400303) and the National Natural Science Foundation of China (No. 31401512).

## Conflict of interest and funding

The authors have not received any funding or benefits from industry or elsewhere to conduct this study.

## References


1. Yan ZG, Du YJ, Zhao QY, Fan RF, Guo WL, & Ma RD, et al. Mucosal immune responses against live Newcastle disease vaccine in immunosuppressed chickens. *Pak Vet J* 2011; 31(4): 280–6.
2. Cui ZZ, Meng SS, Jiang SJ, Wei JP. Serological surveys zof chicken anemia virus, avian reticuloendotheliosis virus and avian reovirus infections in white meat-type chickens in China. *Acta Veterinaria Et Zootechnica Sinica* 2006; 37(2): 152–7.
3. Cazaban C. Immunosuppression in chickens – what is it? *Int Poul Prod* 2006; 13(8): 13–14
4. Shini S, Shini A, Kaiser P. Cytokine and chemokine gene expression profiles in heterophils from chickens treated with corticosterone. *Stress* 2010; 13(3): 185–94.
5. Patel DM, Riedel DJ. Fever in immunocompromised hosts. *Emerg Med Clin North Am* 2013; 31(4): 1059.
6. Bagga A, Hari P. Levamisole-induced vasculitis. *Pediatr Nephrol* 2000; 14(10–11): 1057.
7. Joly C, Palisse M, Ribbe D, De CO, & Genevey P. [Acute levamisole poisoning]. *Presse Medicale* 1998; 27(15): 717.
8. Palcoux JB, Niaudet P, Goumy P. Side effects of levamisole in children with nephrosis. *Pediatr Nephrol* 1994; 8(2): 263.
9. Fan Y, Lu Y, Wang D, Liu J, Song X, Zhang W, et al. Effect of epimedium polysaccharide-propolis flavone immunopotentiator on immunosuppression induced by cyclophosphamide in chickens. Cell Immunol 2013; 281(1): 37–43.
10. de Vrese M, Schrezenmeir J. Probiotics, prebiotics, and synbiotics. *Adv Biochem Eng Biotechnol* 2008; 111(8): 1.
11. Goldin BR. Health benefits of probiotics. *Br J Nutr* 1998; 80(4): S203.
12. Galdeano C, Perdigon G. Role of viability of probiotic strains in their persistence in the gut and in mucosal immune stimulation. *J Appl Microbiol* 2004; 97(4): 673.
13. Paturi G, Phillips M, Jones M, & Kailasapathy K. Immune enhancing effects of *Lactobacillus acidophilus* LAFTI L10 and *Lactobacillus paracasei* LAFTI L26 in mice. *Int J Food Microbiol* 2007; 115(1): 115–118.
14. Cross ML. Microbes versus microbes: immune signals generated by probiotic *lactobacilli* and their role in protection against

microbial pathogens. *Fems Immunol Med Microbiol* 2002; 34(4): 245–53.

15. Gill HS, Rutherfurd KJ, Prasad J, Gopal PK. Enhancement of natural and acquired immunity by *Lactobacillus rhamnosus* (HN001), *Lactobacillus acidophilus* (HN017) and Bifidobacterium lactis (HN019). *Br J Nutr* 2000; 83(2): 167–76.
16. Gill HS, Rutherfurd KJ, Cross ML, Gopal PK. Enhancement of immunity in the elderly by dietary supplementation with the probiotic Bifidobacterium lactis HN019. *Am J Clin Nutr* 2001; 74(6): 833.
17. Kirjavainen PV, El-Nezami HS, Salminen SJ, Ahokas JT, Wright PF, et al. The effect of orally administered viable probiotic and dairy *lactobacilli* on mouse lymphocyte proliferation. *Fems Immunol Med Microbiol* 1999; 26(2): 131–5.
18. Nagafuchi S, Takahashi T, Yajima T, Kuwata T, Hirayama K, Itoh K, et al. Strain dependency of the immunopotentiating activity of Lactobacillus delbrueckii subsp. bulgaricus. *Biosci Biotechnol Biochem* 1999; 63(3): 474.
19. Kawashima T, Hayashi K, Kosaka A, Kawashima M, Igarashi T, Tsutsui H, et al. *Lactobacillus plantarum* strain YU from fermented foods activates Th1 and protective immune responses. *Int Immunopharmacol* 2011; 11(12): 2017–24.
20. Kikuchi Y, Kunitoh-Asari A, Hayakawa K, Imai S, Kasuya K, Abe K, Adachi Y, Fukudome S, Takahashi Y, Hachimura S. 2014. Oral administration of Lactobacillus plantarum strain AYA enhances IgA secretion and provides survival protection against influenza virus infection in mice. PLoS One 9, e86416.
21. Rigaux P, Daniel C, Hisbergues M, Muraille E, Hols P, Pot B, et al. Immunomodulatory properties of *Lactobacillus plantarum*, and its use as a recombinant vaccine against mite allergy. *Allergy* 2009; 64(3): 406–14.
22. Rizzo A, Losacco A, Carratelli CR, Domenico MD, Bevilacqua, N. *Lactobacillus plantarum* reduces Streptococcus pyogenes virulence by modulating the IL-17, IL-23 and Toll-like receptor 2/4 expressions in human epithelial cells. *Int Immunopharmacol* 2013; 17(2): 453–61.
23. Yueyue M, Li Z, Guicheng H. Effects of ten strains of *Lactobacillus* on the activity of immune cells *in vitro*. *Sci Technol Food Ind* (in Chinese, 2018; 39(01): 312–317).
24. Jimenez M. Modification of mitogen-driven lymphoproliferation by ceftriaxone in normal and immunocompromised mice. *Int J Antimicrob Agents* 2003; 22(6): 607.
25. Guo Y, Pan D, Li H, Sun Y, Zeng X, Yan B. Antioxidant and immunomodulatory activity of selenium exopolysaccharide produced by Lactococcus lactis subsp. lactis. *Food Chem* 2013; 138(1): 84–9.
26. Grønbaek H, Skjaerbaek C, Orskov H, Flyvbjerg A. Effect of immunosuppression on kidney and serum insulin-like growth factor-I (IGF-I), IGF binding proteins, and renal growth following unilateral nephrectomy in rats. *Metab Clin Exp* 1998; 47(7): 817–23.
27. Xu C, Wang Y, Jin M, Yang X. Preparation, characterization and immunomodulatory activity of selenium-enriched exopolysaccharide produced by bacterium Enterobacter cloacae Z0206. *Bioresour Technol* 2009; 100(6): 2095–7.
28. Yuan H, Song J, Li X, Li N, Dai J. Immunomodulation and antitumor activity of κ-carrageenan oligosaccharides. *Cancer Lett* 2006; 243(2): 228–34.
29. Yuan C, Wang C, Bu Y, Xiang T, Huang X, Wang Z, et al. Antioxidative and immunoprotective effects of Pyracantha fortuneana (Maxim.) *Li polysaccharides in mice. Immunol Lett* 2010; 133(1): 14–18.
30. Ren D, Li C, Qin Y, Yin R, Du S, Liu H, et al. Evaluation of immunomodulatory activity of two potential probiotic *Lactobacillus* strains by *in vivo* tests. *Anaerobe* 2015; 35(Pt B): 22–7.
31. Park YJ, Liu G, Tsuruta Y, Lorne E, Abraham E. Participation of the urokinase receptor in neutrophil efferocytosis. *Blood* 2009; 114(4): 860.
32. Wang H, Wang M, Chen J, Tang Y, Dou J, Yu J, et al. A polysaccharide from Strongylocentrotus nudus eggs protects against myelosuppression and immunosuppression in cyclophosphamide-treated mice. *Int Immunopharmacol* 2011; 11(11): 1946.
33. Yu X, Wang C, Luo J, Zhao X, Wang L, Li X. Combination with methotrexate and cyclophosphamide attenuated maturation of dendritic cells: inducing Treg Skewing and Th17 suppression in vivo. *Clin Dev Immunol* 2014; 2013(1): 238035.
34. Yu Q, Nie SP, Wang JQ, Liu XZ, Yin PF, Huang DF, et al. Chemoprotective effects of Ganoderma atrum polysaccharide in cyclophosphamide-induced mice. *Int J Biol Macromol* 2014; 64: 395–401.
35. Elmadfa I, Klein P, Meyer AL. Immune-stimulating effects of lactic acid bacteria *in vivo* and *in vitro*. *Proc Nutr Soc* 2010; 69(3): 416.
36. Masood MI, Qadir MI, Shirazi JH, Khan IU, et al. Beneficial effects of lactic acid bacteria on human beings. *Crit Rev Microbiol* 2011; 37(1): 91.
37. Won TJ, Kim B, Oh ES, Bang JS, Lee YJ, Yoo JS, et al. Immunomodulatory activity of *Lactobacillus* strains isolated from fermented vegetables and infant stool. *Can J Physiol Pharmacol* 2011; 89(6): 429.
38. Nakamura S, Kuda T, An C, Kanno T, Takahashi H, Kimura B. Inhibitory effects of Leuconostoc mesenteroides 1RM3 isolated from narezushi, a fermented fish with rice, on Listeria monocytogenes infection to Caco-2 cells and A/J mice. *Anaerobe* 2012; 18(1): 19–24.
39. Li CY, Lin HC, Lai CH, Lu JJ, Wu SF, Fang SH. Immunomodulatory effects of *lactobacillus* and *Bifidobacterium* on both murine and human mitogen-activated T cells. *Int Arch Allergy Immunol* 2011; 156(2): 128–36.
40. Li SP, Zhao XJ, Wang JY. Synergy of Astragalus polysaccharides and probiotics (*Lactobacillus* and *Bacillus* cereus) on immunity and intestinal microbiota in chicks. *Poult Sci* 2009; 88(3): 519–25.
41. Campbell C, Chew B, Luedecke L, Shultz T. Yogurt consumption does not enhance immune function in healthy premenopausal women. *Nutrition & Cancer-an International Journal* 2000; 37(1): 27–35.
42. Son EH, Moon EY, Rhee DK, Pyo S. Stimulation of various functions in murine peritoneal macrophages by high mannuronic acid-containing alginate (HMA) exposure *in vivo*. *Int Immunopharmacol* 2001; 1(1): 147.
43. Hoover SK, Barrett SK, Turk TMT, Lee TC, Bear HD, Cyclophosphamide and abrogation of tumor-induced suppressor T cell activity. *Cancer Immunol Immunother* 1990; 31(2): 121–7.
44. Salgame P, Abrams JS, Clayberger C, Goldstein H, Convit J, Modlin RL, et al. Differing lymphokine profiles of functional subsets of human CD4 and CD8 T cell clones. *Science* 1991; 254(5029): 279.
45. Sobota RM, Muller PJ, Khouri C, Ullrich A, Poli V, Noguchi T, et al. SHPS-1/SIRP1 alpha contributes to interleukin-6 signalling. Cell Signal 2008; 20(7): 1385–1391.
46. Letsch A, Scheibenbogen C. Quantification and characterization of specific T-cells by antigen-specific cytokine production

using ELISPOT assay or intracellular cytokine staining. *Methods* 2003; 31(2): 143–9.

47. Sugisaki H, Yamanaka K, Kakeda M, Kitagawa H, Tanaka K, Watanabe K, et al. Increased interferon-gamma, interleukin-12p40 and IL-8 production in Propionibacterium acnes-treated peripheral blood mononuclear cells from patient with acne vulgaris: host response but not bacterial species is the determinant factor of the disease. *J Dermatol Sci* 2009; 55(1): 47–52.
48. Jang SE, Joh EH, Ahn YT, Huh CS, Han MJ, Kim DH. *Lactobacillus casei* HY7213 ameliorates cyclophosphamide-induced immunosuppression in mice by activating NK, cytotoxic T cells and macrophages. *Immunopharmacol Immunotoxicol* 2013; 35(3): 396–402.

***Guicheng Huo**
Institutional Open Access Program (IOAP): Northeast Agricultural University
Department of Food Science
Northeast Agricultural University
No. 59 Mucai Street, Xiangfang District
Harbin 150030, China
Email: gchuo@neau.edu.cn

# 4

# Alignments of endocrine, anthropometric and metabolic parameters in type 2 diabetes after intervention with an Okinawa-based Nordic diet

Bodil Ohlsson[1]*, Gassan Darwiche[1], Bodil Roth[1] and Peter Höglund[2]

[1]Department of Internal Medicine, Skåne University Hospital, Lund University, Malmö, Sweden; [2]Department of Clinical Chemistry and Pharmacology, Skåne University Hospital, Lund University, Lund, Sweden

*Abstract*

***Background:*** An Okinawa-based Nordic diet with moderately low carbohydrate content and high fat and protein content has been shown to improve anthropometry and metabolism in type 2 diabetes.

***Objective:*** The objectives of this study were to measure plasma or serum levels of hormones regulating energy metabolism and metabolic control, that is, cholecystokinin (CCK), Cortisol, C-peptide, ghrelin, glucagon, glucagon-like peptide-1 (GLP-1), glucose-dependent insulinotropic polypeptide (GIP), insulin, leptin, plasminogen activator inhibitor-1 (PAI-1), polypeptide YY (PYY), resistin, and visfatin after this diet intervention, and to determine partial correlations between hormonal levels and anthropometric and metabolic responses.

***Design:*** A total of 30 patients (17 women) with type 2 diabetes, mean age 57.5 ± 8.2 years, and body mass index (BMI) 29.9 ± 4.1 kg/m$^2$ were served the diet for 12 weeks. Fasting hormones were measured by Luminex and enzyme–linked immunosorbent assay (ELISA) before study start and after 12 and 28 weeks, along with anthropometric and metabolic parameters.

***Result:*** The levels of CCK ($P = 0.005$), cortisol ($P = 0.015$), C-peptide ($P = 0.022$), glucagon ($P = 0.003$), GLP-1 ($P = 0.013$), GIP ($P < 0.001$), insulin ($P = 0.004$), leptin ($P < 0.001$), and PYY ($P < 0.001$) were lowered after dietary intervention. These reduced levels only remained for PYY at week 28 ($P = 0.002$), when also ghrelin ($P = 0.012$) and visfatin ($P = 0.021$) levels were reduced. Changes of glucose values correlated with changed levels of C-peptide and PYY ($P < 0.001$), insulin ($P = 0.002$), and PAI-1 ($P = 0.009$); changes of triglyceride values with changed levels of C-peptide, insulin, and PYY ($P < 0.001$) and PAI-1 ($P = 0.005$); changes of insulin resistance with changes of leptin levels ($P = 0.003$); and changes of BMI values with changed levels of C-peptide, insulin, and leptin ($P < 0.001$).

***Conclusions:*** Okinawa-based Nordic diet in type 2 diabetes has significant impact on the endocrine profile, which correlates with anthropometric and metabolic improvements.

Keywords: *adipokines; incretins; gut hormones; Okinawa-based Nordic diet; metabolic control*

High intake of plant-derived foods and a lower intake of red meat, meat products, sweets, salt, high-fat dairy, and refined grains are considered to be important features of a healthy diet (1). There is a growing interest in healthy dietary patterns, such as Mediterranean and Okinawan diets, to improve metabolism, inflammation, and cardiovascular health in the population (2). A modified Okinawan diet has been developed consisting of moderately low carbohydrate content and higher contents of fiber, fat, and protein, with food components suitable for the Nordic population (3). A single meal of this diet to healthy volunteers has been shown to attenuate the postprandial responses of glucose, C-peptide, insulin, and glucose-dependent insulinotropic polypeptide (GIP), leaving the secretion of adipokines, ghrelin, glucagon, glucagon-like peptide-1 (GLP-1), and plasminogen activator inhibitor-1 (PAI-1) unaffected (4). The increased postprandial satiety did not correlate with any hormonal changes (4).

The question remains as to how much of the responses after a single meal are reflected in long-term effects of dietary interventions. Both luminal carbohydrates and fat induce postprandial secretion of the incretins GIP and GLP-1, GIP secretion being more sensitive to carbohydrate stimulation and GLP-1 secretion being more sensitive to fat stimulation (5, 6). Apart from facilitating glucose-stimulated insulin secretion, GIP also has a role in obesity development through increased hydrolysis of circulating triacylglycerides, with subsequent re-esterification of free fatty acids into triacylglycerides in adipocytes (7). GLP-1 is the most potent incretin and it improves glucose homeostasis during meals by increasing insulin secretion and reducing food intake, gastrointestinal motility, secretion of digestive enzymes into the lumen, and glucagon secretion (8, 9). As GLP-1 reduces intestinal motility, this peptide mediates a better proximal fat absorption (5).

Cholecystokinin (CCK) is released in response to fat and protein, and it is an important hormone in the regulation of gastrointestinal motility and satiety (10). Polypeptide YY (PYY) is secreted in response to fat and protein intake and levels appear to be affected by acute exercise, adiposity, and composition of macronutrients (including fiber) and fatty acids from dietary fat (11). The most important effect of PYY is regulation of appetite and body weight, but recent research suggests that PYY also has an impact on beta cell mass, thereby participating in glucose homeostasis (12). Ghrelin plays a role in body energy metabolism and its concentration is greatest in the fasting state, to be suppressed in response to meal intake (13).

Adipokines, that is, leptin, resistin, and visfatin, are hormones released from the adipose tissue and have a central role in the control of energy metabolism, regulation of glucose and lipid metabolism, and insulin sensitivity (14). These hormones are supposed to be involved in the development of obesity, diabetes, inflammation, auto-immunity, and metabolic syndromes (15). Elevated levels of PAI-1 form a link between obesity, insulin resistance, and the risk of cardiovascular events (16). Cortisol is assumed to be involved in the development of metabolic syndrome and type 2 diabetes (17).

Our hypothesis was that the Okinawa-based Nordic diet influences the hormone secretion in type 2 diabetes, in alignment with changes in metabolic and anthropometric parameters. The diet was given to patients with type 2 diabetes for 12 weeks, with a follow-up after another 16 weeks. Blood samples and clinical examinations were taken before the study started, and after 12 and 28 weeks. The beneficial impact on metabolic and anthropometric parameters has been presented in a previous report (3). The primary objective of the present study was to assess changes in plasma levels of hormones regulating satiety and metabolic control, that is, CCK, Cortisol, C-peptide, ghrelin, glucagon, GLP-1, GIP, insulin, leptin, PAI-1, PYY, resistin, and visfatin, during and after a dietary intervention. The secondary objectives were to determine partial correlations between hormonal levels and metabolic responses, blood pressure, body mass index (BMI), weight, and waist circumference.

## Methods and materials

The subjects were treated according to the Declaration of Helsinki and the study was approved by the Regional Ethics Review Board at Lund University (2014/460). All subjects gave their written, informed consent before participating in the study which was monitored by an external monitor and registered at ClinicalTrials.gov data base (NCT02405806).

### *Study population*

Patients with type 2 diabetes, independently of BMI or anti-diabetic treatment regimen, aged between 18 and 70 years, were recruited from diabetes patients at a primary health care center in the southernmost district of Sweden.Patients were to have both parents born in Scandinavia, to avoid possible influence of ethnicity on the study results. Overall, exclusion criteria were severe food allergy, and severe heart, pulmonary, cardiovascular, malignant, or psychiatric diseases. Patients with type 1 diabetes, severe liver insufficiency, defined as spontaneous international normalized ratio (INR) > 1.1, or severe renal insufficiency, defined as estimated glomerular filtration rate (eGFR) < 30 mL/min/1.73m$^2$, as well as patients with a prior major gastrointestinal surgery were excluded. Patients with known alcohol and drug abuse were not considered for inclusion. Participants were initially informed through a mail of the project design and purpose (Supplementary Fig. 1). One week later, all the patients were contacted by phone by one of the three investigators (BO and GD, physicians, or the nutritionist).

### *Study design*

The trial was a clinical prospective interventional study with the patients being their own controls, performed at Skåne University Hospital, Malmö, Sweden, and conducted for 12 weeks with an Okinawa-based Nordic diet, followed by a clinical follow-up after 16 weeks with unrestricted diets. A detailed description of the study design, diet components, and methodology has recently been published in a separate publication (3). Briefly, all tests were performed under standardized conditions and stable temperatures. The study data consisting of blood sampling, assessments of anthropometric data, and completion of questionnaires were obtained at three separate visits: (1) at study start before introduction of the diet; (2) after 12 weeks on the Okinawa-based Nordic diet; and (3) after 16 weeks on unrestricted diet. In addition, two visits after 2 and 6 weeks were performed to assess anthropometric data and complete a protocol to check for compliance (Supplementary Fig. 1). All participants were instructed by a nutritionist on how to prepare their breakfast, based on the data from the nutrition questionnaire. Food for lunch, dinner, and snacks was delivered home in a cooler bag three times a week, free of charge, along with written information and recipes for meal preparation. The participants were in close contact with a nutritionist throughout the study and compliance was registered. The participants were encouraged to maintain their regular physical activity habits throughout the intervention. Blood samples were collected through an intravenous catheter after a 10-h fast. Metabolic parameters were analyzed at once, and plasma and serum were harvested and stored at −80°C until analyzed for hormonal concentrations. The study started on 2 February 2015 and ended on 18 September 2015.

*Diets*

The diet is based on the traditional Okinawan diet (1) but modified to suit the taste and food components suitable for the Nordic population (3). The meal composition is consistent with moderately low carbohydrate content, one of four nutritional recommendations from the Swedish National Food Agency for patients with diabetes (18). These recommendations are in line with international recommendations (American Diabetes Association [ADA], European Association for the Study of Diabetes [EASD]). At the same time, the contents of fiber, fat, and protein are increased, which lead to a bigger meal demanding more mastication and prolonged meal intake (4). The food is based on traditional Nordic raw food, for example, whole grains, vegetables, legumes, root crops, fatty fish, fruits, berries, and nuts, with minimal industrial processing. Furthermore, the amount of dairy products, red meat, and processed meat, as well as sugar and white flour was limited to have a diet with low glycemic index (GI). The diet has a good nutritional supply including a mean calorie intake of around 1,900 kcal/day, which is slightly lower compared with a traditional diet. The participants were allowed to eat three meals a day, including breakfast, lunch, and dinner, and two snacks between meals consisting of a variety of fruits, berries, and seeds. Organic food items were preferred whenever possible. During cravings, the subjects were instructed to eat a third snack (e.g. carrots, boiled eggs, mackerel in tomato sauce, or cottage cheese with berries) to avoid eating fast carbohydrates. Raw vegetables or green salad were to be ingested with the main meals – 100 g at breakfast and 150 g at lunch and dinner, respectively. The participants were instructed always to start with the vegetables and to eat slowly. Nutrition information is given in Supplementary Table 1. Darwiche et al. (3) have described the details of the food composition.

The meals were planned at the kitchen of Igelösa Life Science Lab (Lund University) and delivered to the subjects regularly free of charge, along with written information and recipes for meal preparation. Two breakfast alternatives were ingested which consisted of porridge or fermented milk in combination with bread, depending on their ordinary breakfast, and the subjects had to buy the breakfast themselves.

No dietary supplements such as fish oil, probiotics, or multivitamin drugs were allowed to be introduced during the study period. One visit to a restaurant or for another diet per week was allowed. Journeys or a stay during a longer time period at another place had to be discussed with the investigators. Maximal intake of alcoholic beverages was set at 30 g ethanol/week, using the following formula: volume% × mL volume/100 × 0.8.

During the study period, the nutritionist met the participants at baseline, and at 2, 6, 12, and 28 weeks afterward (Supplementary Fig. 1). At week 2, a dietary follow-up was conducted with the ability to adjust the food composition. Furthermore, the nutritionist emailed information to all participants weekly, and they could reach the nutritionist by email and telephone calls when needed, to support the subjects and enhance compliance as much as possible. They also had the opportunity to provide written feedback to the nutritionist using the returned cooler bag. Participants completed a nutrition questionnaire which was collected at study start, and at week 12 and 28, and also completed a food diary during the 12 intervention weeks, from which they received feedback by the nutritionist. The participants had a good adherence to the diet, as described in detail previously (3).

*Assessment of clinical variables and anthropometry*

The investigations took place under similar conditions by two clinically experienced physicians (BO and GD) at baseline and at 2, 6, 12, and 28 weeks afterward. Physical examination included cardiopulmonary, abdominal, and neurological examinations as well as measurements of blood pressure, pulse, respiratory rate, weight, height, waist circumference, and assessment of BMI. Blood pressure was measured in the supine position. Weight was measured in patients wearing light clothes without shoes. Normal weight was defined as BMI $< 25$ kg/m$^2$, overweight as BMI $\geq 25$ kg/m$^2$ but $<30$ kg/m$^2$, and obesity as BMI $\geq 30$ kg/m$^2$ (19). Waist circumference was measured, midway between the lower border of the rib cage and the superior border of the iliac crest (20). Diabetic complications were registered including autonomic neuropathy (sexual dysfunction, profound sweating, and orthostatic blood pressure), gastrointestinal dysmotility (based on motility examination), levels of albuminuria (measured as albumin/creatinin ratio), macroangiopathy, peripheral neuropathy (examined by patellar and achilles tendon reflexes, vibration sense, and monofilament), and retinopathy (based on fundus photography). The study questionnaire contained questions about socioeconomic factors, medical history, and lifestyle habits, and was completed at baseline and at week 12 and week 28. A more simple protocol was completed at baseline including information on whether the participants already were on ongoing weight-reducing diet; intake of dietary supplements, vitamins, and probiotics; or food allergy. Another protocol including information about changes in medication, physical activity, or routines, as well as any extraordinary events of daily life during the study time was completed at 2, 6, 12, and 28 weeks afterward (Supplementary Fig. 1).

*Blood sampling and chemistry analyses*

All samples consisted of whole blood drained into ethylenediaminetetra-acetic acid (EDTA) glass tubes (BD Microtainer, Franklin Lakes, New Jersey, USA) or serum separation tubes (SST) with coagulation activator and gel (BD Microtainer). Blood was centrifuged at 3,000 rcf for 10 min, and plasma and serum were immediately cooled and stored in −80°C until analyzed for later hormonal analyses. Cortisol, C-peptide, and insulin in serum; glycated hemoglobin A1c (HbA1c) in blood; and glucose, triglycerides, cholesterol, high-density lipoprotein (HDL), and low-density lipoprotein (LDL) in plasma were analyzed by standard methods in the Department of Clinical Chemistry. Homeostasis model assessment for insulin resistance (HOMA2-IR) was calculated using the HOMA2 calculator version 2.2.3 (21), after exclusion of extreme values of fasting plasma glucose and serum C-peptide.

*Hormonal analyses*

The Luminex analyses were performed in all samples at the same time within 9 months. Human diabetes 10-plex panel (Bio-Plex Pro™ Human Diabetes Immunoassay control no 5029560-1 and 5040782, Bio-Rad Laboratories, CA, USA) was performed on the Luminex-200 (Luminex xMAP, Bio-Rad Laboratories) and data were analyzed using Bio-Plex Manager software 6.0 (Bio-Rad Laboratories). Hormones (pg/mL) measured were ghrelin, glucagon, GLP-1, GIP, leptin, PAI-1, resistin, and visfatin.

Analyses were performed blinded according to the manufacturer's instructions. Briefly, samples were diluted 1:4 and incubated with magnetic beads coupled to specific capture antibodies. After a series of washes in a magnetic wash station (Bio-Plex Handled magnetic washer, 171020100, Bio-Rad Laboratories), biotinylated detection antibodies were added to form a sandwich complex. The final detection complex was created with the addition of streptavidin-phycoerythrin (SA-PE) conjugate. Absolute concentrations were measured from standards provided with the kit. Each run included controls with high and low concentrations for each biomarker, and a blank sample. All samples were analyzed in duplicate and the concentration of hormones bound to each bead was proportional to the median fluorescence intensity (MFI) of reporter signal. Standard curves were calculated with nonlinear regression type 5 parameter logistic. Inter-assay and intra-assay coefficients of variation (cv) for controls are presented in Supplementary Table 2.

Human serum CCK and PYY were analyzed with a commercial competitive inhibition enzyme–linked immunosorbent assay (ELISA) (Cloud-Clone Corp. Houston, Texas, USA, CEB802 Hu and CEB067 Hu, respectively) kit according to the manufacturer's instructions. Standards (0, 12.35, 37.04, 111.11, 333.33, and 1,000 pg/mL), serum sample (50 uL/well), and biotin-labelled CCK and PYY, respectively, were pipetted in duplicates into plates pre-coated with a monoclonal antibody specific to CCK or PYY. The unbound conjugate was washed off and avidin conjugated to horseradish peroxidase (HRP) was added. After a second wash and addition of the 3,3′,5,5′-tetramethylbenzidine (TMB) substrate solution, the intensity of color was measured at 450 nm. CCK or PYY in the samples were reversed proportional to the amount of bound HRP. CCK and PYY concentrations in each sample were interpolated from the standard curve. Intra-assay and inter-assay were CV% <10% and <12%, respectively, for both CCK and PYY.

**Statistical methods**

Two hypotheses were raised: (1) Intervention with an Okinawa-based Nordic diet affects the concentration of adipokines, CCK, cortisol, C-peptide, ghrelin, glucagon, incretins, insulin, PAI-1, and PYY, and (2) the hormone concentration correlates with metabolic responses and changes in blood pressure, BMI, weight, and waist circumference.

A power analysis was performed *a priori* based on a previous unpublished pilot study, and we determined that nine subjects were required to demonstrate that a weight reduction of 5–10%, accompanied by lower blood glucose, lower blood pressure, and improved lipid levels, would lead to clinically significant differences in metabolic parameters to reduce cardiovascular risk factors with 80% power at 5% significance level, as postulated in a previous study (22). The variable demanding most subjects to be able to discover was, what we expected, the diastolic blood pressure. We determined that we needed 18 subjects to demonstrate clinically significant differences in diastolic pressure with 80% power at 5% significance level. To be able to compensate for disappearance, we planned to recruit 25–35 subjects. Two of the recruited subjects interrupted the study at 6 weeks on diet, the time point that was considered as end of the intervention, and data collected at that time point was calculated together with data from subjects with 12 weeks of intervention.

We tested the hypotheses with linear mixed effect models to analyze continuous variables, with random intercept and unstructured co-variances for repeated measures within a subject, with visits as nominal fixed effect, using baseline as reference. We assumed that missing observations were unrelated to the observed value, that is, missing at random. In these analyses, predicted mean values and their 95% confidence limits are presented, together with estimates of changes from baseline and 95% confidence limits and $P$-values for the changes between baseline and week 12 and week 28. Descriptive statistics are given as means and standard deviations for continuous variables and as counts or frequencies for categorical variables. Since we had more than one observation from each subject, partial Spearman's correlations, controlling for subject, were calculated. Statistics were done using MATLAB R2015a (Mathworks Inc.). $P < 0.05$ was considered statistically significant in the calculated changes of values. Due to multiple testing between each hormone and anthropometric and metabolic factors, $P < 0.01$ was considered statistically significant in the partial correlations.

## Results

### *Basal characteristics*

In total, 45 patients with diabetes were randomly selected after consideration of inclusion and exclusion criteria. Of these, 30 patients (67%) (17 women), mean age 57.5 ± 8.2 (range 40–67) years, accepted the invitation. Reasons for not being included were unwillingness to participate ($n$ = 11), late autoimmune diabetes in adult (LADA) ($n$ = 1), a history of gastric by-pass surgery ($n$ = 1), pregnancy ($n$ = 1), or already on a diet ($n$ = 1) (Supplementary Fig. 1). The mean diabetes duration was 10.4 ± 7.6 (range 1–30) years. The treatment was metformin (40%), metformin in combination with insulin (27%), insulin solely (13%), metformin in combination with sulfonylurea (7%), diet solely (7%), sulfonylurea (3%), or dipeptidyl peptidase-4 (DPP 4) inhibitors (3%). The most common secondary complication to the disease was autonomic neuropathy and/or peripheral neuropathy (30%), retinopathy (27%), and nephropathy and macroangiopathy (17% in both). Only one patient had a verified gastroparesis.

Sixteen percent had only completed primary school, 57% had completed high school, and 27% had a higher degree of education. The majority, 67%, were employed, whereas 17% were retired. The rest of the patients were on sick leave or unemployed. Twenty of the patients were married or cohabitated, whereas six were divorced or widow/widower, and four were living alone. Smoking and usage of snuff both occurred in 23% of the patients. Half of the patients drank alcoholic beverages once a month or less, 27% drank alcohol 2–4 times a month, 13% drank alcohol 2–3 times a week, and 10% were teetotalers. A moderate but sporadic physical exercise during leisure time was most common (53%), followed by a moderately regular exercise (27%), regular exercise and training (13%), and sedentary leisure time (7%). Antihypertensive medication was prescribed in 63% of patients and lipid-lowering medication in 47%.

### *Changes in anthropometric and metabolic parameters*

The mean BMI at inclusion was 29.9 ± 4.1 kg/m$^2$, and 50% of the patients ($n$ = 15) were obese. During the interventional period of 12 weeks, the body weight was reduced ($P < 0.001$), accompanied by a reduction of BMI ($P < 0.001$) and waist circumference ($P < 0.001$), calculated by linear mixed model (Table 1). At week 12, only 12 patients were classified as obese. At week 28, the mean weight, BMI, and waist circumference remained significantly lower than at baseline ($P < 0.001$) (Table 1). Both systolic and diastolic blood pressures were decreased at week 12, and the diastolic blood pressure remained lower also at week 28, compared with baseline (Table 1). Blood levels of HbA1c, and plasma levels of glucose, triglycerides, cholesterol, and LDL were decreased during the dietary intervention, but only the HbA1c levels were still decreased at week 28, when also the HDL levels were increased, calculated by linear mixed model (Table 2).

Only two patients had diet management as the sole treatment for diabetes. In 15 subjects, the anti-diabetes medication was gradually reduced during dietary intervention, and 2 subjects, 1 on both oral hypoglycemic agents and insulin, had their medication cancelled. Of the other 12 subjects with insulin treatment, 3 had their insulin therapy cancelled and another 8 had their insulin doses reduced.

Many of the patients had irregular meal habits before inclusion in the study, and often omitted breakfast and/or lunch. At the 28-week follow-up, most patients had kept their regular meal order with the same intake of breakfast as during the intervention, and with an increased intake of vegetables and legumes. The composition of lunch and dinner was partly kept. Seven patients were lost at follow-up because of depression ($n$ = 2), family-related problems ($n$ = 2), unwillingness to show up ($n$ = 2), or work-related time constraints ($n$ = 1) (Supplementary Fig. 1).

### *Changes in hormonal concentrations*

At week 12, the plasma or serum levels of CCK ($P = 0.005$), cortisol ($P = 0.015$), C-peptide ($P = 0.022$), glucagon ($P = 0.003$), GLP-1 ($P = 0.013$), GIP ($P < 0.001$), insulin ($P = 0.004$), leptin ($P < 0.001$), and PYY ($P < 0.001$) were significantly lowered compared with baseline, calculated by linear mixed model. There was a non-significant decrease of PAI-1 levels ($P = 0.082$) (Table 3). At week 28, the plasma levels of PYY ($P = 0.002$) were still lowered, in addition to the levels of ghrelin ($P = 0.012$) and visfatin ($P = 0.021$). Serum levels of insulin ($P = 0.089$) and plasma levels of resistin ($P = 0.082$) were non-significantly lowered at week 28 (Table 3).

*Table 1.* Anthropometric parameters in type 2 diabetes before and after a 12-week Okinawa-based Nordic diet intervention

| Variable | Mean value | 95% CI | | Mean change | 95% CI | | *P* |
|---|---|---|---|---|---|---|---|
| | | Lower | Upper | | Lower | Upper | |
| Weight (kg) | | | | | | | |
| Baseline | 89.8 | 84.5 | 95.1 | | | | |
| Week 12 | 83.6 | 78.1 | 89.0 | −6.20 | −7.61 | −4.78 | <0.001 |
| Week 28 | 85.4 | 79.7 | 91.1 | −4.40 | −6.57 | −2.24 | <0.001 |
| BMI (kg/m$^2$) | | | | | | | |
| Baseline | 29.9 | 28.4 | 31.3 | | | | |
| Week 12 | 27.8 | 26.3 | 29.4 | −2.05 | −.52 | −1.57 | <0.001 |
| Week 28 | 28.4 | 26.8 | 30.0 | −1.47 | −2.13 | −0.82 | <0.001 |
| Waist circumference (cm) | | | | | | | |
| Baseline | 107.3 | 103.4 | 111.2 | | | | |
| Week 12 | 100.3 | 96.1 | 104.4 | −7.02 | −8.62 | −5.42 | <0.001 |
| Week 28 | 101.7 | 97.6 | 105.9 | −5.54 | −7.11 | −3.96 | <0.001 |
| Systolic blood pressure (mmHg) | | | | | | | |
| Baseline | 140.17 | 134.72 | 145.61 | | | | |
| Week 12 | 130.55 | 124.39 | 136.71 | −9.62 | −13.30 | −5.93 | <0.001 |
| Week 28 | 139.74 | 133.84 | 145.65 | −0.42 | −3.65 | 2.81 | 0.796 |
| Diastolic blood pressure (mmHg) | | | | | | | |
| Baseline | 82.33 | 78.73 | 85.93 | | | | |
| Week 12 | 74.88 | 71.03 | 78.73 | −2.70 | −3.57 | −1.84 | <0.001 |
| Week 28 | 78.74 | 74.76 | 82.72 | −1.75 | −2.78 | −0.72 | 0.001 |

The mean values and mean changes and 95% confidence interval (CI) with lower and upper limits are presented for anthropometric parameters at inclusion (baseline) ($n = 30$), 12 weeks after diet intervention ($n = 30$), and 16 weeks after the end of diet intervention (week 28) ($n = 23$). Linear mixed model. Comparisons were made between baseline and week 12 and week 28. $P < 0.05$ was considered statistically significant.

*Partial correlations between changes in hormonal levels and anthropometric and metabolic parameters*

The endocrine changes were in alignment with changes of anthropometric and metabolic parameters (Fig. 1). Changes in concentrations of C-peptide and insulin correlated with changes in values of fasting glucose ($r_s = 0.474$, $P < 0.001$ vs. $r_s = 0.344$, $P = 0.002$), triglycerides ($r_s = 0.652$, $P < 0.001$ vs. $r_s = 0.413$, $P < 0.001$), and BMI ($r_s = 0.424$, $P < 0.001$ vs. $r_s = 0.394$, $P < 0.001$), and correlated inversely with changes in levels of HDL ($r_s = -0.509$, $P < 0.001$ vs. $r_s = -0.301$, $P = 0.006$), calculated by partial Spearman´s correlation test. In addition, the changes in C-peptide levels correlated with changes in HbA1c values ($r_s = 0.315$, $P = 0.004$), and the changes in insulin levels correlated with changes in waist circumference ($r_s = 0.340$, $P = 0.006$). Changes in glucagon and GLP-1 levels both correlated inversely with changes in LDL levels, whereas changed GIP levels correlated with changed HbA1c values. Changes in BMI and waist circumference correlated inversely with changes in ghrelin concentrations, and positively with changes in leptin concentrations, the latter also being correlated with changes in insulin resistance. Changes in PAI-1 and PYY levels correlated with changes in glucose and triglyceride levels, and PYY levels also correlated with changes of HbA1c values. Changes in resistin levels correlated with changes in systolic blood pressure (Table 4). There was no correlation between changes in CCK, cortisol, or visfatin levels and any calculated parameters (data not shown).

## Discussion

Based on the study results presented here, we accepted the research hypothesis that intervention with the Okinawa-based Nordic diet affects several hormones released from the gut and pancreas with lower circulating levels of CCK, C-peptide, glucagon, GLP-1, GIP, insulin, and PYY. The concentrations of cortisol and leptin were reduced, and PAI-1 non-significantly reduced, after 12 weeks, whereas visfatin levels were reduced and resistin non-significantly reduced, after 28 weeks. Apart from CCK, cortisol, and visfatin levels, changes in hormonal levels correlated with the improved anthropometric and metabolic parameters. Despite reductions of weight, BMI, and waist circumference, the ghrelin levels were reduced after 28 weeks, compared to baseline.

The majority of the metabolic and anthropometric changes could be correlated with the endocrine profile, as expected from the literature (5, 6, 11, 12, 14, 16). The endocrine changes may be induced by the diet *per se*, secondary to the metabolic changes, or secondary to the weight

*Table 2.* Circulating metabolic biomarkers in type 2 diabetes before and after a 12-week Okinawa-based Nordic diet intervention

| Variable | Mean value | 95% CI | | Mean change | 95% CI | | *P* |
|---|---|---|---|---|---|---|---|
| | | Lower | Upper | | Lower | Upper | |
| Fasting Glucose (mmol/L) | | | | | | | |
| Baseline | 9.71 | 8.54 | 10.87 | | | | |
| Week 12 | 7.91 | 6.55 | 9.27 | −1.80 | −2.63 | −0.96 | <0.001 |
| Week 28 | 9.28 | 7.71 | 10.85 | −0.42 | −1.58 | 0.73 | 0.466 |
| HbA1c (mmol/mol) | | | | | | | |
| Baseline | 61.57 | 56.42 | 66.72 | | | | |
| Week 12 | 49.20 | 44.02 | 54.38 | −12.37 | −16.40 | −8.33 | <0.001 |
| Week 28 | 54.36 | 48.83 | 59.90 | −7.20 | −11.68 | −2.72 | 0.002 |
| HOMA2-IR (U) | | | | | | | |
| Baseline | 3.00 | 2.50 | 3.51 | | | | |
| Week 2 | 2.53 | 1.96 | 3.09 | −0.48 | −0.85 | −0.11 | 0.012 |
| Week 12 | 2.37 | 1.82 | 2.91 | −0.64 | −0.98 | −0.30 | <0.001 |
| Week 28 | 2.61 | 2.05 | 3.16 | −0.40 | −0.75 | −0.05 | 0.025 |
| Triglycerides (nmol/L) | | | | | | | |
| Baseline | 1.79 | 1.41 | 2.16 | | | | |
| Week 12 | 1.49 | 1.09 | 1.89 | −0.30 | −0.52 | −0.08 | 0.009 |
| Week 28 | 1.96 | 1.46 | 2.46 | 0.17 | −0.20 | 0.54 | 0.367 |
| Cholesterol (mmol/L) | | | | | | | |
| Baseline | 4.65 | 4.36 | 4.95 | | | | |
| Week 12 | 4.22 | 3.87 | 4.57 | −0.44 | −0.69 | −0.18 | 0.001 |
| Week 28 | 4.71 | 4.37 | 5.05 | 0.06 | −0.18 | 0.30 | 0.636 |
| HDL (mmol/L) | | | | | | | |
| Baseline | 1.22 | 1.10 | 1.35 | | | | |
| Week 12 | 1.19 | 1.05 | 1.32 | −0.04 | −0.10 | 0.03 | 0.267 |
| Week 28 | 1.34 | 1.20 | 1.47 | 0.11 | 0.04 | 0.18 | 0.003 |
| LDL (mmol/L) | | | | | | | |
| Baseline | 2.92 | 2.62 | 3.22 | | | | |
| Week 12 | 2.68 | 2.33 | 3.03 | −0.24 | −0.48 | −0.01 | 0.041 |
| Week 28 | 2.82 | 2.49 | 3.16 | −0.10 | −0.30 | 0.11 | 0.356 |

The mean values and mean changes and 95% confidence interval (CI) with lower and upper limits are presented for fasting blood levels of glycated hemoglobin A1c (HbA1c) and fasting plasma levels of glucose, triglycerides, cholesterol, high-density lipoprotein (HDL), and low-density lipoprotein (LDL) at inclusion (baseline) ($n$ = 30), 12 weeks after diet intervention ($n$ = 30), and 16 weeks after the end of diet intervention (week 28) ($n$ = 23). Insulin resistance was measured by HOMA2-IR (21). Linear mixed model. Comparisons were made between baseline and week 12 and week 28. $P < 0.05$ was considered statistically significant.

reduction. After a single Okinawa-based Nordic breakfast to healthy subjects, the postprandial response of glucose, C-peptide, insulin, and GIP were attenuated compared with a traditional breakfast (4). The strongest correlations between anthropometric and metabolic parameters and hormone levels in the present study were observed with C-peptide and insulin levels, which suggest that the immediate endocrine response to the diet is crucial for the evolution of further effects. This hypothesis is strengthened by the fact that normalization of blood glucose *per se* did not affect postprandial levels of GLP-1 and GIP (23).

Both orexigenic (ghrelin) and anorexigenic hormone levels (CCK, glucagon, GLP-1, insulin, leptin, and PYY) were decreased in the present study. The overall decrease of hormonal levels reflects a balance in between the hormones; a decrease in one hormone level initiates a process of further influences. A reduction of GLP-1 and endogenous insulin production, as measured by reduced C-peptide levels, may depend on the reduced carbohydrate content and higher protein content in the diet (24), whereas the reduction in glucagon may be ascribed to the introduction of regular meals with shorter meal intervals, thereby improving substrate oxidation beneficially (25). Although the diet had a relatively high fat and protein content, the concentration of CCK and PYY were reduced after the dietary intervention. However, the study

*Table 3.* Circulating hormonal levels in type 2 diabetes before and after a 12-week Okinawa-based Nordic diet intervention

| | Mean | 95% CI | | Mean change | 95% CI | | P |
|---|---|---|---|---|---|---|---|
| | | Lower | Upper | | Lower | Upper | |
| CCK (pg/mL; serum) | | | | | | | |
| Baseline | 27 | 21 | 32 | | | | |
| Week 12 | 20 | 14 | 26 | −7 | −11 | −2 | 0.005 |
| Week 28 | 23 | 16 | 30 | −3 | −9 | 3 | 0.267 |
| Cortisol (nmol/L; serum) | | | | | | | |
| Baseline | 367 | 337 | 397 | | | | |
| Week 12 | 325 | 290 | 360 | −41 | −74 | −8 | 0.015 |
| Week 28 | 348 | 315 | 382 | −18 | −50 | 13 | 0.249 |
| C-peptide (nmol/L; serum) | | | | | | | |
| Baseline | 0.99 | 0.82 | 1.17 | | | | |
| Week 12 | 0.88 | 0.70 | 1.05 | −0.11 | −0.21 | −1.02 | 0.022 |
| Week 28 | 0.88 | 0.68 | 1.09 | −0.11 | −0.24 | 0.03 | 0.131 |
| Ghrelin (pg/mL; plasma) | | | | | | | |
| Baseline | 852 | 608 | 1094 | | | | |
| Week 12 | 798 | 555 | 1041 | −53 | −139 | 32 | 0.219 |
| Week 28 | 728 | 481 | 975 | −123 | −219 | −28 | 0.012 |
| Glucagon (pg/mL; plasma) | | | | | | | |
| Baseline | 1.93 | 1.29 | 2.58 | | | | |
| Week 12 | 1.28 | 0.63 | 1.92 | −0.66 | −1.09 | −0.23 | 0.003 |
| Week 28 | 1.74 | 1.06 | 2.42 | −0.19 | −0.67 | 0.29 | 0.426 |
| GLP-1 (pg/mL; plasma) | | | | | | | |
| Baseline | 2.66 | 1.79 | 3.54 | | | | |
| Week 12 | 1.78 | 0.91 | 2.66 | −0.88 | −1.56 | −0.19 | 0.013 |
| Week 28 | 2.36 | 1.43 | 3.30 | −-0.30 | −1.08 | 0.48 | 0.477 |
| GIP (pg/mL; plasma) | | | | | | | |
| Baseline | 78 | 57 | 99 | | | | |
| Week 12 | 55 | 34 | 76 | −23 | −36 | −10 | <0.001 |
| Week 28 | 75 | 52 | 98 | −3 | −18 | 12 | 0.692 |
| Insulin (mIU/L; serum) | | | | | | | |
| Baseline | 15.53 | 12.67 | 18.40 | | | | |
| Week 12 | 11.67 | 8.80 | 14.53 | −3.87 | −6.43 | −1.30 | 0.004 |
| Week 28 | 12.96 | 9.72 | 16.19 | −2.58 | −5.55 | 0.40 | 0.089 |
| Leptin (pg/mL; plasma) | | | | | | | |
| Baseline | 9,404 | 587 | 1,294 | | | | |
| Week 12 | 5,850 | 199 | 971 | −3,554 | −5,328 | −1,779 | <0.001 |
| Week 28 | 8,553 | 491 | 1,219 | −851 | −2,078 | 376 | 0.171 |
| PAI-1 (pg/mL; plasma) | | | | | | | |
| Baseline | 72,434 | 58,869 | 85,998 | | | | |
| Week 12 | 66,413 | 52,402 | 80,425 | −6,020 | −12,814 | 774 | 0.082 |
| Week 28 | 71,810 | 56,705 | 86,915 | −623 | −9,455 | 8,209 | 0.889 |
| PYY (pg/mL; plasma) | | | | | | | |
| Baseline | 1,937 | 1,802 | 2,073 | | | | |
| Week 12 | 1,510 | 1,360 | 1,660 | −427 | −572 | −282 | <0.001 |
| Week 28 | 1,673 | 1,502 | 1,844 | −264 | −431 | −97 | 0.002 |
| Resistin (pg/mL; plasma) | | | | | | | |
| Baseline | 5,234 | 3,904 | 6,565 | | | | |
| Week 12 | 5,043 | 3,705 | 6,382 | −191 | −1,118 | 736 | 0.683 |
| Week 28 | 4,325 | 2,915 | 5,736 | −909 | −1,938 | 119 | 0.082 |
| Visfatin (pg/mL; plasma) | | | | | | | |
| Baseline | 998 | 732 | 1,264 | | | | |
| Week 12 | 1,115 | 816 | 1,415 | 117 | −78 | 312 | 0.235 |
| Week 28 | 812 | 535 | 1,089 | −186 | −344 | −29 | 0.021 |

Values are presented as absolute mean values or mean changes and 95% confidence interval (CI) with lower and upper limits at inclusion (baseline) ($n$ = 30), 12 weeks after diet intervention($n$ = 30), and 16 weeks after the end of diet intervention (week 28) ($n$ = 23). CCK = cholecystokinin, GLP-1 = glucagon-like peptide-1, GIP = glucose-dependent insulinotropic polypeptide, PAI-1 = plasminogen activator inhibitor-1, PYY = polypeptide YY. Linear mixed model. Comparisons were made between baseline and week 12 and week 28. $P < 0.05$ was considered statistically significant.

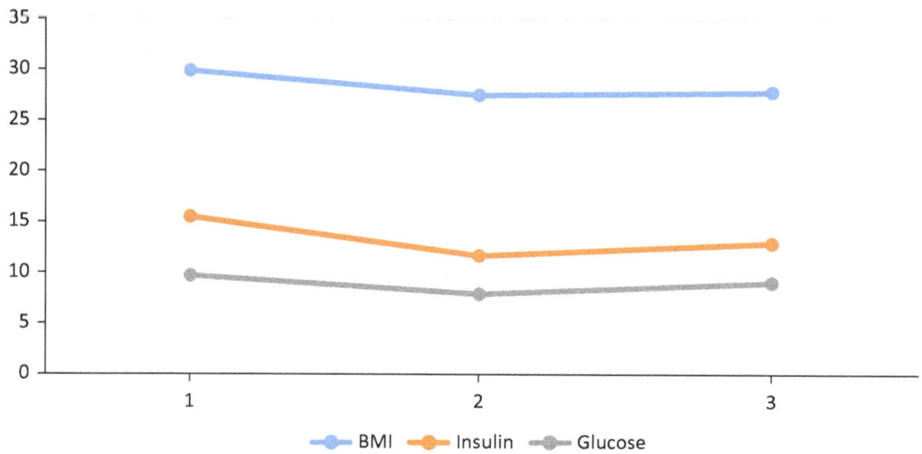


*Fig. 1.* Mean values of body mass index (BMI) (kg/m$^2$) and fasting levels of plasma glucose (mmol/L) and serum insulin (mIU/L) at baseline (1), week 12 (2) and week 28 (3) of the Okinawan-Based Nordic diet intervention in type 2 diabetes.

participant's ordinary food may have had higher total amount of fat and protein than the Okinawa-based Nordic diet.

Although reductions of weight, waist circumference, and blood pressure remained at 28 weeks after study start, the hormonal levels, apart from PYY, had normalized. Noteworthy, ghrelin levels were reduced at follow-up. This is very interesting, since a previous study with a low-energy diet showed that the induced hormonal changes to increase sensation of hunger and encourage weight regain persisted until 1 year later, with elevated levels of ghrelin, which can explain the difficulties to maintain weight loss (26). Lower ghrelin levels render reduced appetite and less hunger (27). By changing the nutritional composition in the Okinawa-based Nordic diet, and not only reducing caloric intake, our participants exhibited lower ghrelin levels and increased or equal satiety with a good ability to maintain the weight loss (4, 28). This delayed effect on ghrelin may suggest a readjustment of appetite regulation and food intake after introduction of a healthier diet. The participants partly withheld the diet between 12 and 28 weeks, which may have contributed to a new balance in the hormonal system. This further suggests that dietary components have a huge influence on the endocrine control, and that the present endocrine alterations do not only depend on weight reduction *per se*. Previous research supports nutrient-specific effects on ghrelin secretion, which may counteract the elevated levels observed after weight loss in other studies (29). However, there may be synergistic effects between a healthy diet, improved metabolism, and weight reduction, but exact mechanisms are difficult to separate. Still, the most important from a clinical point of view is that introduction of a modified diet is correlated with a healthier endocrine profile. The weight loss of 0.5 kg/week was in the same magnitude as observed in previous, similar studies (30).

GIP has specific anabolic effects and enhances insulin secretion and insulin stimulation, which promotes accumulation of fat in adipose tissue (31). It is considered important to diminish the exaggerated GIP secretion, which demands altered chemical and physical food composition, as well as altered eating behaviors (32–34). The present results are in line with the anticipation that an overactive entero-insular axis may play a role in the development of diabetes and obesity (32).

Circulating adipokine levels are increased in obese subjects. Leptin and insulin show a strong relationship, and leptin resistance is accompanied by hyperinsulinemia and insulin resistance (14). The observed reduction of insulin concentration and insulin resistance by the Okinawa-based Nordic diet seem to be interconnected with lower levels of adipokines, although the close relation between resistin and insulin resistance found in other studies could not be confirmed in the present study (14). Resistin levels are elevated in hypertension (35), and, thus, the parallel decrease of systolic blood pressure and resistin in the present study is in alignment with this. Changes in cortisol levels may result from a multitude of factors including both diet (36) and stress in daily life (17).

It remains to determine which of the ingredients in the food are responsible for the observed hormonal and metabolic responses. The physical properties of the food were altered through higher fiber intake demanding more mastication, slower eating, greater gastric volume, and delayed gastric emptying rate. The chemical characteristics were changed with reduction of GI and processed food, lower energy percentage intake of carbohydrates, and higher energy percentage intake of fat and protein. In addition, most subjects had irregular meal habits at inclusion. Only a reduction of meal frequencies, without changes in the nutrition composition, may have great impact on glucose and hormone levels (37). The Ma-Pi 2

*Table 4.* Partial correlations between hormonal, metabolic, and anthropometric changes in type 2 diabetes before and after a 12-week Okinawa-based Nordic diet intervention

| | Correlation coefficient | *P* |
|---|---|---|
| C-peptide | | |
| Glucose | 0.474 | <0.001 |
| HbA1c | 0.315 | 0.004 |
| High-density lipoprotein | −0.509 | <0.001 |
| Triglycerides | 0.652 | <0.001 |
| Body mass index | 0.424 | <0.001 |
| Insulin | | |
| Glucose | 0.344 | 0.002 |
| High-density lipoprotein | −0.301 | 0.006 |
| Triglycerides | 0.413 | <0.001 |
| Body mass index | 0.394 | <0.001 |
| Waist circumference | 0.340 | 0.006 |
| Glucagon | | |
| Low-density lipoprotein | −0.324 | 0.003 |
| GLP-1 | | |
| Low-density lipoprotein | −0.387 | 0.004 |
| GIP | | |
| HbA1c | 0.335 | 0.002 |
| Ghrelin | | |
| Body weight | −0.482 | <0.001 |
| Body mass index | −0.444 | <0.001 |
| Waist circumference | −0.436 | <0.001 |
| Leptin | | |
| Body mass index | 0.507 | <0.001 |
| Waist circumference | 0.465 | <0.001 |
| Insulin resistance | 0.330 | 0.003 |
| PAI-1 | | |
| Glucose | 0.289 | 0.009 |
| Triglycerides | 0.309 | 0.005 |
| Polypeptide YY | | |
| Glucose | 0.431 | <0.001 |
| HbA1c | 0.356 | 0.001 |
| Triglycerides | 0.367 | <0.001 |
| Resistin | | |
| Systolic blood pressure | 0.297 | 0.008 |

GLP-1 = glucagon-like peptide-1, GIP = glucose-dependent insulinotropic polypeptide, PAI-1 = plasminogen activator inhibitor-1, PYY = polypeptide YY. Partial correlations, with the three observational time points, baseline, week 12, and week 28 from each individual, by Spearman's correlation test. $P < 0.01$ was considered statistically significant.

macrobiotic diet has similarities with the Okinawa-based diet regarding a high amount of whole grains, vegetables, and legumes, and no added sugar. In contrast, the daily energy percentages consist of 70 E% carbohydrate, 18 E% fat, and 12 E% protein (38). Still, these two diets have similar effects on type 2 diabetes (3, 38), which support previous suggestion that whole-grain cereals, high fiber intake, and unprocessed food is more important than the relative amounts of nutrients (39, 40). Fibers and whole grains act as prebiotics (41), which has been shown to increase PYY and GLP-1 secretion (38), in contrast to our findings. In epidemiologic studies, mortality was lower in subjects with a high intake of whole-grain products, especially intake of breakfast cereals and nonwhite bread (42). Regular consumption of breakfast cereals, especially whole grains, is associated with less overweight and development and management of diabetes (43). The association between high intake of whole-grain products and overall healthier lifestyle habits may reduce the associations to be markers of healthy habits (44). In the present prospective study, the positive effects by dietary modification were observed without concomitant intervention of other lifestyle factors and independently of socioeconomic factors.

One of the limitations of the present study was that only fasting hormonal levels were analyzed and not the total area under the curve during the day. Varying degrees of diabetic complications may also affect results. In the present study, only one patient had verified gastroparesis, which should not influence the result. More patients suffered from autonomic neuropathy, which is, however, not associated with altered concentration of gut hormones in type 1 diabetes (45). Another limitation is the absence of an external control group, which provides some evidence that changes occurring over time were not the result of natural temporal trends or of unmeasured events that occurred contemporaneously with the study. It is a challenge to construct an appropriate control group in open, nonblinded lifestyle studies. A similar dietary interventional study using a control group advised to follow their habitual diet and physical activity did however not show any changes in the controls during the observational time (30). Instead, the participants were characterized at baseline and followed during and after dietary intervention, thus being their own controls to measure intra-individual differences. When people anticipate eating a scheduled meal, cephalic responses induce an increased secretion of several meal-related hormones before the start of the meal (46). Thus, the very expectancy of entering a lifestyle change should have altered the hormonal profile already at baseline. The alterations found thereafter should be secondary to dietary changes, metabolic alterations, and/or weight reductions.

In conclusion, a 12-week dietary intervention in type 2 diabetes with an Okinawa-based Nordic diet has significant impact on the endocrine profile, which is in alignment with the anthropometric and metabolic improvements.


## Acknowledgements

We thank Igelösa Life Science AB, Lund, whose staff supplied and prepared the meals.

**Financial support**

This study was supported by grants from Hans-Gabriel and Alice Trolle Wachtmeister's Foundation for Medical Research, King Gustaf V's and queen Victoria Free Maison's Foundation, Dir Albert Påhlsson's Foundation, Development Foundation of Region Skåne, and Foundation of Skåne University Hospital.

**Conflict of interest**

The authors have not received any funding or benefits from industry or elsewhere to conduct this study.

**Authors' contribution**

BO, GD, and PH designed the study. BO ran and financed most of the study. BR performed the Luminex and ELISA analyses blinded. BO and PH performed the statistical analyses. BO wrote the manuscript. All authors contributed to the writing of the manuscript by constructive criticism and the final version was approved by all authors.

## References

1. Willcox DC, Scapagnini G, Willcox BJ. Healthy aging diets other than the Mediterranean: a focus on the Okinawan diet. Mech Ageing Dev 2014; 136–137: 148–62.
2. O'Keefe JH, Gheewala NM, O'Keefe JO. Dietary strategies for improving post-prandial glucose, lipids, inflammation, and cardiovascular health. J Am Coll Cardiol 2008; 51: 249–55.
3. Darwiche G, Höglund P, Roth B, Larsson E, Sjöberg T, Wohlfart B, et al. An Okinawan-based Nordic diet improves anthropometry, metabolic control, and quality of life in Scandinavian patients with type 2 diabetes: a pilot trial. Food Nutr Res 2016; 60: 32594.
4. Ohlsson B, Höglund P, Roth B, Darwiche G. Modification of a traditional breakfast leads to increased satiety along with attenuated plasma increments of glucose, C-peptide, insulin, and GIP in human. Nutr Res 2016; 36: 359–68.
5. Yoder SM, Yang Q, Kindel TL, Tso P. Differential responses of the incretin hormones GIP and GLP-1 to increasing doses of dietary carbohydrate but not dietary protein in lean rats. Am J Physiol Gastrointest Liver Physiol 2010; 299: G476–85.
6. Yoder SM, Yang Q, Kindel TL, Tso P. Stimulation of incretin secretion by dietary lipid: is it dose dependent? Am J Physiol Gastrointest Liver Physiol 2009; 297: G299–305.
7. Asmar M, Simonsen L, Madsbad S, Stallknecht B, Holst JJ, Bülow J. Glucose-dependent insulinotropic polypeptide may enhance fatty acid re-esterification in subcutaneous abdominal adipose tissue in lean humans. Diabetes 2010; 59: 2160–3.
8. Holst JJ, Vilsbøll T, Deacon CF. The incretin system and its role in type 2 diabetes mellitus. Mol Cell Endocrinol 2009; 297: 127–36.
9. Gutierrez-Aguilar R, Woods SC. Nutrition and L and K-enteroendocrine cells. Curr Opin Endocrinol Diabetes Obes 2011; 18: 35–41.
10. Overduin J, Gibbs J, Cummings DE, Reeve JR Jr. CCK-58 elicits both satiety and satiation in rats while CCK-8 elicits only satiation. Peptides 2014; 54: 71–80.
11. Cooper JA. Factors affecting circulating levels of peptide YY in humans: a comprehensive review. Nutr Res Rev 2014; 27: 186–97.
12. Persaud SJ, Bewick GA. Peptide YY: more than just an appetite regulator. Diabetologia 2014; 57: 1762–9.
13. Chu S, Schubert ML. Gastric secretion. Curr Opin 2013; 29: 636–41.
14. AL-Suhaimi EA, Shehzad A. Leptin, resistin and visfatIn: the missing link between endocrine metabolic disorders and immunity. Eur J Med Res 2013; 18: 12.
15. Tilg H, Moschen AR. Role of adiponectin and PBEF/visfatin as regulator f inflammation: involvement in obesity-associated diseases. Clin Sci 2008; 114: 275–88.
16. Nordt TK, Sawa H, Fujii S, Bode C, Sobel BE. Augmentation of arterial endothelial cell expression of the plasminogen activator inhibitor typ-1 (PAI-1) gene by proinsulin and insulin in vivo. J Mol Cell Cardiol 1998; 30: 1535–43.
17. Anagnostis P, Athyros VG, Tziomalos K, Karagiannis A, Mikhailidis DP. Clinical review: the pathogenetic role of cortisol in the metabolic syndrome: a hypothesis. J Clin Endocrinol Metab 2009; 94: 2692–701.
18. Nordic Nutrition Recommendations 2012. Available from: http://www.norden.org/en/theme/nordic-nutrition-recommendation/nordic-nutrition-recommendations-2012. Cited 3 April 2017.
19. World Health Organization. Global database on body mass index; 2015. Available from: http://apps.who.int/bmi/index.jsp?introPage=intro_3.html. Cited 3 April 2017.
20. Clinical Guidelines on the Identification, Evaluation, and Treatment of Overweight and Obesity in Adults–The Evidence Report: National Institutes of Health. Obes Res 2008; 6(Suppl 2): 51S–209S.
21. The Oxford Centre for Diabetes, Endocinology, and Metabolism, Diabetes Trials Unit. The University of Oxford. 2016. https://www.dtu.ox.ac.uk/homacalculator. Cited 12 January 2016.
22. Wing RR, Lang W, Wadden TA, Safford M, Knowler WC, Bertoni AG, et al. Benefits of modest weight loss in improving cardiovascular risk factors in overweight and obese individuals with type 2 diabetes. Diabetes Care 2011; 34: 1481–6.
23. Højberg PV, Vilsbøll T, Zander M, Knop FK, Krarup T, Vølund A, et al. Four weeks of near-normalization of blood glucose has no effect on postprandial GLP-1 and GIP secretion, but augments pancreatic B-cell responsiveness to a meal in patients with Type 2 diabetes. Diabet Med 2008; 25: 1268–75.
24. Smeets AJ, Westerterp-Plantenga MS. Acute effects on metabolism and appetite profile of one meal difference in the lower range of meal frequency. Br J Nutr 2008; 99: 1316–21.
25. Smeets AJ, Soenen S, Luscombe-Marsh ND. Energy expenditure, satiety, and plasma ghrelin, glucagon-like peptide 1, and peptide tyrosine-tyrosine concentrations following a single high-protein lunch. J Nutr 2008; 138: 698–702.
26. Sumithran P, Prendergast LA, Delbridge E, Purcell K, Shulkes A, Kriketos A, et al. Long-term persistence of hormonal adaptations to weight loss. N Engl J Med 2011; 365: 1597–604.
27. Delzenne N, Blundell J, Brouns F, Cunningham K, De Graaf K, Erkner A, et al. Gastrointestinal targets of appetite regulation in humans. Obes Rev 2010; 11: 234–50.
28. Ohlsson B, Darwiche G, Roth B, Bengtsson M, Höglund P. High fiber, fat and protein contents lead to increased satiety, reduced sweet cravings, and decreased gastrointestinal symptoms, independently of anthropometric, hormonal, and metabolic factors. J Diabet Metabol 2017; 8: 3.
29. Lean ME, Malkova D. Altered gut and adipose tissue hormones in overweight and obese individuals: cause or consequence? Int J Obes 2016, 40: 622–32.

30. Adamsson V, Reumark A, Fredriksson IB, Hammarström E, Vessby B, Johansson G, et al. Effects of a healthy Nordic diet on cardiovascular risk factors in hypercholesterolaemic subjects: a randomized controlled trial (NORDIET). J Intern Med 2011; 269: 150–9.
31. Heller RF. Hyperinsulinemic obesity and carbohydrate addiction: the missing link is the carbohydrate frequency factor. Med Hypotheses 1994; 42: 307–12.
32. Yip RG, Wolfe MM. GIP biology and fat metabolism. Life Sci 2000; 66: 91–103.
33. Peracchi M, Santangelo A, Conte D, Fraquelli M, Tagliabue R, Gebbia C, et al. The physical state of a meal affects hormone release and postprandial thermogenesis. Br J Nutr 2000; 83: 623–8.
34. Shimotoyodome A, Fukuoka D, Suzuki J. Coingestion of acylglycerols differentially affects glucose-induced insulin secretion via glucose-dependent insulinotropic polypeptide in C57BL/6J mice. Endocrinology 2009; 150: 2118–26.
35. de Faria AP, Modolo R, Fontana V, Moreno H. Adipokines: novel players in resistant hypertension. J Clin Hypertens 2014; 16: 754–59.
36. Vinales KL, Schlögl M, Piaggi P, Hohenadel M, Graham A, Bonfiglio S et al. The consistency in macronutrient oxidation and the role for epinephrine in the response to fasting and overfeeding. J Clin Endocrinol Metab 2017; 102:279–89.
37. Carlson O, Martin B, Stote KS, Golden E, Maudsley S, Najjar SS, et al. Impact of reduced meal frequency without caloric restriction on glucose regulation in healthy, normal-weight middle-aged men and women. Metabolism 2007; 56: 1729–34.
38. Fallucca F, Fontana L, Fallucca S, Pianesi M. Gut microbiota and Ma-Pi 2 macrobiotic diet in the treatment of type 2 diabetes. World J Diabetes 2015; 6: 403–11.
39. Bakhøj S, Flint A, Holst JJ, Tetens I. Tetens I. Lower glucose-dependent insulinotropic polypeptide (GIP) response but similar glucagon-like peptide 1 (GLP-1), glycaemic, and insulinaemic response to ancient wheat compared to modern wheat depends on processing. Eur J Clin Nutr 2003; 57: 1254–61.
40. Tovar J, Nilsson A, Johansson M, Björck I. Combining functional features of whole-grain barley and legumes for dietary reduction of cardiometabolic risk: a randomised cross-over intervention in mature women. Br J Nutr 2014; 111: 706–14.
41. Zhong Y, Nyman M, Fåk F. Modulation of gut microbiota in rats fed high-fat diets by processing whole-grain barley to barley malt. Mol Nutr Food Res 2015; 59: 2066–76.
42. Johnsen NF, Frederiksen K, Christensen J, Skeie G, Lund E, Landberg R, et al. Whole-grain products and whole-grain types are associated with lower all-cause and cause-specific mortality in the Scandinavian HELGA cohort. Br J Nutr 2015; 23: 1–16.
43. Williams PG. The benefits of breakfast cereal consumption: a systematic review of the evidence base. Adv Nutr 2014; 5: 636S–73S.
44. Egeberg R, Frederiksen K, Olsen A, Johnsen NF, Loft S, Overvad K, et al. Intake of wholegrain products is associated with dietary, lifestyle, anthropometric and socio-economic factors in Denmark. Public Health Nutr 2009; 12: 1519–30.
45. Hammersjö R, Roth B, Höglund P, Ohlsson B. Esophageal and gastrointestinal motility affects glucose homeostasis and plasma levels of incretin and leptin. Rev Diab Stud 2016; 13: 79–90.
46. Drazen DL, Vahl TP, D'Alessio DA, Seeley RJ, Woods SC. Effects of a fixed meal pattern on ghrelin secretion: evidence for a learned response independent of nutrient status. Endocrinology 2006; 147: 23–30.

***Bodil Ohlsson**
Department of Clinical Sciences Skåne University Hospital
Jan Waldenströms street 15, plane 5, SE-205 02 Malmö, Sweden
Email: bodil.ohlsson@med.lu.se

# 5

# Household decision-making around food in rural Tajikistan: a cross-sectional study to help extension workers in the field

Elizabeth A. Wood[1]*, Katharine McNamara[1], Agata Kowalewska[2] and Nargiza Ludgate[3]

[1]Department of Environmental & Global Health, College of Public Health and Health Professions, University of Florida, Gainesville, FL, USA; [2]Department of Food Science & Human Nutrition, College of Agricultural and Life Sciences, University of Florida, Gainesville, FL, USA; [3]Department of Animal Sciences, College of Agriculture and Life Sciences, University of Florida, Gainesville, FL, USA

*Abstract*

This study was conducted to research and develop recommendations for gender transformative approaches that will address misconceptions around food and nutrition, and reducing barriers around dietary diversity within rural Khatlon Province, Tajikistan. Most of the population in Tajikistan live in rural areas and spend a large part of their income on food. While stunting in children under 5 years has decreased, acute malnutrition and the number of underweight children has increased. This is a qualitative, cross-sectional study that involved secondary data analysis, key informant interviews (KIIs), and focus group discussions (FGDs) to gauge appropriate interventions for agricultural extension agents seeking to improve the nutritional outcomes of their communities. In February of 2017, data were collected from 4 KIIs and 15 FGDs that were stratified as mothers with young children, mothers-in-law, and husbands, across 12 different villages. Analysis of the KIIs and FGDs included NVivo software for coding and to uncover the most salient themes and characteristics from each. The participants of this study reported several misconceptions and taboos surrounding certain foods, especially during pregnancy, and food practices for children under the age of 5 years. Results also indicated a household hierarchy of decision-making surrounding food that included who buys, cooks, and decides what to buy. The findings of this study will be used as a springboard to launch gender-responsive and nutrition-sensitive interventions through the local agricultural extension agents.

Keywords: *decision-making; food misconceptions; gender; global health; nutrition*

Tajikistan is a landlocked, mostly mountainous country within Central Asia that borders Uzbekistan, Afghanistan, Kyrgyzstan, and China. The population in 2017 was 8.4 million people, with a 0.99 male to female ratio in 2016 and 73% living in rural areas (1, 2). Since the collapse of the Soviet Union, several countries within Central Asia, including Tajikistan, have experienced the breakdown of their economic system. According to the World Bank (3), inequality, specifically in rural regions of Tajikistan, has increased between 2012 and 2014, with the Gini Coefficient standing at 29 on a national level and 28.4 within rural areas. The gross domestic product (GDP) is gradually improving with a specific emphasis on diversifying the agricultural sector, which accounts for 23% of the GDP and provides approximately 75% of the labor force (4, 5). Despite these improvements, Tajikistan has struggled with having the highest malnutrition rates within Central Asia, with 10% of children under 5 years suffering from acute malnutrition, 26% from chronic malnutrition, and over 75% of the population living within rural Tajikistan still facing food insecurity (6).Tajikistan has four provinces (Sughd, Khatlon, Gorniy-Badakhshan, and the Region of Republican Subordination); however, Khatlon Province was specifically chosen for this study because of its potential for agricultural production, high undernutrition rates, and having the most people living in poverty (5).

The scarcity of jobs in rural Tajikistan drives over 800,000 people, mostly men, to migrate out of Tajikistan in search of employment; over 95% of people that migrate go to Russia specifically (7). Khatlon Province, the site of this study, experiences a higher rate of male migration (38.9%) than the national average (35.7%) (8). The remittances that are sent back account for over half of Tajikistan's economy and are primarily controlled by women within households (3, 7). As a result of men leaving the household in search of job opportunities and higher wages, there has been a feminization of agriculture within rural villages. Some reports have revealed that gendered roles in agriculture, gendered division of labor, and gendered determinants of social status have gradually shifted as a result of this male migration, specifically in Khatlon Province, and have allowed women the opportunity to participate in decision-making within the household as well as control the household income (2, 7). However, other reports have indicated that 'Despite labor migration having expanded women's roles, it does not appear to have affected their status in terms of increased agency and ability to make autonomous personal choices' (9, p. xvii). This gender imbalance has had other negative effects with regard to adolescent girls, aged 15 and 16 years, marrying at an earlier age to ensure that they have a husband (10). Therefore, while male-out migration may be empowering women, specifically mothers-in-law, within the household, it has created a triple burden of responsibilities for young women in terms of domestic, agricultural, and family obligations.

Malnutrition remains a public health problem within Tajikistan. In 2012, the Demographic Health Survey in Tajikistan indicated that 26% of children under 5 years are stunted, 10% are wasted, and 12% are underweight, with Khatlon Province having among the highest percentages in all three indicators (2). Malnutrition and undernutrition is most severe among vulnerable populations, such as women and children. According to a joint report by the World Bank and UNICEF (11), the immediate causes of undernutrition are inadequate dietary intake and disease, driven by inadequate access to food, inadequate care provided to children, and insufficient health and environmental services. This is also perpetuated by gender inequality, underrepresentation of girls within education, and government resource allocations that are unfavorable to the poor (11). Women specifically are more susceptible to anemia and deficiency of vitamin A and iodine which contribute to Tajikistan's high maternal and child mortality (4, 5, 12).

The goal of this study was to research and develop recommendations for gender transformative approaches – addressing gender inequalities and transforming the dynamics between men and women – that will address food misconceptions, perceptions of healthy eating, and reduce barriers surrounding dietary diversity within the rural Khatlon Province of Tajikistan. The Agriculture Extension System (AES) is in a unique position to transmit these practices to the field through existing, community-based programs. AES agents, responsible for delivering information to farmers, have the potential to bridge agriculture, nutrition, and gender by integrating these topics within their ongoing technical trainings. The specific aims of this study were to identify and understand ways to engage husbands and mothers-in-law (who live within or near the same domicile) in household nutrition through extension services and to investigate practices within households around dietary habits and nutritional behavior. These groups were chosen specifically as a result of young women, often young or new mothers, being forced to leave school in order to take on the burden of feeding the household, being the caretaker of children, and managing the household chores, such as collecting water (9). The mother-in-law (which will be abbreviated as MiL since this study was from the perspective of the young, in-married women) plays and important role in food choice due to the hierarchy of the household. Young or new mothers (who will be referred to as in-married women) often live with or near her in-laws where she has limited agency and decision-making power within the household. The household dynamic in rural Tajikistan differs from urban areas in that the average household has 6.9 members compared to 4.9 members in urban households; this again is a result of households in rural areas being traditionally multigenerational with the in-laws living in the same domicile (2). In addition, households within Khatlon Province tend to have the lowest rates of household members who are over the age of 6 years and received any education (2). Therefore, by working within the unique community and household context of rural Tajikistan, efforts to improve nutrition will be more sustainable and have increased impact on the lives of people in the region.

## Methods

In collaboration with in-country partners, fieldwork for this study was completed in February 2017. Researchers from the University of Florida (UF), located in the United States, integrated students from the Masters of Public Health (MPH) program in Gainesville, Florida, United States, in addition to students from the Tajikistan Agrarian University (TAU) in Dushanbe, Tajikistan, to assist in the data collection and fieldwork phase of this study. Both UF and TAU students had public health or agriculture extension knowledge prior to the study and were trained in qualitative research methods before participating in any data collection. UF researchers had background knowledge in global public health and nutrition. A local partner, Tajikistan Agriculture and Water Activity (TAWA), assisted with logistical support, such as lodging, and provided trained, local agriculture extension agents to facilitate focus groups.

### *Participants*

Participants for the KIIs were selected based on their work within the Khatlon Province or their knowledge of the population as it pertains to nutrition, including a clinic director and representatives from international organizations. Participants for the FGDs were purposefully recruited from villages that extension agents work in and have established women's groups. These women's groups, formed by the Women Entrepreneurship for Empowerment Project (WEEP), bring women of reproductive age together to learn skills, specifically related to agriculture, and nutrition-related aspects. TAWA extension agents have been working throughout these rural villages, establishing trust and relationships with the women inhabitants. Both KIIs and FGDs were conducted to triangulate individual and group-level perception on food, nutrition, and household decision-making within Khatlon Province. However, given the experience of the key informants working in nutrition and health in the target area, more emphasis was put on lessons learned from their fieldwork. Prior to initiating the FGDs, the instrument was tested in Yovon, a village within Khatlon, among mothers with children under the age of 10 years. The instrument was revised and adjusted appropriately for cultural sensitivity.

*Study design*

KIIs were conducted in English or Tajik by UF researchers, UF masters students, and TAU students. During both KIIs and FGDs, an UF researcher was present to ensure quality of data collected. The TAU students acted as translators during interviews conducted in Tajik, while also asking relevant probing questions when appropriate. Interviews were open-ended and semi-structured, and content included perceptions of household nutrition and decision-making surrounding food within the rural villages of Khatlon. Verbal informed consent was requested and documented prior to the interview. A total of four KIIs were conducted, which included interviews with the World Health Organization, UNICEF, German Corporation for International Cooperation, and a local health clinic within Khatlon Province. Key informants were initially chosen based on the in-country partners' knowledge of international organizations working in nutrition. Key informants also provided information on best practices for data collection within Khatlon Province and what to expand on from their previous experience and research.

A total of 15 FGDs were conducted with participant groups ranging from 5 to 18 individuals; however, two focus groups were excluded because of size and participant makeup.[1] Focus groups were stratified as young mothers with children (in-married woman), the in-married women's MiL, and husbands of the in-married women, throughout the catchment area. These groups were chosen based on the composition of the household in Khatlon Province. It was strongly recommended by key informants to keep these groups separated for honest responses. Focus groups were asked semi-structured questions regarding decision-making surrounding food and dietary behavior. Each female FGD was facilitated by a trained agriculture extension agent with a UF and TAU student present. Adjacent to the focus group, the TAU student translated the dialogue between the facilitator and the group in real-time so that the research team could transcribe the conversation as well as ask clarifying questions (via the facilitator) to participants. All male FGDs were conducted by a male TAU student with at least one UF student present. Given the high rate of illiteracy within the study population, informed consent for focus group participants was collected verbally before the discussion began and was read in the local language (Uzbek or Tajik). Focus groups took place in 12 different villages throughout Khatlon Province, and were chosen based on differing geographic barriers and socio-economic status within USAID's Zone of Influence (ZOI). Fifteen FGDs were conducted, with 13 being homogenous by sex and age group, and 2 being mixed ages as previously indicated (seven focus groups with in-married women, four with MiLs, two with husbands, and two with mixed MiLs and in-married women).

*Qualitative analysis*

Transcripts from 4r KIIs and 13 out of 15 FGDs were used for data analysis. Researchers carried out the qualitative analysis using the constant comparative method (13) to code transcripts and find emerging themes simultaneously. Grounded theory (14) was used within analysis to contextualize the themes as they materialized in order to develop connections and relationship that were subsequently made into subthemes. Two of the researchers independently read through all of the transcripts for salient themes, subsequently forming a consensus based on frequency of themes and discussion. All transcripts were then coded independently by two researchers to ensure reliability. All of the final manifested themes and subthemes were centered on household decision-making, food beliefs, and health to better understand how to design applicable interventions with the TAWA extension agents. Themes and subthemes were collected from the data deductively and inductively in that certain themes were created *a priori* whereas others, and most subthemes, were identified upon review using QSR International's NVivo 11 software. Once themes and subthemes were identified, they were presented to the UF research team to finalize and establish a consensus.

**Results**

There were a total of 106 participants across 13 FGDs within five districts (Shaatruz, Jomi, Khuroson/Ghozimalik, Sarband, and Vakhsh) of Khatlon Province. The results of the FGDs have been analyzed and presented below according to the following major themes: Decision-making around food (Theme 1), accessibility of food

[1] The two focus groups that were excluded from the analysis were not stratified, including both in-married women and MiL, and had more participants than necessary (14 in one and 18 in the other).

(Theme 2), misconceptions around food (Theme 3), and dietary information (Theme 4). The results of the focus groups of the same participant group (in-married women, MiLs, or husbands) were highly consistent across districts with the exception of husband's responses for Theme 3 and Theme 4. In general, greater diversity was observed in the responses between participant groups than within participant groups. Theme 3 (Misconceptions around food) and Theme 4 (Dietary information) showed the greatest variation in responses between in-married women, MiLs, and husbands (see Tables 1 and 2). Results from the KIIs were used to refine study design based on cultural practices in the region before initiating FGDs as well as to form a consensus among major themes within FGDs.

#### *Theme 1. Decision-making around food*

All participant groups discussed consistent decision-making processes surrounding food, revealing clear gender roles in food preparation and purchase. Three subthemes were identified within Theme 1 including 1) purchasing foods, 2) cooking, and 3) food purchase decisions.

##### Purchasing foods

All three participant groups agreed that men are the primary purchasers of food. Women play a secondary role in food purchasing; women's purchases are dependent on whether the husband is present. If men are unavailable to go to market, women will go to market and purchase food for the family. Women in the household (in-married women and MiLs) stated that men may be unavailable to purchase foods 'if [they] are busy'. In other cases, women explained that seasonal migration of men to Russia has resulted in the increased role of women in food purchasing.

##### Cooking

There was a consensus across the study population that women, either the in-married woman or MiL, prepare food for the family. Furthermore, all three participant groups emphasized the role of the in-married women in food preparation. In this way, younger women fill the majority of cooking needs for the family while MiL plays a supportive role. For example, one MiL reported that when her daughter-in-law visits her family, the MiL takes over responsibility for cooking during that time. According to the combined reports of the MiLs and husbands, men may depend on the MiLs to cook, may eat out, or cook food themselves if the wife is not available to cook.

##### Food purchase decisions

Again, all participant groups agree that women, either the in-married woman or MiL, decide which foods to buy. According to the participants in the MiL sessions, the reason women decide which foods to purchase is that their 'husbands don't know what to buy because [they] cook'. In cases where MiL and in-married women cohabitate, both women play a role in the decision-making process. However, if MiL and in-married woman live separately, each woman decides what foods to purchase for her respective household.

#### *Theme 2. Accessibility of food*

In general, in-married women, MiLs, and husbands showed consistency in their responses regarding accessibility of food. There are some key differences, however, with respect to where food is acquired, when food is available, how it can be obtained, and solutions for navigating challenges regarding food access. Furthermore, strategies for dealing with limited income were mentioned in three out of the four subthemes. Theme 2 has been divided into the following four subthemes: 1) food acquisition, 2) seasonality, 3) obtaining food, and 4) barriers and solutions.

##### Food acquisition

This subtheme is especially relevant because it illustrates where households are getting their food from. In general, the participant groups agreed that the majority of food is purchased at the market. However, MiLs also discussed occasional purchase from neighbors. In-married women emphasize the importance of homestead production for the majority of food needs, utilizing market purchases only for food items not produced on their own land. Cooking basics, including flour, oil, and onions, were among the food items that must be purchased.

##### Seasonality

There was unanimous agreement among in-married women, MiLs, and men that winter is the most challenging month with respect to food access. All participant groups discussed a strong dependence on food purchases during the winter due to the seasonality of home gardens. According to husbands, this was sometimes due to insufficient Fall harvests. Spring was recognized as the second-most difficult season, with some need to purchase foods. Summer and, to a lesser degree, Fall were identified as seasons of surplus in which nearly all food is produced in home gardens, 'so there is no need to go to the market'.

##### Obtaining food

This subtheme indicates how households obtain their food, whether it is through trade, money, or potentially other means. Women (in-married women and MiLs) agreed that food is primarily obtained through monetary purchase. However, in-married women emphasized the importance of informal credit agreements in which they purchase food on account (without transfer of money) and pay the supplier later. This was mentioned as being quite common in village markets; however, in district markets (which were larger and more centralized within a region)

*Table 1.* Misconceptions around food for pregnant women and children under five

| Misconceptio s around food | In-married women | MiLs | Husbands | Outcomes |
|---|---|---|---|---|
| Pregnant women | 'It depends on the state of health; when they have morning sickness they don't eat oily meals'. 'They don't eat *mantou* a lot, noodles; they are told if you eat these kinds of foods or meals you will have difficulty during birth'. 'In order not to get fat and fat on the child, we don't eat too much bread and baked goods'. 'Doctors said that they shouldn't eat'. 'Doctors tell them not to eat nuts, noodles, bread, foods rich with carbohydrates and recommend to eat more fruits and juice'. 'We know that fruits and vegetables have a lot of fertilizer and chemicals'. | 'Women shouldn't eat noodles and foods with carbohydrates while pregnant. It makes [the] baby very big and difficult to give birth'. 'They are told not to eat pistachios and nuts because they think the babies will be fat'. 'They eat meat, but less eggs because they make the babies big'. 'Pregnant women don't eat as much oily food. They eat a lot of dairy and milk'. 'Bakery, the pregnant women they don't eat much baked goods like bread but they eat most legumes, meats, [and] fruit. The baby will be big and they cannot easily deliver [if they eat baked goods]. 'Our pregnant women are afraid to get very big, and they don't eat *osh, noodles, mantou.* They are told that their babies will become very big. Doctors told them'. | 'Pregnant women eat everything. Meat of horse they do not eat. Also meat from rabbits. When the baby is born, they will have holes in their lip; cleft lip or cleft palate' 'Pregnant women don't eat *osh*'. | In-married women, MiLs, and husbands cite restrictions on women's carbohydrate intake during pregnancy. The most common justification for this practice (given by MiLs and in-married women) is that carbohydrates make the baby large and hard to deliver (potentially macrosomia). Both MiLs and in-married women identify doctors as their source of information on avoiding carbohydrates. MiL and in-married women also discuss avoiding oily or 'heavy' foods during pregnancy. MiL and in-married women also note avoiding eating nuts. There is a mixed consensus on egg consumption among MiL, with some recommending egg consumption while others emphasizing meat consumption over eggs. Husbands mention avoiding horse and rabbit meat due to increased risk of cleft palate. Husbands were the only group to say that pregnant women eat everything (in-married women state that some women eat everything during pregnancy, against the advice of others) |
| Children under five | We don't give them tomatoes, cucumbers, watermelons, or grapes because of diarrhea'. 'When we make soup we make the potato and then we make it watery and make the mashed potato and give it to our children. Some women who don't have enough breast milk, they give cow's milk to their children, some women give formula'. 'We don't give fried potatoes to young children and we don't give them *sambusa, osh, mantou*, hard meals, because it's difficult to digest these meals'. 'For example, one of my daughters likes *chakka* (yogurt mixture), I usually give her light meals like noodles and soup but she likes sweets'. 'They don't give spicy foods to children under five because it is not healthy for the stomach and kidney'. 'The water may get them sick'. 'My children don't eat eggs and meat; they just don't like it'. 'Unwashed vegetables they will get sick from greenhouses. [It] gives children diarrhea'. | 'We don't give cucumbers to the children. We don't give boiled eggs because it's very hard for the stomach to digest, it makes them [have] diarrhea. Some of them after they eat cucumber, they drink water (not boiled)'. 'For children under 2 years old, we do not give them *osh*. We do not give them spicy foods or hot meals'. 'Babies who didn't start talking, they shouldn't eat eggs, because it will influence. They will start speaking very late'. | '[Children under 5 don't eat] spicy food. Salty food.' 'Eggs. It has many calories. Fish, because of the small bones.' | There are differing opinions of best child-feeding practices among in-married women, MiLs, and husbands. One consensus, however, is the avoidance of feeding children eggs. Each group cites a different reason for not feeding their children eggs. In-married women and MiLs voice concern over foods that may cause diarrhea; both groups cite cucumbers as a source of diarrhea. In-married women mention additional foods (tomato, watermelon, and grapes) and unwashed vegetables/fruits as potential sources of diarrhea. MiLs and in-married women also agree that children should not be given *osh, mantou*, eggs, or high-oil foods. In-married women strongly emphasize the importance of preparing light meals or foods with soft texture (soaked biscuits, mashed potatoes, soups) for children. In-married women also note the importance of general child health as a determinant for feeding practices (if the child is already healthy, he/she will experience little enteric disease; if he/she is naturally sickly, there will be more frequent diarrhea) and child food preference factors into what the in-married women prepares for her children. These factors were not cited by MiLs or husbands. |

*Table 2.* Dietary information

| Dietary Information | In-married women | MiLs | Husbands | Outcomes |
|---|---|---|---|---|
| Cause illness | 'I don't eat eggs. I have an allergy and it doesn't matter how it's used'. 'She has allergies so she doesn't eat legumes because of the allergy. She doesn't eat eggs; she doesn't eat kidney beans, [because of] allergies on her hands and feet. She went to the doctor but nothing'. 'All of the vegetables and foods which are grown with chemicals and fertilizer, they can affect us and they can make us sick. Some people died from botulism, after they ate the canned product last year there was one case of botulism'. 'Some people when they eat melons they have allergies'. 'In summer [children] when they eat grapes it makes them diarrhea. Or if they eat melons it also makes them diarrhea, or tomatoes'. 'Some people can't eat goat meat, for example, my mother doesn't eat meat at all, and when she eats meat she gets sick'. 'My mother doesn't eat meat either, when she eats beef she gets sick'. 'We don't consume cotton oil, because it has burning effects'. '[We] do not eat eggs because they had hepatitis so they are not recommended to eat eggs as part of [our] diet'. | People that have illness of hepatitis and typhoid, they don't eat plov because it's heavy, they don't eat eggs because they have diet'. 'Some people if they eat lamb or eggs, it makes them sick. People with high blood pressure or heart problems. Goat meat gives us diarrhea'. 'When you drink milk, you may get a headache'. '. Also not boiling water causes illness'. | 'Osh may cause pain in the stomach. When they eat grapes, it may cause bloating. If you eat pumpkin, it may cause burning in the throat'. 'Sheep's meat. It has many oils'. | There is little consistency between the three groups with respect to which foods can cause illness. However, in-married women, MiLs, and husbands all mention oily food as a potential source of illness. The greatest similarity in responses is observed between in-married women and MiLs with respect to spoiled foods, contaminated water, heavy/ oily foods, or increased sensitivity to some foods if an individual has specific health problems. In-married women, in particular, emphasize allergies as a cause of illness. Health problems that increase likelihood of illness that were mentioned by both in-married women and MiLs include: high blood pressure and hepatitis. In-married women and MiLs also noted hepatitis patients and people with high blood pressure have special diets. In-married women reported the greatest diversity of illness-causing foods; mentioning heavy, high-oil foods, eggs, and meat. Interestingly, in-married women also mention foods with chemicals/grown using fertilizers as sources of illness. |
| Health beliefs | 'We don't eat imported chicken'. 'We give children under one cow's milk. Not goat's milk. It's nice; goat's milk is nicer than cow's milk'. 'My baby was four months old, and I gave him cow's milk because I didn't have enough milk'. 'The foods with vitamins, they eat them'. 'The fruits they have vitamins. Cabbage, flour, I dry eggplants in summer, and then I eat it [them] in the winter'. 'Also important are meat and eggs because they are healthy'. 'Oranges, we don't eat it makes the pressure down. Also the canning that is very cold, we don't eat them in the winter'. 'We do compote, we do canning with tomato and cucumber If we have money in the budget we buy meat'. 'A light meal is soup, rice soup, noodles, rice porridge for breakfast'. 'It's important to have them clean, if we wash them properly that's good for health'. 'Using fertilizer less, using compost instead of chemicals'. We don't eat imported chicken; we eat our chicken from our houses but we don't eat imported chicken'. 'If you have a problem with the stomach you shouldn't eat hard meals (like *osh*)'. 'My mother cannot eat *plov* because she has an allergy for rice'. 'I am not in condition to buy formula, but I buy cow milk for my children which may be healthier'. | 'Onion, potato, flour, rice, carrot, beet, radish, sugar, oil, spaghetti, sugar, and salt are all important'. 'Soup and *plov*, with rice radish, turnip, carrot, salads form carrot, we make salad from green radish, beetroot is good'. 'They make salad from beet root as well'. 'Sometimes we have problems buying meat'. | 'Some of them have high blood pressure, so if they have it they may not eat sugar. It depends on the disease'. 'There are meats we do not eat for religious reasons'. | Affordability is mentioned as a barrier to healthy foods. Meat in particular may not be purchased due to affordability, though it is recognized by both MiLs and in-married women as healthy. Husbands, in contrast, state that meat may not be consumed for religious reasons. In-married women specify which foods are high in vitamins (fruits and vegetables). Both in-married women and MiLs cite the same basic foods that are bought at market (sugar, oil, flour, rice, salt...). In-married women in particular mention avoiding imported chicken for consumption. In-married women also detail the use of soft foods and cow's milk for complementary feeding practices of infants. One in-married woman cited the use of cow's milk in lieu of formula due to affordability. Both husbands and in-married women note the need for a modified diet if one has high blood pressure. Out of all of the groups, in-married women most strongly emphasize the consumption of vegetables, fruits, and dairy. The main constant is the mention of vitamins and vegetables and affordability challenges regarding meat between both groups of women. |

*Table 2.* Continued

| Dietary Information | In-married women | MiLs | Husbands | Outcomes |
|---|---|---|---|---|
| General diet | 'Flour is the most important food. [As well as] oil, potato, onion, salt, salt, tomato pasta, beans'. 'Vegetables are also important, cilantro is important, salad is important, cucumber, tomato, carrots, carrot salad, turnip, pepper, eggplant, pumpkin, rice'. 'Pumpkins are healthier than meat'. 'Meat is more nutritious than beans, turnip, herbs, pumpkin; many people have a diet from beans'. 'Dill and cilantro'. 'Salt is also important; tea is important'. 'Banana, kiwi, pineapple, for the holidays'. 'Almonds, walnuts, red beans they are very nutritious'. 'In the past we didn't consume sour cream, 10–15 years ago we didn't make salads, and now in the past years we make salads with beetroot'. 'We didn't have pineapple, kiwi, oranges, banana'. 'We consume eggs in a different way, we boil it, we fry eggplants with eggs and we cook some other different kinds of food with eggs'. 'We didn't used to eat bananas. I tasted [it] this year; I think that our fruits are tastier than the imported fruits. Our apples are tastier because they are ripened in the sun'. 'I learned to can 2 years ago, there was one organization that came and demonstrated how to do it'. | 'Oil, onion, tomatoes, carrots, beans, rice, lentil, kidney bean, mung bean. Meat, sometimes'. 'Grape carrot, persimmon, pomegranate, oranges, bananas. Sometimes we get banana'. 'Rice porridge is good for people who have heart problems'. 'In winter, rice porridge. It is called *shala*'. 'Osh is also good because it makes people strong. Also, different types of fruits have different vitamins'. 'We buy apple, orange, mandarin, date/fig because they are healthy and have vitamins. They are very healthy for pregnant women'. 'Last year, I tried kiwi and banana for the first time. Kiwi for me as well last year. Also, pineapple'. | 'Flour, oil, tomato, onion, leafy vegetables, herbs. Tea. Flour and oil are most important. We eat lots of bread'. 'Milk products. Traditional foods like *osh*. For breakfast [we] prefer milk products. Lunch [we] prefer soup. Dinner [we] like traditional food like sauce or stew'. 'Potato, onion, flour. Oil, sugar, fruits for children. Pasta is also extremely important to us. They are important for preparing daily meals'. 'Milk products. Fruit- apple, cereals. Meat, specifically cow meat'. | Across all three groups, flour, and oil are identified as the two most important staple foods. Next, onions, tomatoes, potato, and 'fruits and vegetables' (in general) are mentioned by all groups. In-married women emphasize the importance of beets, carrots, radish, salt, and sugar. Both groups of women detail various types of fruits and vegetables and methods of preparation. In-married women, in particular, discuss preparation of salad using beets. Furthermore, banana, kiwi, and pineapple appear to be recent additions to the Tajik diet according to two women's focus groups. Root vegetables appear to play particular importance according to women, as well as legumes and beans. In-married women and husbands mention the use of herbs, in-married women giving detail about preference, while MiLs do not. Only husbands cite dairy products as part of the general diet. Furthermore, husbands mention 'traditional foods' as important to the diet. |

this was not acceptable. While food trade is recognized as rare by both in-married women and MiLs, husbands identified trade as the 'typical' means of obtaining food and 'other times [they] pay with money'.These responses reveal gender-based differences in market transactions in which husbands are more likely to trade than women.

#### Barriers and solutions

All three participant groups identified lack of money as a barrier to food security. In-married women and MiLs reported limited employment as drivers of low income. MiLs in particular suggested skill-building workshops for young girls as a potential means of increasing household income. In-married women and husbands additionally focused on limited food due to poor-quality harvests and low autumn yields. In-married women discussed pest management as a potential solution to improving the quality of crops and reducing insect-related damage. Husbands and MiLs emphasized canning and pickling as solutions for minimizing food purchases and maintaining food sales through value-added goods during the winter.

### *Theme 3. Misconceptions around food*

In general, the participant responses regarding misconceptions around food were consistent regarding which foods to avoid. However, the responses were inconsistent regarding the *reasons* for avoiding that food. Inconsistencies were more apparent in the comparison of women and men focus groups; MiLs and in-married women showed greater congruency than husbands. Theme 3 includes two subthemes: Pregnant women and children under five.

#### Pregnant women

All participant groups discussed restrictions in carbohydrate intake as an important strategy for prenatal health. However, these beliefs vary in the way they were presented. For example, in-married women and MiLs emphasized restrictions in carbohydrate consumption by mentioning a wide range of foods that pregnant women should avoid including *mantou*, noodles, bread, baked goods, and *osh*.[2] Husbands illustrated the practice of prenatal limitation of carbohydrates by identifying *osh* as a food that pregnant women avoid. MiLs and in-married women gave a highly consistent reason for avoiding carbohydrates during pregnancy: carbohydrate consumption leads to a heavy birth weight and difficult delivery. Furthermore, in-married women and MiLs identified doctors as the source of this information.

Aside from carbohydrate consumption, both women participant groups agreed that women should monitor their intake of 'heavy' foods including fats, oils, and nuts because these foods can increase morning sickness symptoms. In-married women did not mention meat consumption, while MiLs and husbands recommended meat and eggs for a prenatal diet. Husbands also discussed avoidance of particular meats (rabbit and horse) due to the increased risk of cleft pallet in infants (See Table 1, 'Husbands'), whereas only MiLs discussed the importance of dairy consumption during pregnancy.Interestingly, both women participant groups discuss ideas surrounding 'pure food'. In-married women, for example, referred to avoiding food that was produced using pesticides or fertilizers while MiLs discussed consuming domestic eggs 'but not the imported ones'. MiLs further identified food from China as unhealthy.

#### Children under five

While there are diverse opinions regarding proper young child-feeding practices between in-married women, MiLs, and husbands, all three participant groups agree that children should not receive eggs. However, each group cited a different reason for the practice. For example, MiLs stated that eggs are 'hard for the stomach to digest', while husbands reasoned that eggs contain too many calories. One in-married woman, meanwhile, highlighted her child's taste preference as the primary reason for not feeding her children eggs (See Table 1). Finally, in-married women and MiLs discussed contaminated water and unwashed fruits and vegetables as sources of diarrhea.

In-married women consistently mentioned two ideas concerning children's diets (1) children's diets should include mostly light, soft foods and (2) the ability to consume a diverse diet depends on the child's baseline health, or whether the child is perceived as 'healthy' or 'unhealthy' according to the community standard. With respect to the first idea, in-married women show a preference for feeding their children 'light meals' like 'noodles and soup' because they are perceived to be easier to digest than 'heavy meals', like fatty or oily foods. In addition, in-married women emphasize the need for children's meals to be soft in consistency and texture. In-married women discussed preparation practices for soft foods, such as mashing potatoes, soaking biscuits in water, or pureeing apples. According to in-married women, baseline health affects child consumption patterns because healthy children are able to eat a greater diversity of food items with a reduced risk of becoming ill. Unhealthy children, meanwhile, must eat a more restricted ('soft' or 'light') diet to prevent further illness. In-married women explained that hard and heavy foods are difficult to digest and likely to make unhealthy children sick. In-married women also connected rural living and exercise to the general health of children (See Table 1, *children under five*).

### *Theme 4. Dietary information*

Participants have varying opinions surrounding dietary information, especially with respect to health beliefs and

[2] Mantou (dumpling) and osh (pilaf) are traditional Tajik foods prepared with flour and rice, respectively.

foods that cause illness. Theme 4 has been divided into three subthemes, including foods that cause illness, health beliefs, and general diet.

#### Foods that cause illness

Responses within this subtheme are highly diverse. However, there was a consensus across all three participant groups that oily foods are a source of food-related illness. The greatest similarity in responses is observed between the women participant groups (in-married women and MiLs). For example, both women's groups agreed that spoiled foods, contaminated water, and heavy foods cause illness. Furthermore, both groups noted that individuals with pre-existing health problems[3] and elderly people experience an increased risk of food-related illness and require dietary restrictions to avoid frequent health issues. In-married women listed the greatest diversity of illness-causing foods. Finally, in-married women emphasized the impact of allergies on illness and diet.

#### Health beliefs

Participant groups showed differing opinions with respect to health beliefs. However, all groups mentioned the importance of traditional foods, many of which are high in carbohydrates and utilize either rice or flour as their main ingredient.[4] In general, in-married women and MiLs show the greatest consistency in their responses, citing the importance of vegetables and fruits due to vitamin content. In addition, both MiLs and in-married women discussed affordability as a barrier to purchasing meat, while husbands specifically discuss religion as a barrier to the consumption of certain meats. Husbands and in-married women identified the need for individuals with high blood pressure to have modified diets through lower sugar and carbohydrate consumption.

In this subtheme, in-married women again mentioned avoiding foods produced using fertilizer or chemicals and their preference for domestic chicken and meat. This concept was first discussed by in-married women (fertilizers) and MiL (domestic animal sourced foods) in Theme 3 (Misconceptions around food, *pregnant women*). Interestingly, in-married women emphasize the importance of 'clean' food, stating that 'if we wash [the vegetables] properly, it is good for our health'. In-married women and MiLs first discussed the importance of washing fruits and vegetables within Theme 3, *children under five.*

[3] Heart problems, high blood pressure, allergies, hepatitis, and typhoid were among the health problems mentioned.

[4] Husbands identified these foods by simply stating 'traditional foods' while in-married women and MiLs discussed their preparation in detail. In-married women and MiLs specifically mention preparation of osh, mantou, and shala.

#### General diet

Across all three participant groups, flour and oil are identified as the most important staple foods. In addition, onions, tomatoes, potato, and 'fruits and vegetables' in general were reported by all groups. Both women participant groups detailed various fruits and vegetables along with methods for preparing them. Furthermore, both women's groups participants identified banana, kiwi, and pineapple as recent introductions to the Tajik diet. Lastly, both groups discussed the important role of root vegetables, legumes, and beans in the general diet. In-married women and husbands mention the use of herbs, and in-married women highlighted taste preference as a driver of food choice. Interestingly, only husbands cited dairy products as an integral part of the general diet.

### Discussion

As prior research establishes, malnutrition is a critical public health issue that disrupts the livelihoods of many Tajik people (2). Stunting, iodine deficiency, and maternal and child anemia account for the greatest proportion of negative health outcomes due to undernutrition in Tajikistan (11). Poor diet, characterized by insufficient amounts of nutritious foods consumed at low frequency, has been identified as the primary driver of such conditions (15). Undernutrition is concentrated among women of reproductive age, children, and rural populations, which may lead to immediate and long-term productive and reproductive consequences and hold severe implications for the quality of life in rural areas. The Tajik diet includes inhibitors of nutrient absorption (particularly iron) like black tea and exclusion of absorption enhancers, such as fresh fruit, animal source foods, and vegetables, which are seasonally unavailable or unaffordable according to this study (15, 16). Even so, these findings point to a general knowledge about the health benefits of various fruits and vegetables, especially among women. Participants cited onion, tomato, and potato as essential components of their diet, and placed importance on the health benefits provided by beans and many types of fruits and vegetables. Many women participants (both in-married and MiLs) placed additional emphasis on consuming a healthy diet during pregnancy. Many fruits and vegetables are considered indulgences rather than central components of the Tajik diet, unlike everyday staples. Participants pointed to the high cost associated with imported fruit, such as kiwi, as a major barrier for why they do not include more fruits and vegetables in their diet. As a result, many fruits are exclusively reserved for special occasions – as one participant stated, residents in her village saved 'banana, kiwi, and pineapple for the holidays'. It is customary in Tajikistan to bring food to guests, but there is concern that this expectation for the appearance of wealth leaves less food on the family table, as mentioned in one of the husband focus groups. To encourage greater dietary diversity, it is recommended to promote locally sourced, affordable health options to make healthy choices more commonplace.

Clear gender roles were noted for the following subthemes of Theme 3, Decision-making around food: *Purchasing food*, *cooking*, and *food purchase decisions*. Husbands appear to hold the responsibility of going to market to purchase or trade for food, while women (MiLs and in-married women) make the decisions regarding what type of food to buy. According to women, the responsibility of making food purchase decisions resides with women because they are the primary food preparers. Between the women of the household, it is unclear under what conditions food purchase decisions are allocated to the MiL as opposed to the in-married woman. The responsibility of making food decisions appears variable, in some cases dependent on the availability of the in-married woman and in others based on negotiations between the in-married woman and the MiL. The MiL may also have a transient role in food preparation depending on the availability of the in-married woman. FGDs also indicated that the absence of men within communities as a result of migration impacted daily life and household roles significantly. Although the focus group instrument did not specifically ask questions about male migration, female FGD participants brought up migration several times as it related to other questions surrounding household decision-making. When asked about household responsibilities, such as shopping for food, women as a whole routinely mentioned how the absence of men had shifted the responsibility to them. MiL participation in shopping for food is significant with regard to the household's nutrition status, as it seems to provide a greater opportunity for women to make changes in their diets. Since women are often the ones purchasing (MiL) and cooking (in-married women) food using gender-specific interventions that address diet diversity, specifically by introducing new crops, could prove more successful. Nevertheless, an increase in responsibilities as a result of male migration may not directly impact power within the household.

Based on the FDGs, it appears that migration has affected women's lives to varying degrees, which depends significantly on the circumstances they are in. In addition, in cases where in-married women live with their MiLs, the MiLs were the heads of household when men were not present. Consequently, extension services should attempt to incorporate MiLs into trainings and educational interventions, as they are often the ones with a significant amount of power and time within a household. It is also beneficial to recognize that the amount of agency a mother has within her household will vary based on which family members she lives with.

Perhaps, the most striking findings from this study are the dietary practices and misconceptions about food prescribed to young children and pregnant women. As with previous studies conducted in other geographic regions, food taboos tend to have the greatest impact on the nutrition status of women and children (17). There was a general consensus that pregnant women should avoid carbohydrates and oily foods due to the risk of a difficult labor associated with heavier birthweight and irritation of morning sickness symptoms, respectively. For example, both in-married and MiLs reported that pregnant women should not consume carbohydrate-rich staple foods like *osh* and *mantou*. Husbands echoed these beliefs to a lesser degree, and with mixed opinions. For example, one participant claimed that 'pregnant women eat everything', while another agreed with the beliefs of women's groups stating that 'pregnant women do not eat *osh*'. Still other men reported a wide variety of beliefs incongruent with other participant groups. Women (MiLs and in-married women) appear to be the primary endorsers and implementers of dietary practices that limit carbohydrate consumption as indicated by the high degree of consistency in the food practices reported by women participant groups.

As many staple foods are rich in carbohydrates, women report the exclusion of these items during pregnancy. Exclusion of staple foods may hold significant implications during lean seasons (Winter and Spring) when vegetables and fruits are unavailable and households live on reduced incomes. The FGDs did not reveal whether such limitations on pregnant women's diets are altered during the lean season to accommodate reduced access to alternative foods. While beliefs surrounding carbohydrate intake and heavy birthweight have not been previously investigated in Tajikistan, studies from other geographic regions (Ethiopia and Nigeria) have made similar findings (16, 18, 19). In Nigeria, one study revealed that pregnant women who were not practicing taboos had significantly greater weight gain and gave birth to heavier infants as compared to women practicing food taboos (17). Determining the immediate impact of food taboos on pregnant women in Tajikistan may represent opportunities for improving maternal health outcomes including maternal morbidity and preterm birth complications.

Restriction of oily foods – oily food in the FGDs included certain meats (goat, lamb) as well as foods containing or cooked with vegetable oil – has additional implications on pregnancy outcomes and child development. For example, sources of omega-3 fatty acids (fish, nuts, vegetable oil) and animal source food (meat) are shown to benefit fetal (physical and cognitive) growth and support the increased nutrient demand associated with pregnancy (20). Avoidance of oil during pregnancy appears to be a cultural practice, while exclusion of carbohydrates was learned through counseling with doctors. This may indicate miscommunication or misunderstanding of dietary recommendations between patients and healthcare professionals.

FGDs conducted with women revealed consistent beliefs surrounding child feedings practices. For example, both MiLs and in-married women voiced that children should receive 'light' and 'soft' foods – described as foods containing less fat and carbohydrates, and foods that have been watered down to a soft consistency. Among the foods restricted from children's diets are staple foods like *sambusa*, *osh*, *fatir*, and *mantou*, which are described as 'hard meals'. According to women participants, heavy foods are more 'difficult to digest' and may result in stomach problems. Interestingly, these beliefs were not reflected by FGDs conducted with husbands. Finally, in-married women and, to a lesser degree, MiLs were concerned with diarrheal disease in children. Both reference cucumber and water as sources of diarrhea; In-married women additionally reported that unwashed fruits and vegetables may be a source of diarrhea. Additional research is needed to determine whether the practice of restricting staple foods among children contributes to the prevalence of stunting in Tajikistan.

It was mentioned in several FGDs with in-married women that that they gave infants aged under 6 months cow's milk when they had difficulties with breastfeeding. Various reasons for the use of cow's milk included not having enough breast milk or not having enough money to buy formula. There was a belief that cow's milk was comparable to breast milk and made babies strong. When asked if participants used milk from other sources, such as goats, in-married women indicated that only cow's milk was preferred because of availability and the high cost of formula. Due to the dangers of using unmodified cow's milk for infants aged under 9 months, nutrition-specific interventions should be introduced to address the use of alternative breast milk within the rural regions. In order to reduce breastfeeding cessation, potential interventions could include providing lactation and breastfeeding support.

Due to the small sample size of this study, several limitations need to be considered. Consistency of beliefs around access to foods or food misconceptions may vary according to the participant's proximity to food centers or education status, respectively. Moreover, the geographic distribution of selected villages was shaped around prearranged Women's Economic Empowerment Project (WEEP) group meeting times and consisted mainly of participants from these groups. Also, while the sample population was intended to include more male focus groups, due to the lack of young, adult males in the target areas, researchers were unable to have a more balanced representation.

This study demonstrates the need for gender-responsive solutions using agricultural extension agents to counter barriers to a healthy diet and dietary diversity in Khatlon Province. Results also established a link between emigration of males to Russia for work and changing household social structure. The impact of migration on household decision-making is worth exploring further to offer more mindful approaches for future intervention strategies in the province. This study suggests that women hold the majority of nutritional knowledge and misconceptions surrounding food, both practicing and engaging in food-restrictive taboos alongside a genuine knowledge of healthy eating practices. Overall, men lacked knowledge of nutrition and dietary practices. In order for agriculture extension agents to address nutritional status of their beneficiaries as part of their duties, extension agents must have knowledge of the intra-household decision-making processes between women and men and between MiLs and in-married women that determine what foods are available in the household. In addition, a food recall study may be a comprehensive follow-up to glean a more accurate picture of the dietary patterns in the Khatlon Province. Further investigation may also prove useful in assessing if there exists an effect of village proximity to district markets on food access.

## Acknowledgements

This research was produced as part of the United States Agency for International Development (USAID) and US Government Feed the Future project "Integrating Gender and Nutrition within Extension and Advisory Services" (INGENAES) under the Leader with Associates Cooperative Agreement No. AID-OAA-LA-14-00008. The United States Agency for International Development is the leading American government agency building social and economic prosperity together with the government and people of Tajikistan. The University of Illinois at Urbana-Champaign is the prime awardee, and partners with the University of California-Davis, the University of Florida, and Cultural Practice, LLC. www.ingenaes.illinois.edu

The research was made possible by the generous support of the American people through USAID. The contents are the responsibility of the authors and do not necessarily reflect the views of USAID or the United States government.

The authors thank the Feed the Future Tajikistan Agriculture and Water Activity project that provided facilitators and logistical support, the Feed the Future Tajikistan Health and Nutrition Activity project, and the Tajikistan Agrarian University students as well as the University of Florida Masters in Public Health students for their contributions.

## Conflict of interest and funding

No potential conflict of interest was reported by the authors.

## References

1. Central Intelligence Agency (2017). The World Factbook. Available from: www.cia.gov/library/publications/the-world-factbook/geos/ti.html [cited 5 October 2017].
2. Statistical Agency under the President of the Republic of Tajikistan – SA/Tajikistan, Ministry of Health – MOH/Tajikistan, and ICF International (2013). Tajikistan demographic and health survey 2012. Dushanbe, Tajikistan: SA/Tajikistan, MOH/Tajikistan, and ICF International.

3. World Bank Group (2016). The World Bank – Tajikistan partnership program snapshot. Washington, DC: World Bank; 2016.
4. United States Agency for International Development (2014). Tajikistan: Nutrition Profile. Washington, DC: USAID.
5. United States Agency for International Development (2015). Feed the future Tajikistan. Washington, DC: USAID.
6. World Food Programme Tajikistan (2017). Dushanbe (Tajikistan): World Food Programme. Available from: http://www1.wfp.org/countries/tajikistan [cited 1 April 2017].
7. United States Agency of International Development (2010). Gender assessment USAID/Central Asian Republics. Washington, DC: USAID.
8. World Bank (2013). Tajikistan – reinvigorating growth in the Khatlon oblast. Washington, DC: World Bank. Available from: documents.worldbank.org/curated/en/677671468339631289/Tajikistan-Reinvigorating-growth-in-the-Khatlon-oblast [cited 22 December 2017].
9. Asian Development Bank (2016). Tajikistan country gender assessment. Mandaluyong City, Philippines: Asian Development Bank.
10. Organization for Security and Cooperation in Europe (2015). Labour migration from Central Asia to Russia: economic and social impact on the societies of Kyrgyzstan, Tajikistan, and Uzbekistan. OSCE Academy. Bishkek, Kyrgyzstan.
11. World Bank (2012). Situational analysis: Improving economic outcomes by expanding nutrition programming in Tajikistan. Dushanbe, Tajikistan: World Bank and UNICEF. (no. 69348)
12. Chaparro C, Oot L, Sethuraman K. Overview of the nutrition situation in four countries in south and central Asia. Washington, DC: USAID FANTA III; 2014.
13. Forman J, Damschroder L. Advances in bioethics Volume 11 empirical methods for bioethics: a primer. San Diego, CA: Elsevier; 2008. Section 2, Qualitative Content Analysis; pp. 39–62.
14. Martin PY, Turner BA. Grounded theory and organizational research. J Appl Behav Sci 1986; 22(2): 141–57.
15. Adrianopoli M, D'Acapito P, Ferrari M, Mistura L, Toti E, Maiani G, et al. Improving diets and nutrition: food-based approaches. Rome, Italy: CABI; 2014. Chapter 18, Optimized feeding recommendations and in-home fortification to improve iron status in infants and young children in the Republic of Tajikistan: a pilot project; pp. 230–45.
16. Collings R, Harvey L, Hooper L, Hurst R, Brown T, Ansett J, et al. The absorption of iron from whole diets: a systematic review. Am J Clin Nutr 2013; 98(1): 65–81.
17. Zepro NB. Food taboos and misconceptions among pregnant women of Shashemene District, Ethiopia, 2012. Sci J Public Health 2015; 3(3): 410–16.
18. Ugwa EA. Nutritional practices and taboos among pregnant women attending antenatal care at general hospital in Kano, Northwest Nigeria. Ann Med Health Sci Res 2016; 6(2): 109–14.
19. Zerfu TA, Umeta M, Baye K. Dietary habits, food taboos, and perceptions towards weight gain during pregnancy in Arsi, rural central Ethiopia: a qualitative cross-sectional study. J Health Popul Nutr 2016; 35(22). DOI: 10.1186/s41043-016-0059-8.
20. Greenberg JA, Bell SJ, Van Ausdal W. Omega-3 Fatty Acid supplementation during pregnancy. Rev Obstet Gynecol 2008; 1(4): 162–9.

---

***Elizabeth A. Wood**
Department of Environmental & Global Health College of Public Health and
Health Professions University of Florida
P.O. Box 100182, 1225 Center Drive Gainesville, FL 32610-0182, USA
Email: liz07@phhp.ufl.edu

6

# Use of fungal alpha amylase and ascorbic acid in the optimisation of grain amaranth–wheat flour blended bread

Ruth J. Kamoto, William Kasapila* and Tinna A. Ng'ong'ola-Manani

Department of Food Science and Technology, Lilongwe University of Agriculture and Natural Resources (LUANAR), Lilongwe, Malawi

*Abstract*

Grain amaranth–wheat flour bread was optimised using ascorbic acid (0.03% dry weight basis) and fungal α-amylase (10 ppm) to investigate their effects on sensory properties of the breads. Six formulations were used in the ratios of 5:95, 10:90, 15:85, 20:80 and 25:75 grain amaranth to wheat flour compositions, while the control bread had 100% wheat flour. Consumer acceptability and preference ranking tests were conducted to describe and evaluate preference and acceptability of the breads. Analysis of consumer acceptability data revealed that there were significant differences ($p < 0.05$) for all the samples in all the attributes tested. Overall consumer acceptability results showed no difference at 25% for all improvers. Principal component analysis for descriptive tests performed by a trained panel demonstrated variations among the breads in graininess, elasticity, crumb colour, stickiness and crumb moistness regardless of the improvers used. The study concludes that using improvers to optimise grain amaranth–wheat flour bread can help improve both the nutritional and organoleptic properties of bread.

Keywords: *improver*; *blending*; *fermentation*; *oven spring*

Amaranth, a plant that grows wildly in many countries of the world, has been underutilised for years. A 1977 article by Jean L. Marx in the journal *Science* has already described amaranth as 'the crop of the future (1)'.

Amaranth is nutritious, stuffed with vitamins, folic acid (vitamin B9), minerals and protein. The plant is edible from tender stems through leaves, flowers and grains. Cooked leaves can be used variously as simple green side dishes, in quiches, pies, toppings and soups. Amaranth grains can be boiled and used to make candies, herbs and pressed seed oil with commercial uses besides toasting much like popcorn and mixed with honey, molasses and chocolate.

In Malawi and other countries in Africa, amaranth leaves are merely eaten as side dishes or relish for maize, rice and banana meals. The grains are left on the plant and consumed by birds or blown away by wind to far-flung areas from people's homes, further making it wild.

Culturally, people in Africa consider this grain inedible, and the problem is compounded by lack of recipes, processing techniques and knowledge of how to incorporate it into the current diets. According to the Educational Concerns for Hunger Organization (ECHO), amaranth contains anti-nutritional factors, including oxalates, nitrates, saponins and phenolic compounds that are reduced in content and effect by cooking (2).

Yet, as befits its weedy life history, amaranth grains grow rapidly and, in most of the wild species, their large seed heads can weigh up to 1 kg and contain a half-million small seeds (3). The grains are very small, about 1 mm in diameter, and difficult to harvest into meaningful volumes for commercial use.

Recently, there has been growing interest in the production of grain amaranth due to its potential in improving nutrition, food security and rural incomes. For example, from the late 1990s, the Indigenous Vegetables Research Project at Bunda College of Agriculture in Malawi has been breeding amaranth predominantly for its grains. The improved grains are golden in colour, lenticular and relatively larger (up to 1.7 mm diameter) than those from wild varieties. A number of humanitarian organisations have been distributing seeds for these varieties to rural households for them to grow in home gardens as part of nutrition interventions.

The United Nations Children's Fund and Food and Agriculture Organization (4) have already identified Malawi as one of the 34 countries (22 from Africa) that account for 90% of the global burden of stunting, with

37 in every 100 children being short for their ages, and called for innovative techniques to improve the nutritional content of foods.

This study used flour from improved grain amaranth as an ingredient in wheat bread to promote its adoption and utilisation in diets.

Breads are an important staple food and suitable for nutritional improvement.

Amaranth grain is high in linoleic acid, protein and lysine, an amino acid found in low quantities in many grains (5), including maize, sorghum, rice and bananas. Amaranth grain is deficient in essential amino acids such as leucine and threonine – both of which are present in wheat germ (5). These variations and complementarities that can be achieved make blending of amaranth and wheat flours all the more important.

Amaranth grain does not contain gluten, which makes it a viable grain for people with gluten intolerance.

However, blending amaranth grain flour with wheat affects the rheological properties of wheat, which, in turn, limits the baking characteristics and quality of the final bread. This study blended best proportions of grain amaranth and wheat flour besides using fungal α-amylase (FA) and ascorbic acid (AA) as improvers to produce good quality and nutritious bread.

Gluten is a composite of storage proteins termed prolamins and glutelins and stored together with starch in the endosperm of various cereal grains, in particular wheat, barley, rye and oats (6, 7). It gives elasticity to dough, helping it rise and keep its shape, and often gives the final product a chewy texture. Gluten is prepared from flour by kneading the flour under water, agglomerating the gluten into an elastic network, a dough, and then washing out the starch.

The results of this study can benefit nutrition practitioners, researchers, rural communities and the food industry to explore ways of commercialising the grains from amaranth and diversify selection of breads.

## Materials and methods

### *Sample acquisition*

Grain amaranth (*Amaranthus hypochondriacus*) was purchased from the horticulture department at Lilongwe University of Agriculture and Natural Resources (LUANAR) and stored in a sack to allow for aeration. Wheat flour, manufactured by Capital Foods, Sunfoil vegetable cooking oil (sunflower oil), Anchor instant yeast, table salt and white sugar were purchased from local shops in the country. Ascorbic acid was supplied by Lab Supplies, and fungal α-amylase enzyme (EN01 Bakezyme P500) manufactured by Lallemand, Montreal, Canada, was purchased from Anchor Yeast, South Africa.

Grain amaranth was sorted to remove physical objects like stones, washed several times to remove dust with clean tap water and dried in the food dryer in the Foods Laboratory at Bunda campus until all the grains were fully dried. It was then ground into flour using a blender (high horse power XTY-767, Taiwan Technical, Taiwan, China) sieved (0.5 mm) several times until almost all the grains were fine. The flour was kept at room temperature in an airtight plastic container until use.

### *The bread making process*

The bread making recipe was adopted from Tang et al. (8), with a few alterations due to the addition of improvers. The basic formula was 400 g flour, 6 g yeast, 30 g white sugar, 4 g salt, 32 g vegetable cooking oil and 230 g water. Grain amaranth flour substitution levels were from 5 to 25%. Ascorbic acid 0.03% (dry weight basis) was used as an improver, while 10 ppm FA was incorporated in each formulation following the manufacturer's instructions. A series of trials were done to standardise the recipe based on the preliminary sensory tests carried out. Bread making processes proposed by Igbabul, Num and Amove (9) were followed (see Fig. 1). The processes in bold were included for maximum manipulation of dough.

The ingredients (wheat flour, grain amaranth flour, sugar, salt, yeast and improvers) were blended for 5 min in a mixer (KitchenAid, Model 5K5SS, MI, USA) and mixed with water and vegetable oil to develop dough. The dough was turned onto a flat clean surface and kneaded manually for 8 min. After kneading, the dough was allowed to rest for 20 min for the first fermentation at 25°C and 72% relative humidity (indoor thermometer and hygrometer, TH101, Mingle, China) using Gallenkamp Hotbox oven size 2. Punching was then done to further develop gluten and redistribute the nutrient supply for yeast, resulting in increased rates of fermentation and gas production (10). The dough was kneaded again for 5 min after which it was divided, moulded and placed in baking pans (21×10×7 cm³). Proofing was done for 40 min at 38 °C and 79% relative humidity, and then baking was done at 230 °C for 20–25 min. Breads were removed from the pans and cooled for 1 h and stored at room temperature for 16 h before sensory evaluation.

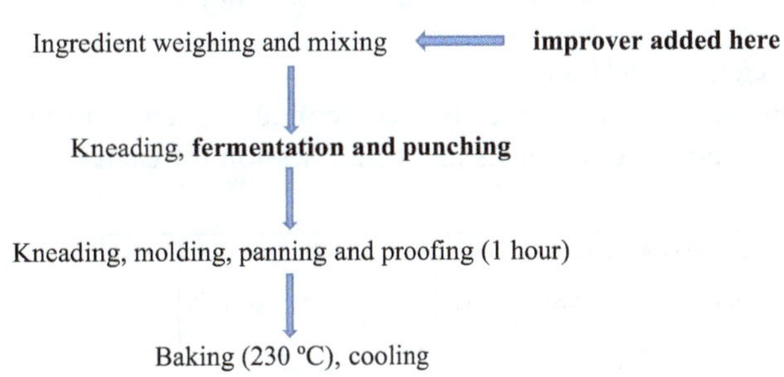


*Fig. 1.* Flow diagram for bread production.

### Ethical consideration

This study was approved by the Ethics Committee of the Lilongwe University of Agriculture and Natural Resources. Actual participation in the study was based on full consent from the students and the headmistress. The researcher informed the students that participation was voluntary and that they had the right to withdraw from the study anytime if they wished so. All the responses given were kept confidential and the forms used for data collection were not shared with anyone outside the team.

### Sensory evaluation

#### *Consumer acceptability test*

Test breads were evaluated by 80 day scholars, 39 females and 41 males aged between 14 and 18 years, from Mkwichi Secondary School. The criterion for inclusion was that the testers must make an informed decision and give consent to participate in the study. The testers were also required to be familiar with sensory qualities of bread to be included in the study. A 9-point hedonic scale (Fig. 2), also known as the degree–of-liking scale, was used by the testers to indicate the extent to which they liked or disliked each bread sample. The scale ranged from 1 'like extremely' to 9 as 'dislike extremely'.

The study was conducted in two spacious, quiet and well-lit classrooms accommodating 20 testers each. The tests were conducted in three sessions. Samples of 5, 10, 15, 20 and 25% amaranth and 100% wheat flour with ascorbic acid as an improver were presented in the first session. Bread samples improved with FA and a combination of ascorbic acid and fungal α amylase (AFA) were tasted in the second and third sessions respectively. All six samples were served at room temperature and presented all at once with a questionnaire in their respective sessions. Consumers were asked to rate each sample on appearance, taste at first bite, aroma, roughness or graininess, aftertaste and overall acceptability. The tests were done at mid-morning when the testers were neither too full nor too hungry. The samples were presented at room temperature in small white plates and were coded and presented randomly using 3 digits. The testers were instructed to taste the samples from left to right in the given order, and no re-tasting was allowed. Clean tap water was provided in disposable cups for palate cleansing before the testers moved on to the next sample (11, 12).

#### *Preference ranking tests*

Preference ranking tests were conducted concurrently with acceptability tests in a single session for each batch.

| Like extremely | Like very much | Like moderately | Like slightly | Like or dislike | Dislike slightly | Dislike moderately | Dislike very much | Dislike extremely |
|---|---|---|---|---|---|---|---|---|

*Fig. 2.* Representation of a 9-point hedonic scale.

After tasting all the six samples in consumer acceptability test, the testers were instructed to rank them from 1 to 6, where 1 referred to the 'most preferred' and 6 the 'least preferred' sample. No ties were allowed in this regard (Fig. 3). The consumers were given a gift as a token of appreciation at the end of each session.

#### *Descriptive test*

Descriptive analysis was conducted by a trained panel of students and staff members at LUANAR in which they described the sensory properties of grain amaranth–wheat blended bread optimised by ascorbic acid, FA and a mixture of the two.

### Screening and selection of study subjects

Food science and technology students responded to an invitation made through notice boards for a screening exercise. A triangle test was used to screen panelists who volunteered to participate in the study. In this regard, the panelists were presented with three sets of samples to assess their accuracy in determining sweetness, saltiness and bitterness. Each set of samples for one panelist had one reference sample with similar formulation to one of the two remaining samples on the tray. For sweetness, besides the reference sample, the two samples had 0.1 and 0.15 molar sugar solutions, while the second set was made of 0.1 and 0.15 molar salt solutions. The third set was for the bitterness test, and two of the three samples contained 0.05 and 0.1 molar of quinine. Finally, 10 panelists were selected based on their ability to discriminate small test differences in terms of sweetness, saltiness and bitterness in the exercise.

### Training of panelists

The researcher briefed the selected panellists about the study and trained them at LUANAR for 4 weeks, with three 1-h sessions per week. The training started with

**Preference Ranking Test**

**Name..................................... Sex M/F Date.....................**

Please taste and rank the samples from most preferred (1) to least preferred (6):

**No ties are allowed**

**Samples**

494 ......

735 ......

287 ......

939 ......

142 ......

677 ......

*Fig. 3.* Preference test questionnaire.

language development where the panellists generated descriptors to be used for the sensory attributes of breads. Proper definitions for the descriptors were generated by the panellists after reaching a consensus. A total of 17 descriptors were generated under appearance, aroma, taste and texture items. Standard references were used for some of the descriptors, and a 15-point line scale was used in which 1 was rated 'none or weakest' and 15 was described as 'extremely intense' for a particular attribute. The descriptive test was conducted on fresh samples every other day in triplicate. Serving of the samples was done in small Ziploc bags to prevent dryness and sequential effect on some of the attributes, for example, crispiness. Crust and crumb colour, earthy smell, yeasty smell, sweetness, alveolus size and regularity were some of the attributes examined. An assessment of panel consistency was done using panel check V 1.4.2 (13). The assessors who were not consistent were provided with further training.

### Determination of physical characteristics of bread

Oven spring was estimated from the difference in height of the dough before and after baking. Loaf weight was measured 30 min after the loaves were removed from the oven using a laboratory scale, and the readings were recorded in grams (14). Loaf volume was measured using the rapeseed displacement method (15). Thus, a box of fixed dimensions ($15\times18\times30$ cm$^3$) was placed in a tray, half filled with sorghum grains, shaken vigorously four times, and then overfilled slightly to allow the overspill fall into the tray. The box was shaken again twice before a straight edge was used to press across the top of the box once to give a level surface. The grains were decanted from the box into a receptacle and weighed. The procedure was repeated three times, and the mean value for grain weight was noted in grams.

A weighed loaf was placed in the box, and weighed grains were used to fill the box; it was levelled off as before. The weight of the grains around the loaf and the volume of grain displaced by the loaf were calculated using the following formula:

Seeds displaced by loaf (L) = C (g) + overspill weight – weight of seeds (g), where C is the mean value for seed weight (Equation 1)

$$\text{Volume of loaf (V)} = \frac{(\text{Seeds displaced by loaf (L)} * \text{Volume of bucket or box})}{\text{Weight of seeds}}$$

(Equation 2)

### Calculation of bread nutrient composition

The nutrient composition of bread was determined by calculating yield factors (YFs) and retention factors (RFs) as stipulated by the European Food Information Resource (16). The nutrient levels in the dish were calculated by first finding the values from the United States Department of Agriculture (USDA) food composition tables (17).

Yield factors were calculated using the following formula:

$$\text{YF} = \frac{\text{Prepared dish, editable part (g)}}{\text{Total quantity ingredients (ready - to - cook)(g)}}$$

(Equation 3)

Retention factors were calculated to find the amount of nutrients retained after preparation (18). Weight YFs were included in the experimental determination of the nutrient RFs, and the following formula was used:

$$\text{RF} = \frac{\text{Nutrient content per 100g dish, edible part}}{\text{Nutrient content per 100g of ingredients (ready - to - cook), edible part}} * \text{YF}$$

(Equation 4)

### Data analysis

Data entry and data analysis were done using SPSS version 20. Two-way analysis of variance (ANOVA) was used to generate the means and determine levels of significance for the results. Principal component analysis (PCA) was performed to determine sensory attributes of importance in grain amaranth–wheat bread.

## Results

#### *Comparison of choice of bread samples based on gender*

Six samples of bread improved with ascorbic acid were given to each of the male and female testers. Data presented in Table 1 show results of how the testers made their choices. The testers showed no significant difference ($p < 0.05$) in their choice of the bread samples.

### Recipe standardisation

After several trials of baking and random preliminary sensory evaluation done by students and staff members,

*Table 1.* Effect of gender on choice of the bread samples improved with ascorbic acid, fungal α-amylase and a combination of the two with different levels of grain amaranth flour

| Improver | Gender | 0% | 5% | 10% | 15% | 20% | 25% | Sig. |
|---|---|---|---|---|---|---|---|---|
| AA | Male | 7 | 8 | 8 | 9 | 6 | 3 | 0.38 |
| | Female | 11 | 11 | 9 | 4 | 3 | 1 | |
| AFA | Male | 10 | 5 | 2 | 14 | 4 | 6 | 0.90 |
| | Female | 12 | 6 | 1 | 12 | 4 | 4 | |
| FA | Male | 12 | 5 | 17 | 1 | 3 | 3 | 0.99 |
| | Female | 12 | 4 | 18 | 2 | 2 | 1 | |

AA, ascorbic acid; AFA, combination of ascorbic acid and fungal α-amylase; FA, fungal α-amylase.

sugar was reduced to 30 g based on the recommendations received, while the rest of the ingredients remained the same. The initial 60 g of sugar as indicated in the adopted method by Tang et al. (8) made the breads sweeter than what the random testers are used to eating. The use of butter presented operational challenges; therefore, it was replaced with the same amount (32 g) of vegetable oil.

Fermentation times were also altered from 15 to 20 min for the first fermentation to improve dough leavening. The second fermentation was reduced from 90 to 45 min because it was observed that the dough that was fermented for 90 min was too sloppy and did not achieve oven spring once put in the oven. This could be attributed to the addition of AA and FA that provided optimal acidic conditions and degraded molecules for fermentation by yeast to occur faster. This led to the yeast being overspent; therefore, it was unable to continue to ferment in the first few minutes the dough was placed in the oven (19), resulting in the production of flat bread. Therefore, the times were changed to still have yeast working in the oven to produce a good bread shape.

The advantage of baking grain amaranth–wheat blended bread is that it does not require sophisticated technology. The use of makeshift ovens with controlled heating is enough to produce high-quality bread that consumers can equally enjoy.

### *Consumer acceptability*

In this study, consumer acceptability tests were used to assess the appearance, aroma, taste at first bite, graininess, aftertaste and overall acceptability of the test breads. The results indicated that there were significant differences ($p < 0.05$) for all bread samples on all the attributes tested for breads improved with ascorbic acid (AA) (Table 2).

Similar trends were observed for bread samples improved with FA and the combination of ascorbic acid and fungal α-amylase (AFA). Overall acceptability showed that ascorbic acid performed better for 10 and 15%, while FA gave better results for 5 and 20% formulations. The combination of the two worked better for the control bread, although it was not very different with the others at 25% blending (Fig. 4).

*Table 2.* Degree of liking of grain amaranth–wheat flour breads with various grain amaranth flour per cent compositions improved with ascorbic acid

| Sample | Appearance | Smell/Aroma | Taste at first bite | Roughness | Aftertaste | Overall acceptability |
|---|---|---|---|---|---|---|
| 0AA | $2.21 \pm 1.33^{a}$ | $2.41 \pm 1.30^{b}$ | $1.48 \pm 0.54^{a}$ | $3.01 \pm 2.03^{ab}$ | $2.52 \pm 1.56^{b}$ | $2.84 \pm 1.84^{ab}$ |
| 5AA | $2.09 \pm 1.18^{a}$ | $2.16 \pm 1.37^{a}$ | $2.26 \pm 1.45^{ab}$ | $2.32 \pm 1.50^{b}$ | $2.29 \pm 1.47^{b}$ | $2.43 \pm 1.49^{b}$ |
| 10AA | $2.43 \pm 1.20^{a}$ | $2.00 \pm 1.65^{a}$ | $2.64 \pm 1.70^{b}$ | $3.65 \pm 2.03^{a}$ | $3.60 \pm 2.16^{a}$ | $2.82 \pm 1.60^{ab}$ |
| 15AA | $1.59 \pm 0.66^{b}$ | $2.63 \pm 1.55^{b}$ | $2.91 \pm 1.51^{c}$ | $2.33 \pm 1.30^{b}$ | $2.63 \pm 1.64^{b}$ | $2.96 \pm 1.75^{ab}$ |
| 20AA | $2.60 \pm 1.65^{a}$ | $3.30 \pm 2.41^{c}$ | $3.55 \pm 1.23^{c}$ | $3.72 \pm 2.17^{a}$ | $3.66 \pm 2.17^{a}$ | $3.48 \pm 2.12^{a}$ |
| 25AA | $2.70 \pm 1.82^{a}$ | $2.83 \pm 1.63^{bc}$ | $2.86 \pm 1.63^{cc}$ | $4.01 \pm 2.34^{a}$ | $3.74 \pm 2.36^{a}$ | $3.59 \pm 2.21^{a}$ |
| *p*-value | 0.000 | 0.000 | 0.000 | 0.000 | 0.000 | 0.001 |

Values in the table are means ± standard deviations.
Means with different superscript in the same column were significantly different ($p < 0.05$).
Hedonic Rating Scale used; 1 = like extremely to 9 = dislike extremely.
AA, ascorbic acid.

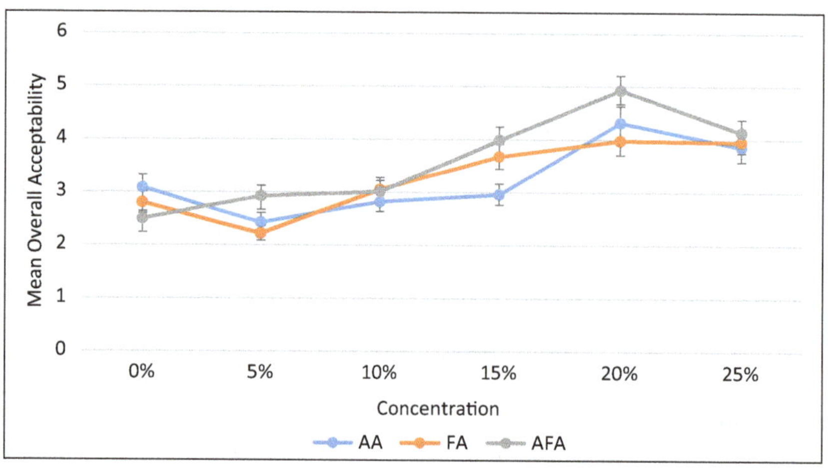


*Fig. 4.* Comparisons of the overall acceptability of the three types of bread samples improved with ascorbic acid, fungal α-amylase and a combination of the two at different per cent compositions of grain amaranth flour.

AA, Ascorbic acid; FA, fungal α-amylase; AFA, combination of ascorbic acid and fungal α-amylase.

*Preference ranking test*

Preference ranking test showed that consumers preferred 15AFA, 5FA and bread baked with 100% wheat flour regardless of the improvers used. Despite better mean scores for 5 and 10% breads in overall consumer acceptability, 5% grain amaranth bread improved with FA and 15% bread improved with AFA were the most preferred of the test breads (Fig. 5).

*Results for descriptive test*

A total of 17 descriptors were generated to describe the appearance, taste, aroma and texture of the breads. These descriptors included brownness of upper crust, brownness of lower crust, crumb colour, alveolus size, alveolus regularity, overall aroma, earthy smell, yeasty smell, saltiness, sweetness, aftertaste, chewiness, crust crispiness, crumb moistness, elasticity, roughness or graininess, and stickiness. Out of the seventeen descriptors mentioned above, nine showed significant differences ($p < 0.05$). PCA indicated the ability of the panel to discriminate the bread samples as presumed.

*Bread improved with ascorbic acid and fungal alpha amylase*

Attributes that were significantly different were further analysed by the PCA. The results obtained showed that the panel described 88.71% of the variation and perceived 5AFA and 10AFA, 20AFA and 25AFA to have similarities in the tested attributes based on their proximity with each other in the map. It perceived the control bread to be totally different from the rest of the test breads (Fig. 6).

*Physical characteristics of breads*

Average weight after cooling indicated that there was an increase in weight with increased amaranth substitutions in all the test breads (Fig. 7). Oven spring and loaf showed significant differences ($p < 0.05$); they were higher in breads that had lower levels of grain amaranth flour (Table 3).

*Nutrient composition*

Table 4 shows the calculated nutrient composition of the breads. Calculations used 0.90 and 1 as yield and retention factors (18), respectively. The results were based on the recipe that was used throughout the study. The varying nutrient contents of the blended bread were an indication that addition of grain amaranth flour assisted in increasing the nutrient content of the breads. Carbohydrate content decreased with increased grain amaranth additions. Micronutrients were only available in very small amounts.

*Discussion*

Wheat flour used in Malawi for bread production is imported from South Africa. Hence, the importation and associated production costs make bread expensive, especially to the rural masses in the country the majority of whom live on less than US$1a day. There is a huge need to use locally available raw food stuffs in the bakery of bread to increase the variety and utilisation. The present study

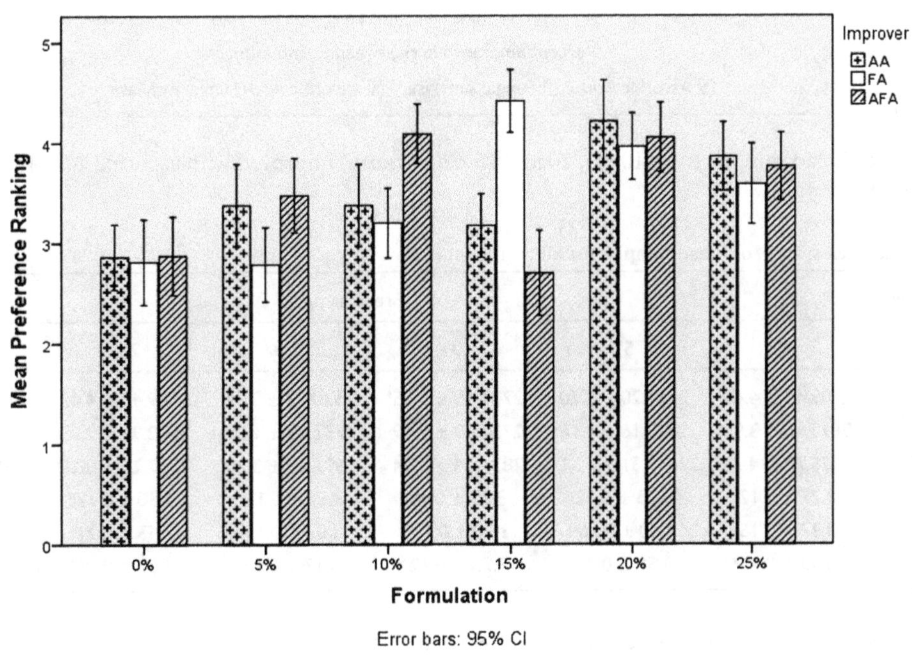


*Fig. 5.* Comparison of preference rankings for different breads.

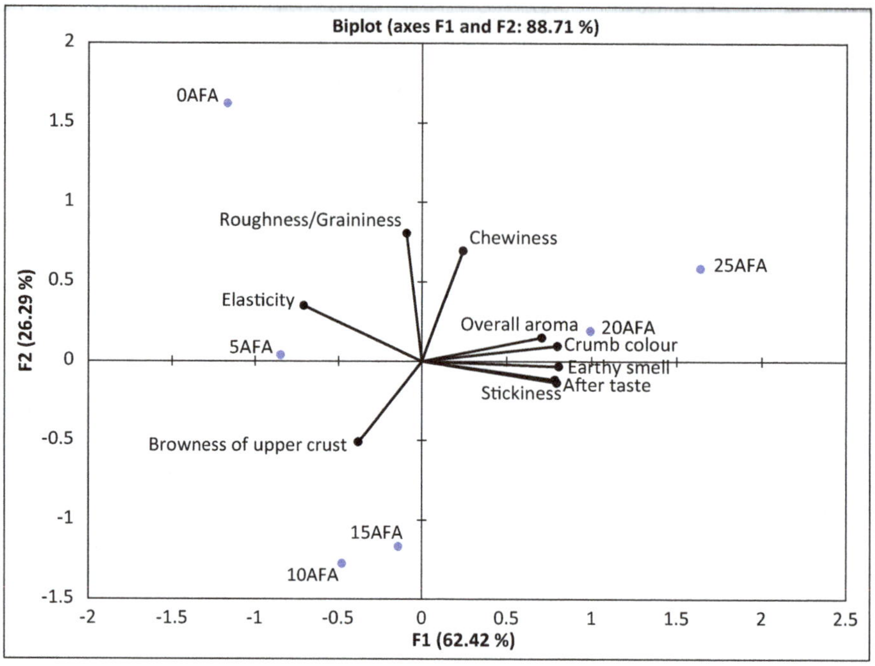


*Fig. 6.* Projection of the bread samples 0AFA, 5AFA, 10AFA, 15AFA, 20AFA and 25AFA on PCA plots. AFA, Bread samples improved with a combination of ascorbic acid and fungal α-amylase.

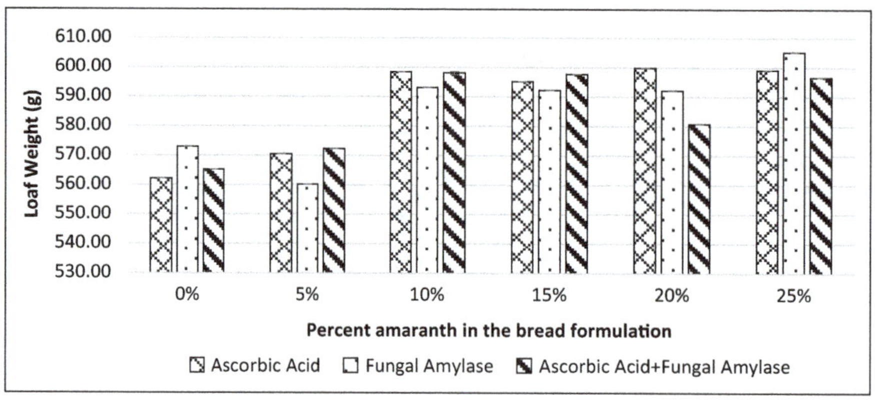


*Fig. 7.* Average weight of bread samples (0, 5, 10, 15, 20 and 25% amaranth) improved with ascorbic acid, fungal α-amylase and a combination of the two.

*Table 3.* Loaf volume and oven spring for bread samples for all treatments

| Attribute | Treatment | Bread samples | | | | | | |
|---|---|---|---|---|---|---|---|---|
| | | 0% | 5% | 10% | 15% | 20% | 25% | *p* |
| Loaf volume | AA | 2709.47 ± 4.47$^{b}$ | 2691.20 ± 3.20$^{c}$ | 2721.65 ± 3.65$^{a}$ | 2520.72 ± 3.72$^{f}$ | 2569.43 ± 4.43$^{e}$ | 2605.96 ± 0.04$^{d}$ | 0.00 |
| | FA | 2879.95 ± 3.95$^{a}$ | 2825.16 ± 4.16$^{b}$ | 2752.09 ± 2.09$^{c}$ | 2752.09 ± 1.09$^{c}$ | 2538.99 ± 2.99$^{e}$ | 2605.96 ± 2.96$^{d}$ | 0.00 |
| | AFA | 3275.72 ± 4.72$^{a}$ | 2849.51 ± 0.51$^{b}$ | 2831.24 ± 3.24$^{c}$ | 2691.20 ± 3.20$^{d}$ | 2557.25 ± 0.25$^{e}$ | 2685.12 ± 2.12$^{d}$ | 0.00 |
| Oven spring | AA | 3.27 ± 0.12$^{a}$ | 3.23 ± 0.12$^{a}$ | 3.13 ± 0.15$^{a}$ | 2.67 ± 0.12$^{bc}$ | 2.30 ± 0.17$^{b}$ | 2.37 ± 0.15$^{c}$ | 0.00 |
| | FA | 3.37 ± 0.15$^{a}$ | 3.30 ± 0.26$^{ab}$ | 3.10 ± 0.10$^{ab}$ | 3.03 ± 0.15b | 2.43 ± 0.21$^{c}$ | 2.37 ± 0.06$^{c}$ | 0.00 |
| | AFA | 3.53 ± 0.15$^{a}$ | 3.50 ± 0.20$^{a}$ | 3.23 ± 0.12$^{b}$ | 3.17 ± 0.12$^{b}$ | 2.67 ± 0.06$^{c}$ | 2.53 ± 0.12$^{c}$ | 0.00 |

Values in the table are means ± standard deviation.
Means with different superscript in the same column are significantly different ($p < 0.05$).
AA, bread improved with ascorbic acid; FA, bread improved with fungal α-amylase; AFA, bread improved with a combination of ascorbic acid and fungal α-amylase.

*Table 4.* Calculated results for nutrient contents of wheat–grain amaranth bread

| Nutrient | Amaranth in bread flours | | | | | | GA |
|---|---|---|---|---|---|---|---|
| | 5% | 10% | 15% | 20% | 25% | 0% | 100% |
| Protein (g) | 6.65 | 6.76 | 6.86 | 6.96 | 7.06 | 6.55 | 13.56 |
| Lysine g/16gN | 7.95 | 8.73 | 9.37 | 10.00 | 10.64 | 7.46 | 5.95 |
| Fat (g) | 6.19 | 6.37 | 6.544 | 6.72 | 6.89 | 6.02 | 7.02 |
| Carbohydrate (g) | 46.06 | 45.81 | 45.56 | 45.31 | 45.07 | 46.31 | 65.25 |
| Fe (μg) | 3.0 | 3.0 | 3.3 | 3.4 | 3.5 | 3.1 | 7,600 |
| Zn (μg) | 0.75 | 0.81 | 0.87 | 0.92 | 0.98 | 0.70 | 2,900 |
| Ca (mg) | 0.01 | 0.02 | 0.02 | 0.03 | 0.03 | 0.00 | 159 |
| Mg (mg) | 0.03 | 0.04 | 0.04 | 0.05 | 0.06 | 0.02 | 248 |

Source: Dokok et al. (19)
Values for lysine: 5.95g/16gN and 2.90g/16gN for grain amaranth and wheat flours, respectively.
GA, 100g grain amaranth flour.

modified wheat bread by adding grain amaranth flour as an ingredient. Amaranth grows wildly in rural area and is culturally eaten as relish for different staples. Paradoxically, the amaranth grain which is equally nutritious is not edible in any form and therefore neglected. The findings of this study can help provide valuable information for consumers, health care practitioners, the government and humanitarian organisations working to improve nutrition in the country.

One key finding of the study was that there were no significant differences in the choice of breads by male and female testers (Table 1). Even though taste sensitivity differs between males and females in real-life situations (20), our results showed that the choice of bread samples was not gender dependent. Analysis of descriptive data from sensory tests showed that testers accepted and preferred bread with 5–15% grain amaranth flour. Acceptability of the test breads decreased as the amaranth flour in the bread increased. The dark colour of the breads, which is typical of grain amaranth, was mild at the aforesaid concentrations compared to when 20–25% additions were used. For instance, testers could easily detect sensory deviations from the common wheat bread when the latter substitutions were added. Control bread had the highest mean score for taste at first bite, which can be attributed to the taste of wheat flour bread that the testers were used to. Lower scores with higher amaranth levels were due to the grain amaranth flour interfering with the actual taste of wheat flour bread. The aftertaste of the bread samples increased in breads with high levels of grain amaranth flour, attributed to the slight bitter taste of grain amaranth (7).

The study used AA and FA enzyme as improvers to enhance the acceptability of the test breads. It hypothesised that breads with up to 25% grain amaranth flour can enhance the utilisation of the grain and be equally preferred by the testers. However, based on the results presented, even with improvers, the addition of amaranth flour as an ingredient to bread and probably other foods should not exceed 15%. The use of improvers helped raise 5, 10 and 15% breads close to the control, while 20 and 25% formulations had reduced oven spring and loaf volume. The explanation for this result is that the improvers degraded complex molecules in 5, 10 and 15% blends, but in the 20 and 25% flours combinations insufficient material was produced for gas production by yeast. Consumers are used to eating bread that is more porous, meaning that higher amounts of grain amaranth flour in bread will not be favoured at all.

Table 4 shows the nutrient composition of the test breads. The addition of amaranth flour contributed protein, in particular, lysine – an essential amino acid necessary for human health. There were also slight increases in iron, zinc and magnesium. Frequent consumption of the test breads, as a staple or co-staple, would assist in curbing micronutrient deficiencies that are of public health concern in Malawi and other developing countries. Taken together, using grain amaranth flour in bread is cheaper than commercial powders and enhancers currently used by the food industry. The increase in the micronutrients as grain amaranth flour is increased can also help commercialise and raise popularity of this ethnic crop (21).

In Malawi, the government and humanitarian organisations promote production of dark green leafy vegetables in home gardens as one way of addressing micronutrient deficiencies among women and under-five children. Grain amaranth could be successfully used in cookery of different foods besides bread to make them more nutritious.

Investigations on the value of adding grain amaranth have remained scanty in Malawi and other countries in Africa. For example, in Malawi, only Gonani (6) has developed bread from amaranth and the work remains unpublished. The other study (7) conducted elsewhere developed biscuits. Nevertheless, both studies reported results similar to those found in the present study. Bread and biscuits with higher amounts of grain amaranth flour were darker in colour and less acceptable by the study subjects, confirming the need to use grain amaranth in lower amounts in foods to enhance acceptability. Given the disparities in cookery and consumer preferences and in light of the paucity of studies undertaken to date, there is a need for more research in the vast majority of countries to understand better the physiochemical, antioxidant and functional properties of the grain.

More so, physical characteristics of breads indicated that values for average weight (Fig. 7) for the control bread and that substituted with 5% grain amaranth flour were close to each other. The compact network in bread dough with higher amounts of grain amaranth flour resulted in less evaporation of the water during baking, leading to heavy bread. However, the addition of AA and FA improved the volume of the breads since they aid in gas production (22). Loaf volume is related with oven spring. When oven spring is higher, the volume of bread is also higher.

The study had some limitations. The rising of the breads was affected as grain amaranth flour substitutions increased due to reduced effect of gluten. During sensory evaluation, no carrier (e.g. tea and bread spread) was used. Notwithstanding these limitations, the study concludes that grain amaranth can be used in breads and examined in other products to enhance diversity and nutrition.

## Acknowledgements

This research was financially supported by USAID through World Learning. The researcher prepared the draft and the other authors reviewed it.

## Conflict of interest and funding

The authors declare no conflict of interest. They have not received any funding or benefits from the industry or elsewhere, besides World Learning, to conduct this study.

## References

1. Marx JL. Speaking of science: amaranth: a comeback for the food of the Aztecs? Science 1977; 198(4312): 40.
2. O'Brien GK, Price ML. Amaranth grain and vegetable types. ECHO Technical Note. 1983. http://www.echonet.org/ [cited 20 May 2018].
3. Tucker J. Amaranth: the once and future crop. Bioscience 1986; 36(1): 9–13.
4. Food and Agriculture Organization (FAO) of the United Nations. Malawi Nutrition Profile. FAO, Rome. 2008.
5. Alvarez-Jubete L, Arendt EK, Gallagher E. Nutritive value and chemical composition of pseudocereals as gluten-free ingredients. Int J Food Sci Nutr 2009; 60: 240–57.
6. Gonani L. Quality of bread from different wheat and Grain amaranthus blends, MSc Thesis, University of Malawi, Bunda College, 2004.
7. Bhuvaneswari G, Sharada GS. Acceptability of grain amaranth substituted bakery products and weaning food. Karnataka J Agric Sci 2003; 17: 775–80.
8. Tang L, Yang R, Hua X, Yu C, Zhang W, Zhao W. Preparation of immobilized glucose oxidase and its application in improving bread making quality of commercial wheat flour. Food Chem 2014; 161: 1–7.
9. Igbabul B, Num G, Amove J. Quality evaluation of composite bread produced from wheat, maize, orange fleshed sweet potato flours. Am J Food Sci Technol 2014; 2: 109–15.
10. Amendola J, Rees N. Understanding baking: the art and science of baking. 3rd ed. New Jersey: John Wiley & Sons, Inc; 2003, pp. 162–164.
11. Lawless HT, Heymann H. Sensory evaluation of food principles and practices. 2nd ed. New York: Springer; 2010.
12. Kemp ES, Hollowood T, Hort J. Sensory evaluation, a practical handbook. 1st ed. John Wiley & Sons Ltd; 2009, pp. 66–136.
13. Tomic O, Luciano G, Nilsen A, Hyldig G, Lorensen K, Næs T. Analysing sensory panel performance in a proficiency test using the PanelCheck software. Eur Food Res Technol 2009; DOI: 10.1007/s00217-009-1185-y.
14. Makinde FM, Akinoso R. Physical, nutritional and sensory qualities of bread samples made with wheat and black sesame (*Sesamum indicum Linn*) flours. IFRJ 2014; 21: 1635–40.
15. Giami SY, Amasisi T, Ekiyor G. Comparison of breadmaking properties of composite flour from kernels of roasted and boiled African breadfruit (*Treculia africana*) seeds. J Raw Mater Res 2004; 1: 16–25.
16. European Food Information Resource. Recipe calculation: food composition course; England: Emerald Group Publishing Limited; 2012.
17. United States Department of Agriculture (USDA) Food Composition Databases. Available from: https://www.google.com/?gws_rd=ssl#q=usda+nutritional+database [cited 8 December 2017].
18. Bognar A. Tables on weight yield of food and retention factors of food constituents for the calculation of nutrient composition of cooked foods (dishes). Karlsruhe, Germany: Bundesforschungsanstalt fur Ernahrung (BFE); 2002. ISSN 0933 – 5463.
19. Dokok L, Modhir AA, Buchtova V, Halasova G, Polacel I. Importance and utilization of amaranth in food industry. 2. Composition of amino acids and fatty acids. Karlsruhe, Germany: Bundesforschungsanstalt fur Ernahrung; 1997.
20. Ton Nu C, MacLeod P, Barthelemy J. Effects of age and gender on adolescents' food habits and preferences. Food Qual Prefer 1996; 7: 251–62.
21. Khokar S, Garduno-Diaz SD, Marletta L, Shahar RD, Ireland JD, Vliet MJ et al. Mineral composition of commonly consumed foods in Europe. Food Nutr Res 2012; 56: 17665. DOI: 10.3402/fnr.v56i0.17665
22. Cauvain S, Young L. Baking problems solved. Woodhead Publishing Limited CRS Press 2001.

***William Kasapila**
Department of Food Science and Technology
Lilongwe University of Agriculture and Natural Resources (LUANAR)
Bunda Campus, P.O. Box 219, Lilongwe, Malawi
Email: wkasapila@yahoo.co.uk

# 7

# Effects of dietary palm olein on the cardiovascular risk factors in healthy young adults

Chenyan Lv[1†], Yifei Wang[1†], Cui Zhou[1], Weiwei Ma[1], Yuexin Yang[2], Rong Xiao[1*] and Huanling Yu[1*]

[1]School of Public Health, Beijing Key Laboratory of Environmental Toxicology, Capital Medical University, Beijing, China;
[2]National Institute for Nutrition and Health, Chinese Center for Disease Control and Prevention, Beijing, China

*Abstract*

***Background:*** Dietary saturated fatty acids are always being hotly debated. Palm olein rich in saturated fatty acids (45.98%) is often considered as being atherogenic nutritionally. There is a lack of information on effects of dietary oil by partially replacing with palm olein on human health.
***Methods:*** A randomized controlled trial with 88 participants has been conducted to elucidate the effect of palm olein on cardiovascular risk factors.
***Results:*** By comparing the soybean oil group (saturated fatty acids amounted to 23.31%) with the cocoa butter group (saturated fatty acids amounted to 93.76%), no significant difference was found ($p > 0.05$) in physiological parameters, serum oxidative stress levels, inflammatory factor, glucose metabolism, and lipid profiles of subjects, which are all cardiovascular risk factors. Although results showed that intervention time can influence the cardiovascular risk factors significantly ($p < 0.05$), there is no relationship between intervention time and dietary oil type.
***Conclusion:*** Therefore, partial replacement of dietary oil by palm olein may not affect cardiovascular risk factors in healthy young adults. There are differences between our research and previous researches, which may be due to the different amount of palm olien in diet. Our research will provide a solid foundation for the application of palm olein in human diets and in the food industry.

Keywords: *palm olein; saturated fatty acids; dietary intervention; replacement; lipid metabolism*

Fat and oil are important components in nutrition for animals and human beings. Dietary fats and oils perform a variety of functions. They provide energy and certain nutrients such as lipid-soluble vitamin, and maintains your core body temperature (1). Recently, several researches have indicated that poly-unsaturated fatty acids (PUFA) have affected many aspects of immune system, including antibody production by B cell and better health of gut-associated lymphoid tissue (2). PUFA has been proved to reduce the production of low-density lipoprotein cholesterol (LDL-C) and increase the production of high-density lipoprotein cholesterol (HDL-C) (3). Meanwhile, both the lipid content and the type of fatty acids can cause alterations both in liver and white adipose tissues. In contrast to unsaturated fatty acids, dietary saturated fatty acids (SFA) have been proved to affect the body health. For example, once the 18:2 fatty acids were replaced by 16:0, the total cholesterol level and LDL–HDL ratio increased slightly, indicating the adverse effect of saturated fatty acids (4). Several animal experiments and controlled feeding studies in humans have demonstrated increases in fasting levels of TC and LDL-C after SFA consumption (5). Moreover, the North Karelia study has demonstrated that reduction of SFA in diet can decrease the serum cholesterol and result in substantial reduction of cardiovascular disease (CVD) risk (6). However, recent systematic reviews on prospective cohort studies have questioned the relationship between dietary SFA and CVD. The observational studies indicated that overall SFA intake does not increase the risk for stroke (7). Another cohort study on Dutch population has indicated that higher SFA intake was not associated with higher

†These authors contributed equally to this work.

ischemic heart disease (8). Therefore, the relationship between dietary SFA and cardiovascular risk factors needs to be further identified. Both the type and the amount of dietary SFA may be key factors for CVD.

Palm olein, a vegetable oil obtained from the palm tree fruits, is composed of ~50% palmitic acid, 40% oleic acid, and 10% linoleic acid. Palm olein with a high content of the SFA (palmitic acid) and a low content of unsaturated fatty acid has been proved to increase the serum cholesterol concentrations in humans since 1960s (9). It has been demonstrated that there is no clear health benefit of replacing saturated fatty acids with starchy food, whereas replacement with unsaturated fatty acids reduced the risk of CVD (10). A decrease as slight as 5% in dietary saturated fatty acid amounted to 13% decrease in CVD occurrence and 26% decrease in deaths (11). On replacing the 'red oil' (palm oil) with the 'white oil' (branded vegetable oil), the saturation of dietary oil will be reduced by about 30% (12). However, a randomized 30-d/30-d crossover study comparing the effect of palm olein and olive oil on plasma lipids has indicated that palm olein is not always a plasma cholesterol-raising fatty acid (13). Similarly, a recent meta-analysis has indicated that the favorable and unfavorable changes in coronary heart disease (CHD)/CVD risk markers are both observed when palm oil constitutes the main dietary SFA intake (14). Recently, a randomized trial of the effects of hybrid palm oil supplementation on human plasma lipid patterns has provided additional support for the concept that hybrid palm oil can be seen as the 'tropical equivalent of olive oil' (15). These studies indicated that the health effect of palm oil is still controversial. Whether partially replacing the dietary oil such as soybean oil with palm olein will affect the body health or not remains unknown. The association between palm olein intakes with CVDs needs further identification, especially for the healthy young adults.

In this study, a single-blind, randomized parallel feeding intervention trial has been employed to determine the influence partially replacing dietary oil with palm olein on the cardiovascular risk factors and further investigate whether the dietary oil composition and the high ratio of saturated fatty acids can affect healthy young adults.

## Materials and methods

### *Materials*

Palm olein used in this study was purchased from Tianjin julong jiahua investment group co., Ltd., China. Cocoa butter was purchased from Zhejiang Qili xingguang cocoa products Corp., Ltd., China. Soybean oil was purchased from Shanghai Liangyou Haishi oils & fats industry co., Ltd., China. All the dietary oils met the national standards (Soybean oil, GB1535-2003; palm olein, GB15680-2009; Cocoa butter, GB/T 22000-2006) and production licenses were obtained. Vacuum blood needle and related materials used in this study were purchased from Becton, Dickinson and Company, USA.

### *Justification of sample size*

A sample size of 108 participants was proposed by using PASS 11.0.7; we conducted a post hoc power calculation and estimated that a sample size of 108 participants would enable the detection of a minimum between palm olein and high oleic sunflower (HOS), in cholesterol of 0.2% (80% power, $\alpha = 0.05$) (16). Our sample size was reasonable according to similar studies of palm olein intervention (17–19).

### *Subjects*

A convenience sample of 108 students from Capital Medical University (50 men and 58 women; age 21.59 ± 0.39; body mass index [BMI] 21.03 ± 0.37; mean ± S.E) was selected to participate in the study. The volunteers with underlying diseases have been ruled out ($n = 15$).

The subjects were randomly allocated to three groups and they were treated with different diets. Data regarding 88 of the volunteers who completed the entire study are included in this report. All of the volunteers were recruited from Capital Medical University by the recruiting announcement in February, 2016. The criteria for inclusion and exclusion are listed below in detail. (1) Inclusion criteria: Adult males or females aged 20–40 years; BMI (18.5–23.9); subjects without a history of atherosclerotic disease or hypertension; subjects must understand the study and then agree to participate; subjects must adhere closely to prescribed food consumption as per research protocol. (2) Exclusion criteria: Abnormal liver function test (elevated transaminases – alanine transaminase [ALT], aspartate transaminase [AST])/abnormal kidney function test (elevated plasma creatinine [CR]); history of type 2 diabetes mellitus, cancer, stomach ulcers, drug abuse or alcoholism; smokers; on lipid/blood pressure-lowering medication/supplements; blood pressure > 140/90 mm Hg; fasting cholesterol (CHO) > 6.2 mmol/L; fasting triglyceride (TG) > 2.0 mmol/L; candidates who are going abroad during the planned schedule for the dietary intervention; subject must not be allergic to intervention; pregnancy and breastfeeding; subjects taking nutritional supplements or on any weight-loss programs; female subjects who are on oral contraceptives; subjects with a history of hypo- and hyperthyroidism; subjects with constipation/bowel movement problems. Finally, 93 subjects were randomized and divided into three groups according to BMI using simple randomization adjusted with sex and ages.

This study was conducted according to the Declaration of Helsinki and was approved by the Ethics Committee for Clinical Research in Chinese Nutrition Society (Approval No. CNS2016001). All of the subjects signed the informed consent document once they learned of the purpose, procedures, and risks of this study. This study has

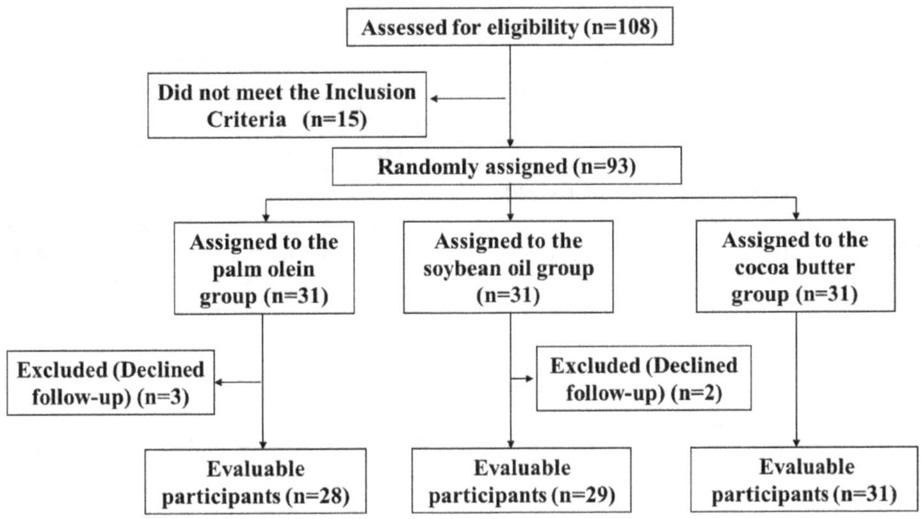


*Fig. 1.* Study flow diagram.

been registered on the Chinese Clinical Trial Registry and the registry number is ChiCTR-IIR-16008733.

*Experimental design*

This study was a single-blind, randomized parallel feeding intervention trial. The subjects were randomly assigned to three groups (cocoa butter group, palm olein group, and soybean oil group) (Fig. 1). This study was conducted for 16 weeks (from April, 2016, to July, 2016). Subjects were then randomized to one of the three treatments for a period of 16 weeks in parallel. The study consisted of an initial stabilization period of 1 week and intervention period of 16 weeks. During the stabilization period, all subjects consumed the basal diet. The basal diet consisted of vegetables, meat, and rice, and only soybean oil was used to prepare the basal diet. As for the intervention period, subjects from three groups were intervened with test fats.

All food (vegetables and staple food) in the diet was cooked with soybean oil. And the oil used for staple food (walnut cake, ujube cake, or Cantonese sponge cake) was partially replaced with cocoa butter and palm olein. The compositions of staple food are shown in Table S1. Due to the different amounts of oil used for making walnut cake, ujube cake, and Cantonese sponge cake, test meals were served as breakfast (for walnut cake) or breakfast (for ujube cake) and lunch (for Cantonese sponge cake). The macronutrient compositions of the test diets were identical (e.g. % of energy as carbohydrates, protein, and fat). Based on the dietary survey of the subjects before intervention, intake amounts of fatty acid from the diet of subjects are 30–36 g/day. In this study, we have replaced 20–22 g oil in the diet with test fatty acids, which is about 1/5 of the total dietary fat. The fatty acid compositional analysis is shown in Table 1. The ratio of saturated fatty acids of cocoa butter, palm olein, and soybean oil is about 4:2:1. And subjects were provided with uniform calorie meals prepared with fats 5 working days a week. At the weekends, meals were not provided to the subjects, instead dietary advice was given including the restricted intake of snacks. All the test meals were provided by the canteen and all the subjects took the meals in the canteen, which were supervised by us. After the meal, we weighed the remaining amount of test meals of subjects to guarantee the intake of calories was equal.

*Table 1.* The compositional analysis of palm olein, soybean oil, and cocoa butter

| Fatty-acid composition[a] | | Palm olein (%) | Soybean oil (%) | Cocoa butter (%) |
|---|---|---|---|---|
| Saturated fatty acid | sn-1,3 | 45.98 | 23.31 | 93.76 |
| | 12:0 | 0.3 | 0 | 0 |
| | 14:0 | 1.1 | 0 | 0.08 |
| | 16:0 | 29.4 | 11.1 | 26.2 |
| | 18:0 | 3.4 | 3.8 | 37.1 |
| | 20:0 | 0.3 | 0.4 | 1.1 |
| | 22:0 | 0 | 0.6 | 0 |
| Mono-unsaturated fatty acid | sn-1,3 | 44.43 | 27.73 | 5.8 |
| | 16:1 | 0.4 | 1.5 | 0 |
| | 18:1 | 50.3 | 22.4 | 36.0 |
| | 20:1 | 0 | 0.1 | 0 |
| | 22:1 | 0 | 0.7 | 0 |
| Poly-unsaturated fatty acid | sn-1,3 | 9.59 | 48.96 | 0.44 |
| | 18:2 | 14.5 | 51.7 | 2.0 |
| | 18:3 | 0.3 | 6.7 | 0 |

[a]Concentration of fatty acids were performed by % by wt.

*Table 2.* Daily energy intake from three calorigenic nutrients during dietary intervention

| Energy/ calorigenic nutrients | Palm olein | Soybean oil | Cocoa butter |
|---|---|---|---|
| Total energy (kcal) | 1807.58 ± 316.43 | 1749.28 ± 445.37 | 1786.09 ± 323.83 |
| Protein (% of energy) | 15.57 ± 1.69 | 15.53 ± 2.45 | 16.03 ± 2.68 |
| Lipid (% of energy) | 35.56 ± 3.86 | 35.42 ± 4.96 | 35.90 ± 4.43 |
| Carbohydrate (% of energy) | 48.87 ± 4.33 | 49.04 ± 5.73 | 48.07 ± 5.51 |

*Diets*

The mean daily calorigenic nutrient intakes from the cocoa butter, palm olein, and soybean oil diets during the intervention periods are shown in Table 2. Nutrient intake from test fat was similar for both the stabilization and intervention periods. The test meals provided about 35% energy as fat, 49% as carbohydrates, and 16% as proteins.

*Blood sampling*

Before the study was started, every subject received a random inclusion number that was used for identification and labeling of blood and serum tubes. Blood samples were drawn after an overnight fast immediately before breakfast at the end of each period. Baseline samples were collected during the stabilization period. Serum was separated by centrifugation after sampling to avoid hemolysis and then stored at −80°C until analyzed. Sample treatments were blinded to the analysts.

*Laboratory methods*

The energy of test diets was calculated according to the China Food Composition. Blood from overnight fasting subjects was collected by antecubital venipuncture into vacutainer tubes containing EDTA for lipid profile determinations and no anticoagulant for apolipoprotein determinations once 4 weeks. The fasting serum CHO, high-density lipoprotein cholesterol (HDL-C), low-density lipoprotein cholesterol (LDL-C), and triglyceride (TG) were measured using commercial kits (Ying-Ke-Xin-Chuang Science and Technology Ltd, Xiamen, China) on an automatic biochemical analyzer. ApoA, ApoB, ApoE, Lp(a), and hsCRP were determined by immunoassay. Nonesterified fatty acids (NEFA) were determined by colorimetry. CR, ALT, and AST were tested by enzymatic methods. The oxidative stress parameters (malondialdehyde [MDA], glutathione peroxidase [GSH-px], total antioxigenic capacity [T-AOC], glutathione [GSH], and oxidized glutathione [GSSG]) were determined by the test kits from Nanjing Jiancheng Bioengineering Institute. Plasma concentrations of insulin and leptin were measured using ELISA kit (R&D Company, Germany and Phoenix pharmaceuticals Inc., USA).

*Data analysis*

All the data were analyzed by SPSS 22.0. Due to the study design, we have tested the index with various time points. Herein, the data were analyzed by analysis of variance for repeated data. All the data were shown as mean ± SE. Probability values less than 0.05 were considered to indicate a significant difference.

## Results

*The effects of dietary palm olein on physiological parameters of the subjects*

The BMI of the subjects (41 men, 47 women) in the three groups ranged from 20 to 22, which is within the normal range of the Chinese standard (18.5–23.9). The BMI in palm olein group has not changed significantly during the 16-weeks intervention, similar to the cocoa butter group and the soybean oil group. There is no significant difference ($p > 0.05$) among three groups as well (Table 3). Similar to BMI, no obvious change has been observed for the body fat rate (BFR) in palm olein group during intervention (Table 3), which is the same for soybean oil group and cocoa butter group.

The results for CR level are shown in Table 3. The serum CR level in palm olein group increased slightly (from 60 μmol/L to 66 μmol/L) after 8 weeks' intervention. There is a significant difference among the CR levels at different time points ($p < 0.05$). There is no interaction between the time and grouping factors. There is no significant difference ($p > 0.05$) among three groups (Table 3) and the grouping is not the influencing factor for CR levels. The levels of liver function indicators ALT and AST are shown in Table 3. The ALT level has not changed significantly along with time. There is no interaction between time and grouping factors. However, the AST level increased significantly after 8 weeks' intervention, and then decreased after 16 weeks' intervention (Table 3), which means time is an influencing factor for AST level. There is no significant difference ($p > 0.05$) among three groups (Table 3) due to ALT and AST.

*The effects of dietary palm olien on the levels of serum oxidative stress and inflammatory factors*

In order to elucidate whether dietary palm olein can affect the oxidative stress response, the levels of GSH-px, GSH, GSSG, MDA, and T-AOC have been identified. There is a significant difference among the GSH-px levels at different time points ($p < 0.05$) (Table 4). There is no interaction between the time and grouping factors ($p = 0.19 > 0.05$). The result of soybean oil group is the same as palm olein group. Grouping has not affected the GSH-px level significantly ($p = 0.28 > 0.05$).

*Table 3.* The changes of BMI, BFR, CR, ALT, and AST level during intervention and the effect of palm olein on them

| Index | Time (week) | Group[a] | | | $P_{(Time)}$ | $P_{(Group)}$ |
|---|---|---|---|---|---|---|
| | | Cocoa butter (*n* = 31) | Palm olein (*n* = 28) | Soybean oil (*n* = 29) | | |
| BMI (kg/cm²) | 0 | 21.12 ± 0.30 | 21.50 ± 0.46 | 20.48 ± 0.35 | 0.000 | 0.246 |
| | 8 | 21.22 ± 0.28 | 21.52 ± 0.44 | 20.71 ± 0.30 | | |
| | 16 | 21.03 ± 0.29 | 21.06 ± 0.45 | 20.44 ± 0.31 | | |
| BFR (%) | 0 | 22.72 ± 1.28 | 23.02 ± 1.56 | 21.60 ± 1.36 | 0.000 | 0.775 |
| | 8 | 21.55 ± 1.35 | 22.09 ± 1.50 | 20.56 ± 1.29 | | |
| | 16 | 21.91 ± 1.32 | 21.69 ± 1.41 | 20.76 ± 1.31 | | |
| CR (μM) | 0 | 60.81 ± 2.07 | 61.68 ± 2.37 | 61.10 ± 2.17 | 0.000 | 0.742 |
| | 8 | 60.26 ± 1.96 | 62.32 ± 2.47 | 60.38 ± 2.07 | | |
| | 16 | 66.29 ± 2.37 | 69.5 ± 2.89 | 65.76 ± 2.17 | | |
| ALT (U/L) | 0 | 11.77 ± 1.15 | 13.39 ± 1.69 | 10.93 ± 0.78 | 0.175 | 0.527 |
| | 8 | 11.48 ± 1.16 | 11.75 ± 1.57 | 9.79 ± 0.66 | | |
| | 16 | 11.71 ± 1.16 | 12.14 ± 1.64 | 11.17 ± 0.99 | | |
| AST (U/L) | 0 | 14.48 ± 1.33 | 15.93 ± 1.20 | 21.60 ± 1.36 | 0.000 | 0.434 |
| | 8 | 20.03 ± 0.99 | 22.04 ± 2.51 | 20.56 ± 1.20 | | |
| | 16 | 13.81 ± 1.38 | 14.14 ± 1.22 | 20.76 ± 1.06 | | |

[a]The data were shown as mean ± SE.

*Table 4.* The effects of palm olein on the oxidative stress levels (GSH-PX; GSH; GSSG; GSH/GSSG; MDA; T-AOC; hsCRP) during dietary intervention

| Index | Time (week) | Group[a] | | | $P_{(Time)}$ | $P_{(Group)}$ |
|---|---|---|---|---|---|---|
| | | Cocoa butter (*n* = 31) | Palm olein (*n* = 28) | Soybean oil (*n* = 29) | | |
| GSH-px (U/ml) | 0 | 277.01 ± 25.13 | 218.95 ± 26.93 | 218.55 ± 14.97 | 0.001 | 0.283 |
| | 8 | 253.02 ± 15.20 | 236.70 ± 14.97 | 265.75 ± 17.73 | | |
| | 16 | 194.59 ± 14.53 | 202.62 ± 16.44 | 216.79 ± 13.86 | | |
| GSH (μM) | 0 | 3.25 ± 0.31 | 3.53 ± 0.25 | 2.71 ± 0.20 | 0.707 | 0.787 |
| | 8 | 3.17 ± 0.25 | 2.81 ± 0.22 | 3.15 ± 0.24 | | |
| | 16 | 3.12 ± 0.24 | 3.01 ± 0.22 | 2.91 ± 0.24 | | |
| GSSG (μM) | 0 | 2.47 ± 0.11 | 2.16 ± 0.10 | 2.46 ± 0.09 | 0.000 | 0.884 |
| | 8 | 2.31 ± 0.12 | 2.58 ± 0.10 | 2.41 ± 0.12 | | |
| | 16 | 3.06 ± 0.12 | 3.16 ± 0.12 | 3.11 ± 0.10 | | |
| GSH/GSSG | 0 | 1.57 ± 0.229 | 1.90 ± 0.21 | 1.23 ± 0.14 | 0.157 | 0.268 |
| | 8 | 1.65 ± 0.20 | 1.22 ± 0.14 | 1.53 ± 0.18 | | |
| | 16 | 1.40 ± 0.40 | 1.23 ± 0.31 | 1.03 ± 0.12 | | |
| MDA (μM) | 0 | 5.16 ± 0.23 | 6.52 ± 0.43 | 5.00 ± 0.28 | 0.237 | 0.092 |
| | 8 | 5.33 ± 0.26 | 4.97 ± 0.20 | 5.27 ± 0.30 | | |
| | 16 | 5.03 ± 0.31 | 5.25 ± 0.46 | 5.09 ± 0.35 | | |
| T-AOC (U/ml) | 0 | 12.77 ± 0.42 | 12.82 ± 0.58 | 12.18 ± 0.61 | 0.000 | 0.261 |
| | 8 | 15.18 ± 0.40 | 15.58 ± 0.53 | 15.14 ± 0.51 | | |
| | 16 | 13.36 ± 0.51 | 14.73 ± 0.72 | 12.77 ± 0.38 | | |
| hsCRP (mg/L) | 0 | 3.52 ± 0.70 | 4.66 ± 0.71 | 3.32 ± 1.05 | 0.000 | 0.296 |
| | 8 | 0.36 ± 0.06 | 1.09 ± 0.41 | 0.48 ± 0.06 | | |
| | 16 | 1.81 ± 0.33 | 1.36 ± 0.26 | 1.36 ± 0.19 | | |

[a]The data were shown as mean ± SE.

There is no significant difference ($p = 0.46 > 0.05$) between the GSH levels in palm olein group and soybean oil group (Table 4), and the GSH levels didn't change significantly along with time ($p = 0.71 > 0.05$). On the contrary, the GSSG levels increased significantly in palm olein group along with intervention time ($p < 0.05$) (Table 4). There is a significant interaction between time and grouping factors. Grouping is not an influencing factor for GSSG levels either ($p > 0.05$). In order to better know the antioxidant ability, we have calculated the GSH/GSSG. As shown in Table 4, the GSH/GSSG level in palm olein group decreased significantly after 8 weeks' intervention. Whereas, the GSH/GSSG level in cocoa butter group and soybean oil group increased slightly after the 8 weeks' intervention and decreased after the 16 weeks' intervention (Table 4).

MDA as a metabolite of PUFA has been identified and the results are shown in Table 4. After 16 weeks' intervention, all of three groups didn't change significantly along with intervention time. However, there is an interaction between intervention time ($p < 0.05$) and the type of dietary fatty acids and there is no significant difference in MDA among three groups ($p > 0.05$). In addition, the T-AOC level changed significantly along with time ($p < 0.05$), which increased during the first 8 weeks' intervention and decreased slightly after another 8 weeks' intervention. There is no interaction between intervention time and the types of dietary oil ($p > 0.05$) and there is no significant difference in T-AOC level among these three groups ($p > 0.05$) (Table 4).

hsCRP as an inflammation marker has been identified to know the effect of palm olein on body's inflammatory response. As shown in Table 4, the hsCRP level in the palm olein group decreased significantly after 8 weeks' intervention and then increased slightly. Similar to almost all of the results, there is no significant difference among these three groups ($p > 0.05$), indicating that the type of dietary oil may not affect the hsCRP level.

*The effects of dietary palm olein on the glucose metabolism*

To evaluate the effect of palm olein intake on the glucose metabolism, the levels of fasting blood-glucose, insulin, and leptin have been determined and the results are shown in Table 5. The fasting blood-glucose level in palm olein group changed significantly during the intervention period ($p < 0.05$). There is no interaction between the intervention time and the type of dietary oil ($p > 0.05$). No significant difference was observed among these three groups (Table 5). Similarly, the insulin levels in the three groups decreased significantly along with time ($p < 0.05$) and there is no significant difference among three groups ($p > 0.05$) (Table 5). The results for homeostasis model assessment of insulin resistance (HOMA-IR) were shown in Table 5. The HOMA-IR ranged from 0.9 to 1.7 which is within the normal range and the trends for HOMA-IR are the same as the trends for insulin. Similarly, as shown in Table 5, the leptin level changed significantly along with time ($p < 0.05$). No significant difference has been observed among different groups ($p > 0.05$).

*The effects of dietary palm olein on the serum lipid profiles*

Dietary fatty-acid composition and type can regulate lipids and lipoprotein metabolism. To know whether the dietary palm olein (rich in saturated fatty acids) can affect the blood lipid metabolism, the serum CHO, TG, LDL-C, and HDL-C have been determined every 4 weeks.

*Table 5.* The effects of palm olein on the glucose/energy metabolism (fasting blood-glucose; insulin; HOMA-IR; leptin) during dietary intervention

| Index | Time (week) | Group[a] | | | $P_{(Time)}$ | $P_{(Group)}$ |
|---|---|---|---|---|---|---|
| | | Cocoa butter (*n* = 31) | Palm olein (*n* = 28) | Soybean oil (*n* = 29) | | |
| GLU (mM) | 0 | 4.51 ± 0.05 | 4.67 ± 0.09 | 4.60 ± 0.06 | 0.000 | 0.514 |
| | 8 | 4.84 ± 0.07 | 4.89 ± 0.08 | 4.86 ± 0.06 | | |
| | 16 | 4.30 ± 0.13 | 4.36 ± 0.13 | 4.24 ± 0.12 | | |
| INS (μIU/ml) | 0 | 8.16 ± 0.52 | 7.62 ± 0.48 | 7.69 ± 0.64 | 0.000 | 0.883 |
| | 8 | 5.67 ± 0.45 | 4.85 ± 0.42 | 5.03 ± 0.44 | | |
| | 16 | 6.41 ± 0.62 | 6.10 ± 0.49 | 6.78 ± 0.76 | | |
| HOMA-IR | 0 | 1.64 ± 0.11 | 1.58 ± 0.11 | 1.60 ± 0.15 | 0.000 | 0.748 |
| | 8 | 1.22 ± 0.10 | 1.05 ± 0.10 | 1.08 ± 0.10 | | |
| | 16 | 1.26 ± 0.14 | 1.21 ± 0.11 | 1.27 ± 0.13 | | |
| Leptin (ng/ml) | 0 | 9.66 ± 1.45 | 8.98 ± 1.31 | 9.59 ± 1.77 | 0.004 | 0.742 |
| | 8 | 7.71 ± 1.22 | 7.12 ± 1.13 | 7.50 ± 1.25 | | |
| | 16 | 11.04 ± 1.42 | 8.31 ± 1.10 | 8.74 ± 1.74 | | |

[a]The data were shown as mean ± SE.

*Table 6.* The effects of palm olein on the serum lipid profiles (CHO; TG; HDL-C; LDL-C; Apo A1; ApoB; ApoE; NEFA; Lp(a)) during dietary intervention

| Index | Time (week) | Group[a] | | | $P_{(time)}$ | $P_{(group)}$ |
|---|---|---|---|---|---|---|
| | | Cocoa butter ($n$ = 31) | Palm olein ($n$ = 28) | Soybean oil ($n$ = 29) | | |
| CHO (mM) | 0 | 4.74 ± 0.12 | 4.55 ± 0.80 | 4.39 ± 0.12 | 0.000 | 0.104 |
| | 4 | 4.78 ± 0.12 | 4.44 ± 0.74 | 4.56 ± 0.14 | | |
| | 8 | 4.63 ± 0.12 | 4.27 ± 0.68 | 4.40 ± 0.13 | | |
| | 12 | 4.65 ± 0.12 | 4.22 ± 0.49 | 4.59 ± 0.14 | | |
| | 16 | 4.29 ± 0.12 | 4.30 ± 0.56 | 3.96 ± 0.11 | | |
| TG (mM) | 0 | 0.91 ± 0.07 | 0.88 ± 0.08 | 0.77 ± 0.05 | 0.009 | 0.08 |
| | 4 | 0.94 ± 0.07 | 1.13 ± 0.17 | 0.88 ± 0.05 | | |
| | 8 | 0.90 ± 0.05 | 0.98 ± 0.08 | 0.73 ± 0.04 | | |
| | 12 | 0.93 ± 0.07 | 0.89 ± 0.08 | 0.76 ± 0.04 | | |
| | 16 | 0.96 ± 0.09 | 0.87 ± 0.08 | 0.73 ± 0.04 | | |
| HDL-C (mM) | 0 | 1.69 ± 0.06 | 1.65 ± 0.06 | 1.69 ± 0.06 | 0.000 | 0.672 |
| | 4 | 1.66 ± 0.06 | 1.60 ± 0.06 | 1.69 ± 0.06 | | |
| | 8 | 1.80 ± 0.06 | 1.69 ± 0.06 | 1.73 ± 0.06 | | |
| | 12 | 1.42 ± 0.04 | 1.39 ± 0.04 | 1.40 ± 0.05 | | |
| | 16 | 1.46 ± 0.04 | 1.44 ± 0.05 | 1.45 ± 0.06 | | |
| LDL-C (mM) | 0 | 2.49 ± 0.09 | 2.36 ± 0.13 | 2.24 ± 0.09 | 0.000 | 0.031 |
| | 4 | 2.38 ± 0.10 | 2.35 ± 0.10 | 2.23 ± 0.08 | | |
| | 8 | 2.47 ± 0.10 | 2.31 ± 0.09 | 2.15 ± 0.07 | | |
| | 12 | 1.95 ± 0.08 | 1.87 ± 0.09 | 1.72 ± 0.05 | | |
| | 16 | 2.21 ± 0.10 | 2.24 ± 0.11 | 2.00 ± 0.08 | | |
| ApoA1 (g/L) | 0 | 1.44 ± 0.06 | 1.39 ± 0.05 | 1.38 ± 0.05 | 0.010 | 0.354 |
| | 8 | 1.48 ± 0.06 | 1.40 ± 0.05 | 1.37 ± 0.05 | | |
| | 16 | 1.38 ± 0.04 | 1.37 ± 0.04 | 1.29 ± 0.05 | | |
| ApoB (g/L) | 0 | 0.75 ± 0.02 | 0.71 ± 0.03 | 0.68 ± 0.03 | 0.000 | 0.309 |
| | 8 | 0.70 ± 0.02 | 0.64 ± 0.03 | 0.61 ± 0.02 | | |
| | 16 | 0.62 ± 0.03 | 0.68 ± 0.05 | 0.62 ± 0.04 | | |
| ApoE (mg/dL) | 0 | 4.51 ± 0.20 | 4.51 ± 0.33 | 4.39 ± 0.22 | 0.000 | 0.515 |
| | 8 | 4.90 ± 0.21 | 4.57 ± 0.28 | 4.41 ± 0.23 | | |
| | 16 | 4.11 ± 0.20 | 4.05 ± 0.27 | 3.66 ± 0.21 | | |
| NEFA (μM) | 0 | 329.19 ± 28.59 | 297.61 ± 31.51 | 306.07 ± 32.09 | 0.000 | 0.397 |
| | 4 | 339.55 ± 42.98 | 290.11 ± 27.97 | 304.14 ± 24.01 | | |
| | 8 | 391.35 ± 21.77 | 387.71 ± 20.93 | 435.58 ± 23.19 | | |
| | 12 | 271.00 ± 32.00 | 238.61 ± 22.46 | 351.93 ± 40.46 | | |
| | 16 | 345.03 ± 27.48 | 361.46 ± 38.49 | 360.55 ± 37.01 | | |
| LP(a) (mg/L) | 0 | 219.42 ± 40.77 | 202.96 ± 41.89 | 181.38 ± 37.82 | 0.021 | 0.811 |
| | 4 | 190.94 ± 34.09 | 217.61 ± 44.67 | 171.17 ± 38.77 | | |
| | 8 | 197.16 ± 37.30 | 189.00 ± 38.78 | 187.39 ± 44.78 | | |
| | 12 | 225.32 ± 41.26 | 191.50 ± 39.99 | 159.03 ± 34.43 | | |
| | 16 | 161.84 ± 28.17 | 167.61 ± 37.17 | 149.10 ± 31.54 | | |

[a]The data were shown as mean ± SE.

As shown in Table 6, the intervention time may affect the CHO levels significantly ($p < 0.05$). However, no interaction has been observed between the intervention time and the dietary oil type. There are no significant differences in CHO level among cocoa butter, palm olein, and soybean oil groups either ($p > 0.05$). In contrast, the TG level did not change significantly along with time ($p > 0.05$) and the palm olein in the diet may not affect the TG level significantly ($p > 0.05$) (Table 6). Similarly, by the ANOVA of repeated data, the serum HDL-C and LDL-C level have changed significantly during 16 weeks' intervention ($p < 0.05$) (Table 6). A significant difference ($p < 0.05$) has been observed for LDL-C levels among three groups. However, the difference may be due to the grouping factor at the beginning of the study. The trends during intervention are almost the same for three groups and there is no significant difference in HDL-C among them ($p > 0.05$). No interaction has been observed between the intervention time and different dietary oils in diets.

The serum ApoA1, ApoB, and ApoE levels are shown in Table 6. Through ANOVA of repeated data, the intervention time has affected the levels of ApoA1, ApoB, and ApoE significantly ($p < 0.05$). Similar to the results for CHO, dietary palm olein intervention has not affected the ApoA1 level. The serum ApoA1 and ApoB levels decreased along with time after intervention (Table 6). In addition, the ApoE level in palm olein group was almost the same during 8 weeks' intervention and then decreased slightly after that (Table 6). As for normal population aged 20–40, we have not observed significant changes in ApoA1, ApoB, and ApoE levels among cocoa butter group, palm olein, and soybean oil groups ($p > 0.05$).

As shown in Table 6, the NEFA level increased slightly during 8 weeks' intervention and then decreased until 12 weeks, indicating that the intervention time can affect the NEFA level significantly ($p < 0.05$). There is no obvious difference in NEFA level among three groups ($p > 0.05$), which is similar to results for TG, CHO, LDL-C, and HDL-C. Meanwhile, after 4 weeks' intervention, Lp(a) level in palm olein group is higher than the level of soybean oil group and cocoa butter group. Nevertheless, the Lp(a) level of palm olein group is between the level of cocoa butter group and soybean oil group after 12 weeks' intervention. Thus, there is no significant difference ($p > 0.05$) among these three groups.

## Discussion

Dietary fatty acids have been regarded as the key risk factors for several chronic diseases, such as obesity, coronary heart diseases, and atherosclerosis. Several studies have shown that the composition of dietary oil may affect the blood lipid profiles (20), but the directions of the effects were inconsistent. In order to elucidate the effect of dietary oil with high ratio of saturated fatty acids on the cardiovascular risk factors, we have identified the physiological parameters, oxidative stress, inflammatory factors, glucose metabolism, and the serum lipid profiles during palm olein intervention.

Firstly, we have not observed the change of BMI and BFR among three groups, results of which indicate that the dietary oil partially replaced with palm olein may not affect the body weight and fat deposition. Analogously, there is no effect on the level of CR, AST, and ALT, suggesting that the dietary oils have not affected the function of kidney and liver. However, these results are contrary to the animal study of atherogenic diet based on saturated fat, which has shown a weight gain effect in rats and elevated AST and ALT level of rats (21), which can be attributed to the different amounts of saturated fat.

Previous research has suggested that oxidative stress plays a significant role in the decrease in beta-cell secretory function by exposure to free fatty acids for a long time (22). Meanwhile, the palm olein has been proved to exhibit protective effects on cardiovascular systems by attenuating the free radicals and then decreasing the oxidative stress (23). However, the oxidative stress indices exhibited no change during dietary intervention, indicating that palm olein and cocoa butter high in saturated fatty acids have no effect on the oxidative stress status for human body. This difference may be from different study subjects and intervention times. Interestingly, palm olein rich in tocotrienol fractions has been proved to reduce the levels of oxidative stress markers, which can be attributed to the effect of tocotrienol (24). Therefore, dietary palm olein may not have an adverse effect on oxidative stress relating to CVD. In addition, C-reactive protein (CRP) is associated with CVD and inflammation in apparently healthy individuals. Our study suggested that palm olein in diet has no significant effect on the hsCRP level ($p > 0.05$). This result is similar to a recent research on cocoa butter, which stated that dietary cocoa butter does not alter the inflammatory markers such as postprandial hsCRP in healthy women (25). Thus, dietary oil partially replaced with palm olein rich in saturated fatty acids has not affected the inflammation status of human body. In addition, the hsCRP levels after 8 weeks and 16 weeks of intervention are lower than the level before intervention, which may be due to the diet low in salt and oil.

What's more, the fasting blood-glucose level has not been affected by palm olein, indicating that partially replacing dietary oil with palm olein may have little effect on the glucose metabolism. In addition, the insulin level and HOMA-IR decreased along with time, which may be due to the healthy dietary pattern (a regular diet low in salt, and with energy balance) during intervention. This result is in accordance with previous researches that palm based oil diets did not affect the markers of insulin resistance and glucose tolerance in overweight Malaysian adults (26). Thus, we can speculate that the moderate level of saturated fatty acids in diet has no relationship with insulin resistance. Similarly, palm olein replacement has not influenced the leptin level, indicating the palm olein intervention may not affect the energy metabolism.

Generally, no significant difference was observed for the blood lipid profiles during intervention for cocoa butter, palm olein, and soybean oil groups. In addition, CHO, TG, HDL-C, and LDL-C have not changed obviously during 16 weeks' intervention. Previous researches on different vegetable oils have indicated that the CHO level in all treated rats for 8 weeks were within the normal range and there was no significant difference in CHO, which is similar to our results (27). However, the TG levels in palm olein group were significantly increased compared to control group (27), which is contradictory to our results. This can be explained by different objects and intervention time. At the same time, HDL-C and LDL-C as possible risk factors for coronary heart disease have not changed as well. This result is consistent with the results from positional distribution of fatty acids on dietary TGs, which showed that the ratio of HDL-C to LDL-C cholesterol and serum TG concentration of human body were unchanged after 3 weeks' intervention (28). On the contrary, previous studies on the fats with a higher proportion of palmitic acid in the sn-2 position have indicated to decrease postprandial lipemia in healthy subjects (29). This can be attributed to the difference in intervention time.

As we have not observed the change in lipid profiles, whether the intervention can affect the apolipoprotein needs to be further identified. ApoA1 has been proved to negatively relate with HDL-C, and ApoB was negatively correlated with LDL-C (30, 31). Thus, results for ApoA1 and ApoB are similar to the results of HDL-C and LDL-C. Dietary intervention with cocoa butter, palm olein, and soybean oil has not affected the serum ApoE level. It has been proved that APOE3 is associated with the potential to more efficiently harvest dietary energy and to deposit fat in adipose tissue, while APOE4 carriers tend to increase fatty-acid mobilization and utilization as fuel substrates especially under high-fat intake (32). As a consequence, the dietary intervention has no effect on fat deposition and fatty-acid utilization.

The dietary intervention with palm olein has not affected the serum NEFA levels, possibly indicating that the high ratio of saturated fatty acid has not affected the adipose fat deposition. Similarly, previous results have shown that alterations in the dietary lipid intake of rats affected the composition but not the amount of myocardial NEFAs (33). Whereas pervious study has reported that Omega-3 supplementation caused a significant reduction in NEFA in the intervention group compared with the placebo group (34). Therefore, the composition of dietary fatty acids is vital for the levels of NEFA.

Meanwhile, Lp(a) as a low-density lipoprotein particle with a specific protein attached to it is hardly influenced by diet (e.g. low-caloric, low-fat, or high-cholesterol diets), which is in accordance with our results. However, previous reports on hydrogenated fish oil, partially hydrogenated soybean oil and butter have indicated the unfavorably effect on lipid risk indicators for coronary heart disease, especially the serum lipoproteins and Lp(a) in men ($p < 0.02$) (35). This may be due to the various intervention time and methods.

In this study, we have not observed the significant difference among three groups. The possible reasons for this observation may be that the sample size of 108 may be underpowered to detect a difference of 10% in the index. In other words, replacing 1/5 of the dietary oil may not affect the cardiovascular risk factors theoretically.

## Conclusions

In conclusion in our study, there are no significant differences in the cardiovascular risk factors after dietary intervention with palm olein. Considering the composition of dietary oil, we can conclude that palm olein with high ratio of saturated fatty acids in dietary oil may not affect the lipid profiles, the insulin resistance, and the function of liver and kidney, especially the oxidative stress level. However, there are still several limitations in this study. Firstly, the intervention time is 16 weeks, which is not long enough to observe the long-term influence of palm olein. And convenience sampling has been used in this study; therefore the results may not be suitable for all adults. Secondly, the sample size may not be powerful to observe the difference between three groups and we will enlarge the sample size to further investigate the effect of palm olein in the follow-up study. Furthermore, it is still contradictory on dietary saturated fatty acids and needs further investigation.

## Acknowledgements

We are grateful to the canteen of Capital Medical University for providing the diets. This work was supported by Mutual fund of the Chinese Nutrition Society and Malaysian palm bureau [Project 2].

## Conflict of interest

The authors have no conflicts of interest to declare.

## References

1. Calder PC. Functional roles of fatty acids and their effects on human health. JPEN J Parenter Enteral Nutr 2015; 39(1 Suppl): 18S–32S.
2. Calder PC, Yaqoob P, Thies F, Wallace FA, Miles EA. Fatty acids and lymphocyte functions. Biochem Soc T 1995; 87(2): 302–9.
3. Zuliani G, Galvani M, Leitersdorf E, Volpato S, Cavalieri M, Fellin R. The role of polyunsaturated fatty acids (PUFA) in the treatment of dyslipidemias. Curr Pharm Des 2009; 15(36): 4087–93.
4. Hayes KC, Pronczuk A, Lindsey S, Diersenschade D. Dietary saturated fatty acids (12:0, 14:0, 16:0) differ in their impact on plasma cholesterol and lipoproteins in nonhuman primates. Am J Clin Nutr 1991; 53(2): 491–8.
5. Iggman D, Riséérus U. Role of different dietary saturated fatty acids for cardiometabolic risk. Clin Lipidol 2011; 6(2): 209–32.
6. Valsta LM, Tapanainen H, Sundvall J, Laatikainen T, Mannisto S. Explaining the 25year decline of serum cholesterol by dietary changes and use of lipidlowering medication in Finland. Public Health Nutr 2010; 13(6A): 932–8.

7. Micha R, Mozaffarian D. Saturated fat and cardiometabolic risk factors, coronary heart disease, stroke, and diabetes: a fresh look at the evidence. Lipids 2010; 45: 893–905.
8. Praagman J, Beulens JW, Alssema M, Zock PL, Wanders AJ, Sluijs I, et al. The association between dietary saturated fatty acids and ischemic heart disease depends on the type and source of fatty acid in the European Prospective Investigation into Cancer and Nutrition-Netherlands cohort. Am J Clin Nutr 2016; 103: 475–82.
9. Keys A, Anderson JT, Grande F. Serum cholesterol response to changes in the diet. IV. Particular saturated fatty acids in the diet. Metabolism 1965; 14: 776–87.
10. Malachi O. Palm oil: an over – acclaimed cooking oil in Nigeria. Annu Res Rev Biol 2015; 7(3): 133–43.
11. Hooper L, Summerbell CD, Higgins JPT, Thompson R, Clements G, Capps N, et al. Reduced or modified dietary fat for preventing cardiovascular disease (Cochrane Review). J Cardiovasc Nurs 2013; 28(3): 204–5.
12. Jakobsen MU, O'Reilly EJ, Heitmann BL, Pereira MA, Balter K, Fraser GE, et al. Major types of dietary fat and risk of coronary heart disease: a pooled analysis of 11 cohort studies. Am J Clin Nutr 2009; 89(5): 1425–32.
13. Tholstrup T, Hjerpsted J, Raff M. Palm olein increases plasma cholesterol moderately compared with olive oil in healthy individuals. Am J Clin Nutr 2011; 94(6): 1426–32.
14. Fattore E, Fanelli R. Palm oil and palmitic acid: a review on cardiovascular effects and carcinogenicity. Int J Food Sci Nutr 2013; 64(5): 648–59.
15. Lucci P, Borrero M, Ruiz A, Pacetti D, Frega NG, Diez O. Palm oil and cardiovascular disease: a randomized trial of the effects of hybrid palm oil supplementation on human plasma lipid patterns. Food Funct 2016; 7(1): 347–54.
16. Filippou A, Teng KT, Berry SE, Sanders TA. Palmitic acid in the sn-2 position of dietary triacylglycerols does not affect insulin secretion or glucose homeostasis in healthy men and women. Eur J Clin Nutr 2014; 68: 1036–41.
17. Tholstrup T, Hjerpsted J, Raff M. Palm olein increases plasma cholesterol moderately compared with olive oil in healthy individuals. Am J Clin Nutr 2011; 94: 1426–32.
18. Voon PT, Ng TK, Lee VK, Nesaretnam K. Diets high in palmitic acid (16:0), lauric and myristic acids (12:0 + 14:0), or oleic acid (18:1) do not alter postprandial or fasting plasma homocysteine and inflammatory markers in healthy Malaysian adults. Am J Clin Nutr 2011; 94: 1451–7.
19. Hall WL, Brito MF, Huang J, Wood LV, Filippou A, Sanders TA, et al. An interesterified palm olein test meal decreases early-phase postprandial lipemia compared to palm olein: a randomized controlled trial. Lipids 2014; 49: 895–904.
20. Wei MY, Jacobson TA. Effects of eicosapentaenoic acid versus docosahexaenoic acid on serum lipids: a systematic review and meta-analysis. Curr Atheroscler Rep 2011; 13(6): 474–83.
21. Hammad KSM, Hallabo SA, Galal SM. Protective effect of linseed oil and walnuts against hypercholesterolemia induced by atherogenic diet in rats. J Food Nutr Res 2015; 3: 653–60.
22. Oprescu AI, Bikopoulos G, Naassan A, Allister EM, Tang C, Park E, et al. Free fatty acid-induced reduction in glucose-stimulated insulin secretion: evidence for a role of oxidative stress *in vitro* and *in vivo*. Diabetes 2007; 56: 2927–37.
23. Bayorh MA, Abukhalaf IK, Ganafa AA. Effect of palm oil on blood pressure, endothelial function and oxidative stress. Asia Pac J Clin Nutr 2005; 14: 325–39.
24. Budin SB, Othman F, Louis SR, Bakar MA, Das S, Mohamed J, et al. The effects of palm oil tocotrienol-rich fraction supplementation on biochemical parameters, oxidative stress and the vascular wall of streptozotocin-induced diabetic rats. Clinics 2009; 64: 235–44.
25. Tholstrup T, Teng KT, Raff M. Dietary cocoa butter or refined olive oil does not alter postprandial hsCRP and IL-6 concentrations in healthy women. Lipids 2011; 46: 365–70.
26. Norhaizan ME, Lee ST, Voon PTNg, Ng TKW, Hazizi AS, Supeng L, et al. Palm based high-oleic cooking oil and extra virgin olive oil diets do not affect markers of insulin resistance and glucose tolerance in overweight adults. J Food Nutr Disord 2016; 5: 5.
27. Dauqan E, Sani HA, Abdullah A, Kasim ZM. Effect of different vegetable oils (red palm olein, palm olein, corn oil and coconut oil) on lipid profile in rat. Food Nutr Sci 2011; 2: 399–403.
28. Zock PL, de Vries JH, de Fouw NJ, Katan MB. Positional distribution of fatty acids in dietary triglycerides: effects on fasting blood lipoprotein concentrations in humans. Am J Clin Nutr 1995; 61: 48–55.
29. Sanders TA, Filippou A, Berry SE, Baumgartner S, Mensink RP. Palmitic acid in the sn-2 position of triacylglycerols acutely influences postprandial lipid metabolism. Am J Clin Nutr 2011; 94: 1433–41.
30. San MMI, Collado YL, Cuadrado Cenzual MÁ, Ciudad Cabañas MJ, Mendive DP. Role of apoa1 on high-density lipoproteln: an intervention with plant sterols in patients with hypercholesterolemia. Nutr Hosp 2014; 31: 494–9.
31. Matthan NR, Welty FK, Barrett PH, Harausz C, Dolnikowski GG, Parks JS, et al. Dietary hydrogenated fat increases high-density lipoprotein apoA-I catabolism and decreases low-density lipoprotein apoB-100 catabolism in hypercholesterolemic women. Arterioscl Throm Vas 2004; 24: 1092–7.
32. Huebbe P, Dose J, Schloesser A, Campbell G, Gluer CC, Gupta Y, et al. Apolipoprotein E (APOE) genotype regulates body weight and fatty acid utilization-Studies in gene-targeted replacement mice. Mol Nutr Food Res 2015; 59: 334–43.
33. Charnock JS, Abeywardena MY, Mclennan PL. The effect of different dietary lipid supplements on the nonesterified fatty acid composition of normoxic rat hearts: a link between nutrition and cardiac arrhythmia. Nutr Res 1992; 12: 1491–502.
34. Farsi PF, Djazayery A, Eshraghian MR, Koohdani F, Saboor-Yaraghi AA, Derakhshanian H, et al. Effects of supplementation with omega-3 on insulin sensitivity and non-esterified free fatty acid (NEFA) in type 2 diabetic patients. Arq Bras Endocrino 2014; 58: 335–40.
35. Almendingen K, Jordal O, Kierulf P, Sandstad B, Pedersen JI. Effects of partially hydrogenated fish oil, partially hydrogenated soybean oil, and butter on serum lipoproteins and Lp[a] in men. J Lipid Res 1995; 36: 1370–84.



***Rong Xiao and Huanling Yu**
School of Public Health
Beijing Key Laboratory of Environmental Toxicology
Capital Medical University
No.10 Xitoutiao, You An Men
Beijing 100069, China
Email: xiaor22@ccmu.edu.cn; yuhlzjl@ccmu.edu.cn

# 8

# National nutrition surveys in Europe: a review on the current status in the 53 countries of the WHO European region

Holly L. Rippin[1]*, Jayne Hutchinson[1], Charlotte E. L. Evans[1], Jo Jewell[2], Joao J. Breda[2] and Janet E. Cade[1]

[1]Nutritional Epidemiology Group (NEG), School of Food Science and Nutrition, University of Leeds, Leeds, United Kingdom; [2]Division of Noncommunicable Diseases and Promoting Health through the Life-Course, World Health Organization Regional Office for Europe, UN City, Marmorvej 51, 21000 Copenhagen, Denmark

*Abstract*

***Objectives:*** The objectives of this study were (1) to determine the coverage of national nutrition surveys in the 53 countries monitored by the World Health Organization (WHO) Regional Office for Europe and identify gaps in provision, (2) to describe relevant survey attributes and (3) to check whether energy and nutrients are reported with a view to providing information for evidence-based nutrition policy planning.

***Design:*** Dietary survey information was gathered using three methods: (1) direct email to survey authors and other relevant contacts, (2) systematic review of literature databases and (3) general web-based searches. Survey characteristics relating to time frame, sampling and dietary methodology and nutrients reported were tabled from all relevant surveys found since 1990.

***Setting:*** Fifty-three countries of the WHO Regional Office for Europe, which have need for an overview of dietary surveys across the life course.

***Subjects:*** European individuals (adults and children) in national diet surveys.

***Results:*** A total of 109 nationally representative dietary surveys undertaken post-1990 were found across 34 countries. Of these, 78 surveys from 33 countries were found post-2000, and of these, 48 surveys from 27 countries included children and 60 surveys from 30 countries included adults. No nationally representative surveys were found for 19 of 53 countries, mainly from Central and Eastern Europe. Multiple 24hr recall and food diaries were the most common dietary assessment methods. Only 22 countries reported energy and nutrient intakes from post-2000 surveys; macronutrients were more widely reported than micronutrients.

***Conclusions:*** Less than two-thirds of WHO Europe countries have nationally representative diet surveys, mainly collected post-2000. The main availability gaps lie in Central and Eastern European countries, where nutrition policies may therefore lack an appropriate evidence base. Dietary methodological differences may limit the scope for inter-country comparisons.

Keywords: *national diet surveys*; *WHO European region*; *dietary assessment methodologies*; *scoping review – gaps*; *multi-criteria analysis*; *nutritional epidemiology*

**Graphical Abstract: National diet surveys identified**

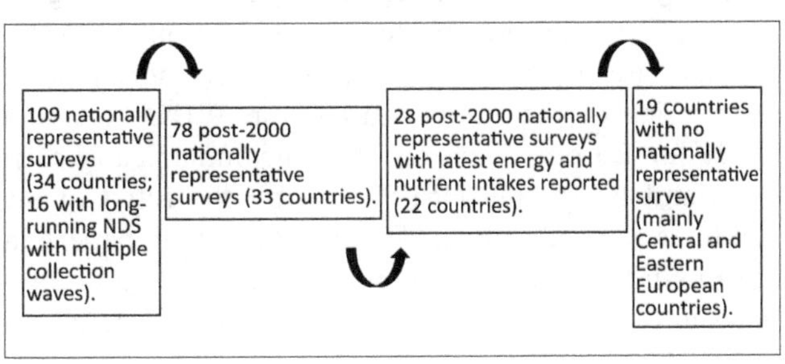


The World Health Organization (WHO) European Food and Nutrition Action Plan aims to 'significantly reduce the burden of preventable diet-related noncommunicable diseases, obesity and all other forms of malnutrition still prevalent in the WHO European Region' and improve diet and nutrition in the European population (1). An unhealthy diet is one of the four major behavioural risk factors for non-communicable diseases (NCDs) in all WHO regions (2), with the European region proportionately suffering the greatest NCD burden. Other risk factors include alcohol, tobacco misuse and physical inactivity (2). In Europe, the four most common NCDs account for 77% of disease and almost 86% premature mortality (1).

NCDs and related conditions, including overweight and obesity, have significant and growing economic and social costs (1), which traditional clinical approaches are increasingly unable to address (3). Mozaffarian et al. (3) call for a shift in emphasis from such pharmacological treatments to primary prevention through addressing lifestyle risk factors such as dietary patterns in order to reduce cardiovascular risk and NCD-associated problems.

Dietary surveys thus have an important role in assessing dietary patterns in the whole population. Nutrition and health surveys formed the main source of information for dietary risk factors and physical inactivity in a systematic analysis of disease risk in 21 regions worldwide across two decades (4). Such surveys can provide a means of monitoring trends, identifying areas of concern and inequality and evaluating policy impact, thereby ultimately contributing to the promotion of best practice across the region (1). The WHO European Food and Nutrition Action Plan (1) explicitly encourages member states to 'strengthen and expand nationally representative diet and nutrition surveys'.

Many western European countries currently have established dietary surveys that assess food and nutrient intake. A global review of country-specific surveys from 1990 to 2010 only reported dietary fat and oil intake (5). A comprehensive, updated review of total nutrient and food intakes across different populations and subgroups in Europe is needed, the results of which could identify where in Europe there is a need to improve diets and whether inequalities exist. This paper makes the first step in this regard, establishing which countries have nationally representative dietary surveys and highlighting gaps in nutrition survey provision across Europe.

This review aims to identify which of the 53 countries in the WHO European region have conducted nationally representative dietary surveys of whole diets at an individual level and those that have not. It identifies key characteristics, centred on time frame, sampling and dietary methodology, of known surveys undertaken since 1990 for adults and children and aims to lay the foundations in establishing a clear picture of the current situation. Following this, future papers will examine energy and nutrient intakes in different population groups across Europe to better assess where both gaps in knowledge and dietary inadequacies lie. Information from dietary surveys can be used as a means for governments and health bodies to monitor and reduce the diet-related risk of NCDs and related conditions across Europe, thereby contributing to the goals set out in the WHO action plan.

## Methods

We used three key approaches to identifying national diet surveys: (1) contacting authors of surveys, (2) systematic literature review and (3) general web-based searches.

### *Identifying authors of national diet surveys*

We identified authors of national surveys within the WHO Europe remit using listed contact names and other information from two main reports of national dietary surveys (5, 6). If no response was obtained from those authors, Internet searches of nutrition organisations by country and the survey titles listed in the review of 1990–2010 surveys (5) and the European Food Consumption Survey (6) were carried out to find other potentially useful contact details. For countries where this approach did not yield usable contact details, Internet searches using various search terms were performed on organisations specialising in nutrition, including known government and public health agencies. WHO also provided contact details for some of those countries for which they had relevant associates. Contacts identified were asked to complete a questionnaire (Appendix 1) to provide information on nationally representative dietary surveys conducted at an individual level since 1990, including links or references to relevant reports.

### *Systematic database search*

For countries where no contact could be identified, systematic searches were undertaken across Web of Science, Medline and Scopus for nationally representative dietary surveys that collected data at an individual level from 1990 to June 2016. The following query terms were run without language restrictions: (survey* OR research* [TS]) AND (nutrition* OR diet* OR food* [TS]) AND (list of countries).

The title of each paper generated by the database searches was screened for relevance according to the criteria in Table 1; those that are not relevant were excluded. The remaining papers were screened by title and abstract, and full article where available, and their appropriateness for inclusion was checked by a second reviewer. Further surveys, related papers and nutrition expert contact names were gathered by general Internet searching to capture any recently released information, targeting known government and public health agencies using various search term combinations in order to maximise returns. Although there were no language restrictions in the initial search, the WHO Regional Office for Europe, Division of Noncommunicable Diseases and Promoting Health through the Life-Course, conducted an additional database search of papers in the Russian language as an extra check to maximise returns in the 12 Central and Eastern European countries where Russian is an official or widely spoken language

*Table 1.* Survey inclusion and exclusion criteria

| Included | Excluded |
|---|---|
| Surveys conducted at an individual level | Surveys collected at group, that is, household level |
| Nationally representative surveys | Non-nationally representative, regional only surveys |
| Results of surveys reported by published and unpublished reports, academic journals and websites | Surveys with data collected prior to 1990 |
| Surveys that included individuals >2 years | Surveys with samples exclusively <2 years |
| Surveys based on whole diet rather than specific food groups | Surveys with incomplete food group coverage |
| | Surveys with small sample sizes ($n$ < 200) |

(Armenia, Azerbaijan, Belarus, Georgia, Kazakhstan, Kyrgyzstan, Moldova, Russia, Tajikistan, Turkmenistan, Ukraine and Uzbekistan). However, no papers or reports that met the inclusion and exclusion criteria were found. The databases searched were PubMed, Web of Science and Google Scholar, using the search terms mentioned above, translated into Russian. Further searches with these terms were undertaken in three specific Russian language databases: Kazakh Academy of Nutrition; 1st Moscow Medical Academy named after Sechenov and Electronic Scientific Library in Russian.

*Database extraction*

Where long-running surveys had multiple collection waves, for example, the French INCA 1 and INCA 2 or UK NDNS 2000–1 and NDNS 2008–12, each collection wave was counted as a separate survey (see Table 2). Survey characteristics were extracted and tabled from the relevant publications, which were accessed in various forms, including summary reports, academic articles and completed questionnaires (see Table 2). The survey characteristics included the following: country name, survey name, year of survey (data collection), information source, sample size and age range, dietary methodology, nutrient composition database and reference. The availability of energy and selected nutrients from the latest surveys collected after 2000 are listed in Appendices 1 and 2.

## Results

*Data extracted*

A total of 109 nationally representative surveys that obtained data on whole diets (rather than focusing only on certain foods) at an individual level since 1990 were found for 34 out of the 53 countries in the WHO office region. Table 2 shows the characteristics of these surveys and that the majority of countries with national dietary surveys (NDS) had conducted multiple surveys. Of the 34 countries with NDS, almost half ($n$ = 16) had long-running surveys with waves conducted over various years; 10 of these also had stand-alone surveys (Table 2). Countries for which relevant survey characteristics were gathered are Andorra, Austria, Belgium, Bulgaria, Cyprus, Czech Republic, Denmark, Estonia, Finland, France, Germany, Greece, Hungary, Iceland, Ireland, Israel, Italy, Kazakhstan, Latvia, Lithuania, the Netherlands, Norway, Poland, Portugal, Romania, Russian Federation, Slovakia, Slovenia, Spain, Sweden, Switzerland, the former Yugoslav Republic of Macedonia, Turkey and the United Kingdom.

Of the 109 nationally representative surveys found, 78 were conducted since 2000, covering 33 countries – those listed previously, excluding Slovakia. Reports of energy and nutrient intakes were not found for each of these surveys. Only 28 surveys from 22 countries were found with post-2000 survey reports of energy and nutrient intakes.

The majority of the surveys were found via Internet searches or emailing contacts gathered by the methods discussed. Current contact details were found for the following 30 countries: Austria, Belgium, Bulgaria, Croatia, Cyprus, Czech Republic, Denmark, Estonia, Finland, France, Germany, Greece, Hungary, Iceland, Ireland, Israel, Italy, Latvia, Lithuania, Malta, the Netherlands, Poland, Portugal, Romania, Russian Federation, Slovenia, Spain, Sweden, Switzerland and the United Kingdom. WHO provided details for Andorra, Kazakhstan and the former Yugoslav Republic of Macedonia. Contact details were not available for the following 20 countries: Albania, Armenia, Azerbaijan, Belarus, Bosnia and Herzegovina, Georgia, Kyrgyzstan, Luxembourg, Monaco, Montenegro, Republic of Moldova, San Marino, Serbia, Slovakia, Slovenia, Tajikistan, Turkey, Turkmenistan, Ukraine and Uzbekistan. For countries where no contact could be identified, the original systematic literature search returned 6,654 papers across the three databases, but only eight of these met the inclusion criteria. Of the 78 surveys undertaken since 2000, 30 papers or reports relating to them were acquired through email contacts, 4 from information extracted by WHO from the WHO Global Nutrition Policy Review 2017, 35 via Internet searching, 2 via the systematic literature search, 18 via the Micha review (5) and 1 from the EFCOSUM survey (6); 11 reports had multiple sources. See Fig. 1 for the full dietary survey screening and Table 2 for the characteristics of all dietary surveys conducted since 1990.

*Table 2.* National diet surveys across the WHO Europe remit 1990–2016

| Country* | Survey name | Survey year | Source ** | Sample size | Sample age | Dietary methodology | Nutrient reference database† | Energy intake graphed Y/N‡ | Reference |
|---|---|---|---|---|---|---|---|---|---|
| Albania | None found | | | | | | | | |
| Andorra | Evaluation of the nutritional status of the Andorran population | 2004–2005 | 6 | 900 | 12–75 | 24hr recall (×2 for 35% sample), FFQ. Face-to-face and phone interview. | CESNID. *Tablas de composición de alimentos.* Barcelona: Edicions Universitat de Barcelona-Centre d'Ensenyament Superior de Nutrició i Dietètica, 2002 | Y | (32) |
| Armenia | | | | | | | | | |
| Austria* | Austrian nutrition report 2012 (OSES) | 2010–2012 | 3 | 1,002 | 7–14; 18–80 | 3-day diary (consecutive) (children); 2×24hr recall (adults). Face-to-face and phone interview. | Analysis run with software '(nut.s) science' based on Bundeslebensmittelschlüssel 3.01/Goldberg cut-offs for data cleaning. | Y | (33) |
| | Austrian study on nutritional status 2007 | 2007 | 4 | 2,472 | 7–100 | Single dietary diary. | | N | (34) |
| | Austrian study on nutritional status (ASNS) | 1993–1997 | 5 | 2,065 | 19–95 | 24hr recall, diet history. | | N | (35) |
| | Austrian study on nutritional status (ASNS) | 1991–1994 | 5 | 2,173 | 6–18 | 7-day diary. | | N | (36) |
| Azerbaijan | None found | | | | | | | | |
| Belarus | None found | | | | | | | | |
| Belgium* | Belgium national food consumption survey (BNFCS) 2014 | 2014–2015 | 2/3 | 3,146 | 3–64 | 2×24hr recall. Face-to-face electronic interview. | The NIMS Belgian Table of Food Composition (Nubel); Dutch NEVO | Y | (37, 38) |
| | Belgium national food consumption survey (BNFCS) | 2004 | 3/4 | 3,245 | 15–100 | 2×24hr recall. Face-to-face interview. FFQ. | | N | (39) |
| Bosnia and Herzegovina | None found | | | | | | | | |
| Bulgaria | National survey on nutrition of infants and children under 5 and family child rearing, 2007 | 2007 | 3 | 1,723 | 0–5 | 2×24hr recall via mother (non-consecutive). Face-to-face interview with the mother. | FCTBL_BG (Food Composition Tables – Bulgaria) | Y | (40–42) |
| | National nutrition survey | 2004 | 4 | 853 | 20–100 | Single dietary diary. | | N | |
| Croatia | None found | | | | | | | | |
| Cyprus | A study of the dietary intake of Cypriot children and adolescents aged 6–18 years | 2009–2010 | 3 | 1,414 | 6–18 | 3-day food record (consecutive inc 1 weekend). Self-completed. | USDA Nutrient Database for Standard Reference and Research | Y | (43) |

*Continued*

*Table 2.* Continued

| Country* | Survey name | Survey year | Source ** | Sample size | Sample age | Dietary methodology | Nutrient reference database† | Energy intake graphed Y/N‡ | Reference |
|---|---|---|---|---|---|---|---|---|---|
| Czech Republic | Individual food consumption study (SISP04) | 2003–2004 | 2 | 2,590 | 4–90 | 2×24hr recall. Face-to-face interview. | | N | (44, 45) |
| | Czech Post-MONICA Study | 1997–1998 | 4 | 2,158 | 19–64 | Single dietary diary. | | N | |
| Denmark* | Danish national survey of diet and physical activity (DANSDA) 2011–2013 | 2011–2013 | 3 | 3,946 | 4–75 | 7-day diary (consecutive). Self-completed. | Danish Food Composition Databank | Y | (46) |
| | Danish national survey of diet and physical activity (DANSDA) 2003–2008 | 2003–2008 | 3 | 4,431 | 4–75 | 7-day diary (consecutive). Self-completed. | | N | (47) |
| | Dietary Habits of Denmark 2000–2002 | 2000–2002 | 4 | 4,120 | 4–75 | 7-day diary. | | N | (48) |
| | National dietary survey | 1995 | 5 | 3,098 | 1–80 | 7-day diary | | N | (49) |
| Estonia | National dietary survey | 2014–15 | 2 | 4,906 | 4 months to 74 years | 2×24hr recall (age >10); 2×24hr food diary (age <10); FFQ (age >2). Face-to-face electronic interview. | | N | Not yet available. |
| | Nutrition and lifestyle in the Baltic Republics | 1997 | 1/4 | 2,015 | 16–64 | 24hr recall + questionnaire | | N | (50, 51) |
| Finland* | The National FINDIET 2012 survey | 2012 | 3 | 1,708 | 25–74 | 48hr recall. Face-to-face interview. | Fineli 7 Food Composition Database | Y | (52) |
| | FINDIET 2007 | 2007 | 2/3/4 | 2,039 | 24–74 | 48hr recall. Face-to-face interview. | | N | (53, 54) |
| | FINDIET 2002 | 2002 | 3 | 13,437 | 25–34, 35–44, 45–54, 55–64, 65–74 | 48hr recall. Face-to-face interview. | | N | (55) |
| | FINDIET 1997 | 1997 | 5 | 3,152 | 25–74 | 24hr recall | | N | (56) |
| | FINDIET1992 | 1992 | 4/5 | 1,861 | 25–64 | 3-day diary | | N | (57) |
| France* | ESTEBAN | 2015–16 | 2 | 3,617 | Children 6–17 1,108; adults 18–74 2,509. | 3×24hr recall | | N | Not yet available. |
| | Enquête Nutri-Bébé 2013 | 2013 | 3 | 1,184 | 15 d–35 m | 3-day weighed diary (non-consecutive). Face-to-face interview. | | N | (58) |
| | Individual national food consumption survey (INCA2) | 2006–2007 | 3 | 4,079 | 3–79 | 7-day diary (consecutive). Self-completed. | Food Composition Database of CIQUAL of Afssa. | Y | (59) |

*Continued*

*Table 2.* Continued

| Country* | Survey name | Survey year | Source ** | Sample size | Sample age | Dietary methodology | Nutrient reference database† | Energy intake graphed Y/N‡ | Reference |
|---|---|---|---|---|---|---|---|---|---|
| | Etude nationale nutrition sante (ENNS); National nutrition and health survey | 2006–2007 | 2/4 | 4,780 | Children 3–17 1, 665; adults 18–74 3,115. | 3×24hr recall (non-consecutive) | | N | (60) |
| | Enquête Nutri-Bébé 2005 | 2005 | 3 | 706 | 1–36 m | 3-day weighed diary (non-consecutive inc weekend). Face-to-face interview. | | N | (61) |
| | Individual national food consumption survey (INCA) | 1998–1999 | 5 | 1,0181,985 | 3–1415+ | 7-day diary. | | N | (62) |
| | Enquête Nutri-Bébé 1997 | 1997 | 3 | 660 | 0–30 m | 3-day weighed diary. Face-to-face interview. | | N | (63) |
| | National food consumption survey (ASPCC) | 1993–1994 | 5 | 1,500 | 2–85 | 7-day diary. | | N | (64) |
| Georgia | None found | | | | | | | | |
| Germany | German national nutrition survey (Nationale Verzehr-studie) II (NVSII) | 2005–2007 | 2/4 | 15,371 | 14–80 | DISHES diet history interview, 24hr recall, diet weighing diary (2×4 days). Face-to-face electronic interview. | Bundeslebensmittelschlüs-sel (BLS) | Y | (65, 66) |
| | Der Kinder- und Jugendge-sundheitssurvey (KiGGS) | 2003–2006 | 3 | 17,641 | 0–17 | Questionnaire. | | N | (67) |
| | German nutrition survey 1998 | 1997–1999 | 4/5 | 3,861 | 20–79 | FFQ | | N | (68) |
| Greece | HYDRIA – Greek national diet and health survey | 2013–14 | 2 | 4,011 | 18+ | 2×24hr recall; food propensity questionnaire. Face-to-face interview. | | N | (69, 70) |
| | Nutrient intakes of toddlers and pre-schoolers in Greece: The GENESIS study | 2003–2004 | 3 | 2,374 | 1–5 | 3-day diary (includes nutrient data). Face-to-face interview. | | N | (71) |
| Hungary* | Hungarian diet and nutri-tional status survey (OTÁP 2014) | 2014 | 2 | 857 | 18–34, 35–64, 64+ | 3-day diary (non-consecutive). Self-completed. | | N | Not yet available. |
| | Hungarian diet and nutri-tional status survey (OTÁP 2009) | 2009 | 2 | 1,165 | 18–34, 35–64, 64+ | 3-day diary (non-consecutive), Self-completed. | Nutricomp. | N | (72) |
| | Hungarian dietary survey 2009 | 2009 | 3 | 3,077 | 19–30, 31–60, 60+ | 3-day diary (non-consecutive), FFQ, self-completed. | Új tápanyagtáblázat. | Y | (73, 74) |

*Continued*

*Table 2.* Continued

| Country* | Survey name | Survey year | Source ** | Sample size | Sample age | Dietary methodology | Nutrient reference database† | Energy intake graphed Y/N‡ | Reference |
|---|---|---|---|---|---|---|---|---|---|
| | 3rd National Hungarian survey | 2003 | 4 | 3,633 | 18–100 | Multiple dietary diary. | | N | (75) |
| | 2nd National Hungarian survey | 1992–1994 | 4/5 | 2,559 | 18–100 | 3×24hr recall + FFQ | | N | (76) |
| Iceland* | The diet of Icelanders – a national dietary survey 2010–2011 | 2010–2011 | 2 | 1,312 | 18–80 | 2×24hr recall + FFQ. Telephone interview. | Icelandic Database of Food Ingredients (ÍSGEM); Public Health Institute for Raw Materials in the Icelandic Market. | Y | (77–79) |
| | The diet of Icelanders, dietary survey of the Icelandic nutrition council 2002 | 2002 | 4 | 1,118 | 15–80 | Single dietary diary. | | N | (80) |
| | Dietary survey of the Icelanders | 1990 | 4/5 | 1,240 | 15–80 | Diet history. | | N | (81) |
| Ireland* | National pre-school nutrition survey | 2010–2011 | 2 | 500 | 1–4 | 4-day weighed food diary (consecutive). Self-completed (by carer). | McCance and Widdowson's The Composition of Foods 5&6 editions | Y | (82) |
| | National adult nutrition survey 2011 (NANS) | 2008–2010 | 2 | 1,500 | 18–90 | 4-day semi-weighed food diary (consecutive). Self-completed. | McCance and Widdowson's The Composition of Foods 5&6 editions | Y | (83, 84) |
| | Survey of lifestyle, attitudes and nutrition in Ireland (SLAN), 2007 | 2007 | 3/4 | 9,223 | 18+ | FFQ. Face-to-face interview. | | N | (85, 86) |
| | National teens' food survey | 2005–2006 | 2 | 441 | 13–17 | 7-day semi-weighed food diary (consecutive). Self-completed. | McCance and Widdowson's The Composition of Foods 5&6 editions | Y | (87) |
| | National children's food survey. | 2003–2004 | 2 | 594 | 5–12 | 7-day weighed food diary (consecutive). Self-completed. | McCance and Widdowson's The Composition of Foods 5&6 editions | Y | (88) |
| | SLAN 2002 | 2002 | 3 | 5,992 | 18+ | Semi-quantitative FFQ. | | N | |
| | SLAN 1998 | 1998 | 3 | 6,539 | 18+ | Semi-quantitative FFQ. | | N | |
| | North-South food consumption survey | 1998 | 5 | 1,379 | 18–64 | 7-day diary. Self-completed. | | N | (89) |
| | Irish national nutrition survey | 1990 | 5 | 1,214 | 8–18+ | Diet history. | | N | (90) |

*Continued*

*Table 2.* Continued

| Country* | Survey name | Survey year | Source ** | Sample size | Sample age | Dietary methodology | Nutrient reference database† | Energy intake graphed Y/N‡ | Reference |
|---|---|---|---|---|---|---|---|---|---|
| Israel* | Mabat national health and nutrition survey of the Elderly (Zahav) | 2005–2006 | 4 | 1,782 | 65–100 | Single dietary diary. | | N | |
| | Mabat first Israeli national health and nutrition survey | 1999–2001 | 4 | 3,240 | 25–64 | Single dietary diary. | | N | |
| Italy | The third Italian national food consumption survey INRAN-SCAI 2005-2006 | 2005–2006 | 3 | 3,323 | 0.1–97.7 | 3-day diary (consecutive). Self-completed. | Banca Dati di Composizione degli Alimenti. INRAN-DIARIO 3.1 | Y | (91) |
| | INN-CA 1994–1996 | 1994–1996 | 4/5 | 2,734 | 0–94 | 7-day weighed diary. Self-completed. | | N | (92) |
| Kazakhstan | Nutritional and health status survey of the population in Kazakhstan | 2008 | 6 | 3,526 | 15–59 | 2×24hr recall | | N | |
| Kyrgyzstan | None found | | | | | | | | |
| Latvia | National diet survey 2012–14 | 2012–2014 | 2 | 3,418 | 0–74 | 2×24hr recall (non-consecutive), FFQ, dietary diary | | N | Results not yet available |
| | Latvian national food consumption survey 2007–2009 | 2008 | 2 | 1,949 | 7–64 | 2×24hr recall (non-consecutive), FFQ. Face-to-face interview. | Latvian National Food Composition Data Base 2009 | Y | (93) |
| | Nutrition and lifestyle in the Baltic Republics | 1997 | 1/4 | 2,299 | 19–64 | 24hr recall + questionnaire | | N | (50, 51) |
| Lithuania | Study of actual nutrition and nutrition habits of Lithuanian adult population | 2013–2014 | 2 | 2,513 | 19–75 | 24hr recall + questionnaire. Face-to-face interview, | EuroFIR Food Classification | Y | (94) |
| | Food consumption survey in adult Lithuanian population | 2007 | 1/2 | 1,936 | 19–65 | 24hr recall. | | N | (95, 96) |
| | Nutrition and lifestyle in the Baltic Republics | 1997 | 1/4/5 | 2,094 | 20–65 | 24hr recall + questionnaire | | N | (50, 51) |
| Luxembourg | None found | | | | | | | | |
| Malta | None found | | | | | | | | |
| Monaco | None found | | | | | | | | |
| Montenegro | None found | | | | | | | | |
| Netherlands* | Dutch national food consumption survey 2012–2016 (DNFCS 2012–16) | 2012–2016 | 2 | 4,340 | 1–79 | 2×24hr recall and 1-day food diary (some age groups), FFQ. | | N | Not yet available: (97) |

*Continued*

*Table 2.* Continued

| Country* | Survey name | Survey year | Source ** | Sample size | Sample age | Dietary methodology | Nutrient reference database† | Energy intake graphed Y/N‡ | Reference |
|---|---|---|---|---|---|---|---|---|---|
| | Dutch national food consumption survey 2007–2010 (DNFCS 2007–10) | 2007–2010 | 2/3 | 3,819 | 7–69 | 2×24hr recall. Telephone (adults)/face-to-face (children) interview, FFQ. | Dutch Food Composition Database (NEVO) | Y | (98–100) |
| | Dutch national food consumption survey – young children (DNFCS 2008) | 2005–2006 | 2 | 1,279 | 2–6 | 2-day diary (non-consecutive). Self-completed (by adult), FFQ. | Dutch Food Composition Database (NEVO) | Y | (101) |
| | Dutch national food consumption survey (DNFCS 2003) | 2003 | 2/4 | 750 | 19–30 | 2×24hr recall (non-consecutive, telephone). | | N | (102) |
| | Dutch national food consumption survey (DNFCS-3) 1997–1998 | 1997–1998 | 2/4/5 | 6,250 | 1–97 | 2-day diary. | | N | (103) |
| | Dutch national food consumption survey (DNFCS-2) 1992 | 1992 | 2/4/5 | 6,218 | 1–92 | 2-day diary. | | N | (103) |
| Norway* | UNGKOST 3 | 2015–2016 | 2 | 1,721 | 4–13 | 4-day online diary plus FFQ (consecutive). Self-completed via web. | The Norwegian Food Composition Tables | Y | (104, 105) |
| | Norwegian national diet survey NORKOST3 | 2010–2011 | 3 | 1,787 | 18–70 | 2×24hr recall and FFQ. Telephone interview. | The Norwegian Food Composition Tables | Y | (106) |
| | Sub-sample of NOWAC (component of EPIC) | 2002 | 1 | 2,000 (female) | 46–75 | FFQ | | N | (107) |
| | UNGKOST-2000 | 2000 | 3 | 3948151,009 | 4, 9 and 13 | 4-day diary, self-completed. | | N | (108) |
| | Norwegian national dietary survey (NORKOST 1997) | 1997 | 4/5 | 2,672 | 16–79 | FFQ | | N | (109) |
| | Norwegian national diet survey (NORKOST 1993–1994). | 1993–1994 | 1/5 | 3,144 | 16–79 | FFQ | | N | (110) |
| | UNGKOST-1993 | 1993 | 5 | 1,7051,564 | 1318 | FFQ | | N | (111) |
| | Pilot study | 1992 | 1 | 1,200 | 16–79 | FFQ | | N | (110) |
| Poland* | WOBASZ II study | 2013–2014 | 3 | 6,170 | 20+ | 24hr recall and FFQ. Face-to-face interview. | | N | (112) |
| | WOBASZ-national multicentre health survey | 2003–2005 | 4 | 6,661 | 20–74 | Single dietary diary | | N | |
| | Sub-sample of the household food consumption and anthropometric survey | 2000 | 4/5 | 4,200 | 1–100 | 24hr recall, face-to-face interview. | | N | (113) |

*Continued*

*Table 2.* Continued

| Country* | Survey name | Survey year | Source ** | Sample size | Sample age | Dietary methodology | Nutrient reference database† | Energy intake graphed Y/N‡ | Reference |
|---|---|---|---|---|---|---|---|---|---|
| | Dietary habits and nutritional status of selected populations | 1991–1994 | 5 | 1,1262, 1934,945 | 11–141820–65 | 24hr recall. | | N | (114, 115) |
| Portugal | National food and physical activity survey (IAN-AF) | 2015–2016 | 6 | 4,221 | 3 m–84 y | 2×24hr recall (non-consecutive) and FPQ (electronic interview), 2-day food diary for children <10 years. Face-to-face electronic interview. | Portuguese Food Composition Table (INSA) | Y | (116, 117) |
| | Dietary calcium and body mass index in Portuguese children | 2002–2003 | 3 | 4,511 | 7–9 | 24hr recall, face-to–face interview. | | N | (118) |
| Republic of Moldova | None found | | | | | | | | |
| Romania | National synthesis, 2006 | 2006 | 4 | 1,036 | 19–100 | FFQ | | | |
| Russian federation* | The Russia longitudinal monitoring survey – higher school of economics (RLMS-HSE) | 2011–2012 | 2/3 | 21,686 | 0–102 | 24hr recall. | | N | (119) |
| | The Russia longitudinal monitoring survey – higher school of economics (RLMS-HSE) | 1994, 1995, 1996, 1998, 2000, 2001, 2002, 2003, 2004, 2005 | 2 | 1994–11,295, 1995–10,632, 1996–10,448, 1998–10,663, 2000–10,969, 2001–12,100, 2002–12,489, 2003–12,634, 2004–12,639, 2005–12,228. | 0–102 | 24hr recall. | | N | (120) |
| San Marino | None found | | | | | | | | |
| Serbia | None found | | | | | | | | |
| Slovakia‡‡ | Nutrient intake in the adult population of the Slovak Republic | 1991–1994 & 1995–1999 | 1 | 4,018 | 19–80 | 24hr recall. Face-to-face interview. | | N | (121, 122) |
| | Nutrient intake in children and adolescents in Slovakia | 1991–1999 | 5 | 3,3374,556 | 11–1415–18 | 24hr recall and FFQ. | | N | (122) |
| Slovenia | Dietary intake of macro – and micronutrients in Slovenian adolescents | 2012 | 3 | 2,224 | 15–16 | FFQ, self-completed. | | N | (123) |

*Continued*

*Table 2.* Continued

| Country* | Survey name | Survey year | Source ** | Sample size | Sample age | Dietary methodology | Nutrient reference database† | Energy intake graphed Y/N‡ | Reference |
|---|---|---|---|---|---|---|---|---|---|
| | Dietary habits of the adult population Slovenia in health protection | 2007–2008 | 2 | 1,193 | 18–65 | 2×24hr recall (non-consecutive), FFQ. Face-to-face interview, | | N | (124) |
| Spain* | ENALIA 2 study | 2014–2015 | 3 | 933 plus 157 pregnant women. | 18–74 | 2×24hr recall, FFQ. Face-to-face electronic interview. | | N | (125)Nutrient intake data not yet available. |
| | ENALIA study | 2012–2014 | 3 | 1,780 | 6 m–17 | 2×1-day diary (<11 years); 2×24hr recall (11+); FFQ (all). | | N | (126)Nutrient intake data not yet available. |
| | ANIBES study | 2013 | 3 | 2,285 | 9–75 | 3-day diary + 24hr recall (consecutive). Face-to-face interview, telephone (interview), tablet and camera (self-report). | Tablas de Composición de Alimentos, 15ª ed | Y (children only) | (28–30) |
| | ENIDE study (Sobre datos de la Encuesta Nacionalde Ingesta Dietética) | 2009–2010 | 3 | 3,000 | 18–24; 25–44; 45–64 | 3-day diary + 24hr recall (consecutive). Interview and self-completed. | Base de Datos Española de Composición de Alimentos – RedBEDCA | Y | (127–130) |
| | The Catalan nutrition survey (ENCAT 2002–2003) | 2003 | 4 | 1,923 | 10–100 | 2×24hr recall (non-consecutive), face-to-face interview, FFQ. | | N | |
| | EnKid study | 1998–2000 | 3 | 3,534 | 2–24 | 24hr recall (×2 in 25% sample), face-to-face interview. FFQ. | | N | (131, 132) |
| Sweden* | Riksmaten adolescents | 2016–2017 | 2 | ? | 11–12; 14–15; 17–19 | 2×24hr recall. | | N | Data collection not yet completed. |
| | Riksmaten 2010–2011 Swedish adults dietary survey | 2010–2011 | 3 | 1,797 | 18–80 | 4-day food diary (consecutive). Self-completed via web. | NFA Food Composition Database | Y | (133) |
| | Riksmaten-barn 2003 Swedish children's dietary survey | 2003 | 3 | 590, 889, 1,016 | 4 y, 8–9, 11–12 | 4-day food diary (consecutive), self-completed >4 years, by adult 4 years. | | N | (134) |
| | Riksmaten 1997–1998 | 1997–1998 | 4/5 | 1,214 | 18–74 | 7-day diary. | | N | (135) |
| Switzerland | MenuCH | 2014–15 | 2 | | | | | N | |
| | National nutrition survey Switzerland (NANUSS). Pilot for MenuCH. | 2008–2009 | 2 | | | | | N | |
| Tajikistan | None found | | | | | | | | |

*Continued*

*Table 2.* Continued

| Country* | Survey name | Survey year | Source ** | Sample size | Sample age | Dietary methodology | Nutrient reference database† | Energy intake graphed Y/N‡ | Reference |
|---|---|---|---|---|---|---|---|---|---|
| The former Yugoslav Republic of Macedonia | First Macedonian food consumption survey | 2015 | 6 | 504 | 16+ | 2×24hr recall. Interview. | | N | Report not yet available. |
| Turkey | Turkey nutrition and health survey 2010 (TNHS) | 2010 | 3 | 14,248 | 0–100 | 24hr recall, FFQ. Face-to-face interview. | BEBS Nutritional Information System Software; Turkish Food Composition Database | Y | (136, 137) |
| Turkmenistan | None found | | | | | | | | |
| United Kingdom* | National diet and nutrition survey rolling programme Y5–6 (NDNS RP 2012–2014 ) | 2012–2014 | 3 | 2,546 | 1.5–94 | 4-day diary (consecutive). Self-completed. | | N | (138) |
| | National diet and nutrition survey rolling programme (NDNS RP 2008–2012) | 2008–2012 | 3 | 6,828 | 1.5–94 | 4-day diary (consecutive). Self-completed. | McCance and Widdowson's The Composition of Foods integrated dataset | Y | (139) |
| | Low income diet and health survey (LIDNS) | 2003–2005 | 4 | | 2–100 | 4×24hr recall. | | N | (140) |
| | NDNS 2000–2001 adults | 2000–2001 | 4 | 1,724 | 19–64 | 7-day weighed dietary diaries. | | N | (141) |
| | NDNS 1997 children | 1997 | | 1,701 | 4–18 | 7-day weighed dietary diaries. | | N | (142) |
| | NDNS 1994–1995 65 years and over | 1994–1995 | 4 | 1,275 | 65–100 | Single dietary diary. | | N | (143) |
| Ukraine | None found | | | | | | | | |
| Uzbekistan | None found | | | | | | | | |

*Countries conducting long-running surveys comprising of multiple collection waves.

**1 = database searches; 2 = email contacts; 3 = general Internet searches; 4 = Micha et al. (5); 5 = European Food Consumption Survey 2001 (6); 6) WHO Global Nutrition Policy Review 2017 extracted information.

†Information regarding nutrient composition databases has been added for those surveys for which energy and nutrient intakes were reported and graphed.

‡Y = energy intakes were taken from the latest survey for which they were reported; N = energy and nutrient intakes were either not reported or were not extracted because intakes for that country were available in a later survey.

‡‡The Slovakian surveys were not truly nationally representative, but were country-wide and designed to 'recruit a diverse sample of subjects of different age categories and socio-economic background' (121).

NB – The EFSA guidance for the standardised collection of national food consumption data was released in 2009.

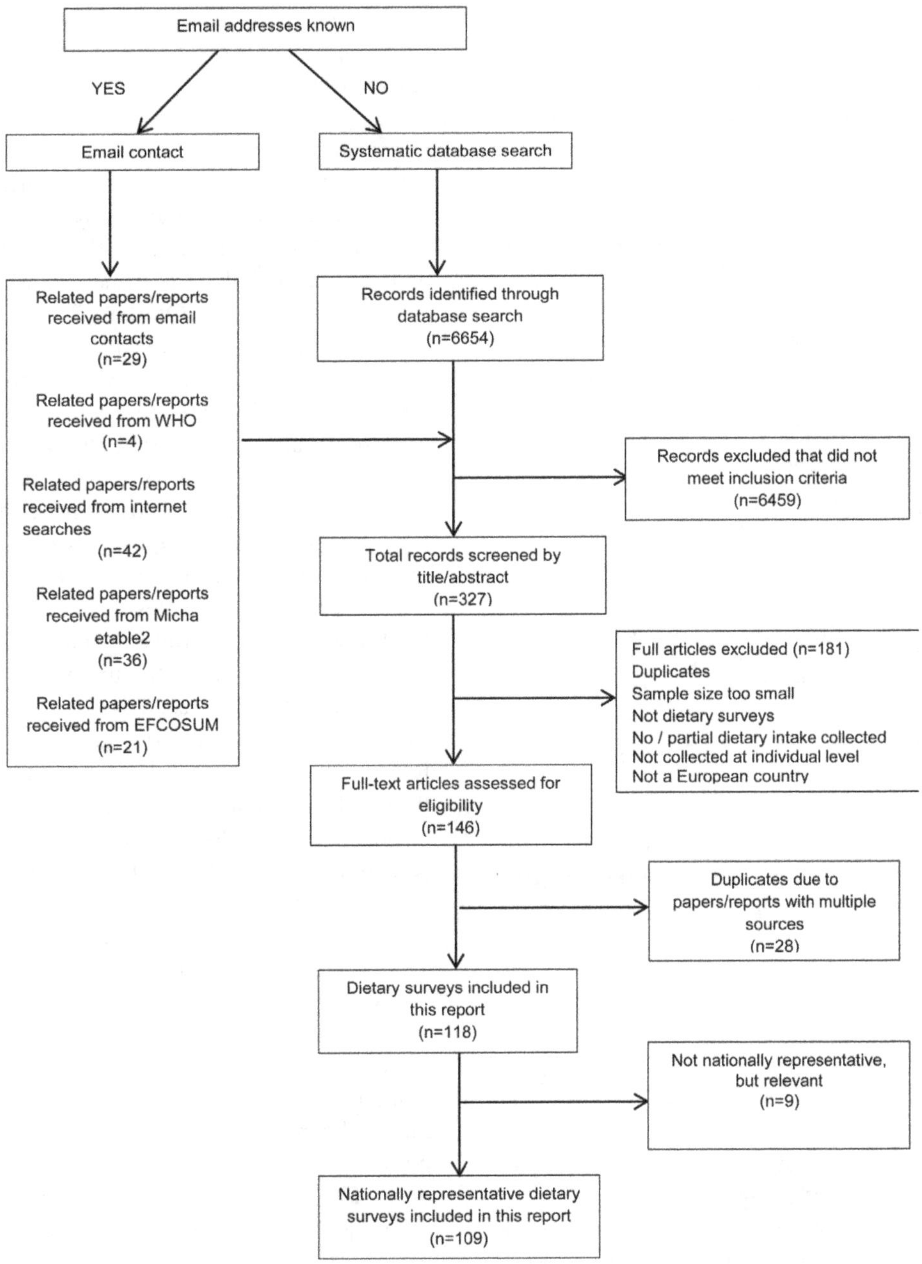


*Fig. 1.* Screening and selection of national dietary surveys.

No nationally representative surveys were found by any method that collected dietary intake of whole diets at individual level for 19 European countries (see Table 3 and Fig. 2). Although one survey of children was found for Croatia, it was not nationally representative (7). In addition, no nationally representative surveys have been found for Slovakia that have been conducted since 2000, and none for Bulgaria and Czech Republic since 2005. In Western Europe, no surveys have been found for Italy or Israel conducted since 2006, or for Andorra since 2005.

Of the 109 nationally representative surveys, 45 obtained dietary information on both adults and children, a further 41 surveys collected dietary information on adults aged 18+ only and 23 on children aged <18 only. For the 86 surveys that included adults, 60 across 30 countries were conducted since 2000. Of the 68 surveys that included children, 48 were conducted since 2000 and spanned 27 countries. Nationally representative surveys for children were missing in nine countries: Croatia, Finland, Hungary, Israel, Lithuania, Luxembourg, Romania, Slovakia and Switzerland. Further gaps were found for Andorran children aged <12 years; Bulgarian children aged above 5 years; Icelandic, Kazakh and Slovenian children aged <15 years; Macedonian children aged

*Table 3.* Level of nationally representative survey provision by country

| Countries with no surveys | Countries with pre-2000 surveys only | Countries with post-2000 surveys without reports of energy and nutrient intakes | Countries with post-2000 survey plus energy and nutrient intakes |
|---|---|---|---|
| Albania | Slovakia | Czech Republic | Andorra |
| Armenia | | Estonia | Austria |
| Azerbaijan | | Greece | Belgium |
| Belarus | | Israel | Bulgaria |
| Bosnia and Herzegovina | | Kazakhstan | Cyprus |
| Croatia | | Poland | Denmark |
| Georgia | | Romania | Finland |
| Kyrgyzstan | | Russian Federation | France |
| Luxembourg | | Slovenia | Germany |
| Malta | | Switzerland | Hungary |
| Monaco | | The former Yugoslav Republic of Macedonia | Iceland |
| Montenegro | | | Ireland |
| Republic of Moldova | | | Italy |
| San Marino | | | Latvia |
| Serbia | | | Lithuania |
| Tajikistan | | | The Netherlands |
| Turkmenistan | | | Norway |
| Ukraine | | | Portugal |
| Uzbekistan | | | Spain |
| | | | Sweden |
| | | | Turkey |
| | | | United Kingdom |

<16 years; Polish children post-2000 and Spanish micronutrient intake in children of all ages.

Non-nationally representative dietary surveys were found for eight countries (Croatia, Czech Republic, Germany, Greece, Iceland, Luxembourg, Russia and Switzerland), but because of our exclusion criteria they were not included in the list of nationally representative surveys in Table 2. Additionally, 16 studies conducted in Central and Eastern European countries were returned from the systematic literature search in English and 49 from the WHO Russian language database search and were not included in any tables; common reasons for rejection were no or partial dietary intake collected, data not collected at individual level, duplicate and sample size too small (<200). Eight countries completed the WHO STEPwise approach to noncommunicable disease risk factor surveillance (STEPS) adult survey (8–15). However, although these were nationally representative population-based surveys with large sample sizes, they were not included in this review because they only covered specific food groups, not whole diets, and as such did not meet our inclusion criteria.

### *Dietary methodologies*

The most common dietary assessment methodologies used across the 109 nationally representative surveys were the 24hr recall and food diary. Of these surveys, 45 used 24hr recall, 35 of which were surveys conducted since 2000 (Table 2). Of the 45 surveys using 24hr recall, the range of daily recalls was 1–4; 29 surveys used *multiple* 24hr recalls, 26 of which were conducted post-2000. Table 2 illustrates that where countries used both 24hr recall and food diaries, this was a combination of methodological changes in waves of long-running surveys, different surveys using different methodologies or both methods being employed within the same survey for different population groups, for example, adults and children. A 2×24hr recall is the method recommended by the European Food Safety Authority (EFSA) for adults' NDS (16). Countries with surveys conducted post-2000 using multiple 24hr recall were Austria, Belgium, Bulgaria, Czech Republic, Estonia, Finland, France, Greece, Iceland, Kazakhstan, Latvia, the Netherlands, Norway, Portugal, Slovenia, Spain, Sweden, the former Yugoslav Republic of Macedonia and the United Kingdom. Spain calculated usual nutrient intake from 24hr recall and a 3-day dietary diary.

Food diaries were used as a primary method by 47 surveys, 33 of which were conducted post-2000. The range of diary days per survey was 1–7. Thirty-eight surveys used *multiple* day diaries as the primary method, and 26 of these were conducted post-2000 from the following countries: Austria, Cyprus, Denmark, France, Greece, Hungary, Ireland, Italy, the Netherlands, Norway, Sweden and the United Kingdom. The majority of these were performed over consecutive days. Weighed diaries were used as the sole method by some surveys in France, Ireland, Italy and the United Kingdom, but also as a primary method by one survey in Germany.

Food frequency questionnaires (FFQs) were used by 12 surveys, 5 of which were conducted post-2000 (Estonia, Ireland, Norway, Romania and Slovenia). FFQs were used by Ireland, Norway and Slovenia in pre-2000 surveys and as a supplementary, rather than primary, dietary assessment tool by other countries (Andorra, Belgium, Greece, Hungary, Iceland, Latvia, Lithuania, the Netherlands, Poland, Slovakia, Spain and Turkey).

Of the 28 surveys that reported energy and nutrient intakes (see Table 2 for older NDS approaches where available), 10 used interviews – these were primarily ($n$ = 8) face-to-face rather than telephone-based, and 3 of these were electronic, for example, computer or tablet-based.

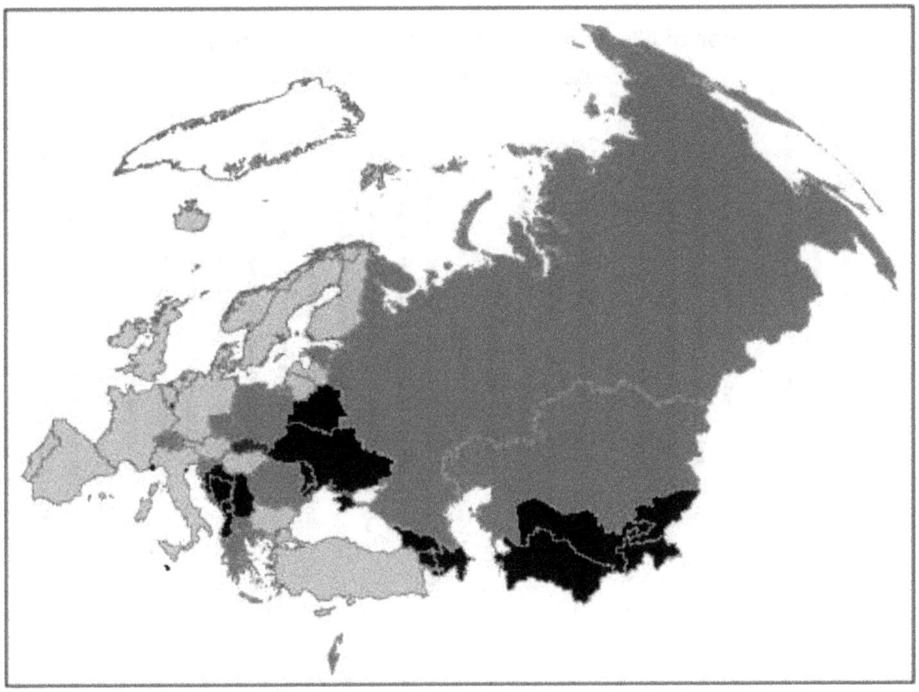

*Fig. 2.* Map of national dietary survey provision by country. Light grey – Post-2000 survey plus nutrient intakes (28 surveys in 22 countries). Medium grey – Post-2000 survey (78 surveys in 33 countries). Medium-dark grey – Pre-2000 survey (3 surveys in 1 country). Dark grey – No survey (19 countries). White – countries not in the WHO Europe remit.

Respondents self-completed in 11 surveys, which were all food diaries. Electronic resources were utilised in five surveys, just two of which were web-based. Five surveys used multiple approaches – these were mainly a combination of face-to-face and telephonic interviews with the exception of Spain, which used both interview forms plus a tablet and camera-photos.

### *Energy and nutrient coverage*

Of the 22 countries that had post-2000 nationally representative survey reports of energy and nutrient intakes, 20 countries reported data for adults and 16 countries for children. This was provided by 28 of the latest post-2000 surveys that reported energy and nutrient data for these countries; 13 surveys included both adults and children, 8 surveyed adults only and 7 sampled children only (3 being separate surveys of children in Ireland). Table 2 identifies these 28 surveys and illustrates their differing methodological approaches.

All 28 surveys included energy and also carbohydrate, fibre, fat and protein intakes. Most surveys ($n$ = 25) included intake data on saturated fat (Germany and the Irish child and teen surveys did not): MUFAs ($n$ = 25) (Germany, Irish child and teen surveys did not) and PUFAs ($n$ = 24) (Germany, Irish child and teen surveys, and the Dutch DNFCS young children did not). See Appendix 2 and Fig. 3 for tabular and graphical summaries of the macronutrients included by each survey. The majority of surveys ($n$ = 21) included intake levels of sugars in some form, either as total sugars or as added sugars or sucrose. However, Cyprus, Germany, the Irish child and teen surveys, Latvia, the Spanish ENIDE survey and Turkey included neither. Given current concerns about sugar consumption, this is an important gap. Few surveys ($n$ = 6) included data on starch intakes and less than half ($n$ = 9) included trans-fatty acid (TFA) intakes (see Appendix 2).

All surveys with the exception of the Spanish ANIBES study included some micronutrients of interest (see Appendix 3 and Fig. 4). However, none of the micronutrients investigated was reported by every survey. Vitamin A, riboflavin, thiamine, vitamin B6, vitamin B12, vitamin C, vitamin D, calcium, magnesium and iron were reported by 26 or more surveys. Copper (13), iodine (13), selenium (11) and fluoride (1 – not tabled) were reported by fewer than half the surveys.

## Discussion

### *Data collection*

This report details the initial findings of a review into dietary surveys across the 53 countries within the WHO Europe remit (17). Nationally representative surveys which collected data on whole diets at individual level

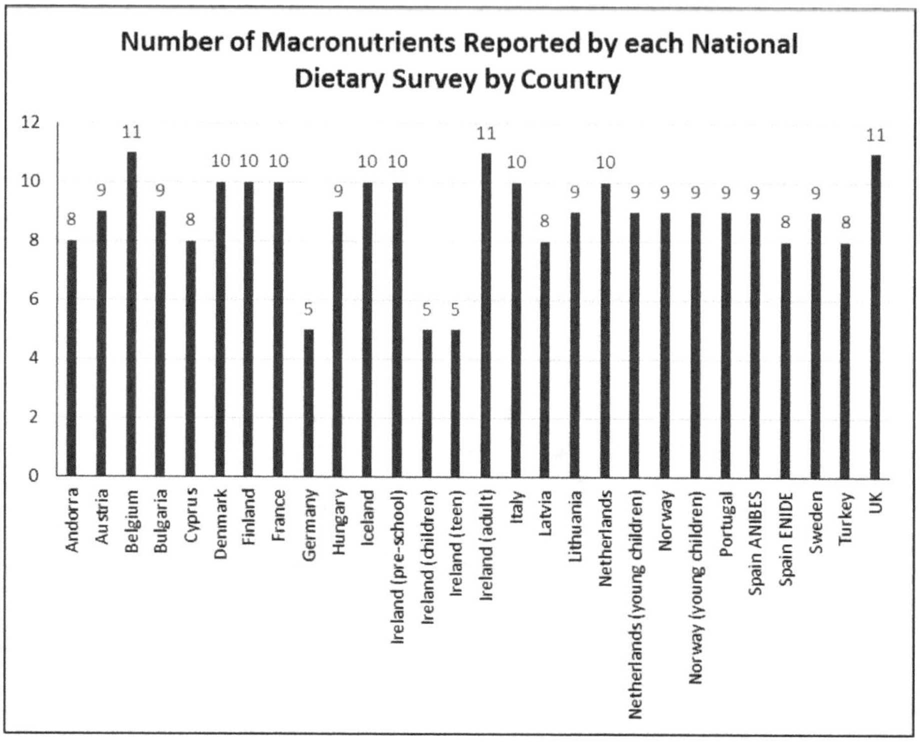


*Fig. 3.* Number of macronutrients reported by each national dietary survey by country*: *Where 12 is the maximum potential number of selected macronutrients of interest being reported in NDS reports: energy, protein, carbohydrate, sugars, sucrose, starches, fibre, total fat, saturated fat, monounsaturated fatty acids (MUFA), polyunsaturated fatty acids (PUFA) and trans-fatty acids (TFA).

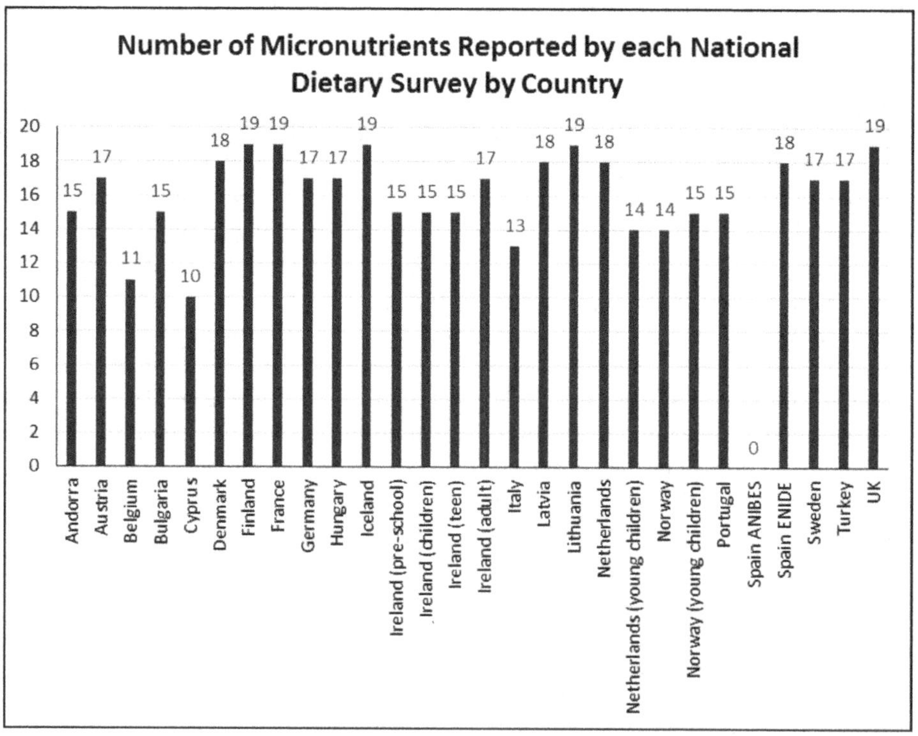


*Fig. 4.* Number of micronutrients reported by each national dietary survey by country*: *Where 19 is the maximum potential number of selected micronutrients of interest being reported in NDS reports: folate (B9), niacin (B3), vitamin A, riboflavin (B2), thiamine (B1), vitamin B12 (biotin), vitamin B6 (pyridoxine), vitamin C, vitamin D, vitamin E, calcium, magnesium, potassium, sodium, iron, copper, iodine, selenium and zinc.

since 1990 were found for only 64% of countries, the main gaps clearly lying in 17 countries in the Central and Eastern European region of the WHO Europe remit. Although eight countries without NDS had recently completed a comprehensive WHO STEPS survey, including questions on fruit and vegetable intake, salt consumption and use of fats and oils in cooking and eating, the survey does not address whole diets and only included adults; therefore, this represents a knowledge gap. However, non-nationally representative surveys were found in two countries that had no other NDS, which demonstrates that although some countries have no nationally representative surveys, other initiatives are in place and the expertise and fieldwork experience needed to conduct NDS may be present. All Western European countries had published survey information after 2000. Of countries with NDS, 16 conducted long-running surveys with multiple collection waves, which could generate important information for trends analysis. Fewer surveys were available that measured diet in children than adults; again gaps were primarily in Central and Eastern European countries. This implies that nutrition policies in this region are based on limited data, which is of concern, as overweight and obesity have tripled in some of these countries since 1980 and NCD prevalence rates are reaching those of Western Europe (1).

Emailing nutrition experts and general Internet searches were the most successful data gathering methods. A major source for contacts and survey information was a global survey review from 1990 to 2010 (5). Few academic papers met the pre-set inclusion criteria in the systematic database search performed for countries – particularly Central and Eastern countries – with no surveys or contacts mentioned in previous reviews, which also minimises the risk of bias. A possible explanation is that survey results and characteristics may be published as government or other official reports rather than academic papers. However, we also undertook wider web-based searches, targeting known government and public health agencies using various search terms to account for this. Another reason is that dietary assessment in large-scale studies like national diet surveys is costly, due to the labour-intensive nature of study preparation and data collection, and therefore may not be undertaken by some countries (18). This could explain the disproportionate concentration of gaps in survey provision in Central and Eastern European countries, which tend to have lower national incomes (19). This highlights a need to clarify major barriers and work with countries to establish mechanisms to overcome these and subsequently to devise and implement NDS.

### *Dietary methodologies of post-2000 surveys*

The most common methods of collecting dietary intake used in the 78 post-2000 surveys were the 24hr recall and food diary, the majority of which were collected over multiple days. Although 24hr recalls are known for under-reporting (20), their increased use could reflect their advantage in being less onerous for respondents and potentially providing more consistent results across all age and sex groups compared with other methods (21). Retrospective dietary recalls can provide detailed information on eating patterns and exert less influence on food choice than food diaries (22), thereby generating a more accurate and realistic report on population nutrient intake. However, such short-term dietary assessment methods are associated with within-person errors and wider variation of intakes within the population, particularly when intakes of only 1 or 2 days are collected, the latter as recommended by EFSA (16). Although FFQs provide long-term assessment, they nevertheless can present inflated energy and nutrient intakes (21), which could explain why few post-2000 surveys used FFQs as the primary dietary assessment method.

Prospective weighed and non-weighed food diaries allow very detailed information to be gathered on multiple days (22) and are sometimes used to validate other methods using a small sub-sample, but have a high respondent burden and like the 24hr recall, are susceptible to under-reporting (23). Food dairies with weighed intake are particularly burdensome and prone to response bias and respondent fatigue (24) – most likely the reason why fewer studies used it as a primary assessment method and the United Kingdom moved from weighed intake to estimated intake.

Many studies used multiple tools to collect food intake. Of the 22 countries for which energy and nutrient intakes were reported, all surveys that collected dietary intake using more than one tool generated energy and nutrient intake data from a primary method and used the other method(s) as a means of validation and calibration. The exception was Spain, which was the only country that used a truly mixed methods approach. Food diaries and 24hr recalls do not provide insight into usual intakes, whereas FFQs are less accurate in estimating individuals' absolute intakes; combining methods could help rectify these shortcomings (24). Spain, Belgium and the Netherlands estimated 'usual' intakes using the Statistical Program to Assess Dietary Exposure (SPADE), although the Dutch intakes presented by age group in this report reflect the average of actual intakes reported by individuals. Of the other countries employing FFQ as a supplementary method, Greece and Iceland also explicitly stated that this was used to estimate usual intake. This approach is designed to overcome within-person errors and wider intake variations when only 2 days of intake have been collected, although methodological limitations cannot be fully negated.

Of the 23 surveys that sampled children only, over half ($n$ = 15) used some form of food diary. This could be because children are expected to remember less retrospectively, so prospective methods of capturing intake, although subject to under-reporting and the limitations mentioned above, are deemed preferable and more accurate. This also fits with EFSA guidance on the collection of national food consumption data, which recommends countries '...use the dietary record method for infants and children and the 24-hour recall method for adults' (16). EFSA further recommend data be collected on two non-consecutive days and that they be supplemented with a food propensity questionnaire (16). It remains to be seen whether more countries will move towards non-consecutive diaries in future surveys; at present, the majority of multiple food diaries are conducted on consecutive days. More detailed methodological recommendations for NDS of children are available via the Pilot study for the Assessment of Nutrient intake and food Consumption Among Kids in Europe (PANCAKE) project (25).

Of the 28 surveys that reported energy and nutrient intakes, Austria, Estonia, Iceland and Norway moved to 2×24hr recall in the latest NDS, perhaps to comply with the latest EFSA guidance (16). The United Kingdom switched from a 7-day weighed to a 4-day estimated food diary, which is more likely a move to reduce respondent burden. Although methodological changes make comparisons problematic across survey waves, the move towards a common approach will ease comparisons between countries in the long term and should be actively encouraged in line with EFSA recommendations. Although this could be logistically and financially challenging, it would assist in making inter-country comparisons and identifying vulnerable groups, thereby enabling the effective targeting of policy resources.

## Technology in national dietary surveys

Care is needed in any dietary assessment method to minimise measurement error. Many dietary assessment methods require highly skilled interviewers, which increases survey costs and presents a potential barrier to conducting NDS (24). Technology like computer-administered interviews and image-capture could help overcome this obstacle and also promote standardised practices. The European Prospective Investigation into Cancer and Nutrition (EPIC)-Soft software package developed by the EPIC Study provided uniform templates for various aspects of NDS including conducting 24hr recall, which has since been modified by the European Food Consumption Validation (EFCOVAL) Study and renamed 'Globodiet'. It aimed for Europe-wide use, but is limited by the need for professionals to be trained in its use (26).

At present, none of the surveys identified used mobile technologies to collect dietary information; although Belgian, German and Portuguese surveys employed electronic interviews, the Spanish ANIBES used tablets and the Norwegian Ungkost3 and Swedish Riksmaten used a web-based food diary. This current lack of use may be due to the lack of validation or differential usability across population groups. However, web-based dietary assessments with self-administered record or recall methodologies have the potential to reduce data entry expense and allow data collection for large numbers on multiple days over different time periods (27). They could therefore be more cost-effective and encourage countries for which cost has been a significant barrier to undertake surveys. For example, myfood24 is an online 24-hour dietary assessment tool that can be used for either of the EFSA-approved (16) 24hr recall or a food diary methods (27). It employs country-specific food databases and is currently in operation in Denmark, Germany and the United Kingdom. Technologies like this could reduce the onus on researchers by automatically coding food records (27). These benefits could encourage countries that historically lack national diet survey provision to undertake surveys and enable countries that already undertake surveys to implement these at more regular intervals. This would serve to increase the amount of dietary and nutrient intake data available in the WHO Europe remit, directly contributing to the WHO objective of strengthening and expanding nationally representative diet and nutrition surveys WHO (1).

### *Energy and nutrient intakes*

Energy and nutrient intake provision was documented from the *latest* survey collected after 2000 for each country for which we could locate intake data. For some countries, more recent surveys had been conducted (see Table 2), but intake data were not yet available in all cases. An additional limitation on data availability was the range of nutrients each survey covered. Of the countries that specified nutrient intakes, Germany and Belgium were the most likely to have gaps in reported intakes of macro- and micronutrients, respectively, and the Spanish ANIBES survey (28–30) only reported macronutrient data (see Appendix 3). This suggests that the reporting of nutrient intakes is inconsistent, making it harder to assess nutrient coverage and make inter-country comparisons.

Inconsistent age groupings across countries also make inter-country comparisons potentially problematic. In Andorra, the youngest age group spanned adults and children, meaning that although children were sampled, intake levels would not be valid in any comparisons. Future investigation could be undertaken using raw data and consistent age groups to obtain more reliable conclusions.

Differences in dietary methodologies may be a limiting factor when making inter-country comparisons. The relatively low levels seen in Turkish adult and child energy intakes compared to other countries could potentially be explained by methodological differences. The Turkish survey used a single 24hr recall, whereas the Belgian, Danish, German, Hungarian, Dutch, Norwegian and Spanish surveys, whilst using different methodologies (see Table 2), all collected data on multiple days. Collection on a single day is more likely to result in error due to less control over day-to-day variation (31).

Lack of alignment and completeness of national food composition databases and classification systems is a further limitation. For example, some food composition databases may not be updated to account for reformulated products, which could introduce differences and potential error in the energy and nutrient content of foods and therefore population intakes as reported in NDS. Common approaches to food composition databases are set out in more detail in the EFCOVAL study (144). Energy and nutrient intake values will be reported and discussed in more detail in future publications (145).

#### *Strengths and limitations*

The strength of the current review is that it presents a unique, current overview of dietary survey characteristics in all WHO Europe countries since 1990. The existence of newer studies such as Bel-Serrat et al. (146) illustrates the fluidity of the situation and the need for updated, comprehensive reviews. This review includes surveys covering both adults and children; therefore, it provides a full picture of the current state of dietary survey provision across the life course. It also discusses methodologies, enabling insights into common methods and paving the way for future exploration of best practice and policy recommendations.

However, the surveys employed different methodologies, both between surveys and within long-running surveys with multiple collection waves, potentially making the task of comparing countries problematic. Despite this, we feel that there is still a need to use the available information to make inter-country comparisons where possible. Another limitation of the review was that we were unable to establish contact with nutrition experts or government officials who may be working in nutrition in some of the 19 countries where no surveys were found, which were mainly Central and Eastern European countries. Therefore, we cannot ascertain that these countries do not have any relevant dietary surveys. We also cannot assure that there are no other nationally representative surveys in countries where we obtained survey information from contacts. However, it is likely that these contacts would be aware of other surveys in their countries; in the distributed questionnaire, contacts were asked for details of all surveys in their country.

### Conclusion

This review found that less than two-thirds of the 53 countries in the WHO European region conducted national diet and nutrition surveys since 1990, with only 22 countries reporting nutrient intake data since 2000. The main survey gaps for both adults and children lie in the Central and Eastern European countries, where nutrition policies may lack an appropriate evidence base. Differing dietary assessment methodologies may have impact on the ability to make inter-country comparisons; existing efforts to harmonise NDS across all ages, particularly guidelines set by EFSA (16), should be encouraged, including beyond Western Europe. It would therefore be beneficial to target future efforts at standardising methodologies and filling knowledge gaps for the countries that have no surveys post-2000 in order to increase the information available for evidence-based policy planning. By establishing which countries have NDS, this review lays the foundation for a future review and stratified analyses of actual nutrient intakes across population groups in Europe.

### References


1. WHO (2014). European food and nutrition action plan 2015–2020. WHO Regional Office for Europe. Copenhagen.
2. Alwan A. Global status report on noncommunicable diseases 2010. World Health Organization; Copenhagen, 2011.
3. Mozaffarian D, Wilson PW, Kannel WB. Beyond established and novel risk factors lifestyle risk factors for cardiovascular disease. Circulation 2008; 117(23): 3031–8.
4. Lim SS, Vos T, Flaxman AD, Danaei G, Shibuya K, Adair-Rohani H, et al. A comparative risk assessment of burden of disease and injury attributable to 67 risk factors and risk factor clusters in 21 regions, 1990–2010: a systematic analysis for the Global Burden of Disease Study 2010. Lancet 2013; 380(9859): 2224–60.
5. Micha R, Khatibzadeh S, Shi P, Fahimi S, Lim S, Andrews KG, et al. Global, regional, and national consumption levels of dietary fats and oils in 1990 and 2010: a systematic analysis including 266 country-specific nutrition surveys. BMJ 2014; 348: g2272.
6. EFCOSUM (2001). European Food Consumption Survey Method Final report. TNO Nutrition and Food Research: Zeist.
7. Barić IC, Cvjetić S, Šatalić Z. Dietary intakes among Croatian schoolchildren and adolescents. Nutr Health 2001; 15(2): 127–38.
8. WHO (forthcoming). STEPS noncommunicable disease risk factor surveillance Republic of Moldova (2013).
9. WHO (forthcoming). STEPS noncommunicable disease risk factor surveillance Krygyzstan (2013).
10. WHO (forthcoming). STEPS noncommunicable disease risk factor surveillance Turkmenistan (2014).
11. WHO (forthcoming). STEPS noncommunicable disease risk factor surveillance Armenia (2016).
12. WHO (forthcoming). STEPS noncommunicable disease risk factor surveillance Belarus (2017).
13. WHO (forthcoming). STEPS noncommunicable disease risk factor surveillance Georgia (2017).
14. WHO (forthcoming). STEPS noncommunicable disease risk factor surveillance Tajikistan (2017).

15. WHO and Ministry of Health of the Republic of Uzbekistan (2014). Uzbekistan STEPS Survey 2014 Factsheet. WHO: Copenhagen.
16. EFSA (2009). General principles for the collection of national food consumption data in the view of a pan-European dietary survey. Parma: EFSA; 2009.
17. WHO (2013). Available from: http://www.euro.who.int/en/health-topics/disease-prevention/nutrition/country-work [cited 23 October 2016].
18. Ocke M, Brants H, Dofkova M, Freisling H, van Rossum C, Ruprich J, et al. Feasibility of dietary assessment methods, other tools and procedures for a pan-European food consumption survey among infants, toddlers and children. Eur J Nutr 2015; 54(5): 721–32.
19. Eurostat (2016). GDP per capita, consumption per capita and price level indices. Available from: http://ec.europa.eu/eurostat/statistics-explained/index.php/GDP_per_capita,_consumption_per_capita_and_price_level_indices [cited 28 November 2016].
20. Holmes B, Nelson M. The strengths and weaknesses of dietary survey methods in materially deprived households in England: A discussion paper. Public Health Nutr 2009; 12(08): 1157–64.
21. Holmes B, Dick K, Nelson M. A comparison of four dietary assessment methods in materially deprived households in England. Public Health Nutr 2008; 11(05): 444–56.
22. Patterson RE, Pietinen P. Assessment of Nutritional Status in Individuals and Populations, in Public health nutrition. In: Gibney MJ, et al., eds. Oxford: Blackwell Science; 2004, pp. 66–81.
23. Rennie KL, Coward A, Jebb SA. Estimating under-reporting of energy intake in dietary surveys using an individualised method. Br J Nutr 2007; 97(06): 1169–76.
24. Buttriss JL, Welch AA, Kearney JM, Lanham-New SA, eds. Public health nutrition. 2nd ed. The Nutrition Society Textbook Series, ed. T.N. Society. Chichester: Wiley Blackwell; 2018.
25. Ocké M, de Boer E, Brants H, van der Laan J, Niekerk M, van Rossum C, et al. PANCAKE – pilot study for the assessment of nutrient intake and food consumption among kids in Europe. Supporting Publications. Parma: EFSA; 2012.
26. Slimani N, Casagrande C, Nicolas G, Freisling H, Huybrechts I, Ocké MC, et al. The standardized computerized 24-h dietary recall method EPIC-Soft adapted for pan-European dietary monitoring. Eur J Clin Nutr 2011; 65(1): 5–15.
27. Carter MC, Albar SA, Morris MA, Mulla UZ, Hancock N, Evans CE, et al. Development of a UK online 24-h dietary assessment tool: Myfood24. Nutrients 2015; 7(6): 4016–32.
28. Moreiras GV, Ávila JM, Ruiz E. Energy balance, a new paradigm and methodological issues: The ANIBES study in Spain. Nutr Hosp 2015; 31(Suppl 3): 101–12.
29. Ruiz E, Ávila JM, Castillo A, Valero T, Del Pozo S, Rodriguez P, et al. The ANIBES study on energy balance in SpaIn: design, protocol and methodology. Nutrients 2015; 7(2): 970–98.
30. Ruiz E, Ávila JM, Valero T, Del Pozo S, Rodriguez P, Aranceta-Bartrina J, et al. Macronutrient distribution and dietary sources in the Spanish population: Findings from the ANIBES study. Nutrients 2016; 8(3): 177.
31. Merten C, Ferrari P, Bakker M, Boss A, Hearty A, Leclercq C, et al. Methodological characteristics of the national dietary surveys carried out in the European Union as included in the European Food Safety Authority (EFSA) Comprehensive European Food Consumption Database. Food Addit Contam A 2011; 28(8): 975–95.
32. Ministeri de Salut, Benestar Social i Família (2007). Evaluation of the nutritional status of the Andorran population. Available from: http://www.salut.ad/images/microsites/AvaluacioNutricional_04-05/index.html [cited 28 February 2017].
33. Elmadfa I, Hasenegger V, Wagner K, Putz P, Weidl N-M, Wottawa D, et al. Österreichischer Ernährungsbericht 2012. Wien: Institut für Ernährungswissenschaften; 2012.
34. Elmadfa I, Friesling H, Nowak V, Hofstadter D. Austrian nutrition report 2008. Vienna: Federal Ministry for Health; 2009.
35. Elmadfa I, Burger P, Derndorfer E, Kiefer I, Kunze M, König J, et al. Österreichischer Ernährungsbericht 1998. Wien: Bundesministerium für Gesundheit, Arbeit und Soziales; 1999.
36. Elmadfa I, Godina-Zarfl B, Dichtl M, König, JS. The Austrian study on nutritional status of 6-to 18-year-old pupils. Bibl Nutr Dieta 1994; 51: 62–7.
37. Bel S, Van den Abeele S, Lebacq T, Ost C, Brocatus L, Stievenart C, et al. Protocol of the Belgian food consumption survey 2014: objectives, design and methods. Arch Public Health 2016; 74(1): 1.
38. De RidderK. Enquête de consommation alimentaire 2014–2015: la consommation alimentaire, in Rapport 4. Brussels: WIV-ISP; 2016.
39. Temme E, Huybrechts I, Vandevijvere S, De Henauw S, Leveque A, Kornitzer M, et al. Energy and macronutrient intakes in Belgium: results from the first National Food Consumption Survey. Br J Nutr 2010; 103(12): 1823–9.
40. Petrova S, Baikova D, Angelova K, Rangelova L, Duleva V, Ovcharova D, et al. Nutrition in children 1–5 years of age in Bulgaria – energy and macronutrient intake. Bulgarian J Public Health 2010; 2(4): 55–65.
41. Petrova S, Rangelova L, Duleva V, Ovcharova D. Nutrition in children 1–5 years of age in Bulgaria – micronutrient intake. Bulgarian J Public Health 2010; 2(4): 66–73.
42. Petrova S, Rangelova L, DulevaV, Ovcharova D, Dimitrov P, Kalinov K, et al. Design and methodology of national survey on nutrition of infants and children under 5 years of age and family child rearing in Bulgaria. Bulgarian J Public Health 2010; 2(4): 1–11.
43. Tornaritis MJ, Philippou E, Hadjigeorgiou C, Kourides YA, Panayi A, Savva SC. A study of the dietary intake of Cypriot children and adolescents aged 6–18 years and the association of mother's educational status and children's weight status on adherence to nutritional recommendations. BMC Public Health 2014; 14(1): 1–11.
44. Dofkova M, Ruprich J, Jakubikova M, Rehurkova I, Blahova J. Czech national food consumption survey: method and application of results. Arch Public Health 2010; 68(Suppl 1): S24.
45. National Institute of Public Health (2015). Environmental health monitoring system in the Czech Republic: summary report 2014. Prague: National Institute of Public Health; 2015
46. Pedersen A, Christensen T, Matthiessen J, Knudsen VK, Rosenlund-Sorensen M, Biltoft-Jensen A, et al. Danskernes Kostvaner 2011–2013. Hovedresultater. Søborg, Denmark: DTU Fødevareinstitute; 2015.
47. Pedersen A, Fagt S, Groth MV, Christensen T, Biltoft-Jensen A, Matthiessen J, et al. Danskernes Kostvaner 2003–2008. Hovedresultater. Søborg, Denmark: DTU Fødevareinstitute; 2010.
48. Lyhne N, Christensen T, Groth MV, Fagt S, Biltoft-Jensen A, Hartkopp H, et al. Danskernes kostvaner 2000–2002. Hovedresultater. Søborg, Denmark: Danmarks Fødevareforskning; 2005.
49. Andersen N, Fagt S, Groth MV, Hartkopp H, Moller A, Ovesen L, et al. Danskernes kostvaner 1995: Hovedresultater. Søborg, Denmark: Levnedsmiddelstyrelsen; 1996.

50. Pomerleau J, McKee M, Robertson A, Kadziauskiene K, Abaravicius A, Vaask S, et al. Macronutrient and food intake in the Baltic republics. Eur J Clin Nutr 2001; 55(3): 200–207.
51. Pomerleau J, McKee M, Robertson A, Vaask S, Pudule I, Grinberger D, et al. Nutrition and Lifestyle in the Baltic Republics. Copenhagen: European Centre on Health of Societies in Transistion & World Health Organization Regional Office for Europe; 1999.
52. Helldán A, Raulio S, Kosola M, Tapanainen H, Ovaskainen ML, Virtanen S. Finravinto 2012-tutkimus-The National FINDIET 2012 Survey. Raportti: 2013_016. Raportti, Helsinki. 2013.
53. Pietinen P, Paturi M, Reinivuo H, Tapanainen H, Valsta LM. FINDIET 2007 Survey: energy and nutrient intakes. Public Health Nutr 2010; 13: 920–4.
54. Reinivuo H, Hirvonen T, Ovaskainen M, Korhonen T, Valsta LM. Dietary survey methodology of FINDIET 2007 with a risk assessment perspective. Public Health Nutr 2010; 13(6A): 915–19.
55. Männistö S, Ovaskainen M, Valsta LM, Korhonen T, Nissinen K, Pakkala H, et al. Finravinto 2002 – Tutkimus. The National FINDIET 2002 Study. Helsinki: Kansanterveyslaitos (KTL); 2003.
56. FINDIET Study Group et al. The 1997 dietary survey of Finnish adults. Helsinki: Publications of the National Public Health Institute B8; 1998.
57. Kleemola P, Virtanen M, Pietinen P. The 1992 dietary survey of Finnish adults. Helsinki: Kansanterveyslaitos; 1994.
58. Tavoularis G. Nutri-Bébé 2013 Study Part 1. Presentation and methodological considerations. Arch Pédiatr 2015; 22(10): 10S1–S6.
59. Agence française de sécurité sanitaire des aliments (AFSSA) (2009). Étude Individuelle Nationale des Consommations Alimentaires 2 (INCA2) (2006–2007). Rapport. Maisons-Alfort: AFSSA; 2009, pp. 1–28.
60. Castetbon K, Vernay M, Malon A, Salanave B, Deschamps V, Roudier C, et al. Dietary intake, physical activity and nutritional status in adults: the French nutrition and health survey (ENNS, 2006–2007). Br J Nutr 2009; 102(05): 733–43.
61. Fantino M, Gourmet E. Apports nutritionnels en France en 2005 chez les enfants non allaités âgés de moins de 36 mois. Arch Pédiatr 2008; 15(4): 446–55.
62. Volatier J. Enquête INCA Individuelle et Nationale sur les Consommations Alimentaires (National and Individual Survey on Eating Consumptions). AFSSA; Paris. 2000.
63. Boggio V, Grossiord A, Guyon S, Fuchs F, Fantino M. Consommation alimentaire des nourrissons et des enfants en bas âge en France en 1997. Arch Pédiatr 1999; 6(7): 740–7.
64. Rigaud D, Giachetti I, Deheeger M, Borys JM, Volatier JL, Lemoine A, et al. Enquête française de consommation alimentaire. I. Energie et macronutriments. Cahiers Nutr Diététique 1997; 32(6): 379–89.
65. Hartmann BM, Heuer T, Hoffmann I. The German Nutrient Database: Effect of different versions on the calculated energy and nutrient intake of the German population. J Food Compost Anal 2015; 42: 26–9.
66. Nationale Verzehrsstudie II (2008). Ergebnisbericht Teil 1. Karlsruhe: Max Rubner-Institut Karlsruhe.
67. Kurth B-M. Der Kinder-und Jugendgesundheitssurvey (KiGGS): Ein Überblick über Planung, Durchführung und Ergebnisse unter Berücksichtigung von Aspekten eines Qualitätsmanagements. Bundesgesundheitsblatt-Gesundheitsforschung-Gesundheitsschutz 2007; 50(5–6): 533–46.
68. Mensink G, Thamm M, Haas K. Die Ernahrung in Deutschland 1998. Gesundheitswesen 1999; 61(2): S200–6.
69. Hellenic Health Foundation, Greek Ministry of Health, and the Hellenic Center for Disease Control & Prevention. HYDRIA – Health and Nutrition of the Population in Greece. Available from: http://www.hhf-greece.gr/hydria-nhns.gr/index_eng.html [cited 16 March 2017].
70. Trichopoulou A, HYDRIA. Program and targeted action for the health and nutrition of the Greek population: the development and implementation methodology and mapping. Greek Health Foundation; Athens. 2015.
71. Manios Y, Grammatikaki E, Papoutsou S, Liarigkovinos T, Kondaki K, Moschonis G. Nutrient intakes of toddlers and preschoolers in Greece: the GENESIS study. J Am Diet Assoc 2008; 108(2): 357–361.
72. Lugasi A. Sarkadi Nagy E, Zentai A, Bakacs M, Illes E, Baldauf Z, Martos E. Országos Táplálkozás és Tápláltsági Állapot Vizsgálat – OTÁP2009. Budapest: Országos Élelmezés- és Táplálkozástudományi Intézet; 2012.
73. Bíró L, Szeitz-Szabó M, Bíró G, Sali J. Dietary survey in Hungary, 2009. Part II: Vitamins, macro-and microelements, food supplements and food allergy. Acta Aliment 2011; 40: 301–312.
74. Szeitz-Szabó M, Bíró L, Bíró G. & Sali J. Dietary survey in Hungary, 2009. Part I. Macronutrients, alcohol, caffeine, fibre. Acta Aliment 2011; 40: 142–52.
75. Zajkás G, Bíró L, Greiner E. T. 4áplálkozási vizsgálat Magyarországon, 2003–2004. Mikro-tápanyagbevitel: vitaminok [Dietary survey in Hungary, 2003–2004. Micro-nutrient intake: vitamins]. Orvosi Hetilap [Hung Med J] 2007; 148: 1593–1600.
76. Bíró G, Antal M, Zajkás G. Nutrition survey of the Hungarian population in a randomized trial between 1992–1994. Eur J Clin Nutr 1996; 50(4): 201–8.
77. Steingrímsdóttir L, Valgeirsdottir H, Halldorsson TI, Gunnarsdottir I, Gisladottir E, Þorgeirsdottir H, Þorsdottir I. Kannanir á mataræði og næringargildi fæðunnar á Íslandi. Læknablaðið 2014; 100: 659–64.
78. Steingrimsdottir L, Valgeirsdottir H, Halldorsson TI, Gunnarsdottir I, Gisladottir E, Þorgeirsdottir H, et al. National nutrition surveys and dietary changes in Iceland. Læknablaðið 2014; 100(12): 659–64.
79. Þorgeirsdóttir H, Valgeirsdóttir H, Gunnarsdóttir I, Gísladóttir E, Gunnarsdóttir BE, Þórsdóttir I, et al. Hvað borða Íslendingar? Könnun á mataræði Íslendinga 2010–2011 Helstu niðurstöður. Embætti landlæknis, Matvælastofnun, Rannsóknastofa í næringarfræði við Háskóla Íslands, Landspítala-háskólasjúkrahús; Reykjavik. 2011.
80. Steingrímsdóttir L, Þorgeirsdóttir H, Ólafsdóttir A. Hvað borða Íslendingar? Könnun á mataræði Íslendinga 2002. Helstu niðurstöður. Rannsóknir Manneldisráðs Íslands V; Reykjavik. 2002.
81. Steingrimsdottir L. Nutrition in Iceland. Scand J Nutr (Sweden) 1993; 37: 10–112.
82. Irish Universities Nutrition Alliance. The national pre-school food survey. Aviailable from: http://www.iuna.net/?p=169 [cited 27 July 2016].
83. Irish Universities Nutrition Alliance (IUNA) (2011). National adult nutrition survey: summary report on food and nutrient intakes, physical measurements, physical activity patterns and food choice motives. IUNA, Dublin.
84. Li K, McNulty BA, Tiernery AM, Devlin NFC, Joyce T, Leite JC, et al. Dietary fat intakes in Irish adults in 2011: how much has changed in 10 years? Br J Nutr 2016; 115(10): 1798–809.

85. Harrington J, Perry I, Lutomski J, Morgan K, McGee H, Shelley E, et al. SLÁN 2007: Survey of Lifestyle, Attitudes and Nutrition in Ireland. Dietary Habits of the Irish Population. Department of Health and Children. Dublin: TSO; 2008.
86. Morgan K, McGee H, Watson D, Perry I, Barry M, Shelley E, et al. SLAN 2007: survey of lifestyle, attitudes & nutrition in Ireland: main report. Dublin: Department of Health and Children; 2008.
87. Irish Universities Nutrition Alliance. The national teen's food survey (2005–2006). Aviailable from: http://www.iuna.net/?p=29 [cited 27 July 2016].
88. Irish Universities Nutrition Alliance. The national children's food survey (2003–2004). Aviailable from: http://www.iuna.net/?p=27 [cited 27 July 2016].
89. Irish Universities Nutrition Alliance (IUNA). North/South Ireland food consumption survey: summary report on food and nutrient intakes, anthropometry, attitudinal data & physical activity patterns. Dublin: Food Safety Promotion Board; 2001.
90. Lee P, Cunningham K. Irish National Nutrition Survey (INNS). Dublin: Irish Nutrition and Dietetic Institute; 1990.
91. Sette S, Le Donne C, Piccinelli R, Arcella D, Turrini A, Leclercq C. The third Italian National Food Consumption Survey, INRAN-SCAI 2005–06 – Part 1: Nutrient intakes in Italy. Nutr Metab Cardiovasc Dis 2011; 21(12): 922–32.
92. Turrini A, Saba A, Perrone D, Cialfa E, D'amicis A. Original communications-food consumption patterns in Italy: the INN-CA Study 1994–1996. Eur J Clin Nutr 2001; 55(7): 571–88.
93. Joffe R, Ozolinš G, Šantare D, Bartkevics V, Mike L, Briška I. The national food consumption survey of LATVIA, 2007–2009, Nacionalais diagnostikas centrs and P.u.v.d.P. centrs Riga: Zemkopibas ministrija; 2009.
94. Barzda A, Bartkevičiūtė R, Baltušytė I, Stukas R, Bartkevičiūtė, S. *Suaugusių ir pagyvenusių lietuvos gyventojų faktinės mitybos ir mitybos įpročių tyrimas.* Visuomenės sveikata 2016; 72(1): 85–94.
95. Barzda A, Bartkevičiūtė R, Abaravicius JA, Stukas R, Satkute R. Food Consumption survey in adult Lithuanian population: nutrient daily intake. Ann Nutr Metab 2009; 55: 212.
96. Barzda A, Jankauskienė K, Tutkuvienė J, Didžiapetrienė J, Gefenas E, Tamošiūnas A, et al. Study and evaluation of actual nutrition and nutrition habits of Lithuanian adult population. Vilniaus universitetas; Zwolle, Vilnius, 2011.
97. RIVM, National Institue for Public Health and the Environment (2017). Dutch national food consumption survey; Zwolle. Available from: http://www.rivm.nl/en/Topics/D/Dutch_National_Food_Consumption_Survey [cited 16 March 2017].
98. Van Rossum CTM, Fransen HP, Verkaik-Kloosterman J, buurma EM, Ocke MC. Dutch national food consumption survey 2007–2010|Part 6 Micronutrients. Bilthoven: RIVM; 2011.
99. Van Rossum CTM, Fransen HP, Verkaik-Kloosterman J, buurma EM, Ocke MC. Dutch national food consumption survey 2007–2010|Part 5 Macronutrients. Bilthoven: RIVM; 2011.
100. Van Rossum C, Fransen HP, Verkaik-Kloosterman J, Buurma-Rethans EJM, Ocké MC. Dutch national food consumption survey 2007–2010: diet of children and adults aged 7 to 69 years. Bilthoven; RIVM; 2011.
101. Ocke M, van Rossum CTM, Fransen HP, Buurma EM, de Boer EJ, Brants HAM. Dutch national food consumption survey young children 2005/2006. Voedselconsumptiepeiling bij peuters en kleuters 2005/2006. Bilthoven: Rijksinstituut voor Volksgezondheid en Milieu RIVM; 2008.
102. Ocké M, Hulshof K, Van Rossum C. The Dutch national food consumption survey 2003. Methodological issues. Arch Public Health 2005; 63: 227–41.
103. Hulshof K, Brussaard JH, Kruizinga AG, Telman J, Löwik MRH. Socio-economic status, dietary intake and 10 year trends: the Dutch National Food Consumption Survey. Eur J Clin Nutr 2003; 57(1): 128–37.
104. Hansen L, Myhre, Andersen LF, UNGKOST 3 Landsomfattende kostholdsundersøkelse blant 4-åringer i Norge, 2016. Helsedirektoratet. Oslo: Folkehelseninstituttet; 2016.
105. Hansen L, Myhre JB, Johansen AMW, Paulsen MM, Andersen LF. UNGKOST 3 Landsomfattende kostholdsundersøkelse blant elever i 4. -og 8. klasse i Norge, 2015. Helsedirektoratet. Oslo: Folkehelseninstituttet; 2015.
106. Totland T, Melnæs BK, Lundberg-Hallén N, Helland-Kigen KM, Lund-Blix NA, Myhre JB, et al. Norkost 3. En landsomfattende kostholdsundersøkelse blant menn og kvinner i Norge i alderen; Helsedirektoratet, Oslo. 2012, pp. 18–70.
107. Parr CL, Hjartaker A, Scheel I, Lund E, Laake P, Veierod MB. Comparing methods for handling missing values in food-frequency questionnaires and proposing k nearest neighbours imputation: effects on dietary intake in the Norwegian Women and Cancer study (NOWAC). Public Health Nutr 2008; 11(4): 361–70.
108. Øverby NC, Andersen LF, Ungkost 2000. Landsomfattende kostholdundersøkelse blant elever i 2002; 4.
109. Johansson L, Solvoll K. NORKOST 1997. National dietary survey among men and women aged 16–79 years. Report 3/1999. Oslo: National Council on Nutrition and Physical Activity; 1999.
110. Johansson L, Solvoll K, Bjørneboe GE, Drevon CA. Dietary habits among Norwegian men and women. Scand J Nutr Naringsforskning 1997; 41(2): 63–70.
111. Andersen LF, Nes M, Sandstad B, Bjørneboe GE, Drevon CA. Dietary intake among Norwegian adolescents. Eur J Clin Nutr 1995; 49(8): 555–64.
112. Drygas W, Niklas AA, Piwońska A, Piotrowski W, Flotyńska A, Kwaśniewska M. Multi-center National Population Health Examination Survey (WOBASZ II study): assumptions, methods and implementation. Kardiologia Polska 2015; 74(1): 681–90.
113. Szponar L, Sekula W, Nelson M, Weisell R. The household food consumption and anthropometric survey in Poland. Public Health Nutr 2001; 4(5B): 1183–6.
114. Szponar L, Rychlik E. Nutrition mode and nutritional status of boys and men in Poland. Żywienie Człowieka i Metabolizm. Suplement 1996; 23(2): 3–37.
115. Szponar L, Rychlik E. Nutrition mode and nutritional status of girls and women in Poland. Żywienie Człowieka i Metabolizm. Suplement 1996; 23(2): 38–70.
116. Lopes C, Torres D, Oliveira A, Severo M, Alarcão V, Guiomar S, et al. Inquérito Alimentar Nacional e de Atividade Física (IAN-AF), 2015–2016 Part 1 Methodological Report. Porto: University of Porto; 2017.
117. Lopes C, Torres D, Oliveira A, Severo M, Alarcão V, Guiomar S, et al. Inquérito Alimentar Nacional e de Atividade Física (IAN-AF), 2015–2016 Part 2 Report. Porto: University of Porto; 2017.
118. Moreira P, Padez C, Mourao I, Rosado V. Dietary calcium and body mass index in Portuguese children. Eur J Clin Nutr 2005; 59(7): 861–7.
119. Kozyreva P, Kosolapov M, Popkin BM, Data resource profile: The Russia longitudinal monitoring survey – Higher school of economics (RLMS-HSE) Phase II: Monitoring the economic

and health situation in Russia, 1994–2013. Int J Epidemiol 2016; 45(2): 395–401.
120. Zohoori N, Henderson L, Gleiter K, Popkin B. Monitoring health conditions in the Russian Federation: The Russia longitudinal monitoring survey 1992–98. US Agency for International Development; Washington 1999.
121. Babinská K, Béderová A. Changes in nutrient intake in the adult population of the Slovak Republic. J Food Compost Anal 2002; 15(4): 359–65.
122. Babinska K, Bederova A, Bartekova S. Dietary pattern in the adult population from selected areas of Slovac Republic. Eur J Epidemiol 1998; 52: S59.
123. Fidler Mis N, Kobe H, Štimec M. Dietary intake of macro-and micronutrients in Slovenian adolescents: comparison with reference values. Ann Nutr Metab 2012; 61(4): 305–13.
124. Blenkuš, MG, Gregorič M, Tivadar B, Koch V, Kostanjevec S, Turk VF, et al. Prehrambene navade odraslih prebivalcev Slovenije z vidika varovanja zdravja. Pedagoška fakulteta; Ljubljana. 2009.
125. Marcos SV, Rubio MJ, Sanchidrián FR, Robledo D. Spanish National dietary survey in adults, elderly and pregnant women. EFSA Support Pub 2016; 13(6): 1–33.
126. Marcos Suarez V, Rubio MJ, Sanchidrián FR, Robledo D. Spanish national dietary survey on children and adolescents. EFSA Support Pub 2015; 12(11): 1–23.
127. AESAN (2011). ENIDE Encuesta Nacional de Ingesta Dietética Española 2011, A.E.d.S.A.y. Nutricion. Madrid: Ministerio de Sanidad, Politica Social e Igualdad.
128. AESAN (2011). Evaluación nutricional de la dieta española. i energía y macronutrientes Sobre datos de la Encuesta Nacional de Ingesta Dietética (ENIDE), A.E.d.S.A.y. Nutricion. Madrid: Ministerio de Sanidad, Servicios Sociales e Igualdad.
129. AESAN (2011). Evaluación nutricional de la dieta española. ii micronutrientes Sobre datos de la Encuesta Nacional de Ingesta Dietética (ENIDE). A.E.d.S.A.y. Nutricion. Madrid: Ministerio de Sanidad, Servicios Sociales e Igualdad; 2011.
130. Estévez-Santiago R, Beltrán-de-Miguel B, Olmedilla-Alonso B. Assessment of dietary lutein, zeaxanthin and lycopene intakes and sources in the Spanish survey of dietary intake (2009–2010). Int J Food Sci Nutr 2016; 67(3): 305–313.
131. Pérez-Rodrigo C, Ribas L, Serra-Majem Ll, Aranceta J. Food preferences of Spanish children and young people: the enKid study. Eur J Clin Nutr 2003; 57: S45–8.
132. Serra-Majem Ll, Ribas L, García A, Pérez-Rodrigo C, Aranceta J. Nutrient adequacy and Mediterranean Diet in Spanish school children and adolescents. Eur J Clin Nutr 2003; 57: S35–9.
133. Amcoff E, Edberg A, Enghardt BH, Lindroos AK, Nälsén C, Pearson M, et al. Riksmaten – vuxna 2010–11 Livsmedels- och näringsintag bland vuxna i Sverige. Livsmedelsverket; Uppsala. 2012.
134. Enghardt B, Pearson M, Becker W. Riksmaten – barn 2003. Livsmedels-och näringsintag bland barn i Sverige. Livsmedelsverket; Uppsala. 2006.
135. Becker W, Pearson M. Riksmaten 1997–1998. Kostvanor och näringsintag i Sverige-Metod-och resultaatanalys. Uppsala: Livsmedelsverket.
136. Güler S, Budakoğlu I, Besler HT, Pekcan AG, Türkyılmaz AS, Çıngı H, et al. Methodology of National Turkey Nutrition and Health survey (TNHS) 2010. Med J Islamic World Acad Sci 2014; 22(1): 7–29.
137. Turkey Ministry of Health (2014). Türkiye Beslenme ve Sağlık Araştırması 2010: Beslenme Durumu ve Alışkanlıklarının Değerlendirilmesi Sonuç Raporu. Türkiye Cumhuriyeti Sağlık Bakanlığı Sağlık. Istanbul.
138. Bates B, Cox L, Nicholson S, Page P, Prentice A, Steer T, Swan G. National diet and nutrition survey results from years 5 and 6 (combined) of the rolling programme (2012/2013–2013/2014). London: Public Health England & Food Standards Agency; 2016.
139. Bates B, Lennox A, Prentice A, Bates C, Page P, Nicholson S, et al. National diet and nutrition survey: results from years 1, 2, 3 and 4 combined of the rolling program (2008/9–2011/12). London: Public Health England; 2014.
140. Nelson M, Erens B, Bates B, Church S, Boshier T. Low income diet and nutrition survey: summary of key findings. London: TSO; 2007.
141. Henderson L, Gregory J, Irving K, Swan G. National diet and nutrition survey: adults aged 19 to 64 years. Volume 2: energy, protein, carbohydrate, fat and alcohol intake. London: TSO; 2002.
142. Gregory J, Lowe S, Bates CJ, Prentice A, Jackson LV, Smithers G, et al. National Diet and Nutrition Survey: young people aged 4 to 18 years; volume 1: report of the diet and nutrition survey. London: Stationery Office; 2000.
143. Finch S, Doyle W, Lowe C, Bates CJ, Prentice A, Smithers G, et al. National Diet and Nutrition Survey: people aged 65 years and over. Volume 1: report of the diet and nutrition survey. London: TSO; 1998.
144. de Boer EJ, Slimani N, van 't Veer P, Boeing H, Feinberg M, Leclercq C, et al. The European Food Consumption Validation Project: conclusions and recommendations. Eur J Clin Nutr 2011; 65: 102–107.
145. Rippin HL, Hutchinson J, Jewell J, Breda JJ, Cade JE. Adult nutrient intakes from current national dietary surveys of European populations. Nutrients 2017; 9(12): 1288.
146. Bel-Serrat S, Huybrechts I, Thumann BF, Hebestreit A, Abuja M, de Henauw S, et al. Inventory of surveillance systems assessing dietary, physical activity and sedentary behaviours in Europe: a DEDIPAC study. Eur J Public Health 2017; 27(4): 747–55.

***Holly L. Rippin**
Nutritional Epidemiology Group (NEG),
School of Food Science and Nutrition,
University of Leeds, Leeds, LS2 9JT, United Kingdom
Email: fshr@leeds.ac.uk

**Appendix 1. Questionnaire concerning nationally representative diet and nutrition surveys and their methodologies**

Please complete one questionnaire *per diet and nutrition survey (DNS)* for questions 1–3; if necessary make multiple copies. If there any questions in sections 1–3 that you cannot answer, please provide contact details of a person(s) who may be able to answer the outstanding questions.

Please email the completed questionnaire(s) to Holly Rippin fshr@leeds.ac.uk at the University of Leeds, who will be collating this information for the European Office of the World Health Organization.

**Country: xxx**

**Contact (please provide the correct contact person if this is incorrect): Prof/Dr. xxx**

1. **For each DNS carried out in your country since 1990 please fill in the below information:**

Please note that any survey to be included should meet the following criteria:

- The survey should collect dietary intakes across all food groups which are then converted into nutrient values.
- The survey uses national population-based samples or representative regional samples.
- The survey should not be restricted to a specific part of the population (e.g. children, occupational groups or patients).
- Preferably there should be plans to repeat the survey later, unless it already has been repeated. You can also record standalone surveys.

Survey name ................................................
Year(s) when survey data collected.............................
Dietary assessment method/tool used..........................
Genders included in sample...................................
Age ranges included in sample...............................
Sample size (N)
National or regional ............................................
Nationally representative (yes/no)...............................
Institute responsible for the survey...........................
Key contact for survey..........................................
Email for contact person listed above........................

2. **Please provide details of any relevant publications e.g. summary reports, user guides (please provide web links)**

3. **Macro and micro nutrients included in your DNS (please tick all that apply):**

Energy
Total carbohydrates
- Sugars
- Sucrose
- Starches
- Fibre

Total fat
- Saturates
- MUFA
- PUFA
- Trans fatty acids

Protein
Vitamins:
- Folic acid
- Niacin
- Retinol equivalents
- Riboflavin
- Thiamine
- B12
- B6

Minerals:
- Calcium
- Magnesium
- Potassium
- Sodium
- Iron
- Copper
- Fluoride
- Iodine
- Selenium
- Zinc

THANK YOU FOR TAKING THE TIME TO ANSWER THESE QUESTIONS.

*Appendix 2.* Macronutrient provision across dietary surveys

| Country | Survey | Year | Energy (MJ and kcal) | Protein (g) | CHO g or % E | Sugars (g) | Sucrose (g) | Starches (g) | Fibre (g) | Total fat (g) | Saturates (g) | MUFA(g) | PUFA(g) | TFA(g) |
|---|---|---|---|---|---|---|---|---|---|---|---|---|---|---|
| Andorra | Evaluation of the nutritional status of the Andorran population | 2004–2005 | Y | Y | Y | Y | | | Y | Y | Y | Y | Y | |
| Austria | Austrian nutrition report | 2010–2012 | Y | Y | Y | | Y | | Y | Y | Y | Y | Y | |
| Belgium | The Belgian food consumption survey 2014–2015 | 2014–2015 | Y | Y | Y | Y | | Y | Y | Y | Y | Y | Y | Y |
| Bulgaria | National survey on nutrition of infants and children under 5 and family child rearing, 2007 | 2007 | Y | Y | Y | Y | | | Y | Y | Y | Y | Y | |
| Cyprus | A study of the dietary intake of Cypriot children and adolescents aged 6–18 years | 2009–2010 | Y | Y | Y | | | | Y | Y | Y | Y | Y | |
| Denmark | Danish dietary habits 2011–2013 | 2011–2013 | Y | Y | Y | | Y | | Y | Y | Y | Y | Y | Y |
| Finland | The national FINDIET 2012 survey | 2012 | Y | Y | Y | | Y | | Y | Y | Y | Y | Y | Y |
| France | INCA2 | 2006–2007 | Y | Y | Y | Y | | Y | Y | Y | Y | Y | Y | |
| Germany | German national nutrition survey II | 2005–2007 | Y | Y | Y | | | | Y | Y | | | | |
| Hungary | Hungarian dietary survey 2009 | 2009 | Y | Y | Y | | Y | | Y | Y | Y | Y | Y | |
| Iceland | The diet of Icelanders – a national dietary survey 2010–2011 | 2010–2011 | Y | Y | Y | Y | | | Y | Y | Y | Y | Y | Y |
| Ireland | National pre-school nutrition survey | 2010–2011 | Y | Y | Y | Y | | Y | Y | Y | Y | Y | Y | |

*continued*

*Appendix 2.* Continued

| Country | Survey | Year | Energy (MJ and kcal) | Protein (g) | CHO@g or %E | Sugars (g) | Sucrose (g) | Starches (g) | Fibre (g) | Total fat (g) | Saturates (g) | MUFA(g) | PUFA(g) | TFA(g) |
|---|---|---|---|---|---|---|---|---|---|---|---|---|---|---|
| Ireland | National children's food survey | 2003–2004 | Y | Y | Y | | | | Y | Y | | | | |
| Ireland | National teens' food survey | 2005–2006 | Y | Y | Y | | | | Y | Y | | | | |
| Ireland | National adult nutrition survey | 2008–2010 | Y | Y | Y | Y | | Y | Y | Y | Y | Y | Y | Y |
| Italy | The third Italian national food consumption survey, INRAN-SCAI | 2005–2006 | Y | Y | Y | Y | | Y | Y | Y | Y | Y | Y | |
| Latvia | Latvian national food consumption survey 2007–2009 | 2007–2009 | Y | Y | Y | | | | Y | Y | Y | Y | Y | |
| Lithuania | Study and evaluation of actual nutrition and nutrition habits of Lithuanian adult population | 2013–2014 | Y | Y | Y | Y | | | Y | Y | Y | Y | Y | |
| Netherlands | Dutch national food consumption survey (DNFCS) 2007–2010 | 2007–2010 | Y | Y | Y | Y | | | Y | Y | Y | Y | Y | Y |
| Netherlands | Dutch national food consumption survey – young children (DNFCS 2008) | 2005–2006 | Y | Y | Y | Y | | | Y | Y | Y | Y | | Y |
| Norway | Norkost3 | 2010–2011 | Y | Y | Y | | Y | | Y | Y | Y | Y | Y | |
| Norway | Ungkost3 | 2015–2016 | Y | Y | Y | | Y | | Y | Y | Y | Y | Y | |
| Portugal | National food and physical activity survey (IAN-AF) | 2015–2016 | Y | Y | Y | Y | | | Y | Y | Y | Y | Y | Y |
| Spain | ANIBES | 2013 | Y | Y | Y | Y | | | Y | Y | Y | Y | Y | |
| Spain | ENIDE 2011 | 2009–2010 | Y | Y | Y | | | | Y | Y | Y | Y | Y | |

*continued*

*Appendix 2.* Continued

| Country | Survey | Year | Energy (MJ and kcal) | Protein (g) | CHO@g or %E | Sugars (g) | Sucrose (g) | Starches (g) | Fibre (g) | Total fat (g) | Saturates (g) | MUFA(g) | PUFA(g) | TFA(g) |
|---|---|---|---|---|---|---|---|---|---|---|---|---|---|---|
| Sweden | Riksmaten 2010–2011 Swedish adult dietary survey | 2010–2011 | Y | Y | Y |  | Y |  | Y | Y | Y | Y | Y |  |
| Turkey | Turkey nutrition and health survey 2010 (TNHS) | 2010 | Y | Y | Y |  |  |  | Y | Y | Y | Y | Y |  |
| UK | National diet and nutrition survey (NDNS) Years 1–4 | 2008–2012 | Y | Y | Y | Y |  | Y | Y | Y | Y | Y | Y | Y |
| Total | 28 |  | 28 | 28 | 28 | 14 | 7 | 6 | 28 | 28 | 25 | 25 | 24 | 9 |

*Appendix 3.* Micronutrient provision across dietary surveys*

| Country | Survey | Year | B9 (μg) | B3 (mg) | VA (μg) | B2 (mg) | B1 (mg) | B12 (μg) | B6 (mg) | VC (mg) | VD (μg) | VE (mg) | Ca (mg) | Mg (mg) | K (mg) | Na (mg) | Fe (mg) | Cu (mg) | I (μg) | Se (mg) | Zn (μg) |
|---|---|---|---|---|---|---|---|---|---|---|---|---|---|---|---|---|---|---|---|---|---|
| Andorra | Evaluation of the nutritional status of the Andorran population | 2004–2005 | Y | Y | Y | Y | Y | Y | Y | Y | Y | Y | Y | Y | Y | Y | Y | | | | Y |
| Austria | Austrian nutrition report | 2010–2012 | Y | Y | Y | Y | Y | Y | Y | Y | Y | Y | Y | Y | Y | Y | Y | | Y | | Y |
| Belgium | The Belgian food consumption survey 2014–2015 | 2014–2015 | Y | | | Y | Y | Y | Y | Y | Y | | Y | | | Y | Y | | Y | | |
| Bulgaria | National survey on nutrition of infants and children under 5 and family child rearing, 2007 | 2007 | Y | Y | Y | Y | Y | Y | Y | Y | Y | Y | Y | Y | | Y | Y | | | | Y |
| Cyprus | A study of the dietary intake of Cypriot children and adolescents aged 6–18 years | 2009–2010 | | | Y | Y | Y | | Y | Y | | | Y | Y | Y | Y | Y | | | | |
| Denmark | Danish dietary habits 2011–2013 | 2011–2013 | Y | Y | Y | Y | Y | Y | Y | Y | Y | Y | Y | Y | Y | Y | Y | | Y | Y | Y |
| Finland | The national FINDIET 2012 survey | 2012 | Y | Y | Y | Y | Y | Y | Y | Y | Y | Y | Y | Y | Y | Y | Y | Y | Y | Y | Y |
| France | INCA2 | 2006–2007 | Y | Y | Y | Y | Y | Y | Y | Y | Y | Y | Y | Y | Y | Y | Y | Y | Y | Y | Y |
| Germany | German national nutrition survey II | 2005–2007 | Y | Y | Y | Y | Y | Y | Y | Y | Y | Y | Y | Y | Y | Y | Y | | Y | | Y |
| Hungary | Hungarian dietary survey 2009 | 2009 | Y | Y | Y | Y | Y | Y | Y | Y | Y | Y | Y | Y | Y | Y | Y | Y | | | Y |

*continued*

*Appendix 3.* Continued

| Country | Survey | Year | B9 (µg) | B3 (mg) | VA (µg) | B2 (mg) | B1 (mg) | B12 (µg) | B6 (mg) | VC (mg) | VD (µg) | VE (mg) | Ca (mg) | Mg (mg) | K (mg) | Na (mg) | Fe (mg) | Cu (mg) | I (µg) | Se (mg) | Zn (µg) |
|---|---|---|---|---|---|---|---|---|---|---|---|---|---|---|---|---|---|---|---|---|---|
| Iceland | The diet of Icelanders – a national dietary survey 2010–2011 | 2010–2011 | Y | Y | Y | Y | Y | Y | Y | Y | Y | Y | Y | Y | Y | Y | Y | Y | Y | Y | Y |
| Ireland | National pre-school nutrition survey | 2010–2011 | Y | Y | Y | Y | Y | Y | Y | Y | Y | Y | Y | Y | | | Y | Y | | | Y |
| Ireland | National children's food survey | 2003–2004 | Y | Y | Y | Y | Y | Y | Y | Y | Y | Y | Y | Y | | | Y | Y | | | Y |
| Ireland | National teens' food survey | 2005–2006 | Y | Y | Y | Y | Y | Y | Y | Y | Y | Y | Y | Y | | | Y | Y | | | Y |
| Ireland | National adult nutrition survey | 2008–2010 | Y | Y | Y | Y | Y | Y | Y | Y | Y | Y | Y | Y | Y | Y | Y | Y | | | Y |
| Italy | The third Italian national food consumption survey, INRAN-SCAI | 2005–2006 | | | Y | Y | Y | Y | Y | Y | Y | Y | Y | Y | Y | | Y | | | | Y |
| Latvia | Latvian national food consumption survey 2007–2009 | 2007–2009 | Y | Y | Y | Y | Y | Y | Y | Y | Y | Y | Y | Y | Y | Y | Y | Y | Y | | Y |
| Lithuania | Study and evaluation of actual nutrition and nutrition habits of Lithuanian adult population | 2013–2014 | Y | Y | Y | Y | Y | Y | Y | Y | Y | Y | Y | Y | Y | Y | Y | Y | Y | Y | Y |
| Netherlands | Dutch national food consumption survey (DNFCS) 2007–2010 | 2007–2010 | Y | | Y | Y | Y | Y | Y | Y | Y | Y | Y | Y | Y | Y | Y | Y | Y | Y | Y |

*continued*

*Appendix 3.* Continued

| Country | Survey | Year | B9 (µg) | B3 (mg) | VA (µg) | B2 (mg) | B1 (mg) | B12 (µg) | B6 (mg) | VC (mg) | VD (µg) | VE (mg) | Ca (mg) | Mg (mg) | K (mg) | Na (mg) | Fe (mg) | Cu (mg) | I (µg) | Se (mg) | Zn (µg) |
|---|---|---|---|---|---|---|---|---|---|---|---|---|---|---|---|---|---|---|---|---|---|
| Netherlands | Dutch national food consumption survey – young children (DNFCS 2008) | 2005–2006 | Y |  | Y | Y | Y | Y | Y | Y | Y | Y | Y | Y |  |  | Y | Y |  | Y |  |
| Norway | Norkost3 | 2010–2011 | Y |  | Y | Y | Y | Y | Y | Y | Y | Y | Y | Y | Y | Y | Y |  |  |  |  |
| Norway | Ungkost3 | 2015–2016 | Y |  | Y | Y | Y | Y | Y | Y | Y | Y | Y | Y | Y | Y | Y |  |  | Y |  |
| Portugal | National food and physical activity survey (IAN-AF) | 2015–2016 | Y | Y | Y | Y | Y | Y | Y | Y | Y | Y | Y | Y | Y | Y | Y |  |  |  | Y |
| Spain | ANIBES | 2013 |  |  |  |  |  |  |  |  |  |  |  |  |  |  |  |  |  |  |  |
| Spain | ENIDE 2011 | 2009–2010 | Y | Y | Y | Y | Y | Y | Y | Y | Y | Y | Y | Y | Y | Y | Y |  | Y | Y | Y |
| Sweden | Riksmaten 2010–2011 Swedish adult dietary survey | 2010–2011 | Y | Y | Y | Y | Y | Y | Y | Y | Y | Y | Y | Y | Y | Y | Y |  |  | Y | Y |
| Turkey | Turkey nutrition and health survey 2010 (TNHS) | 2010 | Y | Y | Y | Y | Y | Y | Y | Y | Y | Y | Y | Y | Y | Y | Y |  | Y |  | Y |
| UK | National diet and nutrition survey (NDNS) Years 1–4 | 2008–2012 | Y | Y | Y | Y | Y | Y | Y | Y | Y | Y | Y | Y | Y | Y | Y | Y | Y | Y | Y |
| TOTAL | 28 |  | 25 | 20 | 26 | 27 | 27 | 26 | 27 | 27 | 26 | 25 | 27 | 26 | 21 | 22 | 27 | 13 | 13 | 11 | 22 |

* Key

| B9 | Folic acid |
|---|---|
| B3 | Niacin |
| VA | Vitamin A (retinol equivalent) |
| B2 | Riboflavin |
| B1 | Thiamine |
| B12 | Vitamin B12 |
| B6 | Vitamin B6 |
| VC | Vitamin C |
| VD | Vitamin D |
| VE | Vitamin E |

| Ca | Calcium |
|---|---|
| Mg | Magnesium |
| K | Potassium |
| Na | Sodium |
| Fe | Iron |
| Cu | Copper |
| I | Iodine |
| Se | Selenium |
| Zn | Zinc |
| | |

# 9

# Evaluation of a short Food Frequency Questionnaire to assess cardiovascular disease-related diet and lifestyle factors

Karianne Svendsen[1]*, Hege Berg Henriksen[1], Beate Østengen[2], David R. Jacobs Jr.[3], Vibeke H. Telle-Hansen[2], Monica H. Carlsen[1] and Kjetil Retterstøl[1,4]

[1]Department of Nutrition, Institute of Basic Medical Sciences, University of Oslo, Oslo, Norway; [2]Faculty of Health Sciences, Oslo Metropolitan University, Oslo, Norway; [3]Division of Epidemiology and Community Health, School of Public Health, University of Minnesota, Minneapolis, USA; [4]The Lipid Clinic, Department of Endocrinology, Morbid Obesity and Preventive Medicine, Oslo University Hospital, Oslo, Norway

*Abstract*

***Background:*** The Vascular lifestyle-Intervention and Screening in phArmacies (VISA) study investigates diet and lifestyle factors associated with risk of cardiovascular disease (CVD). As part of the study methodology, a short Food Frequency Questionnaire (FFQ), the VISA-FFQ, was adapted from the Norwegian NORDIET-FFQ.

***Objective:*** The aim of this study was to evaluate the VISA-FFQ and its ability to estimate intakes of foods and lifestyle factors in screening for elevated risk of CVD. The evaluation included assessment of relative validity of intake of milk fat and assessment of reproducibility of several foods and lifestyle factors.

***Design:*** Relative validity of milk fat estimated from the VISA-FFQ was assessed in 307 participants by comparing estimated dietary intake of the fatty acids pentadecanoic acid (15:0) and heptadecanoic acid (17:0), from milk fat with whole blood biomarkers 15:0 and 17:0. Reproducibility was evaluated in 122 participants by comparing consistency in intakes of different foods and lifestyle factors reported by the VISA-FFQ and administered twice with a 4-week interval.

***Results:*** Dietary 15:0 milk fat estimated from the VISA-FFQ correlated positively with whole blood 15:0 ($r = 0.32$, $P < 0.05$). Men presented higher correlations than women did. Acceptable and consistent reproducibility ($r = 0.44$–$0.94$ and no large difference between test and retest) was observed for most beverages, milk products, spreads on bread and meat (all of which included food items categorised into at least two fat categories) and also for eggs, fruits and vegetables, nuts, pasta and rice, dessert/sweets, smoking and physical activity. Reproducibility did not consistently meet a satisfactory standard ($r \leq 0.41$ or large difference between test and retest) for unsweetened cereals, fatty fish, cakes, oils, white-, bread, crispbread and rice.

***Conclusion:*** The validity of the VISA-FFQ was acceptable for intake of milk fat, and there was an overall satisfactory, though variable, reproducibility for intake of several foods and lifestyle factors in the VISA-FFQ.

Keywords: *Food Frequency Questionnaire; validity; biomarkers; fatty acids; dietary assessment; short-FFQ; milk-fat; saturated fat*

It has been calculated that an unhealthy diet contributes to the largest proportion of disability-adjusted life years globally (1) and is associated with about 45% of all deaths from cardiovascular diseases (CVD) and type 2 diabetes (T2D) in America (2, 3). It is therefore important to assess food and lifestyle factors that can modulate the risk of disease and to use the assessment to recognise individuals and groups who would benefit from dietary changes (4). The Food Frequency Questionnaire (FFQ) is the most common tool in epidemiological studies to assess diet in relation to health outcomes. FFQs are designed to assess usual diet in retrospect, but are often time-consuming to complete (5). Short FFQs are considered less time-consuming (6), which may be of particular importance in any clinical setting where limited time may be an issue (7).

The validated short FFQ, NORDIET-FFQ (8), was developed in an ongoing study of colorectal cancer patients (9). The NORDIET-FFQ was designed to assess adherence to the Norwegian food-based dietary guidelines (10), including estimation of food quantities for the previous 1–2 months (9). Convenient, quantitative assessment of foods and lifestyle associated with CVD was desired in the Vascular lifestyle-Intervention and Screening in phArmacies (VISA) study (11). The Norwegian screener 'SmartDiet' offered such assessment (12), however without estimation of food quantities. Consequently, a study-specific FFQ, the VISA-FFQ, was adapted from the NORDIET-FFQ in order to include assessment of intake of foods and lifestyle factors associated with CVD risk.

The aim was to evaluate the VISA-FFQ's relative validity of estimated intake of milk fat (using biomarker fatty acids pentadecanoic acid [15:0] and heptadecanoic acid [17:0] as references) and reproducibility of intake of foods and lifestyle factors among a group of individuals with moderately high risk of CVD.

## Methods

### *Study design*

The study population was pharmacy customers in 48 pharmacies that were enrolled in the VISA study. The VISA study subsample included 558 participants with moderately elevated risk of CVD who had been screened in the previous year. Of them, 375 participants participated in a 4-week intervention randomised by pharmacy (23 intervention pharmacies and 25 usual care pharmacies) in September 2015 and were for that eligible for this evaluation (Table 1).

During the pharmacy visit (time 1, the beginning of the intervention), participants were asked for consent to obtain extra blood for dried blood spots (DBS) sampling and to complete the VISA-FFQ. If consent was given, participants were also asked to self-sample DBS and complete the VISA-FFQ at home 4 weeks later, at designated time 2 (end of intervention).

The VISA-FFQ and DBS were completed on the same or the next day. For the purpose of this study, data from the VISA-FFQ and fatty acid 15:0 and 17:0 % of Fatty Acid Methyl Ester (FAME) assayed from DBS obtained at time 1 and 2 were utilized to evaluate the VISA-FFQ for relative validity of milk fat and overall reproducibility.

### *DBS sampling*

The DBS is a form of bio-sampling where blood obtained by a finger-prick lancet is blotted on spots on filter paper (DBS-card) (13). DBS sampling was performed by health care providers in pharmacies at time 1 and by each participant (self-sampling) at time 2. Fasting samples were desired but not required. Participants with appointments late in the day, and those who had taken

*Table 1.* Retrospective background characteristics of completers- and non-completers of the VISA-FFQ at study inclusion.

| | Completers ($N$ = 368) | Non-completers ($N$ = 190)[a] | $p$[b] |
|---|---|---|---|
| Men, % ($N$) | 26.1 (96/368) | 32.6 (62/190) | 0.11 |
| Living alone, % ($N$)[c] | 37.8 (139/368) | 36.8 (70/190) | 1.00 |
| Smokers, % ($N$)[d] | 17.2 (54/368) | 22.9 (43/188) | 0.02 |
| Ethnicity outside Nordic countries, % ($N$)[e] | 11.8 (43/365) | 15.7 (29/185) | 0.23 |
| Low education, % ($N$)[f] | 52.4 (184/351) | 59.2 (106/179) | 0.14 |
| Age (years), mean (SD) | 58.1 ± 13.7 | 53.7 ± 15.9 | 0.02 |
| Body mass index (kg/m$^2$), mean (SD) | 27.0 ± 4.4 | 27.2 ± 5.1 | 0.64 |
| Hemoglobin A1c (%), mean (SD) | 5.5 ± 0.3 | 5.5 ± 0.3 | 0.28 |
| Systolic blood pressure (mmHg), mean (SD) | 131.1 ± 16.9 | 131.7 ± 17.6 | 0.72 |
| Diastolic blood pressure (mmHg), mean (SD) | 80.3 ± 9.6 | 81.2 ± 10.5 | 0.33 |
| Total cholesterol (mmol/L), mean (SD) | 6.5 ± 1.2 | 6.4 ± 1.3 | 0.18 |
| HDL-cholesterol (mmol/L), mean (SD) | 1.7 ± 0.5 | 1.7 ± 0.5 | 0.07 |
| LDL-cholesterol (mmol/L), mean (SD) | 3.9 ± 1.0 | 3.9 ± 1.0 | 0.39 |
| Triglycerides (mmol/L), mean (SD) | 2.0 ± 1.1 | 2.1 ± 1.2 | 0.57 |

Data are presented as percentage (%) and numbers (N), or mean and standard deviation (SD). HDL, high density lipoprotein; LDL, low density lipoprotein.
[a]Includes 7 participants that attended the study visit but did not complete the questionnaire.
[b]Chi-square test of independence or independent sample *t*-test.
[c]Not married/no significant other and widow/widower/divorced.
[d]% Yes, daily/Yes, occasionally.
[e]Both or one parent born outside Norway.
[f]Low education ≤13 years of schooling.

omega-3 supplements or had recently eaten fatty fish were excluded from DBS sampling. After completion, the DBS-card was left to dry for 2–4 h before it was put in an airtight aluminium bag and stored in the refrigerator at 1–4°C (14).

DBS samples were returned either to the University of Oslo or directly to the laboratory responsible for the analyses, VITAS AS (Oslo). From DBS, fatty acids in whole blood (plasma and cells) (15) were separated and determined by extracting FAME that were further analysed with gas chromatography – flame ionisation detector (GC-FID) after direct transmethylation by VITAS. The results were given in % of FAME (16).

#### *VISA-FFQ*

The 62-item VISA-FFQ originates from the 66-item NORDIET-FFQ (8). The VISA-FFQ and the NORDIET-FFQ share the features of 15 minutes completion time and of being a semi-quantitative FFQ that covers habitual dietary intake (grams/day) of food and lifestyle factors for the past 1–2 months (8). The questionnaires include both frequency (how often the item was consumed) and amount of the food items. Amounts were expressed as portion sizes, specified according to the food composition and nutrient calculation system (named KBS), version AE-14, developed at the University of Oslo. When different foods were combined into one category (such as high-fat [HF] meat comprising, e.g., hamburger, hot dogs and processed meat, ~17% fats), the average portion size of all the items was estimated from KBS and recorded (8). The VISA-FFQ was optically readable, and the handling of data including missing data followed the same procedure as described earlier by Henriksen et al. (8).

#### Development of the VISA-FFQ

In the development of the 62-items VISA-FFQ, we altered 14 items, added 4 items, deleted 9 items and kept the remaining 44 items unchanged from the original NORDIET-FFQ (8), as presented in Supplementary file 1.

#### Altered items

Fourteen items in the categories beverages (milk), milk products, spreads (cheese and meat) and meat (dinner or hot lunch) were revised in order to provide more comprehensive information on intake of foods that are major contributors to dietary saturated fatty acids (SFA) according to the national food database (17). Milk, milk products, cheese and meat products were categorised according to low-fat (LF), medium-fat (MF) and HF content (majority SFA), using KBS and SmartDiet (12) as references (Supplementary file 1). In later data analysis, MF and LF cheese and meat (dinner or hot lunch) were combined into one single medium/LF item each.

#### Items added, deleted and/or unaltered

Four items associated with the risk of CVD were added to the VISA-FFQ. These were; prevalence of smoking and number of cigarettes per day (18), weekly egg intake (19) and use of cholesterol lowering margarine with added plants sterols (20). Smoking and cholesterol lowering margarine had three fixed response categories: 'no'; 'yes, occasional'; and 'yes, daily' and an additional 'do not know' category for the margarine. Egg intake and number of cigarettes were numeric variables (Supplementary file 1). To preserve the VISA-FFQ as a four-page, 62-item questionnaire, nine items in the NORDIET-FFQ that were considered less relevant for CVD risk, or were redundant with information previously collected in VISA study, were dropped in favour of the new items. These included age, height, weight and gender, and five diet-related items: use of dietary supplements, intake of 'small fruits', 'berries and dried fruit' from the category 'fruit', tomato sauce from the category 'vegetables' and 'tea' from the category 'beverages' (Supplementary file 1).

The VISA-FFQ also includes 44 other items within the categories fruits, nuts, vegetables, cereals, beverages, bread, spreads on bread, fat spreads and oils, fish for dinner, rice and pasta, cakes, dessert and sweets, and physical activity. These were unaltered from the NORDIET-FFQ and have previously been validated in a colorectal cancer sample (8, 21).

#### *Evaluation of VISA-FFQ*

Relative validity of milk was assessed at times 1 and 2 in the pooled intervention and usual care pharmacies. Milk fat in the VISA-FFQ comprised the items whole-fat milk, LF milk, HF and MF milk products, and HF and MF cheese. From KBS, we obtained data on average nutritional content of 15:0 and 17:0 from the milk fat items (Supplementary file 2). These data were utilised to calculate total 15:0 and total 17:0 in consumed milk fat estimated from the VISA-FFQ. Hence, to assess relative validity of milk fat, 15:0 and 17:0 in consumed milk fat (grams/day) estimated from the VISA-FFQ were compared with biomarkers 15:0 and 17:0 % of FAME assayed from DBS.

Completed VISA-FFQs obtained from participants in the usual care pharmacies (in which there had not been any intervention) at time 1 (test) and time 2 (retest) were used to evaluate reproducibility. We assessed reproducibility of the 18 items within several categories that were changed relative to the VISA-FFQ: beverages (whole-fat, LF milk and skimmed milk), milk products (HF, MF and LF milk products), spreads on bread (HF, MF and LF cheese, and HF and LF meat), meat for dinner or hot lunch (HF, MF and LF meat), eggs, cigarettes, smoking and use of cholesterol lowering margarine. Next, we assessed reproducibility of the 44 unchanged items within the categories fruits, nuts, vegetables, cereals, beverages, bread, spreads on bread, fat spreads and oils, fish for dinner, rice and pasta, cakes, dessert and sweets, and physical activity.

### *Statistical analysis*

#### Power calculation

Sample size was estimated following Hulley's calculation (22, 23). A sample size of 41 participants would be sufficient to observe correlation coefficients (r) of 0.50 or higher, with a significance level of 5 and 80% power.

#### Statistical methods

All analyses were performed in SAS software 9.4 for Windows, with the exception of the Bland-Altman plots that were computed in SPSS version 23. The level of significance was set to 5%. Continuous variables considered to be non-normally distributed were presented as median and 25th ($P_{25}$) and 75th ($P_{75}$) percentiles; otherwise, data were presented as mean and standard deviation (SD). Categorical data were presented with percentages and numbers.

For the evaluation of relative validity of milk fat, Spearman's rank order correlation (RHO) was used to explore the relationship between 15:0 and 17:0 in consumed milk fat (grams/day) and biomarker 15:0 and 17:0% of FAME. Correlation coefficients were stratified by sex and adjusted for total intake of foods and drinks (grams/day) computed from summarising all food items (except tap water) from the VISA-FFQ.

Several measures were used to evaluate reproducibility of items between test and retest completion of the VISA-FFQ. Spearman's RHO was used, and correlation coefficients were considered as follows: $r \geq 0.50$ was defined as 'satisfactory or good', $r = 0.30$–$0.49$ were defined as 'fair' and $r < 0.30$ was defined as 'poor' (24). Weighted Kappa correlation coefficient was used to explore the strength of relationship between categorical variables. Bland–Altman plots were used to explore the presence of outliers and degree of agreement between test and retest, including the limits of agreement that comprise 95% (mean difference ± 1.96 SD) of the sample (25). Lastly, the non-parametric options, Wilcoxon signed-rank test and Kruskal–Wallis test, were used to test for significant difference in intakes between test and retest, whereas McNemar test was used for categorical variables.

Background characteristics were obtained approximatly 44 weeks prior to the evaluation. Characteristics were presented as the total sample available for the evaluation, completers of the VISA-FFQ compared to non-completers (who either did not complete the VISA-FFQ at time 1 or were lost to follow-up before time 1).

#### Ethics

Participants gave written informed consent to participate. The VISA study was approved by the National Committee for Research Ethics in Norway (REK) with reference number 2013/1660-/REK South-East and was reported to the Norwegian Center for Research.

## Results

In total, 98.1% ($n$ = 368) of participants at time 1 completed the VISA-FFQ (completers). Males were on average 55.6 ± 13.8 years old, whereas females were 59.3 ± 13.2 years old. Compared to the non-completers, smoking was less frequent (17.2%, $n$ = 54 vs. 22.9%, $n$ = 43), and age was higher (58.1 ± 13.7 years vs. 53.7 ± 15.9 years) in completers. Otherwise, samples seemed similar (Table 1).

The sample utilised to evaluate relative validity of milk fat included 307 participants (79 males, 226 females and 2 with missing gender data) at time 1 who had satisfactorily completed both the VISA-FFQ and the DBS. The corresponding number at time 2 was 237 participants (57 males, 173 females and 7 with missing gender data). The sample utilised to evaluate reproducibility (test–retest) consisted of 122 participants (26 males and 96 females) who completed the VISA-FFQ both at times 1 and 2 (Figure 1).

### *Evaluation of relative validity*

At time 1, intake of 15:0 in consumed milk fat (grams/day), adjusted for total intake of foods and drinks, was significantly correlated with biomarker 15:0 (% of FAME), with $r = 0.32$ ($p < 0.05$) for the total sample. Corresponding correlation between 17:0 in consumed milk fat and biomarker 17:0% of FAME was non-significant ($r = 0.10$). Correlations tended to be slightly higher the first time the biomarker fatty acids were measured, and higher for males than females (Table 2). We also stratified the correlations by age groups. Total food and drinks-adjusted correlations between 15:0 in consumed milk fat and biomarker 15:0 appeared highest for the 57 participants in the age group 18–45 years with $r = 0.56$ ($p < 0.05$). Corresponding correlation in the age group 46–55 years ($n$ = 146) was $r = 0.18$ ($p < 0.05$) and $r = 0.35$ in the age group 66–88 years ($N$ = 104). Overall, Pearson's correlation coefficients were numerically lower than the presented Spearman's RHO coefficients.

### *Evaluation of reproducibility of the altered items*

Measures of reproducibility between the test and retest completion of the VISA-FFQ for the 18 altered or added items are presented in Table 3.

Significant correlations between test and retest results defined as satisfactory or good were observed for 12 out of 18 items (67%). This included eggs ($r = 0.76$) and cigarettes ($r = 0.92$), in addition to LF milk and skimmed milk, HF- and LF-milk products, HF cheese, HF and LF meat (spreads) and HF meat (dinner or hot lunch), smoking and use of cholesterol lowering margarine.

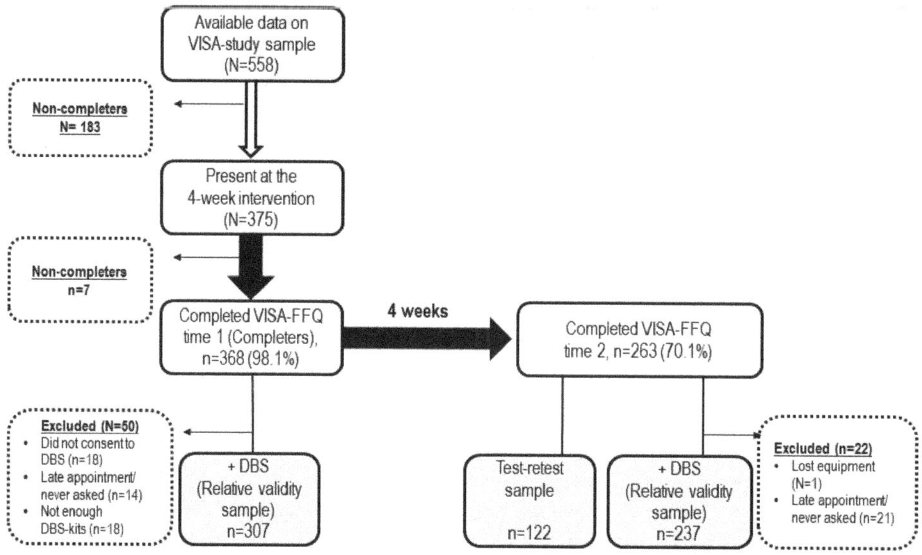


*Fig. 1.* Study design and flow of participants included in the evaluation of the VISA-FFQ.

*Table 2.* Correlations (Spearman's rho) between milk fat estimated from the VISA-FFQ and biomarker saturated fatty acids measured in whole blood at time 1 and 2.

| | Pentadecanoic acid (15:0) % of FAME | | | | | | Heptadecanoic acid (17:0) % of FAME | | | | | |
|---|---|---|---|---|---|---|---|---|---|---|---|---|
| | Time 1[a] | | | Time 2[b] | | | Time 1[a] | | | Time 2[b] | | |
| | Total[c] (N = 307) | Male (N = 79) | Female (N = 226) | Total (N = 237) | Male (N = 57) | Female (N = 173) | Total[c] (N = 307) | Male (N = 79) | Female (N = 234) | Total (N = 237) | Male (N = 57) | Female (N = 173) |
| **Milk (g/day)** | | | | | | | | | | | | |
| Whole-fat milk | 0.16* | 0.17 | 0.16* | 0.14* | -0.08 | 0.20* | 0.06 | 0.16 | 0.02 | 0.10 | 0.02 | 0.13 |
| **Milk products (g/day )**[d] | | | | | | | | | | | | |
| High-fat milk products | 0.20* | 0.24* | 0.18* | 0.18* | 0.29* | 0.12 | 0.05 | 0.15 | 0.01 | 0.05 | 0.01 | 0.04 |
| **Cheese (g/day)** | | | | | | | | | | | | |
| High-fat cheese | 0.24* | 0.36* | 0.21* | 0.24* | 0.52* | 0.14 | 0.11 | 0.08 | 0.13* | 0.10 | 0.34* | 0.03 |
| **Total dietary milk fatty acids**[e] | 0.32* | 0.38* | 0.29* | 0.30* | 0.40* | 0.27* | 0.10 | 0.16 | 0.09 | 0.07 | 0.008 | 0.10 |

VISA-FFQ, Vascular lifestyle-Intervention and Screening in pharmacies- food frequency questionnaire.
FAME = fatty acids methyl esters.
*Correlation coefficient is significant at the 0.05 level (2-tailed). Adjusted for total food and drink intake (except tap water) in grams/day.
[a]Dried blood spot sampling and VISA-FFQ performed in pharmacy.
[b]Dried blood spot sampling and VISA-FFQ performed at home.
[c]Including missing gender.
[d]Cream and yoghurt.
[e]Total dietary milk fatty acids 15:0 and 17:0 were estimated from intakes of from milk, milk products and cheese except low-fat/fat-free and compared to corresponding biomarker fatty acid.

Significant correlations defined as fair were found for the remaining items. Combining MF and LF items for cheese (spreads) and meat (dinner or hot lunch) into a single item each resulted in correlations considered satisfactory/good (Table 3).

Among these 18 items, only typical intake in grams/day of HF cheese, whole-fat milk and use of cholesterol lowering margarine was significantly different between test and retest (Table 3). The Bland–Altman plots in Figure 2 illustrate that the mean difference in intake of HF cheese between test and retest was −2.00 grams/day. Further, that 95% of the observations were within the range of 15.7–19.7 grams/day (limits of agreements), corresponding to about two slices of cheese (Figure 2a). Mean difference in the intake of whole-fat milk was 9.0 grams/day, with limits of agreements of 148.0–157.0 grams/day, corresponding

*Table 3.* Measures of reproducibility for 18 food and lifestyle factors[a] in the test-retest sample ($N$ = 122).

| | Test (time 1)[b] | Retest (time 2)[c] | *P*-value of difference[d] | Correlation coefficient[e] |
|---|---|---|---|---|
| | Total (*N* = 122) | Total (*N* = 122) | Total (*N* = 122) | Total (*N* = 122) |
| | Median ($P_{25}$, $P_{75}$) | Median ($P_{25}$, $P_{75}$) | *p* | *r* |
| **Milk (g/day)** | | | | |
| Whole-fat milk | 0 (0,0)/ 23.8±14.9[f] | 0 (0,0)/ 14.9±52.1[f] | 0.03 | 0.45* |
| Low-fat milk | 58.0 (0, 142) | 50.0 (0, 186) | 0.94 | 0.81* |
| Skimmed milk | 0 (0, 14) | 0 (0, 28) | 0.92 | 0.68* |
| **Milk products (g/day)[g]** | | | | |
| High-fat milk products | 0 (0, 7) | 0 (0, 3.5) | 0.67 | 0.50* |
| Medium-fat milk products | 7.0 (0, 17.8) | 7.0 (0, 14.5) | 0.34 | 0.48* |
| Low-fat milk products | 3.5 (0, 14.5) | 7.0 (0, 23.3) | 0.63 | 0.53* |
| **Spreads (g/day)** | | | | |
| High-fat cheese | 3.6 (1.43, 9.3) | 6.4 (1.4, 9.3) | 0.02 | 0.51* |
| Medium-fat cheese | 0 (0, 3.6) | 0 (0, 3.6) | 0.50 | 0.40* |
| Low-fat cheese | 0 (0, 1.4) | 0 (0, 1.4) | 0.77 | 0.47* |
| Medium/low-fat cheese[h] | 1.4 (0, 6.4) | 0 (0, 6.4) | 0.47 | 0.51* |
| High-fat meat[i] | 1.4 (0, 3.6) | 0 (0, 3.6) | 0.72 | 0.59* |
| Low-fat meat[j] | 3.6 (0, 6.4) | 3.6 (0, 6.4) | 0.82 | 0.59* |
| **Meat dinner or hot lunch (g/day)** | | | | |
| High-fat meat[k] | 10.5 (0, 42.0) | 10.5 (0, 21.0) | 0.14 | 0.52* |
| Medium-fat meat[l] | 15.8 (0, 43.5) | 21.0 (0, 43.5) | 0.09 | 0.44* |
| Low-fat meat[m] | 43.5 (21.0,64.5) | 43.5 (21, 64.5) | 0.43 | 0.46* |
| Medium/low-fat meat[h] | 64.5 (32.3, 87.0) | 64.5 (43.5, 106.5) | 0.06 | 0.50* |
| **Other** | | | | |
| Eggs per week | 4.0 (2, 6) | 3.0 (2, 5) | 0.29 | 0.76* |
| Number of cigarettes | 10.0 (7, 20) | 8.0 (0, 10) | 0.25 | 0.92* |
| Smoking[n] | 0.08 (10/121) | 0.08 (10/122) | 1.00 | 0.94* |
| Cholesterol lowering Margarine[n] | 30.0 (36/120) | 36.7 (44/120) | 0.03 | 0.50* |

VISA-FFQ, Vascular lifestyle-Intervention and Screening in pharmacies- food frequency questionnaire.
*Spearman's rank order correlation (rho) coefficient is significant at the 0.05 level (2-tailed).
[a]These 18 items in the VISA-FFQ were revised relative to the original questionnaire, NORDDIET-FFQ (8).
[b]VISA-FFQ completed at pharmacy.
[c]VISA-FFQ completed at home.
[d]Tested by Wilcoxon Signed-Rank test, McNemar test for smoking and cholesterol lowering margarine.
[e]r = Spearman's rho coefficient or Weighted Kappa coefficient (smoking and cholesterol lowering margarine).
[f]Mean and standard deviation.
[g]Milk products = cream and yoghurt (whole-fat, medium-fat and low-fat according to approximately SFA content).
[h]Not an original category in the VISA-FFQ. Made by combining low-fat and medium-fat alternatives.
[i]High fat meat spreads = salami, liver paste etc.
[j]Low-fat meat spreads = ham, chicken/turkey etc.
[k]High-fat meat = ground meat, sausage, hamburger.
[l]Medium-fat meat = low-fat ground meat, sausage, hamburger.
[m]Low-fat meat = game, pork, chicken filets.
[n]Yes, daily /Yes, occasionally % (n/N).

to a big glass of milk (Figure 2b). No distinct pattern of outliers was observed for any item.

#### *Evaluation of reproducibility of the unaltered items*

Among the unaltered items, significant correlations between test and retest results defined as satisfactory or good were observed for 35 out of 44 items (80%) (Table 4). These included all items in the categories nuts, cereals, beverages, fish for dinner, cakes, dessert and sweets and physical activity. Despite satisfactory correlations, estimated intake of tomato, unsweetened and sweetened cereals, tap water, sodas with no added sugar, fatty fish, cakes and dessert and chips was significantly different in intakes (grams/day) between test and retest. Particularly for

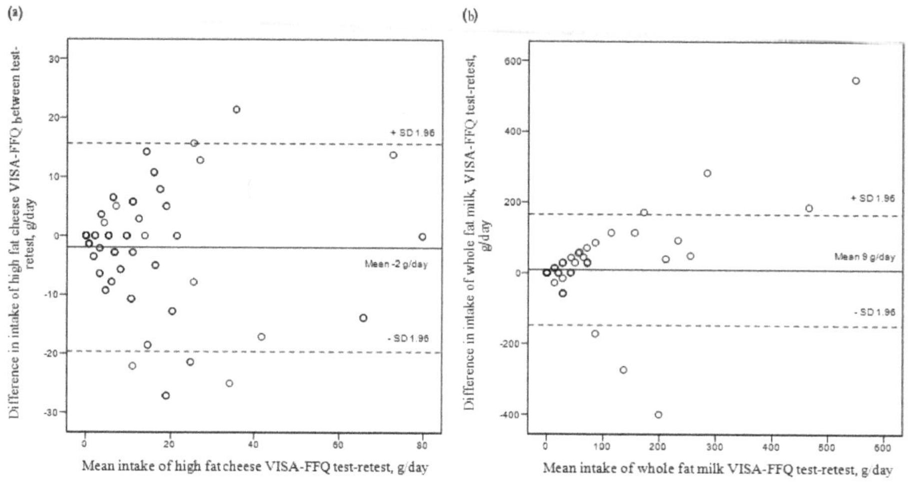

*Fig. 2.* Bland–Altman plot of intake of high-fat cheese (a) and whole-fat milk (b) as estimated from test and retest completion of the VISA-FFQ ($N$ = 122).

*Table 4.* Measures of reproducibility for 44 food and lifestyle factors[a] in the test-retest sample ($N$ = 122).

| | Test (time 1)[b] | Retest (time 2)[c] | *P*-value of difference[d] | Correlation coefficient[e] |
|---|---|---|---|---|
| | Total ($N$ = 122) | Total ($N$ = 122) | Total ($N$ = 122) | Total ($N$ = 122) |
| | Median ($P_{25}$, $P_{75}$) | Median ($P_{25}$, $P_{75}$) | *p* | *r* |
| **Fruits (g/day)** | | | | |
| Large fruit | 57.0 (43.0, 93.0) | 57.0 (39.5, 93.0) | 0.46 | 0.69* |
| Medium-size fruit | 14.5 (6.1, 43.0) | 14.5 (0, 43.0) | 0.45 | 0.46* |
| **Nuts (g/day)** | | | | |
| Unsalted | 5.4 (1.3, 12.6) | 3.6 (0, 11.6) | 0.13 | 0.58* |
| Salted | 0.9 (0, 3.6) | 1.8 (0, 3.6) | 0.73 | 0.53* |
| **Vegetables (g/day)** | | | | |
| Garlic | 0.1 (0, 0.7) | 0.1 (0, 0.6) | 0.49 | 0.81* |
| Onion | 5.8 (2.5, 12.9) | 5.8 (1.4, 8.7) | 0.08 | 0.65* |
| Tomato | 30.2 (18.2, 60.5) | 28.0 (14.0, 55.9) | 0.03 | 0.53* |
| Mixed salad | 28.5(13.2, 49.1) | 28.5 (7.3, 46.5) | 0.14 | 0.47* |
| Other vegetables | 68.4 (34.7, 111.6) | 55.8 (34.8, 104.9) | 0.92 | 0.50* |
| **Cereals (g/d)** | | | | |
| Sweetened cereals | 0 (0, 0)/3.51±10.2[f] | 0 (0, 0)/1.34±5.8[f] | 0.01 | 0.65* |
| Unsweetened | 7.3 (0, 35.5) | 17.8 (0, 46.5) | 0.003 | 0.62* |
| **Beverages (g/d)** | | | | |
| Tap water | 274 (186, 548) | 274 (186, 548) | 0.01 | 0.61* |
| Sodas with no added sugar | 28.0 (0, 114.0) | 28.0 (0, 86.0) | 0.01 | 0.71* |
| Juice | 28.0 (0,86.0) | 28.0 (0, 93.0) | 0.40 | 0.75* |
| Other beverages with no added sugar | 0 (0, 28) | 0 (0, 28) | 0.83 | 0.53* |
| Beer with alcohol | 0 (0, 70.0) | 0 (0, 140.0) | 0.44 | 0.77* |
| Liquor, g/d | 0 (0, 0) | 0 (0, 0) | 0.36 | 0.69* |
| Wine with alcohol | 15.4 (0, 63.8) | 15.4 (0, 63.8) | 0.67 | 0.73* |
| Filtered coffee | 342.5(0, 685.0) | 342.5 (13.1, 465.0) | 0.72 | 0.71* |
| Other coffee (espresso, etc.) | 0 (0, 142.5) | 0 (0, 107.5) | 0.37 | 0.77* |

*Table 4.* Continued

| | Test (time 1)[b] | Retest (time 2)[c] | P-value of difference[d] | Correlation coefficient[e] |
|---|---|---|---|---|
| | Total (N = 122) | Total (N = 122) | Total (N = 122) | Total (N = 122) |
| | Median ($P_{25}$, $P_{75}$) | Median ($P_{25}$, $P_{75}$) | p | r |
| **Bread (g/d)** | | | | |
| Bread (60 % cereals) with 0-25 % wholemeal flour | 0 (0, 0) | 0 (0, 0) | 0.77 | 0.09 |
| Bread (60 % cereals) with 25-50% wholemeal flour | 0.0 (0, 72.0) | 0.0 (0, 72.0) | 0.66 | 0.49* |
| Bread (60 % cereals) with 50-75 wholemeal flour | 60.0 (0 , 180.0) | 60.0 (0, 120.0) | 0.38 | 0.54* |
| Bread (60 % cereals) with 75-100 wholemeal flour | 0 (0, 60.0) | 0 (0, 60.0) | 0.85 | 0.44* |
| White crispbread (0-25% wholegrain) | 0 (0, 0) | 0 (0, 0) | 0.56 | 0.10 |
| Wholemeal crispbread (100% wholegrain) | 14.0 (0, 28.0) | 14.0 (0, 28.0) | 0.83 | 0.62* |
| **Spreads on bread** | | | | |
| Sweetened spreads(g/week) | 20.0 (0, 90.0) | 20.0 (0, 60.0) | 0.56 | 0.59* |
| Fruits and vegetables as spreads (g/day) | 37.5 (0, 75.0) | 37.5 (0, 67.5) | 0.42 | 0.48* |
| Fish spreads (g/ week) | 90 (0, 162) | 90 (0, 162) | 0.82 | 0.66* |
| **Fat spreads and oils % (n/N)** | | | | |
| Oils, margarine, butter or not using any | 97.5 (119/122)[g] | | 0.16 | 0.41* |
| Types of fat spreads or not using any | 93.4 (114/122)[g] | | 0.80 | 0.77* |
| **Fish for dinner (g/day)** | | | | |
| Fatty fish | 42.1 (20.3, 62.4) | 20.3 (20.3, 42.05) | <0.001 | 0.68* |
| Processed fish | 6.3 (0, 25.2) | 25.2 (0, 25.2) | 0.94 | 0.55* |
| Lean fish | 20.3 (0, 42.1) | 20.3 (7.6, 42.1) | 0.79 | 0.55* |
| **Rice and pasta (g/day)** | | | | |
| White rice | 0 (0,14.0) | 0 (0, 22.4) | 0.88 | 0.41* |
| Wholegrain rice | 0 (0,0) | 0 (0,0) | 0.75 | 0.61* |
| White pasta | 0 (0, 17.5) | 0 (0, 17.5) | 0.63 | 0.53* |
| Wholegrain pasta | 0 (0,17.5) | 0 (0, 17.5) | 0.17 | 0.73* |
| **Cake, dessert and sweets (g/d)** | | | | |
| Cakes | 16.8 (0, 25.8) | 17.4 (8.4, 34.8) | 0.01 | 0.52* |
| Dessert | 12.6 (0, 26.1) | 12.6 (0, 25.2) | 0.03 | 0.58* |
| Chocolate/candy | 3.5 (0, 15.3) | 7.3 (0, 14.5) | 0.61 | 0.59* |
| Chips | 0 (0, 6.5) | 0 (0, 8.4) | 0.04 | 0.67* |
| **Physical activity (min/day)** | | | | |
| Moderate intensity | 18.1 (10.8, 35.3) | 18.1 (11.0, 37.6) | 0.69 | 0.57* |
| High intensity | 0.8 (0, 11.0) | 0.5 (0, 11.0) | 0.30 | 0.64* |

VISA-FFQ, Vascular lifestyle-Intervention and Screening in pharmacies- food frequency questionnaire. g/day, grams per day min/day, minutes per day.
*Spearman's rank order correlation (rho) coefficient is significant at the 0.05 level (2-tailed).
[a]These 44 items in the VISA-FFQ were unaltered from the original questionnaire, NORDDIET-FFQ (8).
[b]VISA-FFQ completed at pharmacy.
[c]VISA-FFQ completed at home.
[d]Tested by Wilcoxon Signed-Rank test or McNemars test for fat spreads and oils.
[e]r= Spearman's rho coefficient or Weighted Kappa coefficient fat spreads and oils.
[f]Mean± standard deviation.
[g]Percent and frequency of participants reporting the same category (not using/ using soft margarines/ using butter / using oils) both at test and retest.

sweetened cereals, tap water, sodas with no added sugar, dessert and chips, median and 25th and 75th percentiles were similar between time test and retest, but $p$-value for difference was significant due to small number of users or differences in the extremes of intake.

Furthermore, significant correlations defined as satisfactory or good were observed for the items large fruit (but not medium fruit, $r = 0.46$), all vegetables except for mixed salad ($r = 0.47$), all spreads on bread (except for fruit and vegetables spreads, $r = 0.48$) and all rice and pasta items except for white rice ($r = 0.41$). Correlations for the category bread were more various ranging from $r = 0.49$ for bread with 75–100% wholemeal flour to $r \leq 0.1$ for white bread and crispbreads (0–25% wholemeal flour).

In total 97% responded to the same category for use of oils (or other cooking fats) between test and retest, but correlation was fair with $r = 0.41$ (Table 4).

### Discussion

The VISA-FFQ's ability to give a relatively valid estimate of milk fat was acceptable, displayed as postive correlations between consumed 15:0 milk fat estimated from the VISA-FFQ (grams/day) and biomarker 15:0 (% of FAME). The VISA-FFQ also showed good and consistent reproducibility for intake (in grams/day) or frequency of use of most of the items in the VISA-FFQ.

#### *Relative validity*

Since not all milk products supply the same amount of fat (26), relative validity of milk fat intake was assessed by comparing the approximate, total intake of 15:0 and 17:0 estimated from consumed milk fat in grams/day, with biomarker fatty acids 15:0 and 17:0 % of FAME (27, 28). These fatty acids are assumed to originate mainly from milk fat because they are produced in relatively high levels in ruminants by rumen microbial fermentation and microbial de novo lipogenesis which may again transfer to the host animal (29). Although milk fat is believed to be the primary source of odd-chain fatty acids, a recent study found that humans can also synthesise them as products of gut fermentation, particularly using propionate as a source (30). Moreover, these fatty acids can also be found in lamb, beef, venison and fatty fish (31), but no significant correlations of these foods with these two fatty acids have been observed (28).

Adjusting for total intake of foods (as the questionnaire was judged not to be sufficient to estimate energy intake) increased the correlation between 15:0 in consumed milk fat and biomarker 15:0 from $r = 0.26$ to $r = 0.32$. The agreement between consumed milk fat and biomarker milk fat was comparable to other studies using whole-blood biomarker 15:0 as reference (32, 33). Supported by others (26, 27), we observed that biomarker 15:0 was a better reference for milk fat intake than 17:0, reflecting the nutritional distribution of fatty acids in milk fat (26).

This validation standard is however imperfect because nutrition composition databases for calculations of milk fat are approximate (26, 34). Additionally, perfect agreement cannot be expected when the periods over which intake was assessed were different (35). VISA-FFQ measures diet for the previous 1–2 months, but the fatty acids in whole blood reflect dietary intake from the last hours to several days (36). There might even be lower proportion of fatty acids in whole blood compared to other blood constituents (32). However, similar correlations for the total sample at time 1 ($r = 0.32$) and 2 ($r = 0.30$) strengthen the validity of the results. Fatty acid concentrations in blood are also affected by metabolism, absorption and genetics that differ among individuals (29). These anticipated variations in biomarker fatty acids can also elucidate variation patterns in correlations with fatty acids in consumed milk fat among genders and age groups. Our observed results on gender difference were similar to a comparable study of Swedish adults (28) and could also be due to women being more likely than men to under-report according to social desirability and approval (37).

#### *Reproducibility*

Reproducibility was measured by assessing how consistently reported food intake and lifestyle factors could be repeated in the same participants within 4 weeks (5, 38). Correlations indicate ability to rank individuals according to the items evaluated and whether this ranking was maintained relative to other participants in the test–retest period (7). Previous studies have shown that short FFQs show good ability to rank individuals according to food intake (7, 38). Our results add to this, with significant correlations defined as satisfactory or good ($r \geq 0.50$) for 76% ($n = 47$) of the VISA-FFQ's items (24), whereas the correlation coefficients were less satisfactory ($r = 0.40$–$0.47$) for intake of LF and MF cheese and meat (dinner or hot lunch), in accordance with other studies (39). When LF and MF items aggregated into one item, the correlations increased to $r = 0.50$. We acknowledge that the fat content in LF and MF meat and cheese is too alike to justify the need for three categories of cheese and meat according to fat intake, as suggested elsewhere (40). Nonetheless, 81% ($n = 50$) of the items had non-significantly difference in intakes between test and retest administration of the VISA-FFQ. The majority of the remaining items had small differences, not considered to be of clinical relevance as supported by others (8). Accordingly, only intake of unsweetened cereals, fatty fish, cakes, oils, white rice, white bread and crispbread showed divergent measures of reproducibility. This could be due to either systematic errors in the VISA-FFQ, true changes in food intake, few responders or extreme outliers (13). Our results are consistent with a Norwegian study evaluating reproducibility of large and comprehensive FFQs (41), the NORDIET-FFQ that were validated against 7-days weighed record (8) and a screener assessing ability to rank intake of HF foods among individuals with elevated cholesterol level (42). Since the test–retest sample consisted of only 26 men, we did not have power to stratify the results by gender. However, we performed a sensitivity analysis on gender and the results appeared similar for men and women.

#### *Strengths and limitations*

The 62-item VISA-FFQ was self-administered, and it appeared to be convenient in many ways; it had 98% completion rate in a clinical setting and 70% at home, and it was quick to self-administer and less time-consuming to analyse compared to other questionnaires (6).

However, the skewed distribution of gender may affect the representativeness of the results.

The evaluation was strengthen by the use of objective biomarkers for milk fat intake, twice, which reduces limitations associated with self-report of dietary intake (36). Although the relative validity correlation coefficient was only 0.32, we considered that to show that the diet items and the objective marker were measuring the same construct. We note that biomarkers have their own limitations, and full energy computation of VISA-FFQ was not possible. Since variation in dietary intake can be due to both errors in measurements and true changes in food intake (43) that cannot be separated (5), we attempted to improve the evaluation of reproducibility by using data solitary from participants who did not receive any intervention. However, it is well known that the awareness of being studied in itself can affect behaviour and consciousness of own habits (44). For instance, in line with current national recommendations for CVD prevention (4), intake of HF meat showed a tendency to decrease after 4 weeks, while MF meat increased. In a group of individuals with elevated risk of CVD, there is therefore a high possibility that these changes truly occurred, supporting the evaluation of the VISA-FFQ. Short FFQs can be used to assess changes in diet and lifestyle frequently (6). Such monitoring is likely to be beneficial for people at risk of disease, such as the VISA study sample (11). As the relationships between today's food intake and risk of CVD and T2D still have uncertainties (45), we aim to use VISA-FFQ as a tool to further assess the relationship between food intake and risk of disease. To broaden the use of the VISA-FFQ, the next step would be to evaluate if the VISA-FFQ is suitable for dietary counselling. However, the counsellor should keep in mind that the assessment will be less comprehensive than with longer and more complete FFQs.

## Conclusion

Milk fatty acid 15:0 estimated from the VISA-FFQ showed positive correlations with biomarker 15:0 % of FAME ($r$ = 0.32 and $r$ = 0.30, $P$ <0.05). In this sense, the VISA-FFQ has acceptable validity in its estimation of milk fat intake. Reproducibility of the VISA-FFQ was considered satisfactory, though varied, for intake of foods and lifestyle factors among a group of individuals with moderately high risk of CVD. We therefore suggest that the VISA-FFQ can be a convenient tool for assessment of (but not limited to) diet and lifestyle factors associated with CVD risk, in various settings.

## Acknowledgements

We would like to thank employees in Boots Norge AS for performing the data collection, and to Kjersti W. Garstad, Lisa T. Mørch-Reiersen in Boots Norge AS for significant contributions to study administration and to the design of the VISA-study. Present and previous employees in MILLS DA and Norwegian Health Association are also acknowledged for their contribution to study administration and/or the design of the VISA-study. We are grateful to all volunteers for participating in the study.

## Authors' contributions

KS had the main responsibility for writing the manuscript. KS, KR, VHTH and DRJ were responsible for the design of the VISA study. All authors contributed to analysis and/or interpretation of data, and writing and approval of the final manuscript.

## Conflict of interest and funding

This work was supported by Wendel Jarlsberg Fund and Vita hjertego' (Mills AS). The sponsors had no role in the design, analysis or writing of this article.

## References

1. Global Burden of Disease 2015 Mortality and Causes of Death Collaborators. Global, regional, and national life expectancy, all-cause mortality, and cause-specific mortality for 249 causes of death, 1980–2015: a systematic analysis for the Global Burden of Disease Study 2015. Lancet 2016; 388: 1459–544.
2. Micha R, Penalvo JL, Cudhea F, Imamura F, Rehm CD, Mozaffarian D. Association between dietary factors and mortality from heart disease, stroke, and type 2 diabetes in the United States. JAMA 2017; 317: 912–24.
3. Mozaffarian D, Appel LJ, Van Horn L. Components of a cardioprotective diet: new insights. Circulation 2011; 123: 2870–91.
4. Sacks FM, Lichtenstein AH, Wu JHY, Appel LJ, Creager MA, Kris-Etherton PM, et al. Dietary fats and cardiovascular disease: a presidential advisory from the American Heart Association. Circulation 2017; 136(3): e1–e23.
5. Willet W, Lenart E. Reproducibility and validity of food-frequency questionnaires. Nutritional epidemiology. New York: Oxford University Press; 1998, pp. 101–47.
6. Andersen LF, Johansson L, Solvoll K. Usefulness of a short food frequency questionnaire for screening of low intake of fruit and vegetable and for intake of fat. Eur J Public Health 2002; 12: 208–13.
7. England CY, Andrews RC, Jago R, Thompson JL. A systematic review of brief dietary questionnaires suitable for clinical use in the prevention and management of obesity, cardiovascular disease and type 2 diabetes. Eur J Clin Nutr 2015; 69: 977–1003.
8. Henriksen HB, Carlsen MH, Paur I, Berntsen S, Bøhn SK, Skjetne AJ, et al. Relative validity of a short food frequency questionnaire assessing adherence to the Norwegian dietary guidelines among colorectal cancer patients. Food Nutr Res 2018; 62: 1306.
9. Henriksen HB, Raeder H, Bohn SK, Paur I, Kvaerner AS, Billington SA, et al. The Norwegian dietary guidelines and colorectal

cancer survival (CRC-NORDIET) study: a food-based multicentre randomized controlled trial. BMC Cancer 2017; 17: 83.
10. Nasjonalt råd for ernæring. Kostråd for å fremme folkehelsen og forebygge kroniske sykdommer: metodologi og vitenskapelig kunnskapsgrunnlag. Oslo: Helsedirektoratet; 2011.
11. Svendsen K, Jacobs DR Jr., Røyseth IT, Byfuglien MG, Mørch-Reiersen LT, Garstad KW, et al. Pharmacies offer a potential high-yield and convenient arena for total cholesterol and CVD risk screening Unpublished results. Submitted EJPH. 2018.
12. Svilaas A, Strom EC, Svilaas T, Borgejordet A, Thoresen M, Ose L. Reproducibility and validity of a short food questionnaire for the assessment of dietary habits. Nutr Metab Cardiovasc Dis 2002; 12: 60–70.
13. Edelbroek PM, van der Heijden J, Stolk LM. Dried blood spot methods in therapeutic drug monitoring: methods, assays, and pitfalls. Ther Drug Monit 2009; 31: 327–36.
14. Holen T, Norheim F, Gundersen TE, Mitry P, Linseisen J, Iversen PO, et al. Biomarkers for nutrient intake with focus on alternative sampling techniques. Genes Nutr 2016; 11: 12.
15. Rise P, Eligini S, Ghezzi S, Colli S, Galli C. Fatty acid composition of plasma, blood cells and whole blood: relevance for the assessment of the fatty acid status in humans. Prostaglandins Leukot Essent Fatty Acids. 2007; 76: 363–9.
16. Aued-Pimentel S, Lago JH, Chaves MH, Kumagai EE. Evaluation of a methylation procedure to determine cyclopropenoids fatty acids from Sterculia striata St. Hil. Et Nauds seed oil. J Chromatogr A 2004; 1054: 235–9.
17. Matportalen. Food database (Matvaretabellen). [cited 2018 Apr 9th]; Available from: http://www.matvaretabellen.no/?language=en
18. U.S. Department of Health and Human Services. The Health Consequences of Smoking: 50 Years of Progress. A Report of the Surgeon General. Atlanta, GA: U.S. Department of Health and Human Services, Centers for Disease Control and Prevention, National Center for Chronic Disease Prevention and Health Promotion, Office on Smoking and Health, 2014. Printed with corrections, January 2014.
19. Spence JD, Jenkins DJ, Davignon J. Egg yolk consumption and carotid plaque. Atherosclerosis 2012; 224: 469–73.
20. Pedersen JI, Kirkhus B, Muller H. Serum cholesterol predictive equations in product development. Eur J Med Res 2003; 8: 325–31.
21. Henriksen HB, Berntsen S, Paur I, Zucknick M, Skjetne AJ, Bøhn SK, et al. Validation of two short questionnaires assessing physical activity in colorectal cancer patients. Accepted BMC Sports Sci Med Rehabil, 2018.
22. Hulley SB. Designing clinical research: an epidemiologic approach. 2nd ed. Philadelphia, PA: Lippincott Williams & Wilkins; 2001.
23. UCSF: Clinical & Translational Science Institute. Correlation sample size. [cited 2018 Apr 9th]; Available from: http://www.sample-size.net/correlation-sample-size/
24. Hankin JH, Wilkens LR, Kolonel LN, Yoshizawa CN. Validation of a quantitative diet history method in Hawaii. Am J Epidemiol 1991; 133: 616–28.
25. Bland JM, Altman DG. Statistical methods for assessing agreement between two methods of clinical measurement. Int J Nurs Stud 2010; 47: 931–6.
26. Jenkins B, West JA, Koulman A. A review of odd-chain fatty acid metabolism and the role of pentadecanoic acid (c15:0) and heptadecanoic acid (c17:0) in health and disease. Molecules 2015; 20: 2425–44.
27. Albani V, Celis-Morales C, Marsaux CF, Forster H, O'Donovan CB, Woolhead C, et al. Exploring the association of dairy product intake with the fatty acids C15:0 and C17:0 measured from dried blood spots in a multipopulation cohort: findings from the Food4Me study. Mol Nutr Food Res 2016; 60: 834–45.
28. Warensjö Lemming E, Nälsén C, Becker W, Ridefelt P, Mattisson I, Lindroos AK. Relative validation of the dietary intake of fatty acids among adults in the Swedish National Dietary Survey using plasma phospholipid fatty acid composition. J Nutr Sci 2015; 4: e25.
29. Vlaeminck B, Fievez V, Cabrita ARJ, Fonseca AJM, Dewhurst RJ. Factors affecting odd- and branched-chain fatty acids in milk: a review. Anim Feed Sci Technol 2006; 131: 389–417.
30. Weitkunat K, Schumann S, Nickel D, Hornemann S, Petzke KJ, Schulze MB, et al. Odd-chain fatty acids as a biomarker for dietary fiber intake: a novel pathway for endogenous production from propionate. Am J Clin Nutr 2017; 105: 1544–51.
31. Risérus U, Marklund M. Milk fat biomarkers and cardiometabolic disease. Curr Opin Lipidol 2017; 28: 46–51.
32. Baylin A, Kim MK, Donovan-Palmer A, Siles X, Dougherty L, Tocco P, et al. Fasting whole blood as a biomarker of essential fatty acid intake in epidemiologic studies: comparison with adipose tissue and plasma. Am J Epidemiol 2005; 162: 373–81.
33. Albani V, Celis-Morales C, Marsaux CF, Forster H, O'Donovan CB, Woolhead C, et al. Exploring the association of dairy product intake with the fatty acids C15:0 and C17:0 measured from dried blood spots in a multipopulation cohort: Findings from the Food4Me study. Molecular nutrition & food research. 2016; 60(4): 834–45.
34. Stefanov I, Baeten V, Abbas O, Vlaeminck B, De Baets B, Fievez V. Evaluation of FT-NIR and ATR-FTIR spectroscopy techniques for determination of minor odd- and branched-chain saturated and trans unsaturated milk fatty acids. J Agric Food Chem 2013; 61: 3403–13.
35. Kaaks RJ. Biochemical markers as additional measurements in studies of the accuracy of dietary questionnaire measurements: conceptual issues. Am J Clin Nutr 1997; 65: 1232s–9s.
36. Hedrick VE, Dietrich AM, Estabrooks PA, Savla J, Serrano E, Davy BM. Dietary biomarkers: advances, limitations and future directions. Nutr J 2012; 11: 109.
37. Kuhnle GG. Nutritional biomarkers for objective dietary assessment. J Sci Food Agric 2012; 92: 1145–9.
38. Cade JE, Burley VJ, Warm DL, Thompson RL, Margetts BM. Food-frequency questionnaires: a review of their design, validation and utilisation. Nutr Res Rev 2004; 17: 5–22.
39. Subar AF, Thompson FE, Kipnis V, Midthune D, Hurwitz P, McNutt S, et al. Comparative validation of the Block, Willett, and National Cancer Institute Food Frequency Questionnaires the eating at America's table study. Am J Epidemiol. 2001; 154: 1089–99.
40. Taylor AJ, Wong H, Wish K, Carrow J, Bell D, Bindeman J, et al. Validation of the MEDFICTS dietary questionnaire: a clinical tool to assess adherence to American Heart Association dietary fat intake guidelines. Nutr J 2003; 2: 4.
41. Parr CL, Veierod MB, Laake P, Lund E, Hjartaker A. Test-retest reproducibility of a food frequency questionnaire (FFQ) and estimated effects on disease risk in the Norwegian Women and Cancer Study (NOWAC). Nutr J 2006; 5: 4.
42. Retzlaff BM, Dowdy AA, Walden CE, Bovbjerg VE, Knopp RH. The Northwest Lipid Research Clinic Fat Intake Scale: validation and utility. Am J Public Health 1997; 87: 181–5.
43. Willet W. Nutritional epidemiology. 3rd ed. Oxford: Oxford University Press; 2013.

44. McCambridge J, Witton J, Elbourne DR. Systematic review of the Hawthorne effect: new concepts are needed to study research participation effects. J Clin Epidemiol 2014; 67: 267–77.
45. Schwab U, Lauritzen L, Tholstrup T, Haldorssoni T, Riserus U, Uusitupa M, et al. Effect of the amount and type of dietary fat on cardiometabolic risk factors and risk of developing type 2 diabetes, cardiovascular diseases, and cancer: a systematic review. Food Nutr Res 2014; 58: 25145.

***Karianne Svendsen**
Department of Nutrition, Institute of Basic Medical Sciences
University of Oslo, Blindern
NO- 0317 Oslo, Norway
Email: Karianne.svendsen@medisin.uio.no

# 10

# Metabolomic analysis of serum from rats following long-term intake of Chinese sausage

Minxian Rong[1]†, Pei Wang[2]†, Yuesheng Qiu[1], Yungang Liu[3], Yiyuan Wang[1] and Hong Deng[1]*

[1]Department of Nutrition and Food Hygiene, Guangdong Provincial Key Laboratory of Tropical Disease Research, School of Public Health, Southern Medical University, Guangzhou, China; [2]Wuhan Centers for Disease Prevention and Control, Wuhan, China; [3]Department of Toxicology, Guangdong Provincial Key Laboratory of Tropical Disease Research, School of Public Health, Southern Medical University, Guangzhou, China

*Abstract*

***Introduction:*** Owing to the contamination of chemical pollutants, especially nitrosamines and their precursors, in Chinese sausage, long-term intake of Chinese sausage may have potential health effects.
***Objection:*** This study investigated the effects of long-term intake of Chinese sausage with different contaminations of *N*-nitrosodimethylamine (NDMA) on rat liver and the potential biomarkers in the serum.
***Methods:*** Serum metabolomic analysis was performed by gas chromatography–mass spectrometry at weeks 7, 17, 25, and 33; simultaneously, liver histopathological examination was conducted and its relationship with the serum metabolomics was also investigated.
***Results:*** In the study, long-term intake of Chinese sausage with different NDMA contents induced significant changes in serum metabolites and liver histopathology in rats. Metabonomic analysis showed that seven metabolites – β-alanine, 3-aminoisobutyric acid, aminooxyacetic acid, D-alanyl-D-alanine, pelargonic acid, palmitic acid (PA), and linoleic acid (LA) – in three sausage diet groups were significantly decreased at four time points, where three other metabolites were notably increased, which included putrescine, ethanolamine phosphate, and taurine. Among the various treatments, the NDMA (sausage-free) group demonstrated the most remarkable changes. Phenylalanine was decreased followed by an increase, and tyrosine persistently declined, both of which were elevated in the NDMA group. In addition, the histopathological result was consistent with that of the serum metabolomic analysis, and the changes in serum metabolites in each sausage diet group and the NDMA group were consistently associated with disorders of lipids, amino acid, and energy metabolism.
***Conclusion:*** This work indicates that excessive NDMA content in sausage may cause liver damage.

Keywords: *Chinese sausage; metabolomics; NDMA; liver damage; GC-MS*

Chinese sausage is a famous traditional processed meat in China; the issue of its safety has been attracting more and more attention because of the contamination of chemical pollutants, especially nitrosamines and their precursors (nitrate, nitrite, etc.). In 2015, the International Agency for Research on Cancer (IARC) reported that processed meats had been classified as carcinogenic to humans (Group 1 carcinogen). The statement by the IARC confirmed that every intake of 50 g of processed meat per day might increase the risk of colorectal cancer by 18% (1). Many epidemiological studies indicate that consumption of smoked or processed meats and other nitrite-related foods is associated with increased risk of gastrointestinal, nasopharyngeal, and pancreatic tumors (2, 3). These consequences might be relevant to the presence of carcinogenic substances, such as volatile *N*-nitrosamines (VNAs) (4–6), polycyclic aromatic hydrocarbons (7), and heterocyclic amines produced during meat processing (pickling, smoking, or high temperature heating), in the diet (8).

†These authors contributed equally to this work.

Chinese sausage is different from Western dry fermented sausages in the manufacturing technology, seasoning, microbial ecology, and flavor, and the contamination of nitrosamines and their precursors in the former is supposed to be significant (9). Our previous studies found that the contamination of VNAs (including *N*-nitrosodimethylamine [NDMA], *N*-nitrosodiethylamine [NDEA], etc.) and its precursors in Chinese-style sausage was serious (9). NDMA formed in sausage might be mainly a result of reactions between dimethylamine and nitrite in certain conditions (10). Nitrite (nitrosating agents) is one of the vital precursors for the formation of NDMA. Its level in processed meat is influential on the concentration of NDMA. In addition, many other factors may also be influential on the formation of nitrosamines in sausages, such as the quality of raw meat used (e.g. microbial activity), use of additional additives (e.g. antioxidants and bioactivators), use of spices (e.g. anise and paprika), temperature during smoking processes, storage conditions (e.g. time and mode), and so on (11, 12). However, there is no way to completely prevent the formation of NDMA in sausages, and therefore NDMA in sausages has to be taken seriously in food safety.

In 1978, IRAC classified NDMA as a Group 2A carcinogen (probably carcinogenic to human) (13). The main target organ of toxicity of NDMA is the liver (14–16). NDMA has been administered to rodents in order to generate animal models of chronic hepatic damage and hepatocellular carcinoma (HCC) (14). It was also found that the histological and genetic signatures of NDMA-induced hepatocarcinogenesis are similar to those of human HCC. NDMA is converted into more toxic metabolites by cytochrome P450 enzymes in the liver (17), which simultaneously trigger the production of reactive oxygen species (ROS) as by-products (18, 19). Exposure of organisms to the toxic metabolites and elevated levels of ROS may result in liver damage. Hence, a subtle metabolic change in liver damage monitoring would be of great clinical importance.

The effects of foods on the body are very complex and subtle. It is difficult to accurately detect the bioactive compounds of foods and characterize their effects on the organism by conventional laboratory methods. Emerging platforms in systems biology provide a new methodology to identify subtle metabolic changes. Metabolomics is a particularly attractive technology that focuses on high-throughput identification and quantification of small-molecule (<1,500 Da) metabolites in a cell, organ, or organism (20). This approach has been used to identify serum principal metabolites and investigate the mechanism of exogenous material on organisms (21–24). In animal hepatotoxicity studies, toxic chemicals such as carbon tetrachloride (25), organophosphorus pesticide (26), and NDEA (27) significantly disrupted the level of several metabolites in blood, including arachidonic acid, lysophosphatidyl ethanolamines, and phosphatidylcholine. A metabolomic study of hepatotoxicity induced by chlorpyrifos and cadmium found that chlorpyrifos and cadmium could disrupt the energy, amino acid, and fatty acid metabolism in rat liver (28). A range of metabolites that represent liver dysfunctions have been examined in previous studies, suggesting the usefulness of metabolomics in exploring potential biomarkers of liver diseases caused by toxic chemicals.

Considering the contamination of nitrosamines and the precursors in Chinese sausages and their hepatotoxicity (such as that of NDMA), we speculate that long-term intake of Chinese sausages could cause hepatic damage, which might eventually progress to chronic liver disease, including hepatitis, cirrhosis, and so on. In the present study, the effects were investigated of long-term intake of different amounts of Chinese sausage and different NDMA contents in the sausage on rat liver, in particular at various time points as suggested by a model of NDMA-induced rat HCC. Moreover, a metabolic approach was applied to investigate the metabolic changes of metabolites in the serum of rats administered a sausage diet or NDMA by itself.

## Materials and methods

### *Chemicals and reagents*

All chemicals and solvents were of analytical or chromatographic grade. NDMA (99.0% purity) was obtained from Tokyo Century Chemical Co., Ltd. (Tokyo, Japan). Methanol, acetonitrile, pyridine, n-hexane, methoxylamine hydrochloride (97%), N,O-Bis(trimethylsilyl) trifluoroacetamide (BSTFA) with 1% Trimethylchlorosilane (TMCS) were purchased from CNW Technologies GmbH (Düsseldorf, Germany). L-2-chlorophenylalanine was from Shanghai Hengchuang Bio-technology Co., Ltd. (Shanghai, China).

### *Animals and treatment*

A total of 180 male Sprague Dawley rats weighing 180–220 g were obtained from the Laboratory Animal Center of Southern Medical University (Guangdong, China). All animal handlings were approved by the Animal Ethics Committee of Southern Medical University and were carried out in accordance with current Chinese legislation. All rats were allowed to acclimatize in communal iron cages for 2 weeks prior to treatment. They were kept at a controlled humidity (50–60%) and temperature (22 ± 2°C) with a 12 h light/dark cycle. After acclimatization, the rats were randomly assigned to five groups ($n$ = 36/group): a control group (CON) fed with AIN-93G diet, positive control (NDMA) group fed with AIN-93G diet and 30 μg/kg NDMA in drinking water, and three sausage diet groups fed with sausage diets I, II, and III, respectively, for a treatment period as long as 33 weeks. Sausage diet I was a diet of 1 part Chinese sausage to 5.5 parts certified rat chow, and the concentration of NDMA in the sausage was 1.13 μg/kg, which was lower than the tolerance limit, specifically, 3 μg/kg, as established by the Ministry of Health of China. Sausage diet II was a diet of 1 part Chinese sausage to 5.5 parts certified rat chow, with a concentration of NDMA in the sausage of 7.37 μg/kg, which exceeded the tolerance limit. Sausage diet III was a diet of 1 part Chinese sausage to 2.7 parts certified rat chow, and the concentration of NDMA in the sausage was 7.37 μg/kg. For the NDMA group, NDMA was supplied to rats through drinking water containing 30 μg/kg NDMA for 12 weeks, at which point it was changed to sterile tap water. Other groups were given sterile tap water during the experiment. Sausage diets were modulated on a control diet of AIN-93G, including corn-starch, casein, maltodextrin, sucrose, soybean oil, fiber, mineral mix, vitamin mix, L-cysteine, choline bitartrate and tert-butylhydroquinone (Table 1). No significant energy or nutrient changes were found in any of the experimental group diets ($p > 0.05$). Moreover, all diets were commissioned by the Guangdong Medical Experimental Animal Center and were vacuum packed, cobalt 60 irradiated and sterilized, and stored at 4°C in the dark.

*Table 1.* Ingredients of rat diets per 100 g

| Ingredients (g) | CON diet | Sausage diet I | Sausage diet II | Sausage diet III |
|---|---|---|---|---|
| Sausage* | – | 18.0 | 18.0 | 36.0 |
| Corn starch | 39.7 | 39.7 | 39.7 | 39.7 |
| Casein | 20.0 | 15.6 | 16.2 | 12.4 |
| Soybean oil | 7.0 | 2.7 | 1.9 | – |
| Sucrose | 10.0 | 6.3 | 5.8 | – |
| Maltodextrin | 13.2 | 12.7 | 13.2 | 7.8 |
| Mixed minerals | 3.5 | 3.5 | 3.5 | 3.5 |
| Mixed vitamins | 1.0 | 1.0 | 1.0 | 1.0 |
| L-cystine | 0.3 | 0.3 | 0.3 | 0.3 |
| Choline chloride | 0.25 | 0.25 | 0.25 | 0.25 |
| Fiber | 5.0 | 5.0 | 5.0 | 5.0 |
| Fat | 7.0 | 7.3 | 7.3 | 10.8 |
| Protein | 18.2 | 19.1 | 19.0 | 18.2 |
| Carbohydrates | 60.3 | 63.3 | 62.1 | 57.8 |
| Energy (kcal)** | 377 | 389.3 | 390.1 | 401.2 |
| Fat–energy ratio (%) | 16.7 | 16.9 | 16.8 | 24.2 |
| Protein–energy ratio (%) | 19.3 | 19.6 | 19.5 | 18.1 |
| Carbohydrate–energy ratio (%) | 64.0 | 63.5 | 63.8 | 57.7 |

*Sausage diet I: the concentrations of NDMA in added sausage was 1.13 μg/kg, which did not exceed the tolerance limit of 3 μg/kg established by the Ministry of Health of China. Sausage diet II and sausage diet III: the concentrations of NDMA in added sausage was 7.37 μg/kg, which exceeded the tolerance limit of 3 μg/kg established by the Ministry of Health of China. **1 kcal = 4.184 kJ. NDMA, *N*-nitrosodimethylamine; CON, control.

According to our previous experiments involving a rat HCC model induced by drinking NDMA water, the serial progression of hepatocarcinogenesis in this animal model was divided into four stages: the inflammation stage (weeks 4–8), the fibrosis stage (weeks 9–17), the cirrhosis stage (weeks 18–25), and the HCC stage (weeks 26–33). The time points at week 7, week 17, week 25, and week 33 were the characteristic histological changes of the inflammation, fibrosis, cirrhosis, and HCC stages, respectively. Thus, eight rats from each group ($n = 8$) were randomly selected in the 7th, 17th, 25th, 33rd week after treatment and anesthetized with chloral hydrate via intraperitoneal injection. Blood samples were obtained from the aorta abdominalis before the rats were sacrificed. Serum was obtained through centrifugation at 3,000 rpm for 15 min; it was then transferred into Eppendorf tubes and stored at −80°C for gas chromatography–mass spectrometry (GC-MS) analysis. Specimens of liver were fixed in 10% neutral formaldehyde for histopathology analysis.

*Histopathology examination*

The collected liver samples fixed in 10% neutral formaldehyde were paraffin-embedded, sectioned, and stained with hematoxylin–eosin. A microimaging system (Olympus; Tokyo, Japan) was used to observe the pathological changes. Microscopic examination of all liver tissues was done at the Pathology Laboratory of Southern Medical University. Histopathological scoring was performed in regard to the degree of hepatic inflammation and fibrosis, which was semi-quantified following the Ishak inflammation and fibrosis score system (29) (Tables S1 and S2 in the supplementary materials).

*Sample preparation for GC-MS analysis*

Serum samples stored at −80°C were thawed at room temperature and then divided into aliquots of 50 μL. The sample was mixed with 10 μL of 2-chloro-l-phenylalanine dissolved in methanol as an internal standard and vortexed for 10 s. Subsequently, 150 μL of ice-cold mixture of methanol–acetonitrile (2/1, v/v) was added, and the mixture was vortexed for 1 min, ultrasonicated at ambient temperature (25–28°C) for 5 min, and stored at −20°C for 10 min. The extract was centrifuged at 12,000 rpm, 4°C for 10 min, and the supernatant (150 μL) was collected in a glass vial and dried in a freeze concentration centrifugal dryer. Eighty microliters of 15 mg/ml methoxylamine hydrochloride in pyridine was subsequently added. The resultant mixture was vortexed vigorously for 2 min and incubated at 37°C for 90 min. Finally, 80 μL of BSTFA (with 1% TMCS) and 20 μL n-hexane were added into the mixture, and the samples were vortexed vigorously for 2 min and then derivatized at 70°C for 60 min and placed at ambient temperature for 30 min before GC-MS analysis. To ensure the stability and repeatability of the GC-MS systems, pooled quality control (QC) samples were used. The QC samples were prepared from a mixture of all sample extracts, treated and tested in the same way as the sample analyzed. One QC sample was inserted and analyzed for every 10 samples.

### *GC-MS nontargeted metabolism analysis*

GC-MS analysis was carried out on a gas chromatograph system (Agilent J&W Scientific, Folsom, CA, California, USA, model 7890B) coupled with a mass selective detector (Agilent, model 5977A). A DB-5MS fused-silica capillary column (30 m × 0.25 mm × 0.25 μm; Agilent) was utilized to separate the derivatives. The analysis was performed under the following conditions: helium (>99.999%) was used as the carrier gas at a constant flow rate of 1 ml/min through the column. The injector temperature was maintained at 260°C. Injection volume was 1 μL by splitless mode, and the solvent delay time was set to 5 min. The initial oven temperature was 50°C; it was ramped to 125°C at a rate of 15°C/min, to 210°C at a rate of 5°C/min, to 270°C at a rate of 10°C/min, and to 305°C at a rate of 20°C/min and finally held at 305°C for 5 min. The temperature of the MS quadrupole and electron impact ion source was set to 150°C and 230°C, respectively. Ions were generated by 70 eV electron energy at a full scan mode (m/z 50–60).

### *Data analysis*

Statistical analysis was performed by one-way analysis of variance using SPSS version 20.0 (Beijing Stats Data Mining Co., Ltd., China); $p < 0.05$ was considered statistically significant.

The GC-MS raw data were analyzed by Chroma Time-of-Flight (TOF) software (v. 4.34, LECO, St Joseph, MI, USA) and LECO-Fiehn Rtx5 database for data pretreatment procedures, such as data baseline filtering and calibration, peak alignment, deconvolution analysis, peak identification, and peak area integration. Then metabolites from the GC-MS spectra were identified with a similarity more than 400. The resulting data were imported into SIMCA-P 13.0 (Umetrics, Umea, Sweden) where a nonsupervised principal component analysis (PCA) was used to visualize general clustering change trends or outliers among the observations. To further distinguish the overall differences in metabolic profiles among the groups, orthogonal partial least squares–discriminant analysis (OPLS-DA) models were utilized. The parameters of OPLS-DA ($R^2Y$, $Q^2Y$) were used for the evaluation of the models. The goodness of fit and predictive ability of the models was quantified as the values of $R^2Y$ and $Q^2Y$ (30). Sevenfold cross validation and a response permutation test were applied to guard against OPLS-DA model overfitting (Supplementary materials, Fig. S2).

Potential biomarkers were selected based on the variable importance in the projection (VIP). Those metabolites with a VIP value greater than 1 in the first principal component of the OPLS-DA model were analyzed, among which each comparison with the control yielding a *p*-value by the Student's *t*-test lower than 0.05 defined a differential metabolite. Then the demonstration of these metabolites, as observed in this study, were matched with their structure messages, which were obtained from the Human Metabolome Databases (HMDB). Finally, the

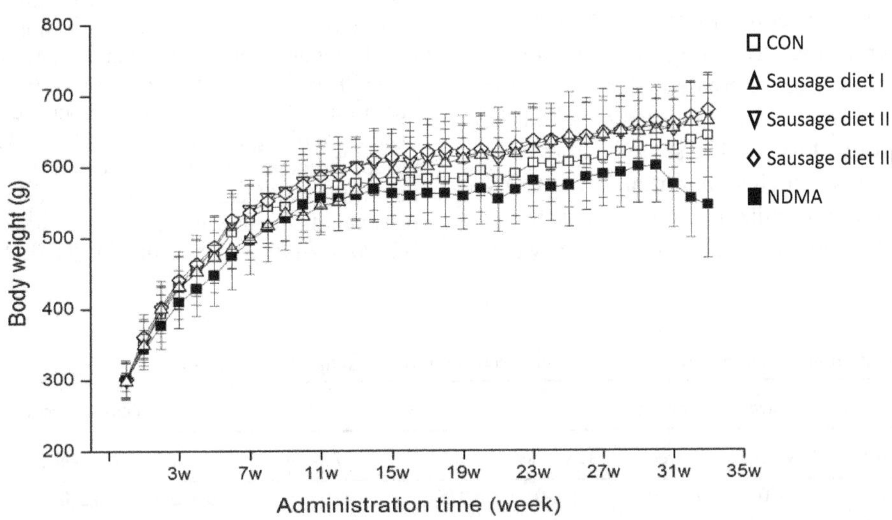


*Fig. 1.* Body weights of rats were measured during the experiment. It's expressed as mean ± S.D. Open square: fed with AIN-93G diet (CON group); regular triangle: fed a granular diet of 1 part Chinese sausage (NDMA content in sausage not exceeding the tolerated limit) to 5.5 parts certified rat chow (sausage diet I); inverted triangle: fed a granular diet of 1 part Chinese sausage (excessive NDMA content in sausage) to 5.5 certified rat chow (sausage diet II); rhombus: fed a granular diet of 1 part Chinese sausage (excessive NDMA content in sausage) to 2.7 parts certified rat chow (sausage diet III); filled square: fed with AIN-93G diet and 30 μg/kg NDMA in drinking water (NDMA group). NDMA, *N*-nitrosodimethylamine; CON, control.

key metabolites were investigated for their metabolism pathways using the databases of Kyoto Encyclopedia of Genes and Genomes (KEGG) (http://www.kegg.jp/) and HMDB (http://www.hmdb.ca).

## Results and discussion

### *Body weights*

The body weights (BWs) of all rats after long-term intake of Chinese sausage were recorded (Fig. 1). The BWs of rats in three sausage diet groups at different time points did not show any significant changes compared with the CON group, as did feeding and water consumption (data not listed). However, changes occurred in BW between NDMA group and the other four groups after 16 weeks ($p < 0.05$): a dramatic decrease was observed in the NDMA group from the 31st week to the end. This showed that drinking water containing 30 μg/kg NDMA impaired the health of rats.

### *Liver histopathology*

Through pathological examination, with semi-quantitative scoring, of the liver tissues from rats in each group, it was evidenced that long-term intake of different amounts of Chinese sausage or intake of sausage with different NDMA contents resulted in varying degrees of liver damage in rats. In the CON group, the hepatic lobules of the rats were complete and clear, the hepatic cords were neat, and hepatocytes were normal during the whole experiment (Fig. 2A). The pathological changes in the liver, including inflammation and fibrosis, both scored as described in Section 2.3, in the three sausage diet groups were specific for the particular feeding time points, the amount of sausage in the feed, and the concentration of NDMA in the sausage, as shown in Fig. 2B through D and Table 2. The liver inflammation score increased along with the elevation of NDMA content in the sausage diet, that is, from sausage diet groups I to III. The score of fibrosis in sausage diet group III was higher than that in the CON group at week 33 ($p < 0.05$), while it was near 0 in sausage diet groups I and II, without statistical significance when

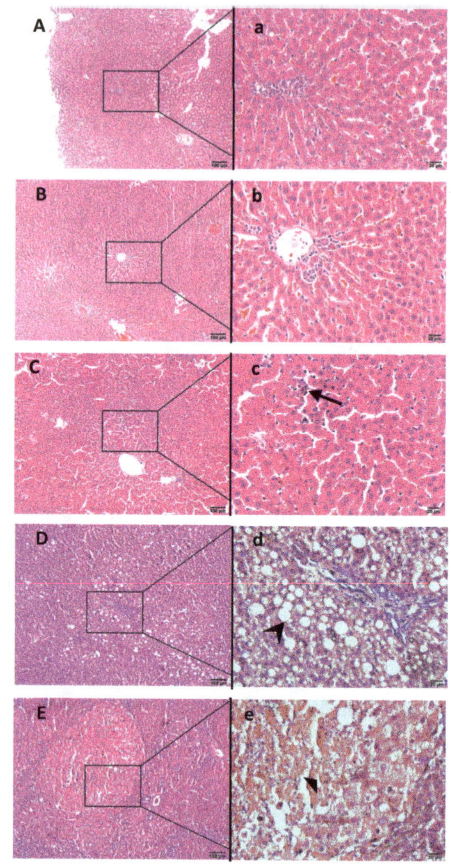


*Fig. 2.* Representative photomicrographs of H&E-stained formalin fixed liver sections from each group rats. During the 33 weeks of feeding, normal liver histology was shown in the control group (A, ×100; a, ×400). A slight hepatic sinusoid was found in sausage diet group I after 25 weeks of feeding (B, ×100; b, 400). In the meantime, a moderate hepatic sinusoidal dilatation, infiltration of a large amount of inflammatory cells (arrow) in hepatic lobules were observed in sausage diet group II (C, ×100; c, ×400). Moreover, fatty degeneration (arrow), fibroblastic proliferation in the portal area, and hepatic lobules were present in sausage diet group III (D, ×100; d, ×400). For the NDMA group, the hepatocyte necrosis (solid triangle), as indicated by the swollen and pale-staining hepatocytes with dilated endoplasmic reticulum, occurred after 25 weeks (E, ×100; e, ×400). NDMA, *N*-nitrosodimethylamine; H&E, hematoxylin–eosin.

*Table 2.* Scores of liver inflammation and fibrosis in each group according to the Ishak score system

| Groups | Liver inflammation score | | | | | Fibrosis score | | | | |
|---|---|---|---|---|---|---|---|---|---|---|
| | 7 weeks | 17 weeks | 25 weeks | 33 weeks | *p* | 7 weeks | 17 weeks | 25 weeks | 33 weeks | *p* |
| CON | 0 ± 0 | 0 ± 0 | 0.5 ± 0.7 | 1.3 ± 0.9 | 0.000 | 0 ± 0 | 0 ± 0 | 0 ± 0 | 0 ± 0 | – |
| Sausage diet I | 0.3 ± 0.7 | 0.3 ± 0.7 | 0.7 ± 0.9 | 2.4 ± 0.9* | 0.000 | 0 ± 0 | 0 ± 0 | 0 ± 0 | 0 ± 0 | – |
| Sausage diet II | 3.9 ± 0.8*a | 7.4 ± 0.8*a | 9.4 ± 0.8*a | 12.6 ± 0.8*a | 0.000 | 0 ± 0 | 0 ± 0 | 0 ± 0 | 0.3 ± 0.9 | – |
| Sausage diet III | 8.0 ± 0.9*b | 10.9±1.0*b | 12.5 ± 1.0*b | 15.9 ± 0.9*b | 0.000 | 0 ± 0 | 0.2 ± 0.7 | 0.7 ± 0.9 | 2.1 ± 0.6* | 0.000 |
| NDMA | 11.1 ± 1.0* | 14.3±0.9* | 15.4 ± 0.9* | 16.9 ± 1.0* | 0.164 | 0 ± 0 | 2.8 ± 0.6* | 3.9 ± 0.7* | 4.7 ± 0.8* | 0.001 |

Values are means ± S.D. Statistical significance was observed when compared with *the CON group, [a]sausage diet group I, and [b]sausage diet group II. NDMA, N-nitrosodimethylamine; CON, control.

compared with the CON group. In the NDMA (sausage-free) group, the pathological changes in the liver were more severe than those in the sausage groups containing NDMA, at lower levels, with the highest scores of liver inflammation and fibrosis as shown in Fig. 2E and Table 2. Clearly, the results of this study suggest that long-term intake of Chinese sausage with excessive NDMA content may cause liver damage.

### *GC-MS analysis*

#### GC-MS fingerprinting and multivariate analysis

All samples were analyzed by GC-MS in full scan mode to obtain serum metabolic profiles containing as many compounds as possible. The typical GC-MS total ion chromatograms (TICs) of rat serum were shown in Fig. S2 in the supplementary materials. In this study, the great stability and reproducibility of the retention time and the intensity of the chromatographic peaks in the QC and all groups indicated that the whole analysis method, including pretreatment and the GC-MS system, was stable and reliable.

After the peak detection and alignment of all TICs, a total of 253 metabolites were enrolled in the final data set for the statistical analysis. To model and evaluate the systemic changes in the metabolites in rat serum, the obtained data were analyzed by PCA and OPLS-DA for each time point. The resultant plots are shown in Fig. S3 in the supplementary materials and Fig. 3a through d. For OPLS-DA plots, the plots for the three sausage diet groups and the NDMA group clearly deviated from that of the CON group in the 7th week (Fig. 3a). And the plots for the three sausage diet groups separated from the NDMA group in the 25th week (Fig. 3c) and completely deviated in the 33rd week of treatment (Fig. 3d). These plots suggested that treatment with long-term intake of Chinese sausage or NDMA induced prominent changes in serum metabolites. The plots for the three sausage diet groups did not completely deviate at week 17 (Fig. 3b), while a clear separation was found at week 25 (Fig. 3c), which suggested that treatment with different amount of sausage in the feed and different concentrations of NDMA in the sausage could induce different changes in serum metabolites. The performance parameters for the classification calculated from the software were $R^2Y = 0.956$, $Q^2 = 0.732$ for 7 weeks of treatment (Fig. 3a); $R^2Y = 0.958$, $Q^2 = 0.786$ for 17 weeks of treatment (Fig. 3b); $R^2Y = 0.928$, $Q^2 = 0.706$

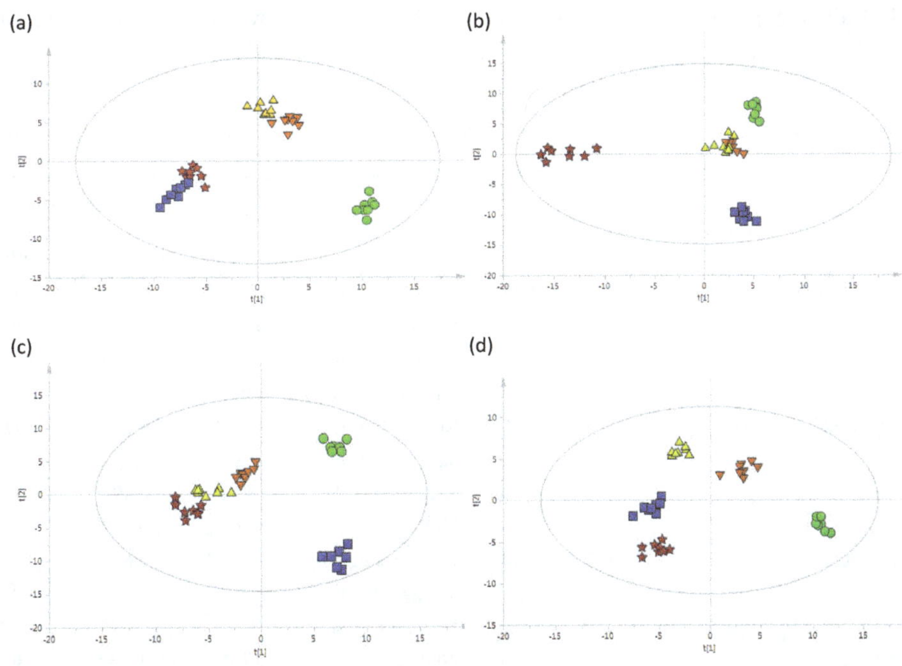


*Fig. 3.* OPLS-DA score plots (a through d) based on the GC-MS data of rat serum treated with sausage and NDMA at different treatment times: (a) rats treated for 7 weeks; (b) rats treated for 17 weeks; (c) rats treated for 25 weeks; (d) rats treated for 33 weeks; $n = 8$ per group. Green filled circles: given the AIN-93G diet (CON group); blue filled squares: fed a granular diet of 1 part Chinese sausage (NDMA content in sausage not exceeding the tolerated limit) to 5.5 parts certified rat chow (sausage diet I); orange filled inverted triangles: fed a granular diet of 1 part Chinese sausage (excessive NDMA content in sausage) to 5.5 parts certified rat chow (sausage diet II ); yellow filled triangles: fed a granular diet of 1 part Chinese sausage (excessive NDMA content in sausage) to 2.7 parts certified rat chow (sausage diet III); red filled pentacles: fed with the AIN-93 diet and 30 μg/kg NDMA in the drinking water group (NDMA group). NDMA, *N*-nitrosodimethylamine; OPLS-DA, orthogonal partial least squares–discriminant analysis; GC-MS, gas chromatography–mass spectrometry.

for 25 weeks of treatment (Fig. 3c); $R^2Y = 0.971$, $Q^2 = 0.73$ for the 33 weeks (Fig. 3d), which indicated that these models had good fitness and predictions. As results of the permutation test, the $R^2Y$-intercept was 0.735, 0.713, 0.621, 0.789; and the $Q^2$-intercept was −0.436, −0.452, −0.44, −0.468 (Supplementary materials, Fig. S1). Apparently, no overfitting of the data was present in our study.

*Differential metabolites*

Serum metabolites in rats changed significantly during the early feeding stage (week 7) in the three sausage groups, including sausage diet I, which contained low amounts of sausage with low content of NDMA in the feed. However, no pathological changes in rat liver were observed in the early stage (week 7) in the three sausage groups, except the NDMA group. Thus, the changes of serum metabolites might be more sensitive than the liver histopathological examination in detecting physiological response to toxicants. The metabolic profiles of the treated groups and the CON group deviated clearly via OPLS-DA (Fig. 3), changes that followed exposure to different amount of sausage and different concentrations of NDMA at different time points. Thirteen metabolites that notably contributed to this discrimination were identified (Table 3). β-Alanine, 3-aminoisobutyric acid, aminooxyacetic acid, D-alanyl-D-alanine, pelargonic acid, PA, and LA were decreased in the three sausage diet groups and the NDMA group, while putrescine, ethanolamine phosphate, and taurine were increased. Phenylalanine was firstly decreased at week 7 following by an increase in the 33rd week in the three sausage diet groups. Phenylalanine, tyrosine, and α-ketoglutarate were elevated over all time periods in the NDMA group. With metabolomics analysis of serum, some of these metabolites were found to play an important role in the metabolic pathways of lipids, amino acids, and energy. The pathogenesis of liver diseases may be attributable to metabolic changes, reflected by abnormal body lipids, amino acids, and energy metabolism in the serum (31).

Four differential metabolites, including PA, LA, taurine, and ethanolamine phosphate, were identified for the treated groups. These four substances in serum are closely related to the body lipid metabolism, suggesting that exposure to Chinese sausage or NDMA could affect the lipid metabolism of rats. PA and LA declined in the 7th week in sausage diet group III and the NDMA group, while they decreased in the 17th week both in sausage diet group I and sausage diet group II. Both of them are free fatty acids (FFA). It has been reported that changes of FFA have damaging effects, such as affecting cell proliferation, significantly increasing hepatotoxicity characterized by liver degeneration, inflammatory cell

*Table 3.* Change in the serum metabolites from rats treated with sausage and NDMA compared with control group for different time points and doses

| Number | Metabolites | Molecular formula | Mass[a] | RT[b] | Groups | Fold change[c] | | | |
|---|---|---|---|---|---|---|---|---|---|
| | | | | | | 7th week | 17th week | 25th week | 33rd week |
| 1 | β-Alanine | $C_3H_7NO_2$ | 102 | 5.17 | Sausage diet I | 0.50** | 0.36** | 0.50** | 0.52** |
| | | | | | Sausage diet II | 0.77* | 0.67** | 0.61* | – |
| | | | | | Sausage diet III | 0.59* | 0.53** | 0.50** | 0.65** |
| | | | | | NDMA | 0.49** | 0.45** | 0.56** | – |
| 2 | 3-aminoisobutyric acid | $C_4H_9NO_2$ | 102 | 5.68 | Sausage diet I | 0.73** | 0.67** | 0.59** | – |
| | | | | | Sausage diet II | 0.66** | 0.63** | 0.50* | 0.75** |
| | | | | | Sausage diet III | 0.43** | 0.49** | 0.39** | 0.57** |
| | | | | | NDMA | 0.23** | 0.25** | – | 0.24 |
| 3 | Aminooxyacetic acid | – | 160 | 6.12 | Sausage diet I | – | 0.67** | – | – |
| | | | | | Sausage diet II | – | – | 0.71* | – |
| | | | | | Sausage diet III | – | – | 0.64* | 0.76* |
| | | | | | NDMA | 0.75* | 0.73* | 0.65* | 0.48** |
| 4 | D-alanyl-D-alanine | $C_6H_{12}N_2O_3$ | 96 | 7.51 | Sausage diet I | – | 0.77* | – | 0.54* |
| | | | | | Sausage diet II | – | – | – | – |
| | | | | | Sausage diet III | – | – | 0.72* | 0.83* |
| | | | | | NDMA | – | 0.81* | 0.62* | 0.63* |
| 5 | Pelargonic acid | $C_9H_{18}O_2$ | 118 | 9.38 | Sausage diet I | – | 0.68* | – | – |
| | | | | | Sausage diet II | 0.68* | – | – | 0.79* |
| | | | | | Sausage diet III | – | 0.72* | – | 0.68* |
| | | | | | NDMA | 0.69* | 0.49* | 0.71* | 0.66* |

*Table 3.* Continued

| Number | Metabolites | Molecular formula | Mass[a] | RT[b] | Groups | Fold change[c] | | | |
|---|---|---|---|---|---|---|---|---|---|
| | | | | | | 7th week | 17th week | 25th week | 33rd week |
| 6 | Putrescine | $C_4H_{12}N_2$ | 86 | 11.54 | Sausage diet I | 3.95** | 2.81** | 4.44** | 3.73** |
| | | | | | Sausage diet II | 2.19** | 1.68** | 0.00** | 1.29* |
| | | | | | Sausage diet III | 2.79** | 2.26** | 1.48** | 1.60* |
| | | | | | NDMA | 3.76** | 2.93** | 1.92** | 2.04** |
| 7 | α-Ketoglutarate | $C_5H_6O_5$ | 203 | 13.51 | Sausage diet I | – | – | – | 1.42* |
| | | | | | Sausage diet II | – | 0.70** | – | – |
| | | | | | Sausage diet III | – | – | 1.30* | 0.58** |
| | | | | | NDMA | – | 1.03* | 1.83* | 2.37** |
| 8 | Phenylalanine | $C_9H_{11}NO_2$ | 192 | 14.54 | Sausage diet I | – | – | 0.84* | – |
| | | | | | Sausage diet II | – | 0.86** | 0.81* | 1.13* |
| | | | | | Sausage diet III | – | – | 0.85* | 1.12* |
| | | | | | NDMA | – | 1.23** | 1.35** | 1.75** |
| 9 | Ethanolamine phosphate | $C_2H_8NO_4P$ | 299 | 15.22 | Sausage diet I | 2.47* | 3.17* | 3.08* | 3.66* |
| | | | | | Sausage diet II | 1.97* | 1.37* | – | 2.15** |
| | | | | | Sausage diet III | – | 2.28** | 2.11** | 2.53* |
| | | | | | NDMA | 3.63** | 2.95** | 2.86** | 3.97** |
| 10 | Taurine | $C_2H_7NO_3S$ | 188 | 15.34 | Sausage diet I | 2.07** | 2.66** | 1.58* | 1.51* |
| | | | | | Sausage diet II | 1.99** | 1.60** | 1.55* | 1.38* |
| | | | | | Sausage diet III | 2.86** | 1.73* | 2.11** | 1.55* |
| | | | | | NDMA | 2.81** | 2.35** | 2.94** | 2.21** |
| 11 | Tyrosine | $C_9H_{11}NO_3$ | 218 | 20.86 | Sausage diet I | – | 0.84* | 0.75* | 0.83* |
| | | | | | Sausage diet II | 0.83* | 0.79* | 0.81* | 0.76** |
| | | | | | Sausage diet III | 0.86* | 0.79* | 0.77* | 0.81* |
| | | | | | NDMA | – | – | 1.25* | 2.14** |
| 12 | Palmitic acid | $C_{16}H_{32}O_2$ | 118 | 22.89 | Sausage diet I | – | 0.64** | 0.66* | 0.62** |
| | | | | | Sausage diet II | – | 0.76* | 0.76* | 0.72* |
| | | | | | Sausage diet III | 0.63** | 0.71* | 0.60** | 0.72* |
| | | | | | NDMA | 0.58** | 0.71* | 0.67* | 0.73* |
| 13 | Linoleic acid | $C_4H_4O_5$ | 82 | 25.19 | Sausage diet I | – | 0.52** | 0.31** | 0.32** |
| | | | | | Sausage diet II | – | 0.59** | 0.47** | 0.38** |
| | | | | | Sausage diet III | 0.45** | 0.42** | 0.31** | 0.35** |
| | | | | | NDMA | 0.69* | – | – | – |

[a]Calculation mass; [b]RT: retention time (minutes); *significantly increased or decreased when compared with the control group at $p < 0.05$; **significantly increased or decreased when compared with the control group at $p < 0.001$; [c]relative concentration of treated rats to the control at the same time. NDMA, N-nitrosodimethylamine; CON, control.

infiltration, and promoting the formation of liver fibrosis (32–34). The decrease of PA and LA may cause lipid metabolism turbulence in the liver and result in lipogenesis in rat hepatocytes. LA is also an essential fatty acid with important physiological functions such as regulating blood lipids and participating in the synthesis of phospholipids. Its reduction may lead to skin damage, liver and kidney diseases, and so on. It has been found that the reduction of LA results in steatosis and lipid metabolism disorders in rat hepatocytes and leads to liver damage (33, 35). In addition, if LA is insufficient, cholesterol will combine with certain saturated fatty acids, causing metabolic disturbances, depositing in the blood vessel wall, gradually leading to atherosclerosis, and triggering cardiovascular and cerebrovascular diseases.

Taurine plays a vital role in the metabolism of bile acid. It can combine anthropodesoxycholic acid under the action of amino acid N-acyltransferase to form taurochenodeoxycholic acid, which is excreted as a component of the bile into the alimentary canal. It functions to promote the digestion and absorption of lipids and fat-soluble vitamins (36). Liver damage, especially chronic liver diseases, can be reflected by an increase of blood bile acids (37). In this study, a significant increase of taurine in rat serum was found following administration of sausage diet or NDMA drinking water, which was consistent with the study of non-alcoholic fatty liver disease (38). Ethanolamine phosphate, a major source of the end-product of sphingosine degradation, was elevated significantly at week 7 after the administration of sausage diets or NDMA drinking water, but the latter changed more dramatically. According to the sphingosine biology pathway, this result might exacerbate hepatic metabolic disorders in the sausage diet groups and NDMA group (39, 40). The liver plays an important role in lipid metabolism, including both the endogenous and exogenous circulation of lipid metabolism and the lipid transport through the serum. Loss of liver function as caused by some hepatotoxicity may disrupt lipid metabolism (41, 42).

In the current study, α-ketoglutarate, phenylalanine, tyrosine, and putrescine were significantly changed in the sausage diet groups and NDMA group compared with the control. Numerous studies have reported the dysregulation of amino acid metabolism in liver disease (43, 44). As an essential catalytic reaction enzyme of amino acid, asparagine aminotransferase (AST) mainly affects the levels of aspartate, α-ketoglutarate, tyrosine, phenylalanine, oxaloacetate, and glutamate. AST preferentially promotes metabolism of aspartate, phenylalanine, tyrosine, cysteine, and so on, serving as $-NH_2$ donors in the transamination of α-ketoglutarate to glutamate (45). It is commonly known that serum AST is a biomarker of liver damage (46). As shown in Fig. S4 (in the supplementary materials), the levels of serum AST in sausage diet group III and the NDMA (sausage-free) group were increased significantly (as compared with the CON group); this is consistent with the changes in serum α-ketoglutarate, phenylalanine, and tyrosine metabolism, as observed in our metabolomics study.

α-Ketoglutarate, a crucial metabolic intermediate of energy production, can be converted to succinyl-coenzyme A (succinyl-CoA) and shunted to the tricarboxylic acid (TCA) cycle. Succinyl-CoA is phosphorylated by succinyl-CoA synthetase accompanied with the hydrolysis of the energy-rich thioester bond for cell growth and proliferation (31). In the present work, α-ketoglutarate was remarkably increased in the NDMA group, suggesting that NDMA-induced liver damage might indirectly lead to imbalance of the TCA cycle; this might be caused by dysregulation of amino acid metabolism in hepatic dysfunction. Another observation related to AST catalysis in the present study was the concentration of phenylalanine and tyrosine, which was changed in both the sausage groups and the NDMA group during the whole experiment. Phenylalanine and tyrosine are aromatic amino acids and their metabolisms are influenced by AST. In the sausage groups phenylalanine went down, followed by a recovery; tyrosine declined persistently, while both amino acids were elevated in the NDMA group. The mechanism and significance of these changes in our study needs further investigation.

Putrescine was significantly increased in the three sausage diet groups as well as in the NDMA group. Putrescine is a polyamine; excessive amounts in vivo are closely related to cell growth and cancer and are likely to be involved in the regulation of genetic processes from DNA synthesis to cell migration, proliferation, differentiation, and apoptosis (47). According to reports in the past, an elevation of putrescine in this study might be related to dysfunction of the liver resulting from NDMA toxicity or polyamines preserved in sausage. However, more insightful research is required to explore how NDMA induces hepatotoxicity by the level of putrescine in vivo.

## Conclusions

In this study, liver damage in rats was observed following long-term exposure to Chinese sausage diets, especially that containing a high level of NDMA. In both the sausage diet groups and the NDMA group the metabolite changes in serum were predominantly disorders of lipids, amino acids, and energy metabolism. The histopathological changes and metabolic signatures related to high level NDMA in sausage were particularly similar to those in the NDMA group. Therefore, excessive NDMA levels in sausage may contribute to liver damage.

## Conflict of interest and funding

The authors have not received any funding or benefits from industry or elsewhere to conduct this study.

## Acknowledgements

This work was financially supported by a grant from the National Natural Science Foundation of China (H. Deng, grant number 81373008) and by the Special Foundation of the President of the School of Public Health, Southern Medical University (grant code GW201706).

## References

1. IARC. IARC monographs evaluate consumption of red meat and processed meat. Lyon, France, 2015.
2. Li F, Duan F, Zhao X, Song C, Cui S, Dai L. Red meat and processed meat consumption and nasopharyngeal carcinoma risk: a dose-response meta-analysis of observational studies. Nutr Cancer 2016; 68(6): 1034–43. doi: 10.1080/01635581.2016.1192200.
3. Larsson SC, Orsini N. Red meat and processed meat consumption and all-cause mortality: a meta-analysis. Am J Epidemiol 2014; 179(3): 282–9. doi: 10.1093/aje/kwt261.
4. Herrmann SS, Granby K, Duedahl-Olesen L. Formation and mitigation of N-nitrosamines in nitrite preserved cooked sausages. Food Chem 2015; 174: 516–26. doi: 10.1016/j.foodchem.2014.11.101.
5. Magee PN, Barnes JM. The experimental production of tumours in the rat by dimethylnitrosamine (N-nitroso dimethylamine). Acta Unio Int Contra Cancrum 1959; 15(1): 187–90.

6. Mitacek EJ, Brunnemann KD, Suttajit M, Martin N, Limsila T, Ohshima H, et al. Exposure to N-nitroso compounds in a population of high liver cancer regions in Thailand: volatile nitrosamine (VNA) levels in Thai food. Food Chem Toxicol 1999;37(4):297–305.
7. Ender F, Havre G, Helgebostad A, Koppang N, Madsen R, Ceh L. Isolation and identification of a hepatotoxic factor in herring meal produced from sodium nitrite preserved herring. Naturwissenschaften 1964; 51(24): 637–8. doi: 10.1007/BF00623677.
8. Li L, Wang P, Xu X, Zhou G. Influence of various cooking methods on the concentrations of volatile N-nitrosamines and biogenic amines in dry-cured sausages. J Food Sci 2012; 77(5): C560–5. doi: 10.1111/j.1750-3841.2012.02667.x.
9. Pei W, Weijun Y, Q Y, Yuesheng Q, Minxian R, Hong D. Levels of nine Volatile N-Nitrosamines in Chinese-Style sausages as determined by Quechers-Based gas chromatography-Tandem mass spectrometry. Ann Public Health Res 2016; 3(4): 1049.
10. Chunlin L, Yongdong L, Rugang Z, Yunhai W. Theoretical studies on the formation of N-nitrosodimethylamine. J Mol Struct: THEOCHEM 2007; 802(1): 1–6. doi: 10.1016/j.theochem.2006.08.045.
11. Herrmann SS, Duedahl-Olesen L, Granby K. Occurrence of volatile and non-volatile N-nitrosamines in processed meat products and the role of heat treatment. Food Control 2015; 48: 163–9. doi: 10.1016/j.foodcont.2014.05.030.
12. Zhang J. The formation and inhibition of nitrosamine in chinese sausage by spice extraction [master]: Northeast Agricultural University, Harbin City, China. 2008.
13. IARC. Relevance of N-nitroso compounds to human cancer: exposures and mechanisms. Proceedings of the IXth International Symposium on N-Nitroso Compounds. IARC Sci Publ 1987; 84: 1–663.
14. Bakiri L, Wagner EF. Mouse models for liver cancer. Mol Oncol. 2013; 7(2): 206–23. doi: 10.1016/j.molonc.2013.01.005.
15. Rajewsky MF, Dauber W, Frankenberg H. Liver carcinogenesis by diethylnitrosamine in the rat. Science 1966; 152(3718): 83–5.
16. Sferra R, Vetuschi A, Pompili S, Gaudio E, Speca S, Latella G. Expression of pro-fibrotic and anti-fibrotic molecules in dimethylnitrosamine-induced hepatic fibrosis. Pathology, Res Pract 2017; 213(1): 58–65. doi: 10.1016/j.prp.2016.11.004. PubMed PMID: 27894619.
17. Lin HL, Parsels LA, Maybaum J, Hollenberg PF. N-Nitrosodimethylamine-mediated cytotoxicity in a cell line expressing P450 2E1: evidence for apoptotic cell death. Toxicol Appl Pharmacol 1999; 157(2): 117–24. doi: 10.1006/taap.1999.8651.
18. Paula SN, Colaco A, Gil DCRM, Manuel OM, Peixoto F, Alexandra OP. N-diethylnitrosamine mouse hepatotoxicity: time-related effects on histology and oxidative stress. Exp Toxicol Pathol 2014; 66(9–10): 429–36. doi: 10.1016/j.etp.2014.07.002.
19. Tasaki M, Kuroiwa Y, Inoue T, Hibi D, Matsushita K, Kijima A. Lack of nrf2 results in progression of proliferative lesions to neoplasms induced by long-term exposure to non-genotoxic hepatocarcinogens involving oxidative stress. Exp Toxicol Pathol 2014; 66(1): 19–26. doi: 10.1016/j.etp.2013.07.003.
20. German JB, Hammock BD, Watkins SM. Metabolomics: building on a century of biochemistry to guide human health. Metabolomics 2005; 1(1): 3–9. doi: 10.1007/s11306-005-1102-8.
21. Coen M. A metabonomic approach for mechanistic exploration of pre-clinical toxicology. Toxicology 2010; 278(3): 326–40. doi: 10.1016/j.tox.2010.07.022.
22. Gomez-Casati DF, Zanor MI, Busi MV. Metabolomics in plants and humans: applications in the prevention and diagnosis of diseases. Biomed Res Int 2013; 2013: 792527. doi: 10.1155/2013/792527.
23. Nicholls AW, Holmes E, Lindon JC, Shockcor JP, Farrant RD, Haselden JN, et al. Metabonomic investigations into hydrazine toxicity in the rat. Chem Res Toxicol 2001; 14(8): 975–87.
24. Yu M, Zhu Y, Cong Q, Wu C. Metabonomics research progress on liver diseases. Can J Gastroenterol Hepatol 2017; 2017: 8467192. doi: 10.1155/2017/8467192.
25. Sadek K, Saleh E. Fasting ameliorates metabolism, immunity, and oxidative stress in carbon tetrachloride-intoxicated rats. Hum Exp Toxicol 2014; 33(12): 1277–83. doi: 10.1177/0960327114527629.
26. Yang J, Sun X, Feng Z, Wu C. Metabolomic analysis of the toxic effects of chronic exposure to low-level dichlorvos on rats using ultra-performance liquid chromatography-mass spectrometry. Toxicol Lett 2011; 206(3): 306–13. doi: 10.1016/j.toxlet.2011.08.012.
27. Qiu P, Sun J, Man S, Yang H, Ma L, Yu P. Curcumin attenuates N-Nitrosodiethylamine-Induced liver injury in mice by utilizing the method of metabonomics. J Agric Food Chem 2017; 65(9): 2000–7. doi: 10.1021/acs.jafc.6b04797.
28. Xu MY, Wang P, Sun YJ, Wu YJ. Metabolomic analysis for combined hepatotoxicity of chlorpyrifos and cadmium in rats. Toxicology 2017; 384: 50–8. doi: 10.1016/j.tox.2017.04.008.
29. Ishak K, Baptista A, Bianchi L, Callea F, De Groote J, Gudat F, et al. Histological grading and staging of chronic hepatitis. J Hepatol 1995; 22(6): 696–9.
30. Trygg J, Holmes E, Lundstedt T. Chemometrics in metabonomics. J Proteome Res 2007; 6(2): 469–79. doi: 10.1021/pr060594q.
31. Beyoglu D, Idle JR. The metabolomic window into hepatobiliary disease. J Hepatol 2013; 59(4): 842–58. doi: 10.1016/j.jhep.2013.05.030.
32. Osman D, Ali O, Obada M, El-Mezayen H, El-Said H. Chromatographic determination of some biomarkers of liver cirrhosis and hepatocellular carcinoma in Egyptian patients. Biomed Chromatogr. 2017; 31(6). doi: 10.1002/bmc.3893.
33. Rosqvist F, Bjermo H, Kullberg J, Johansson L, Michaelsson K, Ahlstrom H, et al. Fatty acid composition in serum cholesterol esters and phospholipids is linked to visceral and subcutaneous adipose tissue content in elderly individuals: a cross-sectional study. Lipids Health Dis 2017; 16(1): 68. doi: 10.1186/s12944-017-0445-2.
34. Gyamfi D, Everitt HE, Tewfik I, Clemens DL, Patel VB. Hepatic mitochondrial dysfunction induced by fatty acids and ethanol. Free Radical Biol Med 2012; 53(11): 2131–45. doi: 10.1016/j.freeradbiomed.2012.09.024.
35. Bernert JT, Jr., Akins JR, Miller DT. Direct determination of the linoleate/oleate ratio in serum cholesterol esters by liquid chromatography. Clin Chem 1982; 28(4 Pt 1): 676–80.
36. Garcia-Canaveras JC, Donato MT, Castell JV, Lahoz A. A comprehensive untargeted metabonomic analysis of human steatotic liver tissue by RP and HILIC chromatography coupled to mass spectrometry reveals important metabolic alterations. J Proteome Res 2011;10(10): 4825–34. doi: 10.1021/pr200629p.
37. Tan Y, Yin P, Tang L, Xing W, Huang Q, Cao D, et al. Metabolomics study of stepwise hepatocarcinogenesis from the model rats to patients: potential biomarkers effective for small hepatocellular carcinoma diagnosis. Mol Cell Proteomics 2012; 11(2): M111.010694. doi: 10.1074/mcp.M111.010694.
38. Li H, Wang L, Yan X, Liu Q, Yu C, Wei H, et al. A proton nuclear magnetic resonance metabonomics approach for biomarker discovery in nonalcoholic fatty liver disease. J Proteome Res 2011; 10(6): 2797–806. doi: 10.1021/pr200047c.
39. Krautbauer S, Eisinger K, Wiest R, Liebisch G, Buechler C. Systemic saturated lysophosphatidylcholine is associated with

hepatic function in patients with liver cirrhosis. Prostaglandins Other Lipid Mediat 2016; 124: 27–33. doi: 10.1016/j.prostaglandins.2016.06.001.
40. Krautbauer S, Wiest R, Liebisch G, Buechler C. Associations of systemic sphingolipids with measures of hepatic function in liver cirrhosis are related to cholesterol. Prostaglandins Other Lipid Mediat 2017; 131: 25–32. doi: 10.1016/j.prostaglandins.2017.06.004.
41. Arain SQ, Talpur FN, Channa NA, Ali MS, Afridi HI. Serum lipid profile as a marker of liver impairment in hepatitis B Cirrhosis patients. Lipids Health Dis 2017; 16(1): 51. doi: 10.1186/s12944-017-0437-2.
42. Mehboob F, Ranjha FA, Masud S. Changes in serum lipid profile among patients suffering from chronic liver disease. Ann KEMU 2007; 13(3): 209–11.
43. Gao R, Cheng J, Fan C, Shi X, Cao Y, Sun B, et al. Serum metabolomics to identify the liver disease-specific biomarkers for the progression of hepatitis to hepatocellular carcinoma. Scientific Rep 2015; 5: 18175. doi: 10.1038/srep18175.
44. Kimura T, Noguchi Y, Shikata N, Takahashi M. Plasma amino acid analysis for diagnosis and amino acid-based metabolic networks. Curr Opin Clin Nutr Metab Care 2009; 12(1): 49–53. doi: 10.1097/MCO.0b013e3283169242.
45. Zou L, Zhao H, Wang D, Wang M, Zhang C, Xiao F. Expression and purification of a functional recombinant aspartate aminotransferase (AST) from Escherichia coli. J Microbiol Biotechnol 2014; 24(7): 998–1003.
46. Qian YY, Peng YR, Shang EX, Ming ZA, Yan L, Zhu ZH, et al. Metabolic profiling of the hepatotoxicity and nephrotoxicity of Ginkgolic acids in rats using ultra-performance liquid chromatography-high-definition mass spectrometry. Chem-Biol Interact 2017; 273: 11–17. doi: 10.1016/j.cbi.2017.05.020.
47. Wang C, Ruan P, Zhao Y, Li X, Wang J, Wu X, et al. Spermidine/spermine N1-acetyltransferase regulates cell growth and metastasis via AKT/beta-catenin signaling pathways in hepatocellular and colorectal carcinoma cells. Oncotarget 2017; 8(1): 1092–1109. doi: 10.18632/oncotarget.13582

***Hong Deng**
Department of Nutrition and Food Hygiene
School of Public Health
Southern Medical University
1838 N. Guangzhou Avenue, Guangzhou
510515, Guangdong, China
E-mail: hongd@smu.edu.cn

11

# A meal concept designed for older adults – Small, enriched meals including dessert

Evelina Höglund[1*], Susanne Ekman[1], Gunnel Stuhr-Olsson[2], Christina Lundgren[2], Berit Albinsson[1], Michael Signäs[3], Christina Karlsson[4], Elisabet Rothenberg[5] and Karin Wendin[5,6]

[1]RISE Research Institutes of Sweden, Agrifood and Bioscience, Göteborg, Sweden; [2]Findus Special Foods, Bjuv, Sweden; [3]Medirest Compass Group AB, Kista, Sweden; [4]ICA Sverige AB, Solna, Sweden; [5]Food and Meal Science, Kristianstad University, Kristianstad, Sweden; [6]Department of Food Science, University of Copenhagen, Copenhagen, Denmark

*Abstract*

***Background:*** The population of older adults is growing and many are at risk of disease-related malnutrition. This is a serious condition which increases the risk for other diseases and distress, human suffering and puts a high load on health care costs. Meal concepts tailored to suit the needs of older adults are required to decrease the incidence of disease-related malnutrition.

***Objective:*** To evaluate sensory perception regarding a concept of small, protein and energy-enriched multi-component meals designed according to the nutritional needs of older adults.

***Design:*** A meal concept of small main courses with complementary desserts and protein and energy-enriched products was evaluated using triangle tests, hedonic evaluation and focus group discussion. Enriched sauces and meals were compared to corresponding commercial products regarding appearance, taste, consistency and overall acceptance.

***Results:*** The concept of a small main course with a complementary dessert was generally perceived as positive by the target group. The acceptance scores for the enriched meals were generally lower than for the commercial meals, mainly owing to the packaging of the enriched meals which required covering the food in sauce. Enriched sauces contained approximately 90% more protein than the commercial sauces. However, protein enrichment affected the sensory properties of the sauces and they were perceived as thicker, creamier and less flavour-intensive.

***Conclusions:*** A concept based on small, protein and energy-enriched meals supplemented with a dessert was considered suitable for increasing the energy and protein intakes of older adults provided that the method of enrichment ensures attractive sensorial properties.

Keywords: *older adults; energy; protein; meals; malnutrition; meal concept*

The population of older adults is growing worldwide due to improved living conditions, health care, nutrition and hygiene (1). However, many older adults in the community are frail, a condition whereby a person has decreased physiologic reserve and resistance to stressors resulting from cumulative declines across multiple systems. This results in vulnerability to adverse outcomes (2) and risk for disease-related malnutrition (DRM) (3–5), a condition associated with muscle loss, weakened immune system, morbidity, mortality and poor quality of life (6–8). The aetiology behind DRM is complex but the major cause is acute and chronic disease leading to inflammation, which in turn causes loss of appetite and muscle wasting. Moreover, mastication problems, dry mouth and throat, olfactory dysfunction and social changes may contribute to the risk of malnutrition in old age (7, 9, 10). Disease-related malnutrition places a high economic burden on health care (11, 12) but could be counteracted through the development of meal concepts, including food products, adapted to the changing needs of those affected.

Poor appetite is strongly associated with poor nutritional intake (3, 5, 13). In order to increase nutritional intake, products customised to the needs of older persons have to be designed in a way that encourages consumption of the entire meal (14). Large portions of food may be overwhelming and discourage intake (15). Moreover, food intake is primarily dependent on the volume of food consumed and not its energy content (16, 17). Therefore, a strategy that can be used for older adults who require increased energy and nutrient intakes is to offer frequent, small servings of food with high energy and nutrient density (18). Formulation and processing of such food is crucial since sufficient energy and nutrients need to be provided in a limited meal volume. Older adults need more protein than younger people to maintain physical function. Those who have, or are at risk of, DRM need even higher levels of protein intake to maintain muscle mass (19). In order to achieve high protein concentration in food products, whey proteins are commonly added. These proteins have properties that stimulate muscle protein synthesis (20–22) and can be added to food products such as sauces, gravies and desserts due to functional properties such as foaming, gelling and water-binding capacity (23). However, protein enrichment of food products is not straightforward since the addition of protein affects flavour as well as consistency. Also, olfactory dysfunction is common in older adults which often leads to a reduced ability to appreciate food (24, 25). Therefore, the sensory attributes of meals designed for older adults require careful attention, underlining the importance of taste and flavour (18). Variety among meal components has been reported to promote intakes of larger quantities of food, partly because satiety can be specific to one type of food (5, 26). Therefore, a concept of small, multi-component meals with high energy and nutrient density, such as a protein-enriched main course supplemented by a dessert, may encourage food intake and reduce the risk of DRM. The aim of this study was to evaluate the concept of small protein and energy-enriched meals designed for older adults using sensory analysis. Enriched meals were compared to corresponding commercial meals with regard to appearance, taste and consistency as well as overall acceptance.

## Material and methods

### *Study setup*

In this study, poor appetite was taken into account and meal size was reduced by 20–30%. The challenge was to reduce the main components of the meals without decreasing the total energy and protein content. In order to compensate for protein reduction in small-sized meals, the sauces and mashed potatoes (when applicable) were protein-enriched. The effects on sensorial properties of protein enrichment of the sauces were evaluated in this study by a discrimination test and hedonic evaluation, while the enrichment of the mashed potatoes was evaluated using only hedonic evaluation.

In order to increase the energy content of the meals, a dessert was added to the main course. The desserts also added variety to the meals which has been suggested to promote food intake. Enriched meals, and their components, were evaluated in a hedonic test concerning appearance, taste, consistency and overall acceptance, and the concept of a small, enriched meal with an attached dessert was discussed in a focus group.

### *Samples*

Six types of ready-to-eat (RTE) meals were manufactured in a pilot plant at Findus Sverige AB, Bjuv, Sweden. Three of the meals were commercial meals available on the consumer market, and the other three were corresponding meals developed and designed according to the nutritional needs of older adults. These meals were of smaller portion size (70–80% (w) of commercial RTEs), protein-enriched with whey powder (sauces and mashed potatoes) and supplemented with a dessert to increase the total energy content of the meal. The composition of the RTE meals and the separate sauces is shown in Table 1. The samples were packed in black paper/plastic trays covered with a transparent plastic film and the desserts were packed in a side tray. All samples were delivered as frozen goods. The day before testing, sauces were thawed at room temperature (approximately 4 h at 20°C) and then in a refrigerator (approximately 16 h at 4°C). About 1 h before the test, the sauces (2.7–3.1 l) were heated to ≥70°C in steel sauce pans on electric hot plates while being continuously stirred, and approximately 40 ml was then poured into coded plastic cups. The RTE meals were heated prior to testing in identical microwaves ovens (700 W) according to the manufacturer's instructions. However, the heating time was adjusted in order to reach a minimum temperature of 65°C throughout in each meal.

### *Respondents*

The inclusion criteria for the respondents (RPs) were: independent living, aged 75+ years, cognitively intact, able to travel to the location where the tests were conducted and willing to eat/like RTE meals. The goal was to recruit both men and women and reach a slightly higher number of women. Ethical approval is not needed for food focus groups; however, the respondents were informed about the products and the terms for participation, which meant voluntary participation, freedom to leave the test without giving a reason, the right to decline to answer specific questions or an assurance that although their answers were recorded, their participation would not affect their future treatment in the health care system in any way.

### *Sensory evaluation*

The sensory evaluations of the meals were carried out at the sensory laboratory at RISE Research Institutes of Sweden, equipped according to ISO 8589:2007. Evaluations were carried out in three steps: (1) a triangle test for detection of differences between commercial and enriched

*Table 1.* Nutritional content of commercial and protein-enriched products

| Product | | Energy (kcal/100g) | Fat (g/100g) | Carbo-hydrate (g/100g) | Protein (g/100g) |
|---|---|---|---|---|---|
| Commercial sauces | Mustard sauce | 124 | 9.1 | 8.3 | 2.3 |
| | Cream sauce | 180 | 15 | 7.6 | 4.4 |
| | Curry sauce | 86 | 5.1 | 7.4 | 2.4 |
| Protein-enriched sauces | Mustard sauce | 132 | 9.6 | 7.3 | 4.1 |
| | Cream sauce | 163 | 12 | 6.6 | 7.2 |
| | Curry sauce | 101 | 5.9 | 6.4 | 5.2 |
| Commercial RTE meals 380–400 g/portion | Fish, mustard sauce* (400 g/portion) | 95 | 3.5 | 9.5 | 5.5 |
| | Meat balls, cream sauce** (400 g/portion) | 160 | 8.5 | 15.0 | 5.0 |
| | Chicken, curry sauce*** (380 g/portion) | 120 | 3.0 | 16.0 | 5.5 |
| Protein-enriched meals 285–310 g/portion | Fish, mustard sauce* (310 g/portion) | 101 | 4.1 | 9.1 | 6.3 |
| | Meat balls, cream sauce** (285 g/portion) | 151 | 7.7 | 14.0 | 6.0 |
| | Chicken, curry sauce*** (285 g/portion) | 121 | 2.4 | 16.0 | 8.2 |
| Concept of protein-enriched meals designed for older adults, including dessert 385 g/portion | Fish, mustard sauce* + Chocolate cake, raspberry cream (Dessert: 75 g/portion) | 146 | 7.5 | 13.0 | 5.9 |
| | Meat balls, cream sauce** + Pancake, strawberry sauce (Dessert: 100 g/portion) | 156 | 7.5 | 16.2 | 5.5 |
| | Chicken, curry sauce*** + Apple cake, custard (Dessert: 100 g/portion) | 174 | 6.7 | 20.0 | 7.8 |

*including mashed potatoes and peas; **including mashed potatoes, lingonberries and peas; ***including rice and broccoli/baby carrots.

sauces, (2) hedonic evaluation to rate the appearance, taste and consistency of commercial and enriched RTE meals, and (3) a focus group discussion to gain a deeper understanding of opinions about RTE meals designed for older adults. The evaluations were carried out over 2 days in the same week. Assessment was made in the following order: mustard sauce, cream sauce and curry sauce (increasing flavour strength).

#### *Hedonic evaluation*

Hedonic evaluation of the RTE meals was conducted on the second test day. The RPs were presented with one meal at a time in the same presentation order: fish with mustard sauce, meat balls with cream sauce and chicken with curry sauce. The commercial meal (with no dessert) was always evaluated before the corresponding enriched meal. The enriched meals included a dessert, which was presented with the main course in order to give the RPs the possibility of giving feedback about the concept of a small main course with dessert. Written information about the name of the meals was provided on the front page of the questionnaire. The test was performed in the sensory laboratory and took 1.5 h. First, the RPs rated the appearance of the meal and its components (mashed potatoes or rice, sauce and protein component) separately before tasting. Finally, all components were considered together to evaluate overall acceptance. The ratings were made on a 9-point hedonic category scale with the ends anchored as 'dislike extremely' and 'like extremely' (27). Furthermore, the RPs were given the opportunity to comment on each assessment in their own words. Sauces and mashed potatoes were the components that were protein-enriched and both taste and consistency were evaluated for these components. The desserts were evaluated with regard to their total acceptance.

#### *Triangle test*

A triangle test, based on ISO 4120 'Sensory analysis, methodology, triangular test' and described by Lawless and Heymann (28), was conducted in order to determine whether older adults (naïve assessors) could detect any difference between commercial and protein-enriched sauces. Each RP was presented with three coded samples, of which two were identical and one different.

The samples were served in random order and the RPs were asked to determine which of the samples was differ-

correct response. Each RP carried out the triangle tests in triplicate. Thus, a total of 36 assessments were carried out for each sauce. Further, the RPs were asked to indicate the reason for their decision. Still water, mineral water, neutral wafers and apple slices were used to rinse the mouth and palate between samples. A break of 5 min was taken between each test replicate of the same sauce. After completing the three test replicates for one sauce, the RPs had a 10-min pause before the next evaluation.

*Focus group*

A focus group discussion was held directly after the hedonic evaluation. A moderator facilitated the discussion which was observed and recorded by an assistant. The focus group was conducted using a semi-structured interview guide and lasted for approximately 1.5 h. The moderator began the focus group by explaining the procedure and asking the RPs to briefly introduce themselves. A semi-structured interview guide was used in order for the focus group to be both structured and at the same time allow follow-up questions and discussion. The frequency and reasons for consuming RTE meals were discussed as well as important attributes of RTE meals. Before starting the next topic for the focus group, the moderator informed the RPs about the meals being evaluated in the hedonic evaluation and the following information was given: the small meals had been protein-enriched in order to meet the increased need for protein among older adults, the enriched meals were of smaller portion size because older adults often have poor appetites, and the small meals contained more energy than the corresponding normal-sized meals. In a subsequent discussion, the RPs were asked to give their opinion of the RTE meals based on the new information they had been given as well as suggest ways for communicating to consumers about meals designed for older adults. Finally, the RPs were asked to give input on improvements of the tested products. The prepared RTE meals were displayed and discussed one at a time.

*Data analysis*

Quantitative data from the hedonic evaluation were transferred to Excel (Microsoft Office, 2010) and qualitative data (comments) were summarised in Word (Microsoft Office, 2010). A pairwise comparison (Student's *t*-test, Microsoft Office Excel, 2010) was performed for each parameter to detect any significant differences ($p \leq 0.05$) between commercial meals and meals designed for older adults.

Data from the triangle test were calculated according to the following equation (29):

$$X = 0.4717z\sqrt{n} + \left[(2n+3)/6\right]$$

X = minimum number of correct/agreeing judgments (X is an integer or closest higher integer)
n = total number of judgments
if $p < 0.05$ z = 1.64

Qualitative data from the focus group were coded using conventional techniques. First, two researchers independently read through the focus group transcripts and the observation field notes and then they performed an initial coding. This coding captured how the respondents perceived the RTE meals and their opinions about them. The initial codes were then merged and discussed among the researchers, and then clustered according to similarity and common features so as to form categories related to perception and opinions of RTE meals. The use of triangulation in the form of different 'investigators' increases the possibility of obtaining credible results (30).

## Results

*Enriched and commercial sauces and meals*

The protein-enriched sauces contained approximately 90% more protein than commercial sauces and the protein-enriched mashed potatoes contained approximately 60% more protein than commercial mashed potatoes. The enriched meals (including dessert) contained approximately 50% more energy than commercial meals for two of the varieties, while one of the meals had a similar energy level for both enriched and commercial meals.

A total of 12 RPs (seven women, five men, aged 75–89 years) conducted the triangle test and hedonic evaluation. Two married couples participated, the other RPs lived alone. Seven RPs (four women, three men, all living alone) participated in the focus group discussion.

*Triangle test*

The enriched sauces contained approximately 90% more protein (mustard sauce 78%, cream sauce 64%, curry sauce 117%) than corresponding commercial sauces (Table 1). However, protein enrichment affected the sensory properties and there was a significant difference in flavour and/or consistency between the commercial and the enriched sauces (Table 2). The differences were larger for the cream sauce (30 correct answers out of 36 assessments in the triangle tests) than the mustard sauce (22 correct answers) and the curry sauce (18 correct answers). Overall, the commercial sauces were perceived as thinner, less creamy, and more flavour-intensive.

*Hedonic evaluation*

In a hedonic evaluation of the commercial RTE and corresponding enriched meals, the scores were higher for the commercial than for the enriched meals for all three dishes and the differences were significant for the meat

*Table 2.* Results of the triangle test (12 respondents and 3 replicates)

| Sauce | Replicate | Number of correct answers | Comments |
|---|---|---|---|
| Mustard | 1 | 8 | Commercial: stronger taste (2), saltier, spicier, more sourEnriched: milder taste, milder citrus flavour, stronger taste |
| | 2 | 6 | Commercial: saltier, sharper, stronger tasteEnriched: milder (3), thicker |
| | 3 | 8 | Commercial: more flavour/spicier/stronger (4), sweeterEnriched: milder (2), saltier, stronger |
| | Total | 22 | |
| Cream | 1 | 10 | Commercial: more pepper (3), spicier, bouillon flavourEnriched: less spicy/pepper (3), milder taste, stronger aftertaste, smoother texture, well thickened |
| | 2 | 10 | Commercial: saltier (2), spicier (2), sweeter, fuller, more flavourEnriched: milder (2), bland, more flavour, creamy, thick |
| | 3 | 10 | Commercial: strong, peppery, sour, mild, thin textureEnriched: milder (3), not so spicy, more sting, salt, thicker |
| | Total | 30 | |
| Curry | 1 | 6 | Commercial: less flavour (2), more tasteEnriched: less flavour (2), spicier |
| | 2 | 5 | Commercial: stronger after taste, more sharpEnriched: less spicy |
| | 3 | 7 | Commercial: less flavour, sweet, more flavour |
| | Total | 18 | Enriched: thick, less flavour |

Eighteen correct answers implied a significant difference ($p \leq 0.05$) between two sauces. Numbers in brackets is number of RPs that gave the same comment.

*Table 3.* Results of the hedonic evaluation

| Hedonic evaluation | | Commercial RTE meals | Enriched meals designed for older adults |
|---|---|---|---|
| Appearance | Fish/mustard sauce | 4.8 | 4.7 |
| | Meat balls/cream sauce | 6.7* | 5.3* |
| | Chicken/curry sauce | 7.5* | 5.3* |
| Mashed potatoes – taste | Fish/mustard sauce | 6.2 | 6.3 |
| | Meat balls/cream sauce | 5.9* | 4.8* |
| Mashed potatoes – consistency | Fish/mustard sauce | 6.8 | 6.2 |
| | Meat balls/cream sauce | 6.8* | 5.0* |
| Sauce – taste | Fish/mustard sauce | 6.8 | 6.5 |
| | Meat balls/cream sauce | 6.4* | 5.1* |
| | Chicken/curry sauce | 5.9 | 5.9 |
| Sauce – consistency | Fish/mustard sauce | 7.2 | 6.3 |
| | Meat balls/cream sauce | 6.7* | 5.8* |
| | Chicken/curry sauce | 6.3 | 6.1 |
| Overall acceptance | Fish/mustard sauce | 5.8 | 5.6 |
| | Meat balls/cream sauce | 6.1 | 5.4 |
| | Chicken/curry sauce | 7.1* | 5.8* |

*significant ($p \leq 0.05$) difference between commercial and enriched meals. RTE, ready-to-eat.

ball and chicken dishes (Table 3). For one of the dishes (meat balls), the enriched mashed potatoes had lower scores regarding taste and consistency compared to the commercial meal, but this was not seen for the fish dish. In the case of the separate mustard and curry sauces, there was no difference in taste or consistency between the commercial and enriched sauces. For the cream sauce, however, the commercial sauce appeared to be accepted to a higher extent than the enriched sauce owing to taste and consistency. The triangle test (Table 2) also showed a significant difference between commercial and enriched cream sauces. No differences were found between commercial and enriched meals regarding the rice or the protein component (data not shown). In terms of the overall acceptance, there were no significant differences between the commercial and enriched meals in the case of the fish and meat ball dishes. However, for the chicken dish, the commercial meal had significantly higher acceptance scores than the enriched meal.

*Focus group discussion*

All respondents in the focus group were used to consuming frozen RTE meals. The majority of the female RPs consumed such meals once a month, while the men in general consumed such meals more often, 1–4 times/week. The reasons for consuming frozen RTE meals were almost the same for men and women, lack of time (because of activities) or lack of inspiration or energy. However, in contrast to the women, several men expressed that, due to cultural reasons, they did not have enough cooking knowledge. The RPs felt that frozen RTE meals were attractive meal solutions, easy to store in the freezer (frequent shopping for food is not needed), and quick to cook.

An important attribute of RTE meals was considered to be an appetising and colourful appearance, to which both a sauce and vegetables should contribute. Several women stated that pieces of fish, chicken, or meat should be visible and presented separately, that is, not hidden in a sauce. The taste was considered to be highly important and the meal should be well-seasoned. They also expressed that the provision of a tasty sauce is especially important.

There was a consensus in the group that designing RTE meals, especially for older adults, and making them more nutrient-dense and protein-rich is a very good idea. The majority were positive to the concept of providing a main course supplemented with a dessert. However, opinions differed regarding the addition of a dessert. Some of the RPs thought that the dessert gave an extra value to the meal by adding variety. Conversely, a pair of female RPs found the desserts unnecessary and would rather eat fresh fruit after the main course. When discussing communication to consumers about RTE meals designed for older adults, most RPs found the words 'protein-rich' and 'energising' both appealing and understandable. However, the word 'energy-dense' was perceived as being cryptic. A photo of the food, as well as the food being visible through the packaging, was considered to make the meals more attractive.

## Discussion

The concept of a small, enriched meal with dessert was evaluated in this study. A deeper understanding of the attitudes towards RTE meals and meals designed for older adults was gained through focus group analysis. Olfactory dysfunction, decreased ability to perceive food flavours, and impaired appetite due to ageing and age-related diseases were discussed. These issues have also been reported in the literature since malnutrition in older adults has been linked to social, physiological, and psychological changes (18). Focus group discussions highlighted the necessity of seasoning being adapted to the preferences of older adults and an attractive sauce, regarding both taste and appearance, was considered positive. Appleton (31) reported that supplementation of meals with sauces can increase energy intake in older adults. In the present study, the protein-enriched sauces contained almost twice the amount of protein than the commercial sauces. However, whey protein enrichment of sauces altered the consistency markedly and led to lower flavour intensity. Hence, protein enrichment significantly affected the sensory properties of the sauces due to the physiochemical properties of whey proteins such as their water-binding capacity and emulsifying properties. When designing protein-rich meals, the protein enrichment should not exceed the level whereby sensory properties are significantly affected, instead these effects need to be addressed in the formulation step by using other ingredients that counteract the effects of protein enrichment. In addition, the physiochemical properties of whey proteins may be altered prior to addition by using thermal, chemical, or physical pre-treatments (32–34) enabling improved functionality in food products.

Overall, commercial RTE meals had a higher acceptance score than the corresponding enriched meal for all dishes. One reason for this may be the packaging as the enriched meals were plated so that most of the meal was covered in sauce, which was not appreciated by the RPs. The consistency of the mashed potatoes in the protein-enriched meals was perceived as poor, which could also be linked to food packaging, resulting in the mashed potatoes being covered with sauce. Hence, plating of the food may be the reason for the lower acceptance scores of enriched meals rather than the actual protein enrichment.

Hughes and Bennett (35) reported that poor cooking skills and low motivation to change eating habits among older men may constitute barriers to improving energy intake and appetite. Frailty and disease increase with age and may lead to a decline in the ability to shop and cook independently (2, 36, 37). There is therefore a need for RTE meals with nutritional content adapted to the needs of older adults. The concept of a small main course with a supplementary dessert was generally perceived as positive, but some of the female RPs preferred fresh fruit after the meal rather than a dessert. However, to reduce the risk of DRM, the food products consumed should have a high energy content (38). Hence, an energy-dense dessert could more easily meet the nutritional demands of many older adults than fresh fruit.

## Limitations

The RPs in the focus group were healthier and more alert than the actual target group of the study (frail older adults at risk of malnutrition). This needs to be considered in relation to the analysis of the focus group discussion. It is difficult to recruit a group of frail and sick older adults for a focus group session. The hedonic evaluation was performed with a limited number of RPs. For a more indicative result, a consumer test with a higher number of RPs should be carried out. However, in order to perform all three types of evaluations, a lower number of RPs was chosen. The results of the study should hence be regarded as indications. Similarly, plating of the commercial and protein-enriched meals would exclude the effects of covering most of the meals in sauce. In the present study, only one level of protein enrichment was used. Testing several levels may have indicated an optimal cut-off point for protein enrichment before any significant effects on sensory properties. Also, pre-treatments of whey powder have the possibility to adapt the physiochemical properties of the powder so that the effects on consistency are reduced. No such pre-treatments were included in the present study.

## Conclusion

A concept of small, protein and energy-enriched RTE meals with dessert was evaluated by older adults in terms of sensory properties and attitudes towards this type of meal. Frozen RTE meals were considered to be convenient meal solutions and an attractive sauce was highlighted as important for consumer acceptance. Protein enrichment of sauces, at levels which doubled the protein content, was feasible but altered the consistency markedly and led to lower flavour intensity. Provided that protein enrichment is carried out in a manner that assures attractive sensorial properties, a protein-enriched sauce qualifies as a suitable component in a meal designed for older adults. Plating of the food turned out to be a key factor regarding visibility of meal components (not covered in sauce) and avoidance of poor consistency due to mixing the sauce with other meal components. The meal concept was perceived as successful in increasing energy and protein intakes in older adults; however, the effects of protein enrichment on sensory properties need to be further investigated in order to design tailored foods intended to decrease age-related DRM.

## Conflict of interest and funding

The authors have not received any funding or benefits from industry or elsewhere to conduct this study.

## References


1. Fund UNP. Aging in the twenty-first century. New York: UNFPA and HelpAge International; 2012.
2. Morley JE, Vellas B, van Kan GA, Anker SD, Bauer JM, Bernabei R, et al. Frailty consensus: a call to action. J Am Med Dir Assoc 2013; 14(6): 392–97.
3. Schlip J, Wijnhoven HAH, H. DDJ, Visser M. Early determinants for the development of undernutrition in an older general population: longitudinal aging study Amsterdam. Br J Nutr 2011; 106: 708–17.
4. Shahar D, Shai I, Vardi H, Fraser D. Dietary intake and eating patterns of elderly people in Israel: who is at nutritional risk? Eur J Clin Nutr 2003; 57: 18–25.
5. van der Meij BS, Wijnhoven HAH, Finlayson GS, Oosten BSH, Visser M. Specific food preferences of older adults with poor appetite. A forced-choise test conducted in various care settings. Appetite 2015; 90: 168–75.
6. Liu L, Bopp MM, Roberson PK, and Sullivan DH. Undernutrition and risk of mortality in elderly patients within 1 year of hospital discharge. J Gerontol 2002; 57A(11): M741–46.
7. Rasheed S, Woods RT. Malnutrition and quality of life in older people: a systematic review and meta-analysis. Aging Res Rev 2012; 12(2): 561–6.
8. Stratton RJ, Elia M. A review of reviews: a new look at the evidence for oral nutritional supplements in clinical practice. Clin Nutr Suppl 2007; 2: 5–23.
9. Attems J, Walker L, Jellinger KA. Olfaction and aging: a mini-review. Gerontology 2015; 61(6): 485–90.
10. Mobley AS, Rodriguez-Gil DJ, Imamura F, Greer CA. Aging in the olfactory system. Trends Neurosci 2014; 37(2): 77–84.
11. Amaral TF, Matos LC, Tavares MM, Subtil A, Martins R, Nazare M. The economical impact of disease-related malnutrition at hospital admission. Clin Nutr 2007; 26: 778–4.
12. Meijers JMM, Halfens R, JG, Wilson L, Schols jMGA. Estimating the costs associated with malnutrition in Dutch nursing homes. Clin Nutr 2012; 31: 65–8.
13. Mudge AM, Ross LJ, Young AM, Isenring EA, Banks MD. Helping understand nutritional gaps in the elderly (HUNGER): a prospective study of patient factors associated with inadequate nutritional intake in older medical inpatients. Clin Nutr 2011; 30: 320–5.
14. Rothenberg E, Wendin K. Texture modification of food for elderly people, in Modifying Food Texture Volume 2: Sensory analysis, Consumer Requirements and Preferences. In Chen J, Rosenthal A, eds. Woodhead Publishing Series in Food Science, Technology and Nutrition: number 284, Cambridge, UK, 2015, 163–85.
15. Huffman GB. Evaluating and treating unintentional weight loss in the elderly. Am Fam Physician 2002; 65(4): 640–50.
16. De Castro JM. Macronutrient and dietary energy density influences on the intake of free-living humans. Appetite 2006; 46: 1–5.
17. Goetze O, Steingoetter A, Menne D, van der Voort IR, Kwiatek MA, Boesiger P, et al. The effect of macronutrients on gastric volume responses and gastric emptying in humans: a magnetic resonance imaging study. Am J Physiol Gastrointest Liver Physiol 2007; 292: G11–7.
18. Nieuwenhuizen WF, Weenen H, Rigby P, Hetherington MM. Older adults and patients in need of nutritional support: review of current treatment options and factors influencing nutritional intake. Clin Nutr 2010; 29: 160–9.
19. Bauer J, Biolo G, Cederholm T, Cesari M, Cruz-Jentoft AJ, Morley JE, et al. Evidence-based recommendations for optimal dietary protein intake in older people: a position paper from the PROT-AGE Study Group. JAMDA 2013; 14(8): 542–59.
20. de Almeida Marques G, de Sao José JFB, Alves Silva D, da Silva EMM. Whey protein as a substitute for wheat in the development on no added sugar cookies. LWT - Food Sci Technol 2016; 67: 118–26.
21. Pennings B, Boirie Y, Senden JMG, Gijsen AP, Kuipers H, van Loon LJC. Whey protein stimulates postprandial muscle protein accretion more effectively than do casein and casein hydrolysate in older men. Am J Clin Nutr 2011; 93: 997–1005.

22. Yang Y, Breen L, Burd NA, Hector AJ, Churchward-Venne TA, Josse AR, et al. Resistance exercise enhances myofibrillar protein synthesis with graded intakes of whey protein in older men. Br J Nutr 2012; 2012: 1780–8.
23. Chung C, Degner B, McClements DJ. Creating novel food textures: modifying rheology of starch granule suspensions by cold-set whey protein gelation. LWT - Food Sci Technol 2013; 54: 336–45.
24. Doty RL, Kamath V. The influences of age on olfaction: a review. Front Psychol 2014; 5(20): 1–20.
25. Duffy VB, Backstrand JR, Ferris AM. Olfactory dysfunction and related nutritional risk in free-living, elderly women. J Am Dietetic Assoc 1995; 95(8): 879–84.
26. Rolls B. Experimental analyses of the effects of variety in a meal on human feeding. Am J Clin Nutr 1985; 42: 932–9.
27. Peryam DR, Girardot NF. Advanced taste test method. Food Eng 1952; 24: 58–, 194.
28. Lawless HT, Heymann H. Sensory evaluation of food. ed. F.S.T. Series. 2010, New York: Springer Science + Business Media.
29. Roessler EB, Pangborn RM, Sidel JL, Stone H. Expanded statistical tables for estimating significance in paired-preference, paired-difference, dou-trio and triangle tests. J Food Sci 1978; 43(3): 940–3.
30. Lincoln YS, Guba EG. Naturalistic inquiry. Beverly Hills, CA: Sage; 1985.
31. Appleton KM. Increases in energy, protein and fat intake following the addition of sauce to an older person's meal. Appetite 2009; 52: 161–5.
32. Lam RSH, Nickerson MT. The effect of pH and temperature pre-treatments on the physiochemical and emulsifying properties of whey protein isolate. LWT - Food Sci Technol 2015; 60: 427–34.
33. Oboroceanu D, Wang L, Magner E, Auty MAE. Fibrillization of whey proteins improves foaming capacity and foam stability of low protein concentrations. J Food Eng 2014; 121: 102–11.
34. Tan MC, Chin NL, Yusof YA, Taip FS, Abdullah J. Improvement of eggless cake structure using ultrasonically treated whey protein. Food Bioprocess Technol 2015; 8(3): 605–14.
35. Hughes G, Bennett KM, Hetherington MM. Old and alone: barriers to healthy eating in older men living on their own. Appetite 2004; 43; 269–76.
36. Johannesson J, Rothenberg E, Dahlin Ivanoff S, Slinde F. Gender differences in practice, knowledge and attitudes regarding food habits and meal patterns among community dwelling older adults. J Aging Res Clin Pract 2016; 5: 220–8.
37. Fried LP, Tangen CM, Walston J, Newman AB, Hirsch C, Gottdiener J, et al. Frailty in older adults: evidence for a phenotype. J Gerontol: Med Sci 2001; 56A(3): M146–56.
38. Collins J, Porter H. The effect of interventions to prevent and treat malnutrition in patients admitted for rehabilitation: a systematic review with meta-analysis. J Human Nutr Diet 2015; 28: 1–15.

***Evelina Höglund**
RISE Research Institutes of Sweden
Agrifood and Bioscience
Box 5401
SE-40229 Göteborg, Sweden
Email:evelina.hoglund@ri.se

# 12

# Implications of Ethiopian Productive Safety Net Programme on household dietary diversity and women's body mass index

Asnake Ararsa Irenso* and Gudina Egata Atomsa

School of Public Health, Haramaya University, Harar, Ethiopia

*Abstract*

***Introduction:*** Poor nutritional status of women remains a critical problem in Ethiopia. Nutrition for women matters not only for the public health relevance of breaking the intergenerational cycle of malnutrition but for its high return in other sectors such as education and health. The Ethiopian Productive Safety Net Programme (PSNP) is a program that protects chronically food-insecure households against food insecurity through cash or food transfer. However, its effect on food access and women's body mass index (BMI) has remained unexplored.
***Objective:*** This study was intended to assess differences in household dietary diversity (HDD) and women's BMI and associated factors among PSNP and non-PSNP households.
***Methods:*** This community-based cross-sectional study was carried out in the Kombolcha District of Eastern Ethiopia from July 1 to 28, 2015. HDD and women's BMI were compared. Ordinal logistic regression was used to identify factors associated with women's BMI.
***Result:*** The prevalence of undernutrition was 27.3% (95% confidence interval [CI]: 23.8–30.9) and 20.2% (95% CI: 17.1–23.5) for women from PSNP and non-PSNP households, respectively. PSNP membership had a significant effect on HDD and minimal effect on women's BMI. Ordinal logistic regression yielded significant associations for medium wealth status, with an odds ratio (OR) of 0.533 (95% CI: 0.339–0.837), uptake of better health care services compared to previous year with an odds ratio (OR) of 0.647 (95% CI: 0.429–0.974) and reduction in selling assets for the sake of buying food with an OR of 1.575 (95% CI: 1.057–2.349).
***Conclusion and recommendation:*** There was high magnitude of chronic energy deficiency among PSNP and non-PSNP households, at 27.3 and 20.2%, respectively, and it was associated with economic status and health care utilization, suggesting the need to promote profitable income-generating activities and nudging for minimum health care as a condition for transfer.

Keywords: *BMI; PSNP; social protection; HDD; Ethiopia; drought; women*

Launched in 2005, the Ethiopian Productive Safety Net Programme (PSNP) is the largest African social protection program to provide predictable transfers. The government launched Phase 4 of the PSNP in 2015 (1). The main objective of the PSNP is to increase livelihoods and resilience to shocks and to improve food security and nutrition for rural households vulnerable to food insecurity. It has public works, direct support and livelihood components directed at heads of household. The program enables households with an able-bodied adult in public works to receive cash or in-kind transfers for 6 months of the year. By contrast, households without labor capacity become permanent, direct support clients; they receive 12 months of unconditional transfers and are linked with social protection services. Beneficiaries are paid in cash equivalent to 15 kg of cereals and 4 kg of pulses per month (adjusted for inflation). The wage rate used to compute the transfer in cash varies according to the purchasing power in different areas. The livelihood component includes skill-related trainings provided by appropriate institutions or conditional capacity building of grassroots institutions such as farmer training centers (1, 2).

Malnutrition has remained a major global issue in the post-Millennium Development Goals era. Ending this problem has continued to receive more attention and commitment for its extraordinary contribution towards the progress of Sustainable Development Goal (SDG) targets (3).

This remains true in Ethiopia, where poor nutritional status of women remains a central problem. According to the Ethiopian Demographic and Health Survey (EDHS) (2), about 27% of women of reproductive age are chronically malnourished (4). Since 2016, the PSNP has been closely connected to the National Nutrition Programme and particularly the Community-Based Nutrition Programme, which focuses on nutrition education for mothers and supplementary food for children and mothers. In this regard, Ethiopia's PSNP has a critical role in advancing and accelerating progress toward improved food and nutrition security mentioned under SDG 1 (5, 6).

Nutrition for women matters not only for the public health relevance of breaking the intergenerational cycle of malnutrition but also for its high return in numerous other sectors such as education and community health. A major current focus of women's nutrition revolves around how to ensure improved decision-making for women and in turn a greater right to food and nutrition security, in addition to maximized improvement in social protection programs (7, 8). Social protection is a nutrition-sensitive development effort aimed at improving nutrition among nutritionally vulnerable populations and individuals (9).

Productive safety nets have a direct impact on consumption and a secondary impact on school attendance, enrolment and retention, utilization of health services, food security, nutrition, and accumulation of assets and building of livelihoods (10). The impetus of PSNP was to deliver a predictable package of support for a number of years that leads to asset accumulation and enable households to cover year-round food needs, in addition to building resilience to moderate shocks (state of graduation) (11). Though it has achieved this goal, improvements thought to achieve better nutrition and health outcomes have been implemented recently (1).

Ethiopia's PSNP has improved nutritional outcomes by addressing the underlying causes of malnutrition (through nutrition-sensitive interventions) such as female empowerment, maternal and child health, infant and young child feeding practices, vaccination campaigns, dietary diversity, and water, sanitation, and hygiene. This work through soft conditionalities means public works clients have co-responsibilities to attend behavior change communication sessions for pregnant and lactating women (PLW) and their young children (1, 12). The program enhances household food consumption and dietary diversity by providing families with cash and increasing purchasing power. Transfers also work by minimizing negative coping mechanisms and empowering women in poverty to focus on specific services. This aids women in making better choices for self- and family care with an anticipated positive influence on the nutritional status of women and children (5, 13–15).

Ethiopia's PSNP relies on meeting eligibility criteria that include being members of the community, having chronic household food insecurity, which is a food gap of 3 months or more per year, in the last 3 years; sudden food insecurity due to severe loss of assets and households with inadequate family support. Clients are selected through community-based targeting, meaning that a community food security task force facilitates client selection through reading client conditions out loud and discussing it against criteria at a public meeting (1). It aims to empower and support vulnerable women among other target groups by improving water security through pond construction or rehabilitation, improved firewood availability through rehabilitated natural environment and nutrition insecurity (16–18).

However, cascades of chronic food insecurity that lead to migration of key household members to towns for work leave women with an immense workload of home subsistence farming (normally more than 50% of women work in agriculture), childcare, and public work of PSNP (17, 19, 20). Provided unequal participation and benefit share from the PSNP, and high burden of agriculture, economic and domestic care work, women's nutrition will continue to be a challenge (1). In addition, a cash-first principle of PSNP in male-headed households may lead to less control over transfer by women; males may misuse these funds, leading to conflicts. In other words, transfers not allocated to women influence intrahousehold resource allocation by leaving women with limited bargaining power. Despite the empowerment component in PSNP, a recent PSNP assessment has recognized women in male-headed and female-headed households as underserved and vulnerable groups (21–23). This is worsened by women's triple burdens of land access; specifically, they account for less than 20% of the landholders, land policy that is based on state ownership of land (state controls land ownership, gives all rights except sale and mortgage) and limited agricultural inputs even when they have access to land (19, 24).

Based on the ethical notion of fairness and limited resources, the government of Ethiopia must use a fair mechanism for separating the population into those eligible and ineligible for social transfers. Ethiopia's PSNP uses a combination of geographic and community-based targeting, with the transfer going to the household head. While it has been shown that community-based targeting effectively identifies the poor, geographic targeting that considers differences among homogenous poor and vulnerable groups remains questionable (25). Specifically, the inclusion of the most deprived and vulnerable people, harmonization with other interventions, and sensitization of all stakeholders on the role of women are far from optimal (26).

Generally, ensuring food and nutrition security at the household level requires investment in nutrition-sensitive interventions, protecting women's rights, and improving their social and nutritional status (19). A key step in understanding the difference PSNP makes is to understand the relationship between poverty levels based on household consumption and the asset-based wealth index, because asset holdings are a critical outcome of PSNP (27). Based on this, an appraisal of the effect of PSNP across geographic areas is of great interest in terms of women's nutritional status and the ability of their households to access an adequate quantity and quality of food to promote positive health outcomes. In addition, it is important to assess whether a combination of women's nutritional status and household dietary diversity (HDD) predicts membership in PSNP and certain wealth groups. Therefore, this study was intended to assess factors associated with differences in HDD and women's body mass index (BMI) among PSNP and non-PSNP households.

## Methods

A community-based cross-sectional study was carried out in the Kombolcha District of Eastern Ethiopia from July 1 to 28, 2015. This period overlapped with failed spring (mid-February to May) rain that affected crop production from the first harvest that would provide 20% of food production followed by the end of 6 months of PSNP cash transfer (28). The district contains 19 *kebeles* (smallest administrative units in Ethiopia next to districts), out of which 10 are non-beneficiary and 9 kebeles (total of 2,375 households) benefit from cash transfers. This translates to about 9,752 people who receive cash in exchange for participating in public works and 1,409 people with direct support. For this study, five PSNP and six non-PSNP kebeles were selected randomly, and only public works participants were included in the study.

Though fairness and transparency is the core principle of PSNP client selection, there are inclusion and exclusion errors. Corrupt officials, clan politics, and quota allocation were the main causes of inclusion and exclusion errors (22, 29). To obtain data with a low bias estimate, firstly, the data collection was carefully planned to include the same variables by using similar data collection tools and procedures for beneficiary and non-beneficiary households. Secondly, outcomes related to program participation were identified using key PSNP-related variables (livestock ownership, household landholding, access to government health post, asset depletion and food aid, and asset losses) that identify outcomes related to women's nutrition and other related variables. This information was obtained from the *kebele* food security task force (KFSTF), which has seven members, including a health extension worker. Thirdly, to attain comparable access to market systems, similar livelihood zones known for khat and vegetable production were selected. These livelihood zones had similar agro-ecology and production patterns of these commercial crops; the participants had common livelihood strategies and comparable access to markets, including distance from the market. In this district, cash was provided because the markets functioned well.

Information about women was collected during the mother's interview for eligible children aged 6 months to 5 years (information on children being processed in another publication). Hence, participants were selected from five randomly selected PSNP and six non-PSNP kebeles. Women eligible for a child interview were identified from lists obtained from the district PSNP office compiled by KFSTF and respective *kebele* health extension workers. Non-PSNP kebeles have similar KFSTFs that follow the same procedure to identify food insecure clients. Both PSNP and non-PSNP household lists are finally ascertained by social networks leaders called *gare* (groups containing 25–30 women). In order to minimize handout expectations and a spillover effect of the transfer, women from non -PSNP beneficiary households were entirely selected from non-beneficiary kebeles. Pregnant women and direct support beneficiaries were excluded from this study.

### *Data collection procedures and quality assurance*

A structured pretested questionnaire was used to assess socioeconomic and demographic characteristics of the households. Nursing students who could speak a local language (Afaan Oromo) were trained to collected data. The tool was pretested on 20 households to determine its suitability to local accent, format, wording, and order. In addition, periodic checking of the weighing scale and repeated measurement were used to assure the data quality.

Ethical clearance was obtained from the Haramaya University College of Health and Medical Science Institutional Health Research Ethics Review Committee. The objective of the study, known benefits, and risks of participant involvement in the research were communicated. Informed written and signed consent was obtained from women before commencing the study.

### Variables

The primary outcome of this study was women's BMI. The secondary outcome was Household Dietary Diversity Score (HDDS). In the statistical analyses, the factor considered as a potential confounder was maternal age. Factors considered as potential effect modifiers were the sex of head of household and PSNP beneficiary status.

### Body mass index

BMI is a proxy indicator of energy status (undernutrition), calculated as weight (kg) divided by the square of height ($m^2$). Women's height was measured to the nearest 0.5 cm without shoes, feet flat, heels together, legs straight using a portable wooden height-measuring board with a sliding head bar following standard anthropometric techniques. Heights <145 cm were classified as stunted. Weight was measured repeatedly to the nearest 100 g using an electronic scale (SECA, Hamburg, Germany). A BMI of 17–18.4 indicates marginal energy deficiency, 16 to <17 moderate energy deficiency, and that of less than 16.0 indicates severe chronic energy deficiency. A BMI of ≥25 signifies overweight, and >30 signifies obesity. Even though a global database on women nutrition is not available, a BMI of 20–25 kg/m$^2$ is recommended for good health and is associated with normal fertility. A weight for height equivalent to a BMI of 18 kg/m$^2$ or lower is considered too low for successful reproductive ability (30).

### Household Dietary Diversity Score

The HDD score is a measure of the total number of different food groups consumed in the last 24 hours by household members with a well-grounded construction of diet quality and accuracy, cross-checked with incomes. HDDS ranges from 0 to 12, the higher the better, and it is a good indicator of both quantity and quality. It is included in the acute food insecurity reference table for household group classification of the Integrated Food Security Phase Classification (IPC). HDDS does not have established categorical cutoffs and is analyzed only as a scale measure. A face-to-face interview was used to administer the tool. For households with unusual food intake in the previous 24 hours, another appointment was made for the interview. Due emphasis was placed on acquiring a response with minimal social desirability bias (31–33).

### Household Wealth Index

Household wealth is a proxy measure of household income for long-term wealth. Principal components analysis was run using 38 items comprising productive assets, livestock, household goods, and consumer durables. It was used as a continuous variable, and each household was classified as being in the lowest, middle, or highest asset category.

### Sample size determination

Analysis was performed on data that were already available for child wasting. Excluding 52 women, the final sample size was 623 women from PSNP and 635 non-PSNP (total 1,258). This sample size is sufficient for the analysis of the data to produce results with sufficient statistical precision.

#### *Statistical methods*

Data were entered in EpiData 3.1 and the software package SPSS version 23 for Windows was used for statistical analysis. To examine whether associations differed across groups, stratification was done based on PSNP and wealth index. Descriptive statistical analysis was conducted to describe the characteristics of participants. For constructing wealth index based on 38 items, the selection of each factors was based on the rotated component matrix of greater than 0.5. One-way Analysis of Variance (ANOVA) was conducted. The independent-samples *t*-test was used to compare mean HDDS across PSNP and other variables. In order to check whether the assumptions of Multivariate analysis of variance (MANOVA) were met, preliminary assumption testing for normality, linearity, univariate and multivariate outliers, homogeneity of variance–covariance matrices, and multicollinearity were conducted. No significant violation was found. Further, an ordinal logistic regression model was used for prediction of women's BMI (dependent variable). The odds ratio (OR) was used as the primary measure of strength and direction of the relationship between each independent variable and the women's BMI values, which were categorized into underweight (BMI<18.4), normal (BMI 18.5–24.9), and overweight (BMI ≥25). In this analysis, OR less than 1 indicated a negative relationship.

## Result

The study included 1,311 women, of whom 39 were pregnant and 14 had out-of-range values, which resulted in a final sample size of 1,258. Table 1 shows the characteristics of participants stratified by PSNP membership, where 50.5% (653) were non-PSNP and 49.5% (623) were PSNP households. There were 146 (11.6%) female-headed households, mainly 57.5% (84) from PSNP households.

The overall prevalence of underweight women (BMI <18.5) was 23.7% (95% confidence interval [CI]: 21.3–26.13). Out of this, the prevalence of BMI severe energy deficiency was 3.2% among PSNP households, which was higher than for non-PSNP households (1.4%) (Fig. 1).

The total mean HDDS was 5.76 ± 1.59 and the mean difference between PSNP and non-PSNP households was statistically significant. The magnitude of the differences in the means as indicated by eta squared was 0.142 (Table 2).

A multivariate analysis of variance was performed to find any group differences based on a linear combination of women's BMI that indicate utilization and HDD that showed the access and quality aspect of food insecurity. Inclusion of both dependent variables in the analyses provided the maximum amount of information regarding the effects of PSNP. Hence a two-way MANOVA was employed in which a 2 PSNP (beneficiary and non-beneficiary) ×3 wealth index (low, medium, and high socioeconomic status) were the between-participant factors. The combined dependent variable was significantly affected by state of PSNP membership, $F(2, 1251) = 40.995$, $p < 0.001$; Wilks' lambda = 0.938, and the wealth index $F(4, 2502) = 8.269$, $p < 0.001$; Wilks' lambda = 0.974, but not by their interaction $F(4, 2504) = 2.2$,

*Table 1.* Characteristics of women from PSNP and non-PSNP households in Kombolcha District of eastern Ethiopia, 2015

| Variables | Non-PSNP (*n* = 635) | PSNP (*n* = 623) | Total (*n* = 1,258) |
|---|---|---|---|
| Head of Household | | | |
| Male | 573 (90.2%) | 542 (86.5%) | 1,114 (88.4%) |
| Female | 62 (9.8%) | 84 (13.5%) | 146 (11.6%) |
| Last pregnancy intentional | | | |
| No | 100 (15.7%) | 170 (27.3%) | 270 (21.5%) |
| Yes | 535 (84.3%) | 435 (72.7%) | 988 (78.5%) |
| Family planning use | | | |
| No | 477 (75.1%) | 422 (67.7%) | 899 (71.5%) |
| Yes | 158 (24.9%) | 201 (32.3%) | 359 (28.5%) |
| Breastfeeding now | | | |
| No | 331 (52.1%) | 371 (59.6%) | 702 (55.8%) |
| Yes | 304 (47.9%) | 252 (40.4%) | 556 (44.2%) |
| Less school attrition | | | |
| No | 372 (58.6%) | 293 (47%) | 665 (52.9%) |
| Yes | 263 (41.4%) | 330 (53%) | 593 (47.1%) |
| More health care services | | | |
| No | 153 (24.1%) | 172 (27.6%) | 325 (25.8%) |
| Yes | 482 (75.9%) | 451 (72.4%) | 933 (74.2%) |
| Reduced selling assets for food | | | |
| No | 449 (70.7%) | 519 (83.3%) | 968 (76.9%) |
| Yes | 186 (64.1%) | 104 (16.7%) | 290 (23.1%) |
| Vegetable garden ownership | | | |
| No | 550 (86.6%) | 546 (87.6%) | 1,096 (87.1%) |
| Yes | 85 (13.4%) | 77 (12.3%) | 162 (12.9%) |
| Wealth index | | | |
| Low | 74 (11.7%) | 341 (54.7%) | 415 (33%) |
| Medium | 196 (47%) | 221 (35.5%) | 417 (33.1%) |
| High | 365 (50.5%) | 61 (9.8%) | 426 (33.9%) |

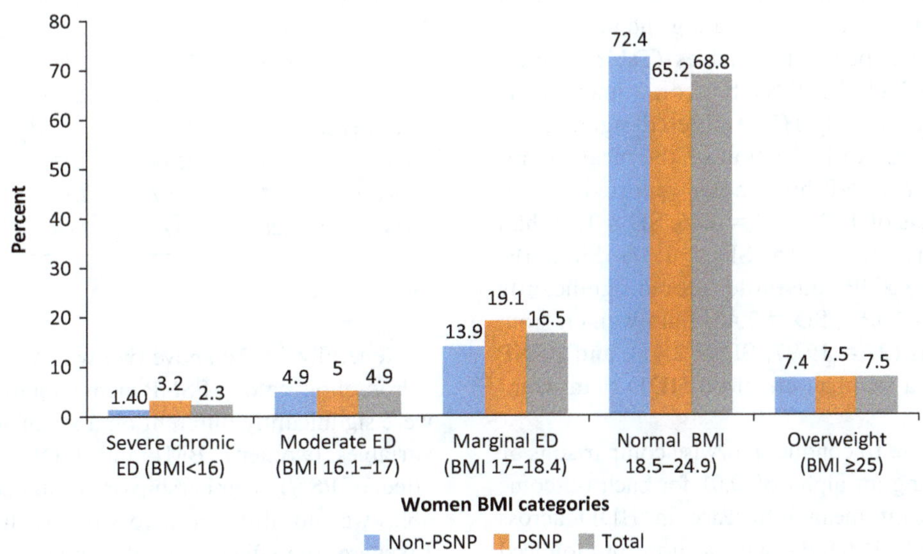


*Fig. 1.* Prevalence of chronic energy deficiency of women from Productive Safety Net Programme (PSNP) and non-PSNP households in Kombolcha District, 2015.

ED: Energy Deficiency.

*Table 2.* Effect of PSNP on characteristics of women from PSNP and non-PSNP households in Kombolcha District, 2015

| | Mean ± SD | | | Mean differences | Eta squared |
|---|---|---|---|---|---|
| | Total | Non-PSNP | PSNP | | |
| HDD | 5.76 ± 1.59 | 6.36 ± 1.5 | 5.15 ± 1.37 | 1.2** | 0.142 |
| Women's BMI | 20.29 ± 2.46 | 20.61 ± 2.46 | 19.97 ± 2.41 | 0.63** | 0.017 |
| Women's age | 28.75 ± 5.85 | 27.98 ± 5.64 | 29.54 ± 5.96 | −1.6** | 0.018 |
| Number of children under five | 1.73 ± 0.69 | 1.69 ± 6.80 | 1.76 ± 0.694 | −0.066 | 0.002 |
| Family size | 6.2 ± 2.2 | 6.18 ± 2.43 | 6.23 ± 1.96 | −0.047 | 0 |
| Land size (ha) | 0.56 ± 0.36 | 0.639 ± 0.412 | 0.470 ± 0.26 | 0.0194** | 0.056 |

**$p < 0.001$. HDD, household dietary diversity.

*Table 3.* Effect of PSNP, wealth index, and their interaction on women's BMI and HDD for PSNP and non-PSNP households in Kombolcha District

| Independent Variables | Dependent variables | Univariate *F* | *df* | Partial $\eta^2$ |
|---|---|---|---|---|
| Wealth index | Women's BMI | 2.9 | 2/1252 | 0.005 |
| | HDD | 13.70** | 2/1252 | 0.021 |
| PSNP | Women's BMI | 9.20** | 1/1252 | 0.007 |
| | HDD | 75.90** | 1/1252 | 0.057 |
| Interaction of PSNP × wealth index | Women's BMI | 0.28 | 2/1252 | 0.000 |
| | HDD | 4.30* | 2/1252 | 0.007 |

*$p < 0.05$, **$p < 0.01$.

$p = 0.993$, $\eta^2 = 0.004$. The result showed association between PSNP and the combined dependent variable ($\eta^2 = 0.062$) and wealth index ($\eta^2 = 0.013$). This indicates that the linear composite of HDD and women's BMI differs significantly with respect to PSNP membership and across wealth levels but not by their interaction (Table 3).

Follow-up ANOVAs for investigating the main effect on the individual dependent variables (Table 4) indicated significant effects for PSNP both on women's BMI and HDD. However, only HDD differed significantly across wealth levels. An inspection of the mean scores indicated that non-PSNP households reported significantly higher levels of HDD ($M = 6.36$, SD = 1.5) than PSNP households ($M = 5.15$, SD = 1.37). Similarly, women from non-PSNP households scored significantly higher BMI ($M = 20.61$, SD = 2.46) than women from PSNP households ($M = 19.97$, SD = 2.41), and PSNP membership had a stronger effect on HDD than women's BMI (Table 2).

Tukey's procedure to conduct pairwise comparisons of women's BMI using an alpha of 0.01 for each outcome showed a significant mean difference in HDD across wealth categories ($p < 0.001$), with a more pronounced mean difference between low and high wealth levels. Hence, non-PSNP households scored higher on both HDD and women's BMI (Table 4).

*Table 4.* Means and standard deviations of women's BMI and HDD as a PSNP and wealth category for PSNP and non-PSNP households in Kombolcha District, 2015

| Group | *n* | Women BMI | | HDD | |
|---|---|---|---|---|---|
| | | *M* | SD | *M* | SD |
| PSNP | | | | | |
| No | 635 | 20.6 | 2.46 | 6.35 | 1.57 |
| Yes | 631 | 19.97 | 2.4 | 5.15 | 1.36 |
| Wealth index | | | | | |
| Low | 415 | 20.16 | 2.47 | 5.09 | 1.48 |
| Medium | 417 | 19.97 | 2.37 | 5.7 | 1.37 |
| High | 426 | 20.72 | 2.46 | 6.4 | 1.6 |

Generally, in the above two-way MANOVA, we asked if households along PSNP membership and wealth index were significantly different on a set of linearly combined variables (women's BMI and HDD). The interaction effect of PSNP membership on combined dependent variables was not different across the wealth index gradient. Likewise, the effect of wealth index on dependent variables was similar for PSNP and non-PSNP households. Hence, the combination of women's BMI and HDD did not predict PSNP or wealth group membership.

*Table 5.* Multivariable ordinal regression model for predicting the risk of higher category of BMI for women from PSNP and non-PSNP households in Kombolcha District, 2015

| | B | SE(B) | *p* | OR | 95% CI |
|---|---|---|---|---|---|
| HDD | 0.067 | 0.065 | 0.307 | 1.069 | 0.941–1.215 |
| Age of mother (years) | −0.008 | 0.020 | 0.665 | 0.992 | 0.954–1.030 |
| Total land size (ha) | −0.240 | 0.221 | 0.279 | 0.787 | 0.510–1.214 |
| Family size | 0.057 | 0.049 | 0.240 | 1.059 | 0.962–1.166 |
| PSNP | | | | | |
| No | 0.165 | 0.218 | 0.450 | 1.179 | 0.769–1.808 |
| Yes (ref) | 0.000 | | | 1.000 | |
| Wealth index | | | | | |
| Low | −0.343 | 0.269 | 0.203 | 0.710 | 0.419–1.203 |
| medium | −0.629 | 0.231 | 0.006 | 0.533 | 0.339–0.837 |
| High (ref) | 0.000 | | | 1.000 | |
| Sex of head of household | | | | | |
| Male | −0.190 | 0.306 | 0.530 | 0.825 | 0.453–1.504 |
| Female (ref) | 0.000 | | | 1 | |
| Breastfeeding now | | | | | |
| No | −0.636 | 0.366 | 0.082 | 0.530 | 0.259–1.084 |
| Yes (ref) | 0.000 | | | 1.000 | |
| Better healthcare services uptake[a] | | | | | |
| No | −0.436 | 0.209 | 0.037 | 0.647 | 0.429–0.974 |
| Yes (ref) | 0.000 | | | 1.000 | |
| Less school attrition[b] | | | | | |
| No | −0.261 | 0.207 | 0.207 | 0.770 | 0.514–1.155 |
| Yes (ref) | 0.000 | | | 1.000 | |
| Reduced selling assets for food[c] | | | | | |
| No | 0.455 | 0.204 | 0.026 | 1.575 | 1.057–2.349 |
| Yes (ref) | 0.000 | | | 1.000 | |
| Intention to have more children | | | | | |
| No | 0.27 | 0.207 | 0.193 | 1.310 | 0.872–1.967 |
| Yes (ref) | 0.000 | | | 1.000 | |

[a]Household members' health services uptake compared to previous year.
[b]School attrition of household members compared to previous year.
[c]Selling more assets to buy food compared to last year.
CI, confidence interval; OR, odds ratio.

### *Predictors of women's nutritional status*

To examine factors associated with nutritional status, women's BMI measurements were categorized as underweight (BMI <18.5), normal (BMI 18.5–25), and overweight (BMI ≥25). Ordinal regression was conducted (Table 5) and yielded significant associations for wealth index, Uptake of better health care service compared to the previous year, and a reduction in selling assets for the sake of buying foods. As the most notable outcome, controlling for the other explanatory variables, women in the middle wealth index (OR = 0.533) had 46.7% lower odds than women from the high wealth index of being in the higher BMI category.

## Discussion

This study was set out to assess the differences in women's nutritional status as determined by BMI and the factors associated with it among PSNP and non-PSNP households. Emphasis was also given to understanding how an asset-based wealth index interacted with PSNP to influence HDD and women's nutritional status.

Previous PSNP-related studies did not examine this issue. Hence, a lack of adequate literature was a challenge and points to the need for further studies in the future. On the other hand, this study is useful in informing PSNP stakeholders how to plan and allocate appropriate resources, especially for women. The study data were collected from PSNP and non-PSNP households only once and generalizability is limited to a similar population definition.

*Difference in women's BMI and HDD*

There were large differences in HDD with respect to PSNP, which was indicative evidence for an effect on household food access. This is consistent with findings from the Democratic Republic of Congo, where similar unconditional cash transfer recipients were free to spend the cash transfer for diverse reasons, and in particular for food items (34). However, the result is counter to evidence on vulnerability to drought and food price shocks in Ethiopia, which points to a greater risk of decreased consumption in drought-prone areas by non-PSNP households compared to PSNP households from price inflation (35).

However, contrary to expectation, PSNP has a minimal effect on women's BMI. This mismatch might indicate the presence of an underlying factor that hinders translation of transfer into better nutrition outcome. Although it might be true that government initiated integration of nutrition into the PSNP late in 2016 (1, 36), the prevalence of underweight women is comparable to national figures. For instance, according to the 2011 EDHS reports, 27% of women were thin. This is comparable to PSNP (27.3%) but lower than non-PSNP (20.2%) household women. However, a figure of 6% overweight or obese is lower than the figure reported by EDHS (4). This contrasts with findings from rural India and Nigeria, where chronic energy deficiency is lower than obesity (37, 38). On the contrary, this study showed lower obesity, with an impending 'food insecurity–obesity paradox', with lack of recognition of the rising rates of overweight and obesity (36).

One notable finding was severe chronic energy deficiency for PSNP (3.2%) and non-PSNP (1.4%) women. Compared to findings from low- and middle-income countries that range between 1.8 and 6.2%, the PSNP result is comparable to Madagascar (3.4%). This level of undernutrition is related to high morbidity, mortality, and poor maternal–fetal outcomes with the potential of perpetuating intergenerational malnutrition (39). This reinforces how addressing conditional minimum preventative health care is mandatory (Brière & Rawlings, 2006). Evidence from Shigutes et al.'s (2013) report showed increased community-based health insurance uptake and retention through increasing demand and risk aversion behavior among PSNP households. This shows the untapped potential of PSNP for being a platform to address the most pressing maternal and child health care issues (40).

Like other similar social protection programs, there was a lower mean HDD among PSNP households that can be explained by the effect of cash transfers where markets are not able to respond to increased demand by increasing supply, thereby pushing up local prices and reducing access to food groups during usual lean transfer seasons (41). This finding is in favor of Sabates-Wheeler and Devereux (2010) work on Ethiopia's PSNP that supports food transfers or a 'cash plus food' scheme as preferable to cash transfers alone in achieving the PSNP's goal. This argument contradicts the cash-first policy of Ethiopia's PSNP (1, 42).

The high magnitude of women's undernutrition and lower HDD among women from non-PSNP is against the key design feature of a good public works program, which is inclusion of poor household as far as the wage rate is not higher than unskilled manual labor that do not attract households who are not poor (43). Taking into account PSNP membership and wealth index together, there was a difference in the mean of the linear combination of the HDD and women's BMI, but with non-significant interaction. This demonstrates that the effect of economic status on the linear combination of the HDD and BMI is not different for PSNP and non-PSNP members.

From follow-up ANOVA, PSNP has a greater effect on HDD than women's BMI. This means the program has a better outcome at household level than on women's nutritional status. This might be a result of interaction within the household such as time use, money, and other resources that influence the nutritional status of women. This is consistent with the 'collective approach' intrahousehold resource allocation theory, which assumes transfer is influenced by the identity of the transfer recipient (man or woman), which in turn affects how this transfer is used and who benefits from it. To put it another way, 86.5% of PSNP beneficiaries are male-headed households and they are the recipients of the transfer. Hence, they influence how the transfer is used for household members as opposed to women recipients (woman-headed households), who tend to use them differently (44). Contrary to this, an analysis of the nutrition impact of Bolsa Família's program found that household expenditure decisions in nutrition from increased bargaining power of women showed no evidence that favors this hypothesis, and impacts were driven by conditionalities that demanded households spend the transfer on health care and education, which recipients are not required to do in the PSNP (45).

*Predictors of women's nutritional status*

Women's BMI results showed undernutrition because of energy deficiency, health status, and a lack of access to health services and sanitation. This study finding showed reduced BMI for middle wealth index women, a finding that aligns with other low- and middle-income countries where the highest wealth quantile is associated with better BMI (46). Nevertheless, for lower wealth index the BMI reduction was not significant. The most likely explanation for this finding is related to control, ownership, and the struggle to retain assets among the middle wealth group. It also raises concerns related to empowerment of women, which is positively associated with calorie availability and dietary diversity at the household level (47). This suggests the need for more attention not only to reproductive, social, and cultural norms but also differentials in income shocks and subsequent poverty (48).

Women from households that did not reduce sale of assets for food were 57.7% more likely to become underweight. A household's distress sale of assets is one outcome indicator for the PSNP public works component in Ethiopia, and it shows the extent of change in a household's short-term vulnerability to shocks. An Irreversible asset decapitalization and income shock reduce uptake of health care services, which subsequently leads to loss in labor productivity (49).

The analysis showed a higher proportion of breastfeeding women in PSNP households than non-PSNP households. Further analysis showed, though non-significant, lactating women had a higher risk of being in lower BMI category. This is congruent with the Ministry of Agriculture's enhanced social assessment and consultation report that acknowledges health and safety risks for PLW participating in public works. As a result, PLW switch to temporary direct support (up to 1 year after birth) with co-responsibilities of attending health care (antenatal care, postpartum health facility visit and immunization) and nutrition services, such as growth monitoring and participation in nutrition-related behavioral change communication (1).

### Conclusion and recommendations

This study has provided evidence of the PSNP's substantial effect on HDD and its minimal effect on women's BMI. The overall mean value of women's BMI was within the normal range. However, there was a high prevalence of female undernutrition and low HDD. The PSNP was born out of decades of emergency food aid that met only emergency nutritional requirements, with no lasting impact. Similarly, mainstreaming nutrition took three phases of PSNP to initiate. Hence, sooner or later strong behavioral interventions and other determinants of nutritional status must be addressed to unleash PSNP's human capital development, especially on nutrition. These efforts should be supplemented through the proper implementation of income-generating opportunities and health-related soft conditionalities directed to women beyond a gender-based quota.

In addition, reassessing strategy to implement a rights-based framework to address chronically food-insecure households residing in non-beneficiary kebeles should be considered. The improvements noted in our study were not only revisiting women who were thought to be the primary target of this intervention, but also including comparative groups exclusively residing in non-beneficiary kebeles. However, the levels of empowerment of women, which is central to the success of the PSNP, need to be established well in future studies.

### Acknowledgments

We would like to thank Haramaya University for funding the entire study.

### Conflict of interest and funding

Asnake Ararsa Irenso and Gudina Egata Atomsa declares that they have no conflict of interest. Authors has received research grant from Haramaya University.

### References


1. Government of Ethiopia. Productive safety net programme phase IV: programme Implementation Manual. Ministry of Agriculture (Ethiopia), Addis Abab; 2014. Available at https://www.usaid.gov/sites/default/files/documents/1866/psnp_iv_programme_implementation_manual_14_dec_14.pdf.
2. Devereux S, Sabates-Wheeler R, Tefera M, Taye H. Ethiopia's Productive Safety Net Programme (PSNP): trends in PSNP transfers within targeted households. Brighton, UK, and Addis Ababa, Ethiopia: Institute of Development Studies and Indak International Pvt LC; 2006.
3. Haddad LJ, Hawkes C, Achadi E, Ahuja A, Ag Bendech M, Bhatia K, et al. Global Nutrition Report 2015: actions and accountability to advance nutrition and sustainable development. Intl Food Policy Res Inst; 2015. http://dx.doi.org/10.2499/9780896298835.
4. CSA and ICF International. Ethiopia demographic and health survey 2011. Addis Ababa, Ethiopia and Calverton, MD: Central Statistical Agency and ICF International; 2012, p. 430.
5. Burchi F, Strupat C. The impact of cash transfers on food security in sub-Saharan Africa: evidence, design and implementation. DIE Briefing Paper; 2016. Available at SSRN: https://ssrn.com/abstract=3089365 or http://dx.doi.org/10.2139/ssrn.30893652016.
6. FAO. Social protection framework promoting rural development for all. Food and Agriculture Organization of the United Nations, Rome; 2017. Available at http://www.fao.org/3/a-i7016e.pdf.
7. Committee on World Food Security (CFS). Policy round table gender, food security and nutrition: Thirty-seventh Session, 17–22 October 2011, Item V: Food and Agriculture Organization of the United Nations, Rome; 2011. Available at http://www.fao.org/cfs/home/products/en/
8. World Health Organization. Proposed global targets for maternal, infant and young child nutrition. Summary of main issues raised and WHO responses. Geneva: World Health Organization; 2012.
9. Alderman H, Elder L, Goyal A, Herforth A, Hoberg YT, Marini A, et al. Improving nutrition through multisectoral approaches. Washington DC: World Bank Group; 2013. Available at http://documents.worldbank.org/curated/en/625661468329649726/Improving-nutrition-through-multisectoral-approaches
10. Beazley R, Vaidya K. Social protection through work in lower-income countries: an assessment framework. International Policy Centre for Inclusive Growth, Brazil; 2015. Available at http://www.ipc-undp.org/pub/eng/OP313_Social_protection_through_work_in_lower_income_countries_an_assessment_framework.pdf.
11. Food Security Coordination Bureau (FSCB). Graduation guidance note. Addis Ababa: Ministry of Agriculture and Rural Development, Government of Ethiopia; 2007.
12. Gross R, Schoeneberger H, Pfeifer H, Preuss H-J. The four dimensions of food and nutrition security: definitions and concepts. SCN News 2000; 20: 20–5.

13. Porter C, Goyal R. Social protection for all ages? Impacts of the Ethiopian national safety net on child nutrition. Soc Sci Med 2015; 159: 92–99.
14. Vir SC. Improving women's nutrition imperative for rapid reduction of childhood stunting in South Asia: coupling of nutrition specific interventions with nutrition sensitive measures essential. Matern Child Nutr 2016; 12: 72–90. https://doi.org/10.1111/mcn.12255
15. Wood RG. Is there a role for cash transfers in climate change adaptation? IDS Bull 2011; 42(6): 79–85. https://doi.org/10.1111/j.1759-5436.2011.00277.x
16. Rispel LC, de Sousa CAP, Molomo BG. Can social inclusion policies reduce health inequalities in sub-Saharan Africa? – A rapid policy appraisal. J Health Popul Nutr 2009; 27(4): 492. https://doi.org/10.3329/jhpn.v27i4.3392
17. World Bank. Coping with Change: how Ethiopia's PSNP & HABP are building resilience to climate change. Natural Resources Management Sector Ministry of Agriculture, Ethiopia; 2013. Available at http://www.ltsi.co.uk/images/M_images/PSNP%20Coping%20with%20Change.pdf
18. Wiseman W, Van Domelen J, Coll-Black S. Designing and implementing a rural safety net in a low income setting: lessons learned from Ethiopia's Productive Safety Net Program 2005–2009. Washington, DC: World Bank; 2010, p. 56.
19. Committee on World Food Security (CFS). Policy recommendations: gender, food security and nutrition. 2011. ISBN 978-92-5-109703-8. Available at www.fao.org/3/a-i7016e.pdf.
20. Harris J. Agriculture, nutrition and health essentials for non-specialist development professionals, IFPRI, Delhi; 2011. Available at https://www.g-fras.org/fr/component/phocadownload/category/96-training-resources.html?download=849:agriculture-nutrition-and-health-essentials-for-non-specialist-development-professionals
21. Devereux S. Can social safety nets reduce chronic poverty? Dev Policy Rev 2002; 20(5): 657–75. https://doi.org/10.1111/1467-7679.00194.
22. Ministry of Agriculture. Productive Safety Net Program Phase 4 (PSNP 4): enhanced social assessment and consultation. Washington, D.C. : World Bank Group; 2014. Available at http://documents.worldbank.org/curated/en/550881499432708125/Enhanced-social-assessment-and-consultation.
23. Tirivayi N, Knowles M, Davis B. The interaction between social protection and agriculture: a review of evidence. Global Food Security 2016; 10: 52–62. https://doi.org/10.1016/j.gfs.2016.08.004
24. Belay K, Manig W. Access to rural land in Eastern Ethiopia: mismatch between policy and reality. JARTS 2004; 105(2): 123–38.
25. FAO. The state of food and agriculture–social protection and agriculture: breaking the cycle of rural poverty. Rome: Food and Agriculture Organization of the United Nations; 2015.
26. FAO. Social Protection Division (ESP): FAO's work in social protection. Food and Agriculture Organization of the United Nations Rome; 2014. Available at http://www.fao.org/social-protection/en/.
27. Hjelm L, Mathiassen A, Wadhwa A. Measuring poverty for food security analysis: consumption-versus asset-based approaches. Food Nutr Bull 2016; 37(3): 275–89. https://doi.org/10.1177/0379572116653509
28. Ethiopia Humanitarian Country Team (EHCT). Ethiopia slow onset natural disaster. UN Office for the Coordination of Humanitarian Affairs; 2015. Available at https://www.unocha.org/.
29. Welteji D, Mohammed K, Hussein K. The contribution of Productive Safety Net Program for food security of the rural households in the case of Bale Zone, Southeast Ethiopia.Agric Food Sec 2017; 6(1): 53. https://doi.org/10.1186/s40066-017-0126-4
30. Frisch RE. Linking body fat and reproduction. In: Caballero B, ed. Encyclopedia of human nutrition, four-volume set. 2nd edn. Oxford: Elsevier; 2005. ISBN: 0 12 150110 8 £496/$995 4 vols. https://doi.org/10.1108/09504120610655547
31. Leroy JL, Ruel M, Frongillo EA, Harris J, Ballard TJ. Measuring the food access dimension of food security: a critical review and mapping of indicators. Food Nutr Bull 2015; 36(2): 167–95. https://doi.org/10.1177/0379572115587274
32. Maxwell D, Vaitla B, Coates J. How do indicators of household food insecurity measure up? An empirical comparison from Ethiopia. Food Policy 2014; 47: 107–16. https://doi.org/10.1016/j.foodpol.2014.04.003
33. Swindale A, Bilinsky P. Household dietary diversity score (HDDS) for measurement of household food access: indicator guide. Washington, DC: Food and Nutrition Technical Assistance Project, Academy for Educational Development; 2006. https://doi.org/10.1016/j.gfs.2017.02.004
34. Aker J. "Cash or Coupons? Testing the Impacts of Cash versus Vouchers in the Democratic Republic of Congo." CGD Working Paper 320. Washington, DC: Center for Global Development; 2013. Available at http://www.cgdev.org/publication/cash-or-coupons
35. Hill RV, Porter C. Vulnerability to drought and food price shocks: evidence from Ethiopia (English). Policy Research working paper; no. WPS 7920. Washington, D.C. : World Bank Group; 2016. Available at http://documents.worldbank.org/curated/en/959471482167974723/Vulnerability-to-drought-and-food-price-shocks-evidence-from-Ethiopia
36. Gillespie S, van den Bold M, Team SoCS. Stories of change in nutrition: an overview. Global Food Security 2017; 13: 1–11. https://doi.org/10.1016/j.gfs.2017.02.004
37. Ene-Obong H, Enugu G, Uwaegbute A. Determinants of health and nutritional status of rural Nigerian women. J Health Popul Nutr 2001; 19: 320–30.
38. Prakruthi B, Prakash J. Nutritional status and dietary pattern of Indian rural women with reference to energy intake and expenditure. J Commun Nutr Health 2013; 2(1): 44.
39. Razak F, Corsi DJ, Slutsky AS, Kurpad A, Berkman L, Laupacis A, et al. Prevalence of body mass index lower than 16 among women in low-and middle-income countries. JAMA 2015; 314(20): 2164–71. https://doi.org/10.1001/jama.2015.15666
40. Shigute Z, Mebratie AD, Sparrow R, Yilma Z, Alemu G, Bedi AS. Uptake of health insurance and the productive safety net program in rural Ethiopia. Social Science & Medicine. 2017 Mar 1; 176:133–41. https://doi.org/10.1016/j.socscimed.2017.01.035
41. Slater R. Holmes R, Mathers N. Food and Nutrition (in-) Security and Social Protection. OECD Development Co-operation Working Papers, No. 15, OECD Publishing, Paris. 2014. http://dx.doi.org/10.1787/5jz44w9ltszt-en.
42. Sabates-Wheeler R, Devereux S. Cash transfers and high food prices: explaining outcomes on Ethiopia's Productive Safety Net Programme. Food Policy 2010; 35(4): 274–85. https://doi.org/10.1016/j.foodpol.2010.01.001
43. Subbarao K. Systemic shocks and social protection: role and effectiveness of public works programs (English). Social Protection discussion paper series; no. SP 0302. Washington, D.C.: The World Bank; 2003. Available at http://documents.worldbank.org/curated/en/659301468771611298/Systemic-shocks-and-social-protection-role-and-effectiveness-of-public-works-programs
44. Haddad L, Hoddinott J, Alderman H. Intrahousehold resource allocation in developing countries: models, methods and policies. American Journal of Agricultural Economics 1991; 81(2): 480–482. https://doi.org/10.2307/1244597

45. Cruz M, Ziegelhofer Z. Beyond the income effect: impacts of conditional cash transfer programs on private investments in human capital (English). Policy Research working paper; no. WPS 6867. Washington, DC: World Bank Group; 2014. Available at http://documents.worldbank.org/curated/en/756371468020374714/Beyond-the-income-effect-impacts-of-conditional-cash-transfer-programs-on-private-investments-in-human-capital
46. Keding GB, Msuya JM, Maass BL, Krawinkel MB. Dietary patterns and nutritional health of women: the nutrition transition in rural Tanzania. Food Nutr Bull 2011; 32(3): 218–26. https://doi.org/10.1177/156482651103200306
47. Johnson NL, Kovarik C, Meinzen-Dick R, Njuki J, Quisumbing A. Gender, assets, and agricultural development: lessons from eight projects. World Dev 2016; 83: 295–311. https://doi.org/10.1016/j.worlddev.2016.01.009
48. GIZ. Quick test of social protection systems on their gender sensitivity and inclusivity. Available from: https://www.giz.de/expertise/downloads/giz2017-en-social-protection-gender-inclusion-quick-test.pdf. 2016
49. De Janvry A, Sadoulet E, Solomon P, Vakis R. Uninsured risk and asset protection: can conditional cash transfer programs serve as safety nets. Social Protection Working Paper.SP discussion paper; no. 604. Washington, DC: World Bank; 2006. Available at http://documents.worldbank.org/curated/en/231231468314079566/Uninsured-risk-and-asset-protection-can-conditional-cash-transfer-programs-serve-as-safety-nets

***Asnake Ararsa Irenso**
School of Public Health
College of Health and Medical Sciences,
Haramaya University
P.O. Box 235, Harar, Ethiopia
Email: abbaabokku@gmail.com

# 13

# Neuroprotective effects of chloroform and aqueous fractions of noni juice against t-Butyl hydroperoxide-induced oxidative damage in SH-SY5Y cells

Jianguo Chen[1†], Xue Shi[2†], Yang Chen[2], Hanqiao Liang[3], Chi Cheng[3*] and Qiyang He[2*]

[1]Inner Mongolia Mengniu Diary Industry Group Co, Ltd, China; [2]Institute of Medicinal Biotechnology, Peking Union Medical College and Chinese Academy of Medical Sciences, Beijing, China; [3] China Center of Industrial Culture Collection, China National Research Institute of Food and Fermentation Industries, Beijing, China

*Abstract*

Oxidative stress is more likely to cause damage to neuronal cells and mediates some neurodegenerative disorders. It is well known that natural antioxidants can prevent oxidative stress damage and become a potential therapeutic strategy. Noni juice obtained from the fruit of the tree *Morinda citrifolia*, as a folk medicine, has been used for over two thousand years. In the current study, the neuroprotective effect and mechanism of noni juice extracts against tert-Butyl hydroperoxide (TBHP)-induced SH-SY5Y cell damage were investigated. The results demonstrated that chloroform fraction (CF) and aqueous fraction (AF) of noni juice protected SH-SY5Y cells against TBHP-induced oxidative stress and the associated apoptosis effectively. CF and AF treatment significantly weakened the TBHP-induced cytotoxicity, reactive oxygen species generation, mitochondrial membrane depolarization, and apoptotic features. CF and AF restored cellular antioxidant enzyme activity; upregulated expression of heme oxygenase-1, catalase, and superoxide dismutase-1; and increased the nuclear accumulation of nuclear factor-erythroid 2 related factor 2 (Nrf2). The antioxidant and neuroprotection potential of CF may account for its high total phenolic and flavonoid content, while AF may be rich in polysaccharides. These results suggest that CF and AF exhibit antioxidant defense through the upregulation of Nrf2 along with endogenous antioxidants and reduce apoptosis via inhibiting the mitochondrial pathway to protect SH-SY5Y cells damaged by TBHP. CF and AF might be developed as agents for neurodegeneration prevention or therapy.

**Keywords:** noni juice; neuroprotective; oxidative stress; Nrf2; apoptosis

Compared with other organs, lower levels of antioxidant enzymes, higher metabolic activity and higher content of polyunsaturated fatty acids in the brain, neurons are more susceptible to oxidative stress (1, 2). The imbalance between oxidants and antioxidants may destroy the redox signal and lead to oxidative stress. Excessive oxidative stress can cause oxidative damage in biomolecules such as DNA, proteins, lipids, and carbohydrates. Many neurodegenerative diseases, such as Alzheimer's disease, Parkinson's disease, Huntington's disease, and amyotrophic lateral sclerosis, may be caused by neuronal damage resulting from intracellular oxidative stress (3–8). Increasing evidence suggests that natural antioxidants may attenuate neurotoxicity and play important roles in prevention and treatment of oxidative stress-induced neurodegenerative diseases (9–12).

Herbal extracts rich in antioxidants, as traditional medications, have potent antioxidant activity and prevent neurodegenerative diseases caused by oxidative stress. *Morinda citrifolia* L. is commonly known as 'noni' and has been extensively used as a folk remedy for 2000 years in Polynesia, Australia, Southeast Asia, and Hawaii. Noni juice, obtained from the fruit of *M. citrifolia*, is reported to have many bioactive phytochemical constituents, such as glycosides, iridoids, anthraquinones, flavonoids, phenolic acid, and coumarins (13–15). It has been proven that noni juice exhibits many pharmacological properties, including antioxidant, anti-inflammatory, and antitumor effects (16–19). Therefore, it is suggested that the antioxidant and anti-inflammatory properties of noni juice can provide a protective effect against oxidative stress-induced neurodegenerative diseases.

[†]These authors contributed equally to this work.

Although protective effects of noni juice against scopolamine, ß-amyloid, and streptozotocin-induced memory impairment caused by focal ischemia and rotenone in animals have been reported (20–21), there is no data available on the neuromodulatory potential and molecular mechanism of noni juice or its extracts on neuronal cell damage. Thus, for the first time, we investigated the neuroprotection and potential mechanism of noni juice extracts against tert-Butyl hydroperoxide (TBHP)-induced neurotoxicity in SH-SY5Y cells.

## Materials and methods

### *Preparation of noni juice extracts*

Noni juice (10 liters) was purchased from Noni Biological Engineering Development (Hainan, China). Noni juice was partitioned successively with chloroform, ethyl acetate, and n-butanol. Each fraction was evaporated in a vacuum to obtain a chloroform fraction (CF, 3.3g), an ethyl acetate fraction (EF, 5.3g), an n-butanol fraction (BF, 60.7g), and an aqueous fraction (AF, 64.8g).

### *Chemicals and reagents*

TBHP and Rhodamine 123 were purchased from Sigma-Aldrich (St. Louis, MO, USA). An annexin V/propidium iodide (PI) double staining kit was purchased from Nanjing KeyGen Biotech Co., Ltd. (Nanjing, China). Catalase (CAT), superoxide dismutase-1 (SOD-1), glutathione peroxidase (GPx), and glutathione reductase (GR) kits were obtained from Nanjing Jiancheng Bioengineering Institute (Nanjing, China). A Cell Counting Kit-8 was purchased from Biotool (Shanghai, China). 5-(and-6)-carboxy-2',7'-difluorodihydrofluorescein diacetate (H2DFFDA) was obtained from Invitrogen (Carlsbad, CA, USA).

### *Animals*

Specific pathogen-free Sprague-Dawley rats were used for the acute oral toxicity tests. Male and female rats (3-week-old) were provided by the Institute of Experimental Animals, Chinese Academy of Medical Sciences (Beijing, China). Animals were housed in the animal house with a controlled temperature of 24 ± 1°C, relative humidity of 60 ± 5%, and a 12-hr light–dark cycle.

### *Cell culture*

The SH-SY5Y human neuroblastoma cell line was purchased from the American Type Culture Collection (Rockville, MD, USA). The cells were cultured in Dulbecco's Modified Eagle Medium/Ham's F-12 (DMEM/F12) supplemented with 10% fetal bovine serum (Gibco, Australia) and maintained at 37°C in a humidified atmosphere with 5% $CO_2$.

### *Acute oral toxicity*

Ten liters of noni juice was freeze-dried to obtain 69.4 g of powder. The noni juice powder was dissolved in distilled water at 375 mg/mL. Toxicity of the noni juice was assessed after a single oral administration in rats. The rats were randomly divided into two groups, each group with five males and five females. The rats were administered noni juice powder at 15,000 mg/kg body weight (BW) or the vehicle control (distilled water). Treatments (20 mL/kg BW) were administered a single dose by oral gavage. The single dose administration on the morning of Day 1 was followed by a 14-day observation period in which mortality or signs of morbidity were recorded for each animal. Animals were weighed immediately on Day 1 and again on Day 15.

### *Bacterial reverse mutation test*

Noni juice powder was assessed by two independent experiments for its potential to induce reverse mutation by the Ames test as described by Dillon GP (22). Genotoxicity was measured in *Salmonella typhimurium* strains TA 97, TA 98, TA 100, and TA 102. NJP was administered at 8, 40, 200, 1,000, and 5,000 μg/plate. All mutagenicity testing was performed in the presence or absence of the postmitochondrial fraction of liver homogenates (S9) from rats pretreated with Aroclor 1254.

### *Determination of total phenolic, flavonoid, and polysaccharide contents*

The total phenolic (TPC) and flavonoid contents were determined according to the method of Wu CR et al. (23). The TPC contained in each sample was expressed as milligrams of gallic acid equivalents (GAE) and flavonoid amount was expressed as milligrams of rutin equivalents (RE). Polysaccharide content was determined by a spectrophotometric method at 485 nm, modified from the method described by Li et al. (24). The amount of polysaccharide contained in each sample was expressed as milligrams of D-glucose equivalents (GE).

### *Cytotoxicity of noni juice extracts and TBHP*

The Cell Counting Kit-8 assay was used to assess cell viability. SH-SY5Y cells were seeded into 96-well plates and allowed to adhere for 24 h. To evaluate the cytotoxicity of TBHP, SH-SY5Y cells were treated by TBHP for 2 h; then the drug was washed out and cells were incubated for 48 h. After adhesion for 24 h, SH-SY5Y cells were treated with noni juice extracts for 48 h, and then the cytotoxicity of noni juice extracts was evaluated. The cell viability was determined using the Cell Counting Kit-8. In brief, 10 μL CCK-8 solution was added to each well of the plate. Then, the plate was incubated at 37°C for an additional 3 h. The absorbance of the WST-8 formazan dye was measured at 450 nm. The half maximal inhibitory concentration ($IC_{50}$) value was calculated from the nonlinear regression analysis.

*Effects of noni juice extracts on SH-SY5Y cells against TBHP-induced toxicity*

To investigate the protective effect of noni juice extracts in TBHP-induced cell death, the cells were incubated with DMEM/F12 for 24 h. After incubation with noni juice extracts for 4 h, cells were treated with TBHP for 2 h and then exposed to noni juice extracts for 48 h. Cell viability was measured by means of the CCK-8 assay.

*Measurement of cellular antioxidant enzymes*

SH-SY5Y cells were seeded into 10-cm culture dishes for 24 h. After pretreatment of noni juice extracts for 4 h, cells were incubated with TBHP for 2 h and then exposed to noni juice extracts for 48 h. SH-SY5Y cells were collected from culture dishes and sonicated on ice. The solution was centrifuged for 15 min at 4°C to eliminate cell debris, and the supernatant was used in enzyme activity assays. Antioxidant enzyme activities including CAT, GPx, GR, and SOD-1 were measured as described by Heng-Yin Ju et al. (25).

*Reactive oxygen species and mitochondrial membrane potential assays*

The method was performed according to the protocol previously published (26). To determine the effect of CF and AF on TBHP-induced reactive oxygen species (ROS) generation, SH-SY5Y cells were seeded into 6-well plates at a density of $3\times10^5$ cells/well and allowed to adhere for 24 h. After incubation with CF or AF for 4 h, cells were treated with TBHP for 2 h and then followed by the addition of various concentrations of CF or AF for 48 h. Then the SH-SY5Y cells for the detection of ROS were incubated with 10 μmol/L 2',7'-dichlorodihydrofluorescein diacetate (H2DCFDA) at 37°C for 30 min in the dark. For the mitochondrial membrane potential assay, the SH-SY5Y cells were incubated with 0.5 mmol/L Rhodamine 123 at 37°C for 30 min in the dark. ROS generation was analyzed by a BD FACSCalibur cytometerwith the CELLQuest program.

*Reverse transcriptase-polymerase chain reaction*

The RNA (500 ng) was reverse-transcribed with the Moloney murine leukemia virus reverse transcriptase (Promega Corp., Madison, WI, USA) and oligo (dT)16 primer (Promega) in 20 μL of reaction mixture. Each PCR primer used in this study was as follows (forward and reverse, respectively): heme oxygenase-1 (HO-1), 5'-CTT GGC TGG CTT CCT TAC C-3' and 5'-CAT TGC CTG GAT GTG CTT T-3'; CAT, 5'-CCG ACG AGA TGG CAC ACT TTGACA-3' and 5'-CGC GAG CAC GGT AGG GAC AGT TC-3'; SOD-1, 5'-CCA TCA ATA TGG GGA CAA TACAC-3' and 5'-ACA CGA TCT TCA ATG GAC AC-3'; GAPDH, 5'-AGT GTA GCC CAG GAT GCC CTT-3' and 5'-GCC AAG GTC ATC CAT GAC AAC-3'.

*Western blot analysis*

The method was performed according to the protocol previously published (27). The level of β-actin was used as a loading control. The antibodies against superoxide dismutase 1 (SOD-1) (#4266), Nrf2 (#12721), cleaved/total poly(ADP-ribose) polymerase-1 (PARP-1) (#9532), and cleaved caspase-3 (#9661) were obtained from Cell Signaling Technology, Inc. (Danvers, MA, USA). The antibody to β-actin (HC201) was obtained from TransGen Biotech (BeiJing, China).

*Detection of apoptotic cells by annexin V-(fluorescein isothiocyanate, FITC)/PI*

SH-SY5Y cells were seeded into six-well plates at a density of $3\times10^5$ cells/well and allowed to adhere for 24 h. After incubation with noni juice extracts for 4 h, cells were treated with TBHP for 2 h, followed by the addition of various concentrations of CF for 48 h. To quantify apoptosis, cells were stained with annexin V and PI using an annexin V-FITC/PI apoptosis kit (BD Biosciences, San Jose, CA, USA), following the protocol provided by the manufacturer. The fluorescence intensity was measured using a BD FACSCalibur flow cytometer according to the protocol previously published (28).

*Statistical analysis*

Results were expressed as the mean ± SD from at least three independent experiments. One-way ANOVA was used to analyze the variance for the means of multiple groups. Student's *t*-test was applied for comparing the means of two groups. Statistical analysis was performed using SPSS 17.0 and significant differences were considered at values of $p < 0.05$.

## Results

*Acute oral toxicity*

During the 14-day single-dose acute toxicity study, no mortality or clinical signs of morbidity occurred in Sprague-Dawley rats with 15,000 mg/kg BW of noni juice powder. Body weights of animals were unaffected by treatment (Table 1) and macroscopic examination of main organs showed no apparent abnormalities.

*Table 1.* Effect on body weight in rats acutely treated with noni juice

| Noni juice powder (mg/kg) | Sex | Number dosed | Body weight (mean ± SD) | |
|---|---|---|---|---|
| | | | Day 1 | Day 15 |
| 0 | M | 5 | 196.4±12.2 | 274.9±11.4 |
| 0 | F | 5 | 193.3±9.8 | 230.4±10.3 |
| 15,000 | M | 5 | 198.5±13.3 | 275.0±18.5 |
| 15,000 | F | 5 | 192.0±11.8 | 228.1±9.9 |

*Bacterial reverse mutation test (Ames test)*

The bacterial reverse mutation tests indicated that noni juice powder did not induce mutagenic activity toward any of the *S. typhimurium* strains with or without S9 activation at concentrations up to 5,000 μg/plate (Table 2).

*TPC, flavonoid, and polysaccharide contents*

TPC, flavonoid, and polysaccharide contents of noni juice extracts were measured systematically by spectrophotometric methods (Table 3). CF contained the highest TPC (284 mg of GAE/g CF) and a higher amount of flavonoids (156 mg of RE/g CF). Each gram of EF contained the highest amount of flavonoids (172 mg of RE) and higher amounts of TPC (255 mg of GAE). However, the amount of polysaccharide (584 mg of GE/g AF) contained in AF was more than other fractions.

*Cytotoxic effects of noni juice extracts and TBHP on SH-SY5Y cells*

To determine doses of noni juice extracts that could be used without adversely affecting cell viability, the latter was determined using the CCK-8 assay and plotted on the survival curves. The $IC_{50}$ values of CF and EF for SH-SY5Y cells were 65.13 and 65.72 μg/mL, respectively (Fig. 1a). No cytotoxicity or changes in cell morphology were observed with 10 μg/mL CF or EF. The $IC_{50}$ values for BF and AF were both greater than 0.5 mg/mL. In order to evaluate the cytotoxicity of TBHP, SH-SY5Y cells were treated with different concentrations of TBHP (5–500 μM) and a dose-dependent cell death was observed (Fig. 1b). Concentrations of TBHP ≥50 μM dramatically decreased cell viability and cell death reached 40% after 50 μM TBHP treatment.

*CF and AF confer protection on SH-SY5Y cells against TBHP-induced toxicity*

In the present study, we evaluated the protective effect of noni juice extracts against TBHP challenge by CCK-8 assay. To determine the protective effects of noni juice extracts against TBHP-induced cytotoxicity, SH-SY5Y cells were preincubated with noni juice extracts for 4 h, treated with TBHP for 2 h, followed by treatment with noni juice extracts for 48 h. With 50 μM TBHP, only 60.6% of cells were viable as compared to the control group. However, as shown in Fig. 2, it was noteworthy that TBHP-induced cell death was significantly ameliorated by CF and AF treatments. Treatment with 10 μg/mL CF markedly improved

*Table 3.* TPC, flavonoid, and polysaccharide contents of noni juice extracts

| | TPC (mg of GAE/g) | Flavonoids (mg of RE/g) | Polysaccharides (mg of GE/g) |
|---|---|---|---|
| CF | 284.84±5.36 | 156.32±10.11 | nd |
| EF | 255.66±8.84 | 172.07±6.89 | nd |
| BF | 38.73±1.25 | 14.0±0.23 | 179.34±8.64 |
| AF | 75.45±4.21 | 8.64±0.18 | 584.64±12.28 |

TPC, total phenolic content; GAE, gallic acid equivalents; RE, rutin equivalents; GE, D-glucose equivalents; CF, chloroform fraction; EF, ethyl acetate fraction; BF, n-butanol fraction; AF, aqueous fraction; nd, not detect.

*Table 2. Salmonella typhimurium* reverse mutation test for noni juice by the direct-plate incorporation method with and without S9 activation

| Noni juice powder (ug/plate) | Number of revertants/plate | | | | | | | |
|---|---|---|---|---|---|---|---|---|
| | TA97 | | TA98 | | TA100 | | TA102 | |
| | - | + | - | + | - | + | - | + |
| Experiment 1 | | | | | | | | |
| 0 | 119.3±14.6 | 116.0±12.5 | 35.7±5.7 | 40.0±3.0 | 141.7±12.6 | 144.3±13.1 | 267.3±16 | 261.3±8.1 |
| 8 | 122.3±17.5 | 121.7±14.6 | 36.0±3.6 | 38.0±5.6 | 147.0±17.1 | 145.0±14.7 | 266.7±15.5 | 265.7±16.6 |
| 40 | 120.3±16.3 | 125.7±10.6 | 36.3±4.5 | 39.0±4.6 | 150.7±13.3 | 144.3±18.5 | 269.7±15.9 | 266.0±13.1 |
| 200 | 120.0±10.0 | 114.7±15.0 | 39.3±3.1 | 37.0±5.0 | 150.3±20.6 | 150.3±13.5 | 267.7±18.0 | 265.3±15.0 |
| 1,000 | 119.0±16.8 | 123.0±12.2 | 37.7±5.7 | 39.7±5.0 | 155.3±15.5 | 154.3±15.0 | 271.3±17.2 | 267.7±12.3 |
| 5,000 | 120.3±10.0 | 125.0±9.2 | 37.7±3.1 | 38.7±4.7 | 156.7±13.3 | 154.3±13.7 | 269.7±13.3 | 163.3±18.2 |
| Positive control | 1,270.0±81.9 | 1,296.7±97.1 | 1,926.7±70.2 | 1,826.7±94.5 | 1,326.7±73.7 | 1,336.7±112.4 | 1,353.3±138.0 | 920.0±60.0 |
| Experiment 2 | | | | | | | | |
| 0 | 117.7±11.6 | 120.0±14.0 | 42.7±4.5 | 41.7±4.2 | 153.0±10.8 | 146.3±12.7 | 264.7±22.0 | 267.7±11.6 |
| 8 | 123.3±10.4 | 122.7±13.0 | 39.0±4.6 | 36.0±5.6 | 158.3±14.7 | 150.7±17.2 | 270.0±11.4 | 262.3±8.6 |
| 40 | 124.7±12.7 | 120.7±11.0 | 36.7±4.7 | 37.7±5.5 | 163.0±12.1 | 152.3±17.8 | 263.7±12.7 | 270.7±13.7 |
| 200 | 120.3±15.6 | 127.3±17.2 | 39.0±2.6 | 37.0±4.0 | 155.0±16.1 | 143.3±12.3 | 271.0±14.5 | 265.7±13.9 |
| 1,000 | 124.7±9.1 | 126.3±13.3 | 39.7±5.5 | 38.0±2.6 | 160.3±16.0 | 146.7±17.2 | 271.7±18.5 | 270.7±14.2 |
| 5,000 | 124.0±10.8 | 119.3±17.8 | 39.3±4.2 | 40.7±4.7 | 164.3±12.1 | 149.7±13.6 | 264.3±18.9 | 270.7±19.0 |
| Positive control | 1,293.3±61.1 | 1,316.7±96.1 | 1,873.3±92.9 | 1,880.0±124.9 | 1,270.0±117.9 | 1,313.3±101.2 | 1,436.7±106.0 | 890.0±70.0 |

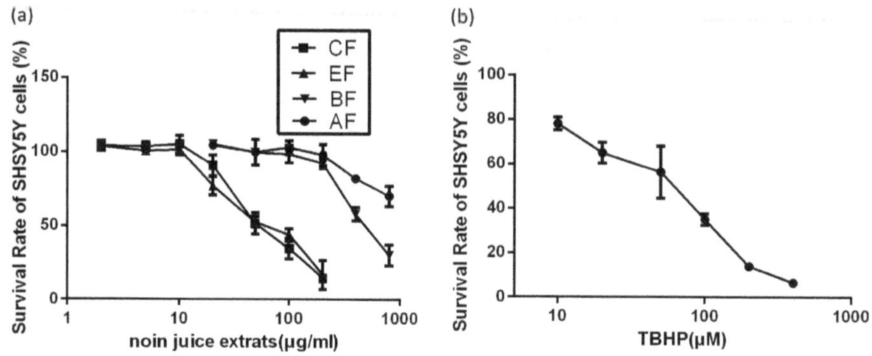


*Fig. 1.* Survival of SH-SY5Y cells treated with noni juice extracts and TBHP. (a) Survival of SH-SY5Y cells that were treated with noni juice extracts for 48 h. (b) Survival of SH-SY5Y cells that were treated with TBHP for 2 h. Data represent the mean ± SD of three independent experiments. TBHP, tert-Butyl hydroperoxide.

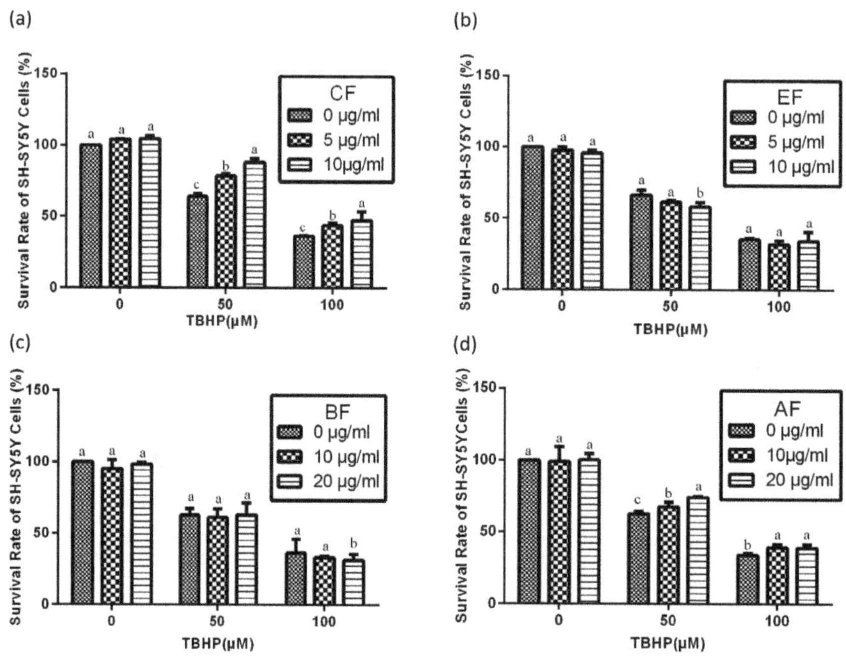


*Fig. 2.* Effects of noni juice extracts on TBHP-treated SH-SY5Y cells. After incubation with noni juice extracts for 4 h, SH-SY5Y cells were treated with TBHP for 2 h and then exposed to noni juice extracts for 48 h. Data are expressed as mean ± SD ($n = 3$). [a–c]The bars with different letters represent significant difference ($p < 0.05$), compared with each control group.

cell survival up to 87.8%, and 20 μg/mL AF reestablished cell viability to 76.4%. However, neither EF nor BF had any significant effect on cell viability.

### *Effects of noni juice extracts on antioxidant enzymes activity in TBHP-treated SH-SY5Y cells*

In order to investigate whether antioxidant enzymes are involved in the removal of free radicals by noni extracts, SOD-1, CAT, GPx, and GR activities in SH-SY5Y cells were measured by the spectrophotometric degradation method. As shown in Table 4, oxidative damage induced by TBHP remarkably reduced the activity of antioxidant enzymes, while noni juice extracts pretreatment restored their activities almost similar to the control group, indicating that active ingredients in noni juice extracts have antioxidant defense ability (Table 4). Moreover, greater restoring capacity for antioxidant enzymes was observed in CF and AF groups, which was consistent with the result that CF and AF treatment conferred protection on SH-SY5Y cells against TBHP-induced toxicity. CF exhibited the best restoring capacity for antioxidant enzymes. It is speculated that higher activity of antioxidant enzymes could attenuate ROS-induced cell damage more efficiently.

### *CF and AF inhibits TBHP-induced ROS generation*

Further, the effects of CF and AF on TBHP-induced ROS generation were investigated. As shown in Fig. 3, compared with the control group, TBHP treatment markedly

*Table 4.* Effects of noni juice extracts on SOD-1, CAT, GPx, and GR activity in SH-SY5Y cells exposed to 50 μM TBHP

| Samples | SOD-1 (U/mg) | Catalase (U/mg) | GPx (mU/mg) | GR (mU/mg) |
|---|---|---|---|---|
| Control | 43.2±2.93** | 1.84±0.16* | 37.3±2.58** | 8.89±0.68** |
| 50 μM TBHP | 18.7±3.79 | 1.01±0.08 | 23.0±2.08 | 3.45±0.58 |
| 5 μg/mL CF+ TBHP | 45.5±2.99** | 2.16±0.17** | 40.8±1.82** | 9.94±0.67** |
| 5 μg/mL EF+ TBHP | 34.1±2.00** | 1.61±0.10* | 30.2±2.42* | 8.9±0.91** |
| 10 μg/mL BF+ TBHP | 37.2±2.38** | 2.26±0.05** | 36.2±3.48** | 4.97±0.89* |
| 10 μg/mL AF+ TBHP | 43.0±3.79** | 2.07±0.06** | 40.1±1.75** | 9.7±1.31** |

After incubation with noni juice extracts for 4 h, SH-SY5Y cells were treated with TBHP for 2h and then exposed to noni juice extracts for 48 h. Data are expressed as mean ± SD ($n$ = 3). *$p$ < 0.05 and **$p$ < 0.01 as compared to TBHP-treated cells.

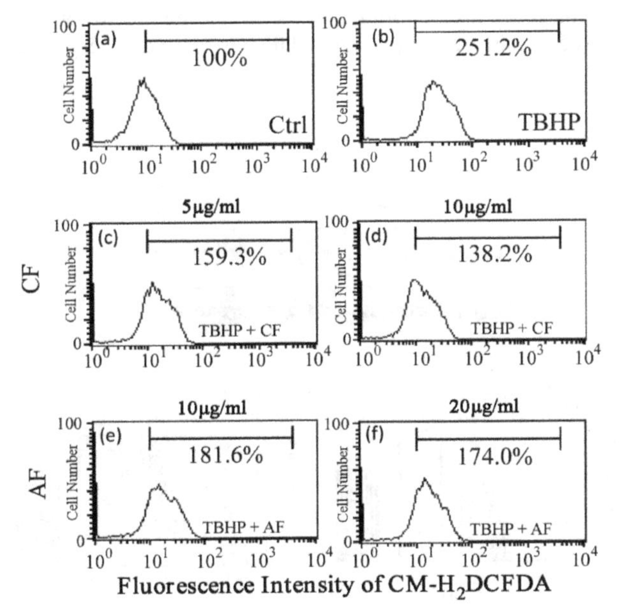


*Fig. 3.* Effect of CF and AF on TBHP-induced ROS generation. SH-SY5Y cells were treated with (a) 0, (b) 50 μM TBHP, (c) 5 μg/mL CF + 50 μM TBHP, (d) 10 μg/mL CF + 50 μM TBHP, (e) 10 μg/mL AF + 50 μM TBHP, (f) 20 μg/mL AF + 50 μM TBHP. After treatment, the cells were stained with H2DCFDAfor 30 min and then analyzed by flow cytometry. CF, chloroform fraction; AF, aqueous fraction; ROS, reactive oxygen species.

increased the fluorescence intensity of SH-SY5Y cells to 251.2%. However, 5 μg/mL CF and 10 μg/mL AF significantly decreased the fluorescence intensity to 159.3 and 181.6%, respectively. The results indicated that CF and AF could eliminate endogenous ROS in SH-SY5Y cells treated with TBHP efficiently.

*Inhibitory effects of CF and AF on TBHP-induced disruption of mitochondrial membrane potential (MMP)*

In order to examine whether the protection of CF and AF on SH-SY5Y cells against TBHP-induced toxicity involves the MMP pathway, measurement of MMP was carried out. Data showed that treatment with TBHP resulted in a marked decrease of MMP to 70.3%, which demonstrated that TBHP induced the mitochondrial damage via depolarization of MMP. However, pretreatment with 5 μg/mL CF and 10 μg/mL AF restored the MMP to 85.5 and 80.2%, respectively. These results indicated that CF and AF potentially suppressed the depolarization of MMP and partially showed the protective effects against TBHP-induced toxicity (Fig. 4).

*Effects of CF and AF on HO-1, CAT, and SOD-1 gene expression*

To explore the molecular mechanism of CF and AF protection on SH-SY5Y cells, gene expression of antioxidants and Phase II detoxifying enzymes such as HO-1, CAT, and SOD-1 were analyzed by Reverse Transcription-Polymerase Chain Reaction (RT-PCR). As shown in Fig. 5a, CF and AF treatment increased the expression of HO-1, CAT, and SOD-1 gene expression. Compared to the control group, treatment with 5 μg/mL CF upregulated HO-1, CAT, and SOD-1 gene expression 2.30-fold, 1.65-fold, and 2.10-fold, respectively, while 10 μg/mL AF upregulated HO-1, CAT, and SOD-1 gene expression 1.28 times, 1.35 times, and 1.47 times, respectively (Fig. 5b through d).

*Effect of CF and AF on Nrf2 nuclear translocation*

The activation of Nrf2/ antioxidant response element (ARE) pathway is well known to confer resistance of cells to oxidative stress. In order to understand whether the upregulation of antioxidant enzymes and Phase II detoxification enzymes by CF and AF were related to activation of Nrf2, the transactivation of Nrf2 in nuclear fractions was examined by Western blotting. As illustrated in Fig. 6a, CF and AF treatment obviously increased Nrf2 accumulation compared to the control group. A 3.16-fold increase in the nucleus Nrf2 was observed in the 10 μg/mL CF treatment group by comparison with 2.35-fold in the 10 μg/mL AF group (Fig. 6b). It is likely that the Nrf2 signaling pathway is an important neuroprotective mechanism of CF and AF against TBHP-induced oxidative damage in SH-SY5Y cells.

*CF inhibited TBHP-induced apoptotic cell death*

To explore whether CF and AF conferring protection on SH-SY5Y cells against TBHP-induced toxicity was

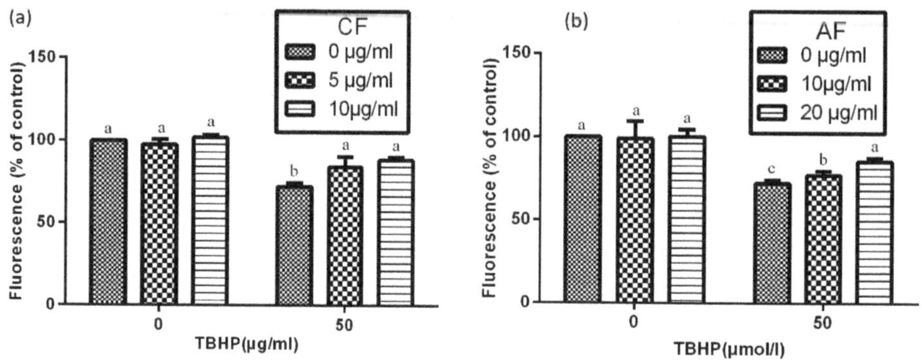


*Fig. 4.* Estimation of mitochondrial membrane potential in SHSY5Y cells. After incubation with CF or AF for 4 h, SH-SY5Y cells were treated with TBHP for 2 h and then exposed to CF or AF for 48 h. After staining with Rhodamine 123 for 30 min, the cells were assayed with a FACSCalibur cytometer. Data are expressed as mean ± SD ($n$ = 3). [a–c]The bars with different letters represent significant difference ($p < 0.05$), compared with each control group.

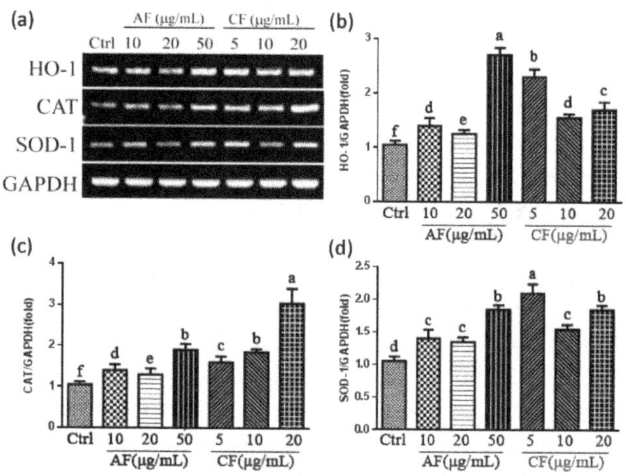


*Fig. 5.* Effects of CF and AF on HO-1, CAT, and SOD-1 gene expression. (a) SH-SY5Y cells were pretreated with AF and CF for 24 h. Gene expression was analyzed by RT-PCR. (b) Quantification of HO-1 gene expression. (c) Quantification of CAT gene expression. (d) Quantification of SOD-1 gene expression. [a–f]The bars with different letters represent significant difference ($p < 0.05$). HO-1, heme oxygenase-1; CAT, catalase; SOD-1, superoxide dismutase-1.

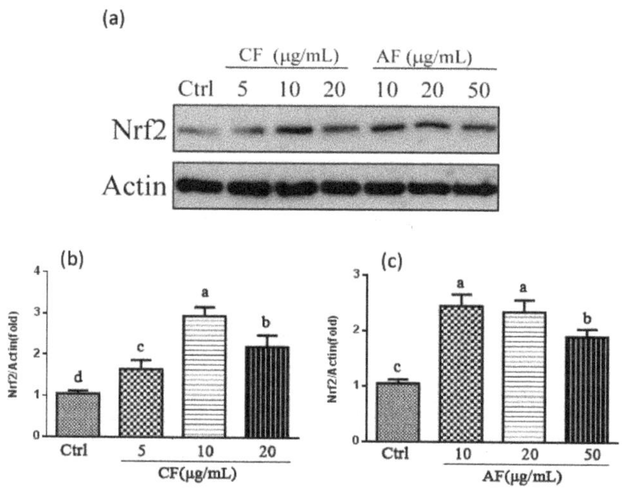


*Fig. 6.* Effect of CF and AF on the nuclear translocation of Nrf2. (a) SH-SY5Y cells were pretreated with CF and AF for 24 h. Nuclear extracts were prepared and analyzed by Western blot. (b) Quantification of Nrf2 protein expression pretreated with CF. (c) Quantification of Nrf2 protein expression pretreated with AF. [a–d]The bars with different letters represent significant difference ($p < 0.05$).

associated with apoptosis, the double-staining method using FITC-labeled annexin V and PI was performed. CF was chosen to investigate the mechanism of its protection on TBHP-induced cell apoptosis. As shown in Fig. 7a, the cell apoptosis rate of the control group was 1.41% and that of the 50 μM and 100 μM TBHP groups was obviously increased to 24.29 and 78.0%. However, 10 μg/mL CF treatment significantly reduced the TBHP-induced cell apoptosis rate of the 50 μM and 100 μM TBHP groups, respectively, to only 9.56 and 33.93%. These results indicated that CF exhibited protective effects against oxidative stress-induced apoptosis.

In the present study, we examined whether THBP-induced cell death was mediated through native caspase-3 cleavage and PARP-1 degradation and further explored the molecular mechanisms of the neuroprotective effect of CF on THBP-induced apoptosis. As shown in Fig. 7b, cleaved caspase-3 protein and degradation of PARP-1 were undetected in the control group but appeared after exposure to TBHP. However, CF significantly prevented the activation of caspase-3 and cleavage of PARP-1, indicating that CF could reverse the TBHP-induced apoptotic cell death efficiently. These results demonstrated that CF exhibited protective effects against TBHP-induced SH-SY5Y cells apoptosis through preventing activation of caspase-3.

## Discussion

Although noni juice is well known as an antioxidant, the anti-oxidation effect and molecular mechanism of its extracts against oxidative damage in neurons are at present

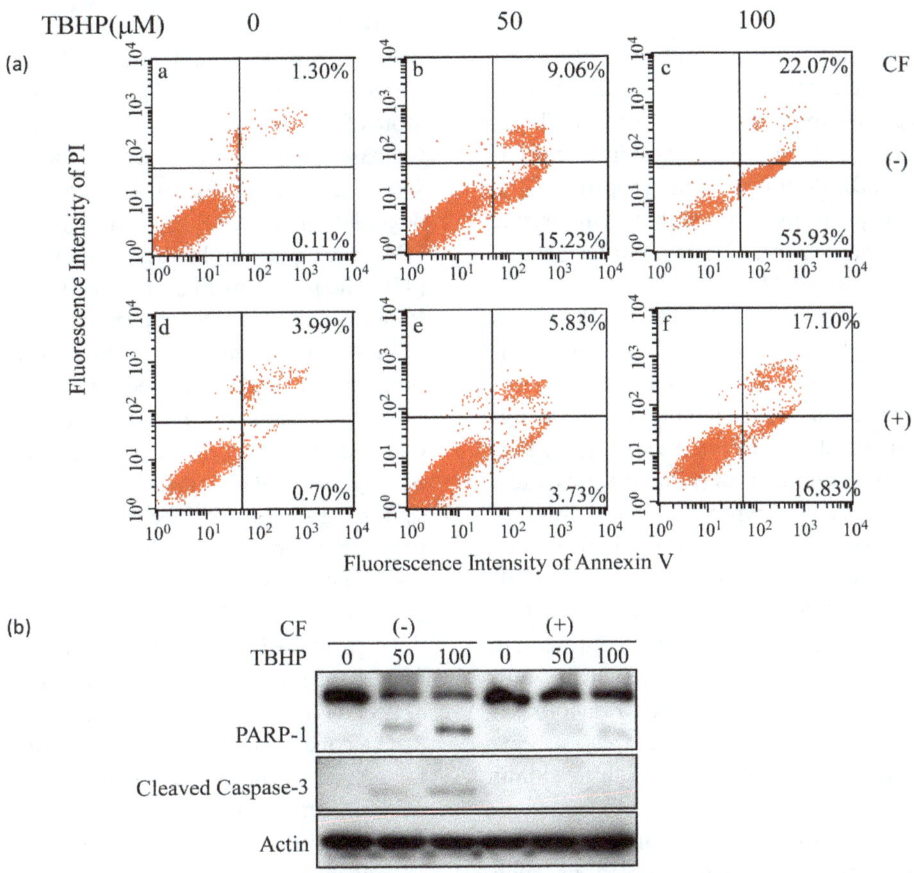


*Fig. 7.* Effect of CF on TBHP-induced apoptosis in SH-SY5Y cells. (a) Apoptotic cells were detected by annexin V and PI double staining and analyzed by flow cytometry. (b) Western blot analysis of the status of PARP-1 and cleaved caspase-3. β-actin was used as a loading control. A representative result of three independent experiments is shown. PARP-1, poly(ADP-ribose) polymerase-1; PI, propidium iodide.

unclear. In this study, SH-SY5Y cells with oxidative damage induced by TBHP were used as a model to explore the antioxidant and neuroprotective effects of noni juice extracts and reveal the underlying mechanism.

The acute oral toxicity and genotoxicity potential of noni juice were investigated. Noni juice did not induce mortality, clinical signs of morbidity, or physiologic abnormalities in Sprague-Dawley rats at a dose of 15,000 mg/kg BW and was also nongenotoxic at concentrations up to 5,000 μg/plate. The results indicated that the maximum tolerated dose of noni juice was > 215.38 mL/kg BW in rats. These results suggest low toxicity of noni juice in acute toxicity studies.

Phenolic compounds and Polysaccharides of valuable plants for health care and medicine have been proven to be the main classes of natural antioxidants and correlated with their antioxidant activities (29–32). Our present study showed that CF contained the highest amount of TPC, while AF had a higher content of polysaccharides than other fractions. Recent reports also indicate that TPC, flavonoids, and polysaccharides are the bioactive compounds present in noni juice, which are responsible for its antioxidant and other pharmacological properties (15–17).

Previous studies revealed that several herbal extracts could inhibit TBHP-induced cell loss efficiently (33, 34). In this study, pretreatment with CF and AF significantly prevented cell loss in a dose-dependent manner. However, EF and BF had no ability to improve cell viability. These results indicated that CF and AF protected SH-SY5Y cells in the presence of TBHP-induced oxidative stress. The high TPC and flavonoid content of CF may account for its antioxidant and neuroprotection potential, while AF may be rich in polysaccharides.

ROS is a major pathological factor that can lead to many serious diseases, including neurodegeneration and cardiovascular diseases. Intracellular ROS production disrupts redox balance or oxidative stress not only in relation to cell proliferation and signal transduction but also to inducing apoptosis (35, 36). Because ROS serves as an initiator of TBHP-induced toxicity, we measured intracellular ROS levels subsequently. Our results showed that CF and AF were able to inhibit TBHP-induced ROS generation, which indicated that the neuroprotective effects of CF and AF may be mediated by blocking ROS overproduction. CF reduced the apoptosis rate caused by TBHP, indicating that changes in ROS levels are essential for CF protection against TBHP-induced cell apoptosis. The results are similar to previous findings that demonstrate the ROS scavenging activity of *Cyperus* extract against $H_2O_2$-induced neuronal stress (37).

Antioxidant enzymes such as CAT, GPx, SOD-1, and GR play important roles in detoxifying ROS and maintaining redox status. Compelling evidence demonstrates that the activities of antioxidant enzymes decrease significantly in many neurodegenerative diseases (38). Perhaps the neuroprotective effects of noni juice extracts were related to antioxidant enzyme action. In order to further confirm the participation of antioxidant status, we examined their activities. CF and AF inhibited TBHP-induced reduction of SOD-1, CAT, GPx, and GR levels. The results demonstrated that the neuroprotective effects of CF and AF may partly be mediated through enhancing the antioxidant enzyme activity. Previous reports also showed that the neuroprotective effects of natural plants are associated with activation of antioxidant enzyme activity (10, 25).

Nrf2 is a major regulator for ARE-driven antioxidant and Phase II detoxifying enzyme expressions, such as NAD(P)H quinone oxidoreductase 1 (NQO1), HO-1, CAT, and SOD-1. Increasing studies reveal that these antioxidant enzymes are regulated by activation of Nrf2 and play an important role in oxidative stress-induced neuronal injury (39–42). Our results showed that CF and AF treatment increased the nuclear translocation of Nrf2, which was also associated with elevated antioxidative enzyme expressions of HO-1, CAT, and SOD-1. In addition, induction of HO-1 expression was higher than that of SOD-1 and CAT, indicating that HO-1 may be a major factor exerting neuroprotective effects. It is hypothesized that promoting antioxidants and Phase II detoxifying enzymes via activating Nrf2 nuclear translocation might be responsible for CF and AF protecting SH-SY5Y cells from TBHP-induced oxidative damage.

A collapse of MMP is associated with several models of apoptosis and used to assess stress-induced apoptotic cell damage (43–45). Mitochondrial damage has been observed in Parkinson's disease by inhibition of Complex I activity, which results in mitochondrial impairment. Our results are in agreement with other reports that oxidative stress induced by TBHP impairs the mitochondrial membrane, resulting in the depolarization of MMP. CF and AF potentially restrained the depolarization of MMP induced by TBHP. In this study, we further explored the possible role of CF in TBHP-induced mitochondrial apoptosis.

TBHP-induced apoptosis mainly occurs via the apoptotic caspase pathway; apoptosis is induced by initiating mitochondrial dysfunction (46). Caspases are important mediators of cell death through the cleavage of many substrates. Caspase-3 is an executioner for the death program in response to various stressors. Activated caspase-3 catalyzes the degradation of PARP-1, which is an important ribozyme in DNA repair, cell proliferation, apoptosis, and transcription (47). The results in Fig. 7b show that CF protected TBHP-induced apoptosis via preventing caspase-3 activation.

In summary, this study demonstrated the antioxidant potential and molecular mechanisms involved in the neuroprotective effects of CF and AF. Our findings suggest that CF and AF can provide neuroprotection for SH-SY5Y cells against TBHP-induced oxidative damage and apoptosis through improving the antioxidant status, maintaining the mitochondrial membrane integrity, and regulating the apoptotic markers. Moreover, CF and AF could elevate antioxidant and Phase II detoxifying enzyme expression through activating the nuclear translocation of Nrf2, which may be the underlying molecular mechanism for protecting SH-SY5Y cells from TBHP-induced oxidative damage. It can be concluded that CF and AF are potential candidates for preventing neuronal-associated disorders mediated by oxidative stress. However, it is necessary to further explore the derivatized compounds in CF and AF with better neuroprotective activity, which should be investigated as a natural remedy for neurodegenerative disorders.

## Acknowledgments

This work was supported by grants from the National Scientific Foundation of China (31471150) and Scientific and Technological Development Project of China, National Research Institute of Food and Fermentation Industries (No. KJ14-BS-02).

## Conflict of interest and funding

The authors have not received any funding or benefits from industry or elsewhere to conduct this study.

## References

1. Friedman J. Why is the nervous system vulnerable to oxidative stress? In: Gadoth N, Gobel HH, eds. Oxidative stress in applied basic research and clinical practice. The Humana Press, New York; 2011, pp. 19–27.
2. Bhat AH, Dar KB, Anees S, Zargar MA, Masood A, Sofi MA. Oxidative stress, mitochondrial dysfunction and neurodegenerative diseases; A mechanistic insight. Biomed Pharmacother. 2015; 74: 101–10.
3. Jiang T, Sun Q, Chen S. Oxidative stress: a major pathogenesis and potential therapeutic target of antioxidative agents in Parkinson's disease and Alzheimer's disease. Prog Neurobiol. 2016; 147: 1–19.
4. Chi-Rei W, Mei-Yueh H, Yung-Ta L, Heng-Yin J, Hui Ching. Oxidative stress and neurodegenerative disease. Neurosciences. 2014; 9(9): 19–23.

5. Zawia NH, Lahiri DK, Cardozo-Pelaez F. Epigenetics, oxidative stress, and Alzheimer disease. Free Radical Biol Med.2009; 46(9): 1241–9.
6. Pringsheim T, Jette N, Frolkis A, Steeves TD. The prevalence of Parkinson's disease: a systematic review and meta-analysis. Mov Disord. 2014; 29(13): 1583–90.
7. Kalonia H, Kumar P, Kumar A. Attenuation of pro-inflammatory cytokines and apoptotic process by verapamil and diltiazem against quinolinic acid induced Huntington's like alteration in rats. Brain Res. 2011; 1372: 115–26.
8. Kalonia H, Kumar P, Kumar A. Licofelone attenuates quinolinic acid induced Huntington's like symptoms: possible behavioural, biochemical and cellular alterations. Prog Neuropsycho pharmacol Biol Psychiatry.2011; 35(2): 607–15.
9. Abushouk AI, Negida A, Ahmed H, Abdel-Daim MM. Neuroprotective mechanisms of plant extracts against MPTP induced neurotoxicity: future applications in Parkinson's disease. Biomed Pharmacother. 2017; 85: 635–45.
10. Peng S, Hou Y, Yao J, Fang J. Activation of Nrf2-driven antioxidant enzymes by cardamonin confers neuroprotection of PC12 cells against oxidative damage. Food Funct.2017; 8(3): 997–1007.
11. Je JY, Lee DB. Nelumbo nucifera leaves protect hydrogen peroxide-induced hepatic damage via antioxidant enzymes and HO-1/Nrf2 activation. Food Funct. 2015; 6(6): 1911–18.
12. Zhang X, Wang L, Wang R, Luo X, Li Y, Chen Z. Protective effects of rice dreg protein hydrolysates against hydrogen peroxide-inducedoxidative stress in HepG-2 cells. Food Funct. 2016; 7(3): 1429–37.
13. Hu MX, Zhang HC, Wang Y, Liu SM, Liu L. Two new glycosides from the fruits of Morinda citrifolia. Molecules. 2012; 17(11): 12651–6.
14. Deng S, West BJ, Palu 'K, Jensen CJ. Determination and comparative analysis of major iridoids in different parts and cultivationsources of Morinda citrifolia. Phytochem Anal.2011; 22(1): 26–30.
15. Bittová M, Hladůkova D, Roblová V, Krácmar S, Kubán P, Kubán V. Analysis of organic acids, deacetyl asperulosidic acid and polyphenolic compounds as a potential tool for characterization of noni (Morinda citrifolia) products. Nat Prod Commun. 2015; 10(11): 1817–20.
16. Z. Mohd Zin , A. Abdul Hamid , A. Osman , N. Saari & A. Misran. Isolation and identification of anti oxidative compound from fruit of noni. Int J Food Properties. 2009; 10(2): 363–73.
17. Lin YL, Chou CH, Yang DJ, Chen JW, Tzang BS, Chen YC. Hypolipidemic and antioxidative effects of Noni (Morinda citrifolia L.) Juice on high-fat cholesterol-Dietary hamsters. Plant Foods Hum Nutr. 2012; 67(3): 294–302.
18. Basar S, Uhlenhut K, Högger P, Schöne F, Westendorf J. Analgesic and anti-inflammatory activity of Morinda citrifolia L. (Noni) fruit. Phytotherapy Res. 2010; 24(1): 38–42.
19. Nualsanit T, Rojanapanthu P, Gritsanapan W, Lee SH, Lawson D, Baek SJ. Damnacanthal, a noni component, exhibits antitumorigenic activity in human colorectal cancer cells. J Nutr Biochem. 2012; 23(8): 915–23.
20. Harada S, Hamabe W, Kamiya K, Satake T, Yamamoto J, Tokuyama S. Preventive effect of Morinda citrifolia fruit juice on neuronal damage induced by focal ischemia. Biol Pharm Bull. 2009; 32(3): 405–9.
21. Harada S, Fujita-Hamabe W, Kamiya K, Mizushina Y, Satake T, Tokuyama S. Morindacitrifolia fruit juice prevents ischemic neuronal damage through suppression of the development of post-ischemic glucose intolerance. J Nat Med. 2010; 64(4): 468–73.
22. Dillon GP, Gaffney MA, Curran CM, Moran CA. Dietary safety of a dual-enzyme preparation for animal feed: acute and subchronic oral toxicity and genotoxicity studies. Regul Toxicol Pharmacol. 2017; 88: 106–17.
23. Chi-Rei W, Mei-Yueh H, Yung-Ta L, Heng-Yin J, Hui Ching. Antioxidant properties of Cortex Fraxini and its simple coumarins. Food Chem.2007; 104: 1464–71.
24. Li S, Shah NP. Characterization, antioxidative and bifidogenic effects of polysaccharides from Pleurotus eryngiiafter heat treatments. Food Chem. 2016; 197(Pt A): 240–9.
25. Ju HY, Chen SC, Wu KJ, Kuo HC, Hseu YC, Ching H, et al. Antioxidant phenolic profile from ethyl acetate fraction of Fructus Ligustri Lucidi with protection against hydrogen peroxide-induced oxidative damage in SH-SY5Y cells. Food Chem Toxicol. 2012; 50(3–4): 492–502.
26. Ou X, Chen Y, Cheng X, Zhang X, He Q. Potentiation of resveratrol-induced apoptosis by matrine in human hepatoma $HepG_2$ cells. Oncol Rep. 2014; 32(6): 2803–9.
27. Chen J, Chen Y, He Q. Action of bleomycin is affected by bleomycin hydrolase but not by caveolin-1. Int J Oncol. 2012; 41(6): 2245–52.
28. Chen Y, Xu R, Chen J, Li X, He Q. Cleavage of bleomycin hydrolase by caspase-3 during apoptosis. Oncol Rep. 2013; 30(2): 939–44.
29. Wu CR, Lin WH, Hseu YC, Lien JC, Lin YT, Kuo TP, et al. Evaluation of the antioxidant activity of five endemic Ligustrum species leavesfrom Taiwan flora in vitro. Food Chem. 2011; 127: 564–71.
30. Zhu F, Cai YZ, Sun M, Ke J, Lu D, Corke H. Comparison of major phenolic constituents and in vitro antioxidant activity of diverse Kudingcha genotypes from Ilex kudingcha, Ilex cornuta, and Ligustrum robustum. J Agric Food Chem. 2009; 57(14): 6082–9.
31. Hernández I, Alegre L, Van Breusegem F, Munné-Bosch S. How relevant are flavonoids as antioxidants in plants? Trends Plant Sci. 2009; 14(3): 125–32.
32. Wang J, Hu S, Nie S. Reviews on mechanisms of in vitro antioxidant activity of polysaccharides. Oxid Med Cell Longev. 2016; 13. doi: 10.1155.
33. Choi BS, Sapkota K, Kim S, Lee HJ, Choi HS, Kim SJ. Antioxidant activity and protective effects of Tripterygium regelii extract on hydrogenperoxide-induced injury in human dopaminergic cells, SH-SY5Y. Neurochem Res. 2010; 35: 1269–80.
34. Lee DS, Keo S, Cheng SK, Oh H, Kim YC. Protective effects of Cambodian medicinal plants on tertbutyl hydroperoxideinduced hepatotoxicity via Nrf2mediated heme oxygenase1. Mol Med Rep. 2017; 15(1): 451–9.
35. Ramyaa P, Padma VV. Ochratoxin-induced toxicity, oxidative stress and apoptosis ameliorated by quercetin--modulation by Nrf2. Food Chem Toxicol. 2013; 62: 205–16.
36. Ramyaa P, Krishnaswamy R, Padma VV. Quercetin modulates OTA-induced oxidative stress and redox signalling in $HepG_2$ cells-up regulation of Nrf2 expression and down regulation of NF-κB and COX-2. Biochim Biophys Acta. 2014; 1840(1): 681–92.
37. Kumar KH, Khanum F. Hydroalcoholic extract of Cyperus rotundus Ameliorates H2O2-Induced Human Neuronal Cell Damage via its anti-oxidative and anti-apoptotic Machinery. Cell Mol Neurobiol. 2013; 33(1): 5–17.
38. Nikam S, Nikam P, Ahaley SK, Sontakke AV. Oxidative stress in parkinson's disease. Indian J Clin Biochem. 2009; 24: 98–101.
39. de Vries HE, Witte M, Hondius D, Rozemuller AJ, Drukarch B, Hoozemans J. Nrf2-induced antioxidant protection: a

promising target to counteract ROS-mediated damage in neurodegenerative disease? Free Radic Biol Med. 2008; 45(10): 1375–83.

40. Chen PC, Vargas MR, Pani AK, Smeyne RJ, Johnson DA, Kan YW. Nrf2-mediated neuroprotection in the MPTP mouse model of Parkinson's disease: critical role for the astrocyte. Proc Natl Acad Sci USA. 2009; 106(8): 2933–8.
41. Rojo AI, Innamorato NG, Martín-Moreno AM, De Ceballos ML, Yamamoto M, Cuadrado A. Nrf2 regulates microglial dynamics and neuro inflammation in experimental Parkinson's disease. Glia. 2010; 58(5): 588–98.
42. Hara H, Ohta M, Adachi T. Apomorphine protects against 6-hydroxydopamine-induced neuronal cell death through activation of the Nrf2-ARE pathway. J Neurosci Res. 2006; 84(4): 860–6.
43. Lin YC, Huang YC, Chen SC, Liaw CC, Kuo SC, Huang LJ. Neuroprotective effects of ugonin K on hydrogen peroxide-induced cell death in human neuroblastoma SH-SY5Y cells. Neurochem Res. 2009; 34: 923–30.
44. Lee CH, Hwang DS, Kim HG, Oh H, Park H, Cho JH, et al. Protective effect of Cyperi rhizoma against 6-hydroxydopamine-inducedneuronal damage. J Med Food. 2010; 13: 564–71.
45. Doi K, Uetsuka K. Mechanisms of mycotoxin-induced neurotoxicity through oxidative stress-associated pathways. Int J Mol Sci. 2011; 12(8): 5213–37.
46. Cai L, Wang LF, Pan JP, et al. Neuroprotective effects of Methyl3,4-Dihydroxybenzoate against TBHP-Induced oxidative damage in SH-SY5Y Cells. Molecules. Molecules. 2016, 21(8):1–14.
47. Hassa, PO, Hottiger, MO. The diverse biological roles of mammalian PARPS, a small but powerful family of poly-ADP-ribose polymerases. Front Biosci. 2008; 13: 3046–82.

***Chi Cheng**
cij123@126.com
China National Research Institute of Food and Fermentation Industries

***Qiyang He**
qiyang_he@vip.163.com
Institute of biomedical technology
Chinese Academy of Medical Scieneces and Peking Union Medical College

# 14

# Activation of macrophage mediated host defense against *Salmonella typhimurium* by *Morus alba* L.

BoYoon Chang[1], BongSeong Koo[2], HyeonCheol Lee[2], Joa Sub Oh[3], SungYeon Kim[1]*

[1]Institute of Pharmaceutical Research and Development, College of Pharmacy, Wonkwang University, Iksan, Jeonbuk, South Korea; [2]ForBioKorea Co., Ltd. Seoul, South Korea; [3]College of Pharmacy, Dankook University, Cheonan, South Korea

*Abstract*

***Background***: The innate immune system plays a crucial role in the initiation and subsequent direction of adaptive immune responses, as well as in the removal of pathogens that have been targeted by an adaptive immune response.
***Objective***: *Morus alba* L. was reported to have immunostimulatory properties that might protect against infectious diseases. However, this possibility has not yet been explored. The present study investigated the protective and immune-enhancing ability of *M. alba* L. against infectious disease and the mechanisms involved.
***Design***: To investigate the immune-enhancing effects of *M. alba* L., we used a bacterial infection model.
***Results and discussions:*** The lifespan of mice infected with a lethal dose of *Salmonella typhimurium* ($1 \times 10^7$ colony forming units – CFU) was significantly extended when they were administered *M. alba* L. Furthermore, *M. alba* L. activated macrophages, monocytes, and neutrophils and induced Th1 cytokines (IL-12, IFN-γ, TNF-α) in mice infected with a sublethal dose ($1 \times 10^5$ CFU) of *S. typhimurium*. *M. alba* L. significantly stimulated the uptake of bacteria into peritoneal macrophages as indicated by increased phagocytosis. Peritoneal macrophages derived from C3H/HeJ mice significantly inhibited *M. alba* L. induced NO production and TNF-α secretion compared with peritoneal macrophages derived from C3H/HeN mice.
***Conclusions***: These results suggest that the innate immune activity of *M. alba* L. against bacterial infection in mice occurs through activation of the TLR4 signaling pathway.

Keywords: *Morus alba L*; *TLR4*; *Salmonella*; *immune defense*; *macrophage*

Bacterial infectious agents are responsible for high morbidity and mortality in humans (1). Antibiotic drugs are used to combat these pathogens; however, the rise in antibiotic-resistant pathogens has led to the development of new therapeutic agents that are effective against these bacteria (2, 3).

The immune system is our natural defense system against pathogens such as viruses, bacteria, and other agents (4). It is composed of the innate immune system and the adaptive immune system. The innate immune system is a primary defense mechanism against invading organisms, while the adaptive immune system acts as a second line of defense. Both aspects of the immune system have cellular and humoral components that mediate their protective functions. Macrophages are the most abundant cells in granulomas and have been shown to play a key role throughout the course of infection in all infected hosts, including humans and non-human primates. Once these bacteria enter a host, Toll-like receptors (TLRs) recognize a variety of microbial products, including bacterial cell wall components and endocytosed nucleic acids, thereby triggering innate immune responses (5–7). Most laboratory studies have focused on the modulation of antimicrobial peptides and innate immune mediators by microbial components (8, 9). However, the effect of herbal plant extracts on immune responses to infectious diseases is not well established. An attempt has been made to identify a potent immunostimulator from plant extracts selected for their immune pharmacological properties. Our previous study showed that *Morus alba* L. had immunostimulatory effects in macrophages (10). In addition, *M. alba* L. might have an indirect anticancer effect by enhancing immune responses through TLR4 signaling (11). However, the protective effects of *M. alba* L. against pathogens have not been examined. In the present study, we investigated the protective effect and macrophage-mediated immune responses of *M. alba* L. in mice challenged with pathogenic *Salmonella typhimurium*.

## Materials and methods

### *Chemical and reagents*

Roswell Park Memorial Institute medium 1640 (RPMI) and fetal bovine serum (FBS) were obtained from GIBCO (Grand Island, NY, USA). A nitric oxide (NO) detection kit was obtained from INTRON Biotechnology (Sungnam, Korea). Trizol was obtained from Invitrogen (Carlsbad, CA, USA). Interleukin (IL) 6, IL-12, interferon gamma (IFN-γ) and tumor necrosis factor alpha (TNF-α) were obtained from R&D Systems (Minneapolis, MN, USA). Penicillin, streptomycin, neutral red, 3-(4,5-dimethylthiaz ol-2-yl)-2,5-diphenyltetrazolium bromide, lipopolysaccharide (LPS), and all other chemicals were obtained from Sigma-Aldrich (St. Louis, MO, USA).

### *Cell culture and animal care*

Peritoneal macrophages were prepared from BALB/c, C3H/HeJ (wild type) and C3H/HeN (TLR4 mutant) mice as described previously (12). RAW264.7 cells were routinely cultured in Dulbecco's Modified Eagle Medium (DMEM; Sigma-Aldrich) supplemented with 2 mM l-glutamine (Sigma-Aldrich) and 10% FBS. Briefly, peritoneal macrophages were harvested from three mice, which had been injected intraperitoneally with 3 mL of thioglycollate broth 3 days before sterile peritoneal lavage with 10 mL of Hank's balanced salt solution. Cells were grown at 37°C in a humidified 5% $CO_2$ incubator. The cells were allowed to adhere to a 96-well culture plate at 37°C in a 5% $CO_2$ incubator for 3 h. Cells were grown in RPMI medium supplemented with 10% heat-inactivated FBS, 100 U/mL penicillin, and 100 µg/mL of streptomycin. *Salmonella typhimurium* was grown on Luria-Bertani (LB) agar or in LB broth, where appropriate, at 37°C under aerobic conditions. Mice were housed in specific pathogen-free (SPF) conditions at 21–24°C and between 40 and 60% relative humidity with a 12 h light-dark cycle. All animals were acclimatized for at least 1 week prior to the start of experiments. All studies were performed in accordance with the guide for animal experimentation by Wonkwang University and approved by the university's institutional animal care and use committee (Approval No. WKU11-21).

### *Preparation of standardized* M. alba *L. extract*

Dried fruits of *M. alba* were purchased from a local herbal market in Jeonbuk, Korea. The fruits were pulverized into powder and extracted twice with hot water (80°C) for 5 h. The solvent was removed under reduced pressure in a RV10 rotary evaporator (IKA, Staufen, Germany) to yield *M. alba* fruit hot water extract (42.8%, *w/w*). The extract was dried to a powder and kept in a closed container until use. To avoid variations in activity for different preparations, sufficient extract was obtained in one batch for use throughout the study. The content of the marker chlorogenic acid in *M. alba* L. was quantitated using high performance liquid chromatography. Results indicated that *M. alba* L. possessed 1.18 mg of chlorogenic acid per 1.0 g of extract (Fig. 1).

### *Induction of* S. typhimurium *infectious model*

SPF male ICR (Institute for Cancer Research) mice (5 weeks old and 25–27 g body weight) were purchased from Hanil Laboratory Animals (Iksan, Korea). The mice were randomly divided into two sets (Fig. 2). The first set contained three groups: a normal group ($n$ = 10), *S. typhimurium*-infected group ($N$ = 10), and 500 mg/kg/day *M. alba* L. + *S. typhimurium*-infected group ($n$ = 10). The second set contained five groups: a normal group ($n$ = 7); *S. typhimurium*-infected group ($N$ = 7); 100, 300, and 500 mg/kg/day *M. alba* L. + *S. typhimurium*-infected group ($n$ = 7, respectively). The normal and *S. typhimurium*-infected groups in these experiments were administered the same volume of distilled water. *M. alba* L. was dissolved in sterile double-distilled water and administered for 5 days consecutively. Twenty-four hours after the last drug administration, the mice of the first set were intraperitoneally injected with a lethal dose of bacterial suspension ($10^7$ colony forming units (CFU)/mouse) to induce peritonitis. The mice in the second set were intraperitoneally injected with a sublethal dose of bacterial suspension ($10^5$ CFU/mouse) to induce peritonitis. The challenged mice were fed a standard diet and water for 8 days and their survival and health were monitored twice per day throughout the experimental period. Any animal that exhibited severe clinical abnormalities, became moribund, or lost 20% of its initial body weight was sacrificed by ethyl ether narcosis and exsanguination. At the end of the experiment, the mice were subjected to ether anesthesia. The blood samples were collected from the central vein.

### *Measurement of cytokines*

Blood and cell culture media were collected and then TNF-α, IL-6, IL-12, and IFN-γ production was measured by the sandwich ELISA method according to the manufacturer's instructions (R&D Systems (TNF-α; DY410, IL-6; DY406, IL-12; DY419), Minneapolis, MN, USA and BD PharMingen (IFN-γ; RUO – 558258), CA, USA)).

### *Hematology test*

Blood samples were collected from the vena cava of all animals under ethyl ether anesthesia at necropsy for hematology. Blood was transferred to a container (EDTA K2; BD Biosciences, South Korea) for WBC (white blood cell), LYM (lymphocyte), MON (monocyte), and NEU (neutrophil) counts using an HORIBA (Edison, NJ, USA).

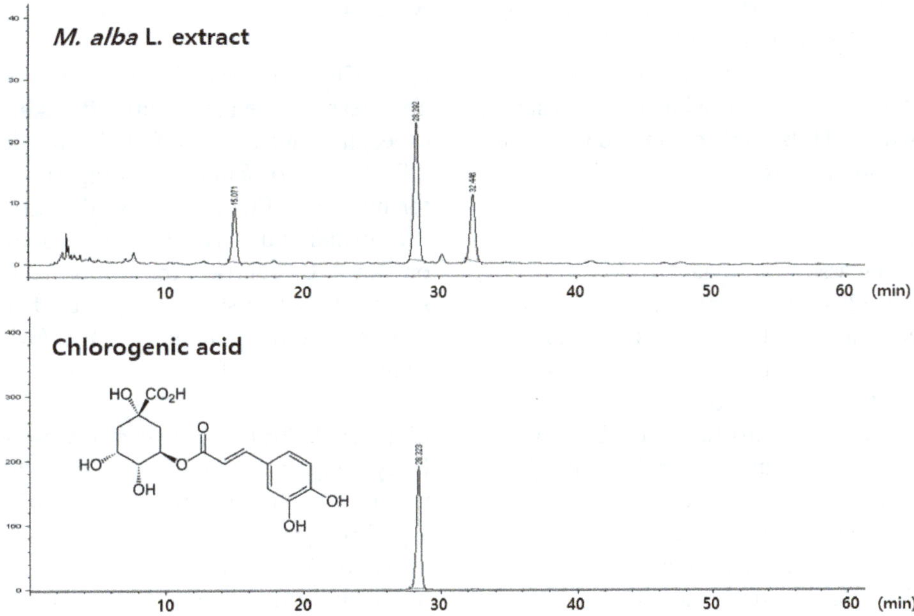


*Fig. 1.* The structure and high-performance liquid chromatography (HPLC) chromatographic profile of chlorogenic acid in *M. alba* L. extract at 340 nm.

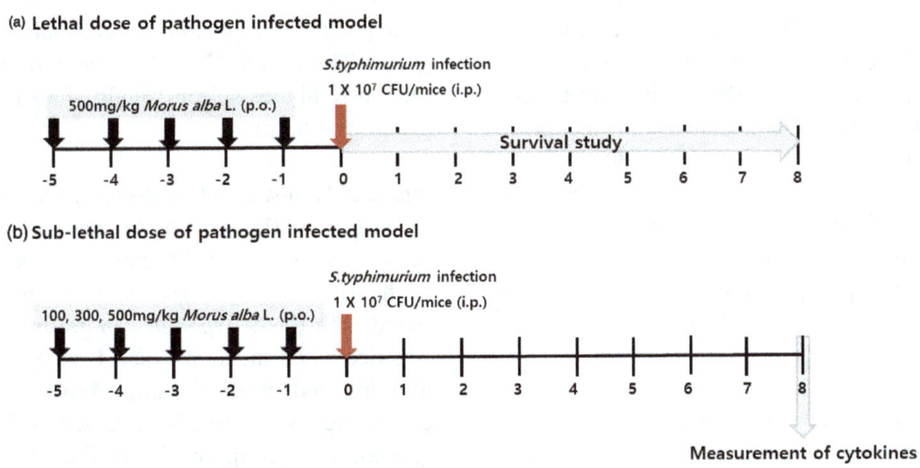


*Fig. 2.* Time schedule of the experimental procedures.

*Assay for peritoneal macrophage phagocytosis*

Phagocytosis assays were performed as described by Han et al. (13). Briefly, opsonization of bacteria fluorescein-labeled *Escherichia coli* wells were opsonized by incubation for 1 h at 37°C with 5% complete mouse serum or with 5% inactivated mouse serum. After opsonization, the serum was removed by centrifugation to eliminate excess opsonins. Fluorescein-5-isothiocyanate (FITC) labeled *E. coli* cells were suspended in Hank's balanced salt solution and added to the adherent phagocytes at a concentration of $5 \times 10^5$ CFU/mL. The final ratios of bacteria to macrophages (multiplicity of infection (MOI) of 50:1) were confirmed in the final volume of 200 μL. After incubation at 37°C for 2 h, phagocytic cells were washed 3 times with phosphate-buffered saline (PBS), which was aspirated to remove non-ingested cell particles. Extracellular fluorescence was quenched by the addition of 100 μL of trypan blue. After 1 min, the FITC bacteria that had not been ingested washed away and the macrophages were rinsed twice with PBS. Next, the macrophages were lysed with lysis buffer (10 mM Tris-HCl, pH 7.5, 130 mM NaCl, 1% Triton X-100, 10 mM $Na_2HPO_4$, 10 mM $Na_4P_2O_7$). The fluorescence intensity (relative fluorescence unit) of bacteria inside the cells was determined at excitation and emission wavelengths of 480 and 520 nm by using a spectrofluorometer (Tecan Infinite F200, Männedorf, Switzerland). The relative phagocytic activity was calculated as the percentage of fluorescence intensity in a sample supplemented with FITC bacteria compared with that with no supplementation (control).

#### *Intracellular killing assay*

The intracellular killing assay was conducted as described by Wu et al. (14). RAW264.7 cells were seeded at a density of 5 × $10^4$ cells/well in a 96-well plate containing 200 µL complete RAW medium and incubated at 37°C for 24 h in an atmosphere of 5% $CO_2$. Three colonies of each *S. typhimurium* strain were inoculated into 10 mL LB broth with appropriate antibiotics and incubated for 16 h at 37°C, with shaking at 200 rpm. Cultures were then centrifuged at 3,000 g for 10 min and resuspended in complete medium to 5 × $10^5$ CFU/mL. The culture medium was removed from the RAW264.7 cells and replaced with 200 µL of this bacterial inoculum per well, to give a MOI of 10:1. This MOI was used as the frequency of infection and was high enough to enable observation of infection events at the single-cell level in subsequent imaging experiments but minimize *Salmonella*-induced macrophage death. The cells were then incubated at 37°C for 30 min in an atmosphere of 5% $CO_2$, after which the supernatant was removed from each well and 200 µL complete RAW medium containing 50 µg/mL gentamicin was added; plates were incubated for either 15 min (T0) or 2 h (T2) at 37°C for 30 min in an atmosphere of 5% $CO_2$. The cells were then washed twice with 200 µL DMEM and lysed in 1% saponin, and the number of intracellular bacteria (CFU) was determined by serial dilution and plating on plate count agar. Intracellular killing percentage was calculated as: [(T0 – T2)/T0] × 100.

#### *NO assay*

Peritoneal macrophages (1 × $10^5$ cells/well) in a 96-well plate were incubated in the presence of three concentrations of *M. alba* L. (10, 30, and 100 µg/mL) for 24 h. NO was measured by determining the concentration of its stable oxidative metabolite nitrite using a microplate assay according to a described method (10). Supernatants (100 µL) were collected and mixed with an equal volume of Griess reagent (1% sulfanilamide and 0.1% N-(1- naphthyl)ethylenediamine dihydrochloride in 5% phosphoric acid) at room temperature for 15 min. The absorbance was read at 570 nm using a microplate reader. $NaNO_2$ was used as a standard.

#### *Statistical analysis*

Data are expressed as the mean ± SD and were examined for their statistical significance of difference by analysis of variance and Student's *t*-test. A *p*-value <0.05 was considered statistically significant.

### Results

#### *Effect of* M. alba L. *on pathogenic* S. typhimurium *in mice*

To determine the therapeutic effects of *M. alba* L. on life expectancy, mice were infected with a lethal dose (1 × $10^7$ CFU) of *S. typhimurium* intraperitoneally and assessed for mortality. Figure 3 shows that the mortality rates in the normal and *S. typhimurium* groups were 100 and 0% on Day 8. By contrast, the groups treated with *M. alba* L. showed 60% had survived on Day 8. These observations demonstrate the potential of *M. alba* L. to protect mice against the lethal effects of *S. typhimurium*.

#### *Effects of* M. alba L. *on body and organ weight*

Body weight was monitored during the experiment to reflect the health status of mice. All the infected groups had significantly greater weight loss compared with normal mice. At Day 5, mice infected with *S. typhimurium* had lost significantly more weight compared with the *M. alba* L. group (Fig. 4). After sacrificing the animals, the organs were removed and weighed. No significant changes in the weights of livers were seen in normal, *M. alba* L. + *S. typhimurium*, or *S. typhimurium* mice (Table 1). However, spleen weights were significantly increased in animals infected with *S. typhimurium* compared with the normal group. The *M. alba* L. + *S. typhimurium* group had a significantly higher spleen weight than the *S. typhimurium* group ($p < 0.05$).

#### *Effects of* M. alba L. *on hematological parameters*

Table 2 shows the effect of *M. alba* L. on the hematological parameters of mice. WBC count was significantly increased in the *M. alba* L. + *S. typhimurium* group ($p < 0.05$) compared with the *S. typhimurium* group. Lymphocyte count was decreased in the *M. alba* L. + *S. typhimurium* group and infected control group. Monocyte and neutrophil counts were significantly increased in the *M. alba* L. + *S. typhimurium* group and infected control group compared with the uninfected control group ($p < 0.05$ for all).

#### *Effect of* M. alba L. *on cytokine production in* S. typhimurium*-infected mice*

To examine the immunomodulatory effect of *M. alba* L. on pathogenic *S. typhimurium* infection, the mice were administered *M. alba* L. (100, 300, and 500 mg/kg) for 5 days, or were not pretreated and were then challenged with 1 × $10^5$ CFU/mouse (sublethal dose) of *S. typhimurium*. After 8 days, the levels of key immune molecules, IFN-γ, TNF-α, IL-12, and IL-6 were measured in serum. The mice fed with *M. alba* L. (300 or 500 mg/kg) had higher IFN-γ, IL-12, and TNF-α production compared with the infected group (Fig. 5a, c, d). However, IL-6 production was not significantly different in the serum of mice in all groups (Fig. 5b).

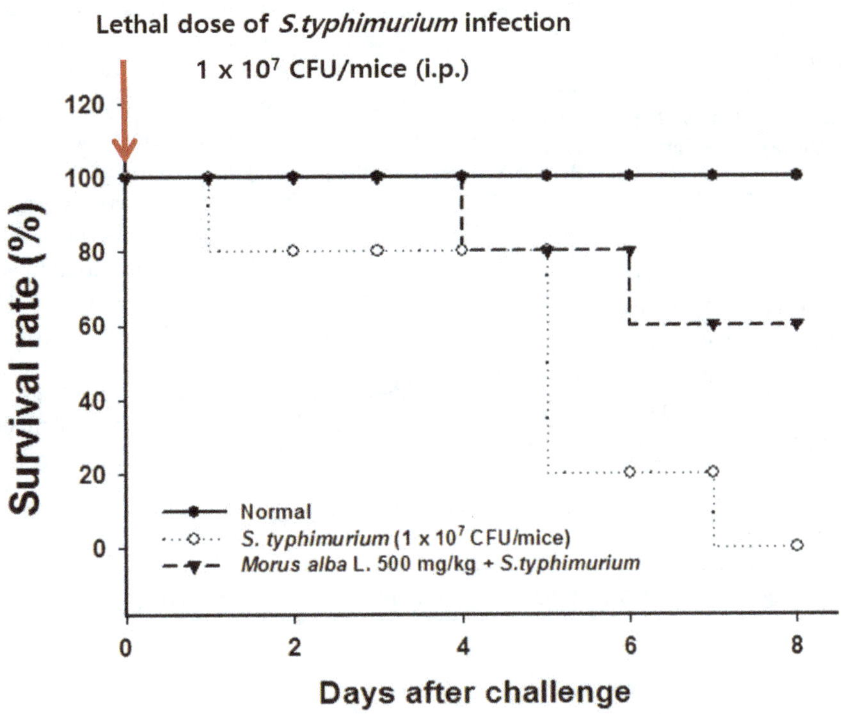


*Fig. 3.* Effects of *M. alba* L. on survival rates in mice challenged with pathogenic *S. typhimurium. Morus alba* L. (500 mg/kg) was orally administered for 5 days to mice, which were then intraperitoneally injected with a lethal dose of a bacterial suspension ($10^7$ CFU/mouse) to induce peritonitis. The challenged mice were kept for 8 days on a standard diet with water and their survival was monitored twice a day throughout the experimental period.

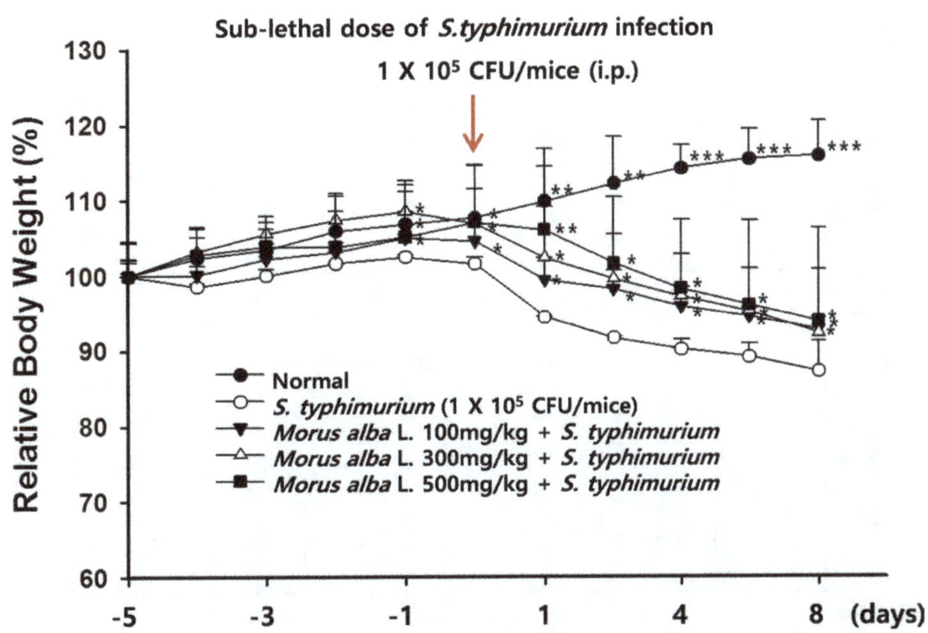


*Fig. 4.* Effects of *M. alba* L. on change in body weight in mice challenged with pathogenic *S. typhimurium. Morus alba* L. (100, 300, or 500 mg/kg) was orally administrated for 5 days to mice, which were then intraperitoneally injected with a sublethal dose of a bacterial suspension ($10^5$ CFU/mouse) to induce peritonitis. The body weight was recorded daily. The values are the means ± S.D. *$p < 0.05$, **$p < 0.01$, ***$p < 0.001$ compared with the *M. alba* L. group.

*Table 1.* Effects of *M. alba* L. on organ weight in mice challenged with pathogenic *S. typhimurium*. The values are the means ± S.D. $*p < 0.05$, compared with the *M. alba* L. group

| Group | Dose (mg/kg) | Body weight (g) | Relative liver weight (%) | Relative Spleen weight (%) |
|---|---|---|---|---|
| ***Normal mice*** | | | | |
| Saline | - | 36.0 ± 1.41 | 5.46 ± 0.08 | 0.35 ± 0.08 |
| ***Mice infected with S. typhimurium (1 × 10$^5$ CFU/mouse)*** | | | | |
| Saline | | 25.8 ± 1.18 | 6.88 ± 0.20 | 1.16 ± 0.08 |
| *Morus alba* L. | 100 | 27.6 ± 0.47 | 7.40 ± 0.64 | 1.41 ± 0.09 * |
| | 300 | 26.4 ± 2.46 | 7.91 ± 0.11 | 1.55 ± 0.11 * |
| | 500 | 27.0 ± 3.57 | 7.40 ± 0.93 | 1.60 ± 0.04 * |

### *Effect of* M. alba *L. on peritoneal macrophage phagocytosis*

*M. alba* L. at the tested concentrations did not affect cytotoxicity (data not shown). Thus, we treated cells with *M. alba* L. at concentrations of 10, 30, and 100 μg/mL during subsequent experiments. To determine the effects of *M. alba* L. on the phagocytic activity of macrophages, the uptake of FITC-labeled *E. coli* particles was compared between *M. alba* L. treated and untreated macrophages. The phagocytosis of macrophages was increased by *M. alba* L. treatment in a dose-dependent manner (Fig. 6a). These results demonstrate that *M. alba* L. enhances macrophage phagocytosis.

### *Effect of M. alba L. on intracellular killing*

The bacteria defense functions of macrophages were further assessed by using a gentamicin protection assay, a

*Table 2.* Effects of *M. alba* L. on hematological parameters in mice challenged with pathogenic *S. typhimurium*. The values are the means ± S.D. $*p < 0.05$, compared with the *M. alba* L. group

| Group | Dose (mg/kg) | WBC (10$^3$/ml) | LYM (%) | MON (%) | NEU (%) |
|---|---|---|---|---|---|
| ***Normal mice*** | | | | | |
| Saline | - | 4.32 ± 0.19 | 76.3 ± 10.28 | 18.4 ± 2.32 | 6.15 ± 3.27 |
| ***Mice infected with S. typhimurium (1 × 10$^5$ CFU/mouse)*** | | | | | |
| Saline | | 1.78 ± 0.24 | 61.3 ± 7.25 | 23.8 ± 1.93 | 16.1 ± 1.27 |
| *Morus alba* L. | 100 | 1.93 ± 0.27 | 62.7 ± 8.93 | 25.4 ± 1.42 | 13.6 ± 1.95 |
| | 300 | 4.22 ± 0.43 * | 55.4 ± 11.75 | 29.5 ± 1.28 * | 22.7 ± 2.95 |
| | 500 | 5.91 ± 1.73 * | 53.4 ± 7.32 | 28.7 ± 1.15 * | 25.1 ± 1.87 * |

WBC, white blood cells; LYM, lymphocytes; MON, monocytes; NEU, neutrophils.

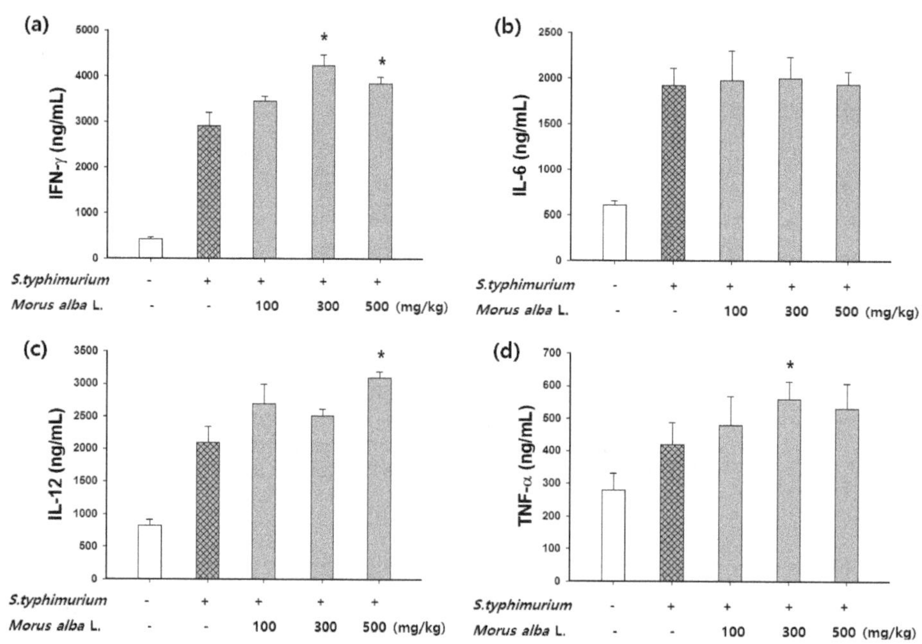


*Fig. 5.* Effect of *M. alba* L. on the production of cytokines in mice challenged with pathogenic *S. typhimurium*. *Morus alba* L. (100, 300, or 500 mg/kg) was orally administrated for 5 days to mice, which were then intraperitoneally injected with a sublethal dose of a bacterial suspension (10$^5$ CFU/mouse) to induce peritonitis. At the end of the experiment, the mice were subjected to ether anesthesia. Serum was collected from the blood of infected mice pre-administered with *M. alba* L. to evaluate the serum levels of (a) IFN-γ, (b) IL-6, (c) IL-12, and (d) TNF-α. The data are the means ± SD, $*p < 0.05$ compared with the *S. typhimurium* group.

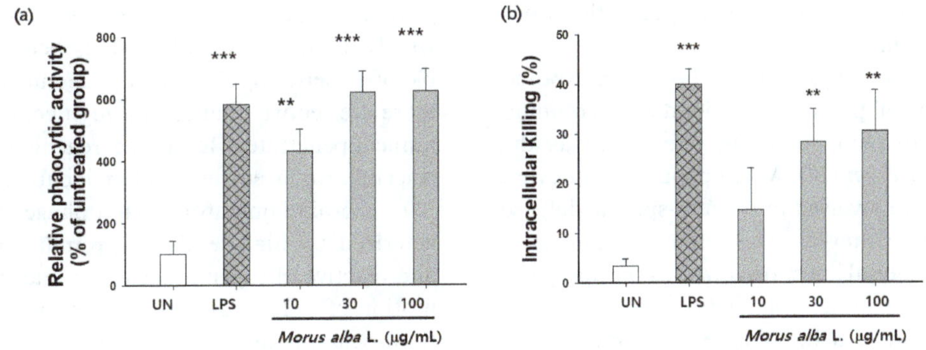


*Fig. 6.* Effects of *M. alba* L. on phagocytic activity and intracellular killing. Peritoneal macrophages derived from BALB/c mice or RAW 264.7 cells were treated with 10, 30, or 100 μg/mL of *M. alba* L. for 24 h, or with LPS (1 μg/mL) as a positive control. (a) After the addition of FITC-labeled *E. coli*, the cells were incubated for 2 h. The supernatants containing unphagocytosed bacteria were removed and then lysed with Triton X-100 containing lysis buffer. Fluorescence intensities of the lysed cells were measured by using a fluorescence microplate reader. (b) After the addition of *S. typhimurium*, the cells were incubated for 2 h. Unphagocytosed bacteria were removed and the cells were lysed with 1% saponin. The number of intracellular bacteria (CFU) was determined by serial dilution and plating on plate count agar (PCA). The values are the mean ± S.D. $^{**}p < 0.01$, $^{***}p < 0.001$ compared with the untreated group.

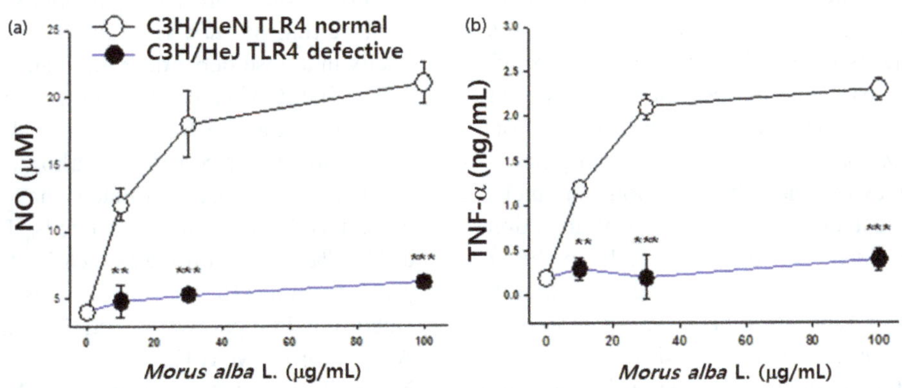


*Fig. 7.* Effects of *M. alba* L. on peritoneal macrophages derived from C3H/HeN and C3H/HeJ mice. Peritoneal macrophages from C3H/HeN and C3H/HeJ mice were stimulated with *M. alba* L. or LPS (1 μg/mL) as a positive control for 24 h. (a) NO and (b) TNF-α levels were determined by ELISA. The values are the means ± S.D. $^{**}p < 0.01$, $^{***}p < 0.001$, compared with C3H/HeN mice.

method commonly used to test intracellular bactericidal activity with live *Salmonella* as the target. The intracellular killing of macrophages was increased by *M. alba* L. treatment in a dose-dependent manner (Fig. 6b), which demonstrated that *M. alba* L. enhanced macrophage intracellular killing.

### *Effects of M. alba L. on peritoneal macrophages from TLR4-deficient mice*

To investigate the involvement of TLR4 signaling in mediating the beneficial effects of *M. alba* L., we compared NO and TNF-α production in peritoneal macrophages from wild-type (C3H/HeN) or TLR4-deficient mice (C3H/HeJ). Significantly increased NO and TNF-α was detected in peritoneal macrophages from C3H/HeN but not C3H/HeJ mice after *M. alba* L. treatment (Fig. 7). Therefore, *M. alba* L. induces the production of proinflammatory cytokines via TLR4.

## Discussion

*Morus alba* L., white mulberry, is a deciduous tree that belongs to the Moraceae family, which is widely distributed in Asia. *M. alba* L. has been used worldwide in traditional medicine for the treatment of various diseases from ancient times to the present (12, 15). Previous studies have indicated that *M. alba* L. possesses various pharmacological properties, including antimicrobial (16), antioxidant (17), antitumor (18), anti-obesity (19), antihypotensive (20), neuroprotective (21, 22), and antidiabetic (23, 24) actions. In addition, our previous studies indicated that the extracts and components of *M. alba* L. fruit water extract were safe (25), immunostimulatory (10, 12, 26), and had indirect anticancer activity by enhancing immune responses mediated by TLR4 signaling (12). However, the effects and mechanisms involved in pathogen defense actions have remained elusive. Therefore, in this study, we examined the pathogen defense properties of *M. alba* L. in mice challenged with pathogenic *S. typhimurium*.

Several studies have suggested that host cells exposed to different groups of pathogens respond with common transcriptional activation programs, referred to as the *core response to infection* (27). Macrophages, monocytes, and granulocytes are involved in the non-specific defense mechanism against pathogens. The common response of macrophages to bacterial infections involves the upregulation of genes involved in M1 polarization (28).

We report that *M. alba* L. enhanced immune activity and resistance to experimental challenge with *S. typhimurium* infection. However, *M. alba* L. did not directly kill *S. typhimurium*. Therefore, the pathogen defense effect of *M. alba* L. is likely to be mediated by potentiation of the host's defense system, such as macrophage activation, rather than by the indirect inhibition of bacterial growth.

We observed hepatomegaly and splenomegaly in *S. typhimurium* infected mice. The present results showed that the killing activity of monocytes and neutrophils was increased in *M. alba* L. treated mice infected with *S. typhimurium*, indicating its potential to enhance non-specific immune responses. Systemic *Salmonella* infection commonly induces splenomegaly in murine or human hosts. The capacity of *Salmonella* to evade killing and replicate within tissue phagocytes means that infection can quickly overwhelm local host defenses at the site of infection. Thus, inflammatory signals produced by cells in the infected tissue rapidly recruit neutrophils and inflammatory monocytes to engulf replicating bacteria. Splenomegaly can cause splenic structure change; splenic tissue structure is correlated with the recruitment and expansion of T and B cells and macrophages (29). The present study provides evidence of the induction of the macrophage phagocytic effect by *M. alba* L.

Furthermore, cytokines such as IL-12, IFN-γ, and TNF-α have a vital role in both innate and adaptive immunity and are responsible for Th1 polarization (30, 31). Because IL-12, IFN-γ, and TNF-α were upregulated in *M. alba* L. treated groups, this suggests it has important immunoregulatory activity by activating macrophages. However, Th2 cytokine production (IL-6) was unaffected. IL-12 is produced primarily by monocytes, macrophages, and other antigen-presenting cells and is essential for fighting infectious diseases and cancer. IL-12 synergizes with TNF-α and other proinflammatory cytokines to stimulate IFN-γ production, as well NK and CD8 T cell cytotoxicity (32). TNF-α is another proinflammatory cytokine and its levels in plasma are directly correlated with the ability of phagocytes to generate superoxide and the activity of iNOS and, thus, NO levels (31). One of the key requirements for the accuracy of the in vitro bactericidal assay is to eliminate the bacteria remaining extracellularly after ingestion by macrophages. For this purpose, gentamicin at a concentration of c. 50 mg/L has been widely used, as this antibiotic is believed to be incapable of penetrating the macrophage membrane. However, there are reports that such a high concentration of gentamicin penetrates HeLa cells, reaching c. 90% of the extracellular concentration after incubation for 72 h. The M1, or proinflammatory, macrophage phenotype is characterized by high levels of proinflammatory cytokines and reactive nitrogen and oxygen intermediates, the promotion of a Th1 response, and strong microbicidal and tumoricidal activity. Phagocytosis is the first step in the macrophage response to invading microorganisms and activation of phagocytosis enhances innate immune responses (33). Phagocytosis by macrophages was increased by *M. alba* L. treatment in a dose-dependent manner. The activation of intracellular killing mechanisms is critical to the antimicrobial activity of phagocytes. The pathogen internalization is followed by the fusion of phagosomes and lysosomes, which exposes the internalized pathogen to antimicrobial proteins and reactive molecules. Results indicate that *M. alba* L. is armed with such a killing capacity in a dose-dependent manner.

The first step in the modulation of cellular events is binding to receptors. TLRs play a central role in macrophage activation and the control of pathogen infections (5).

TLR4 is expressed on macrophages, dendritic cells, B cells, T cells, and endothelial cells. The role of TLR as a *M. alba* L. receptor was clearly demonstrated in our previous study (10, 12). TLR4 binds with *M. alba* L. activated signaling pathways, including MAPKs and NF-κB. Activation of MAPKs is required for the induction of NO as it controls the activation of NF-κB. In this study, the role of TLR4 as an *M. alba* L. receptor was confirmed in macrophages. To investigate this membrane receptor, we examined the effect of *M. alba* L. on primary macrophages isolated from wild-type C3H/HeN and C3H/HeJ mice that have mutant TLR4. *Morus alba* L. induced NO production and TNF-α in macrophages from C3H/HeN, but not from TLR4 mutated C3H/HeJ mice, which suggests that TLR4 is the membrane receptor for *M. alba* L.

In summary, our data suggest that *M. alba* L. activated macrophages via TLR4 to provide protection against *Salmonella* infection, indicating that *M. alba* L. modulates the effector functions of immunocompetent cells.

## Acknowledgements

This work was supported by the Industrial Core Technology Development Program (10067293), funded by the Ministry of Trade, Industry, and Energy (MOTIE, South Korea).

## Authors' contributions

All authors read and approved the final version of the manuscript. S.Y.K. conceived and designed the experiments. B.Y.C. and H.C.L. performed the experiments. B.Y.C., J.S.O., and S.Y.K. analyzed the data. S.Y.K. and B.Y.C. drafted the manuscript. B.Y.C., B.S.K., H.C.L., J.S.O., and S.Y.K. revised the manuscript.

## Conflicts of interest and funding

The authors declare that they have no competing interests.

## References


1. Qu Y, Li R, Jiang M, Wang X. Sucralose increases antimicrobial resistance and stimulates recovery of Escherichia coli mutants. Curr Microbiol 2017; 74(7): 885–8. doi: 10.1007/s00284-017-1255-5.
2. Cherazard R, Epstein M, Doan TL, Salim T, Bharti S, Smith MA. Antimicrobial resistant Streptococcus pneumoniae: prevalence, mechanisms, and clinical implications. *Am J Ther* 2017; 24(3): e361–9. doi: 10.1097/mjt.0000000000000551.
3. Shaker MA, Shaaban MI. Formulation of carbapenems loaded gold nanoparticles to combat multi-antibiotic bacterial resistance: in vitro antibacterial study. Int J Pharm 2017; 525(1): 71–84. doi: 10.1016/j.ijpharm.2017.04.019.
4. Luo A, Leach ST, Barres R, Hesson LB, Grimm MC, Simar D. The microbiota and epigenetic regulation of T helper 17/regulatory T cells: in search of a balanced immune system. *Front Immunol* 2017; 8: 417. doi: 10.3389/fimmu.2017.00417.
5. McClure R, Massari P. TLR-dependent human mucosal epithelial cell responses to microbial pathogens. Front Immunol 2014; 5: 386. doi: 10.3389/fimmu.2014.00386.
6. Gomes MT, Campos PC, de Almeida LA, Oliveira FS, Costa MM, Marim FM, et al. The role of innate immune signals in immunity to Brucella abortus. Front Cell Infect Microbiol 2012; 2: 130. doi: 10.3389/fcimb.2012.00130.
7. Fieber C, Kovarik P. Responses of innate immune cells to group A Streptococcus. Front Cell Infect Microbiol 2014; 4: 140. doi: 10.3389/fcimb.2014.00140.
8. Brito de Assis A, Dos Santos C, Dutra FP, de Oliveira Motta A, Costa FS, Navas CA, et al. Assessing antibacterial potential of components of Phyllomedusa distincta skin and its associated dermal microbiota. J Chem Ecol 2016; 42(2): 139–48. doi: 10.1007/s10886-016-0665-3.
9. Zheng Z, Wei C, Guan K, Yuan Y, Zhang Y, Ma S, et al. Bacterial E3 Ubiquitin Ligase IpaH4.5 of Shigella flexneri targets TBK1 to Dampen the host antibacterial response. J Immunol 2016; 196(3): 1199–208. doi: 10.4049/jimmunol.1501045.
10. Yang XY, Park GS, Lee MH, Chang IA, Kim YC, Kim SY, et al. Toll-like receptor 4-mediated immunoregulation by the aqueous extract of Mori Fructus. Phytother Res 2009; 23(12): 1713–20. doi: 10.1002/ptr.2818.
11. Kim SB, Chang BY, Jo YH, Lee SH, Han SB, Hwang BY, et al. Macrophage activating activity of pyrrole alkaloids from Morus alba fruits. J Ethnopharmacol 2013; 145(1): 393–6. doi: 10.1016/j.jep.2012.11.007.
12. Chang BY, Kim SB, Lee MK, Park H, Kim SY. Improved chemotherapeutic activity by Morus alba fruits through immune response of toll-like receptor 4. Int J Mol Sci. 2015; 16(10): 24139–58. doi: 10.3390/ijms161024139.
13. Han EH, Choi JH, Hwang YP, Park HJ, Choi CY, Chung YC, et al. Immunostimulatory activity of aqueous extract isolated from Prunella vulgaris. Food Chem Toxicol 2009; 47(1): 62–9. doi: 10.1016/j.fct.2008.10.010.
14. Wu J, Pugh R, Laughlin RC, Andrews-Polymenis H, McClelland M, Bäumler AJ, et al. High-throughput assay to phenotype *Salmonella* enterica typhimurium association, invasion, and replication in macrophages. J Vis Exp 2014; 11(90): e51759. doi: 10.3791/51759.
15. Choi JW, Synytsya A, Capek P, Bleha R, Pohl R, Park YI. Structural analysis and anti-obesity effect of a pectic polysaccharide isolated from Korean mulberry fruit Oddi (Morus alba L.). Carbohydr Polym 2016; 146: 187–96. doi: 10.1016/j.carbpol.2016.03.043.
16. Tirupathi RG, Suresh BK, Ujwal KJ, Sujana P, Raoa AV, Sreedhar AS. Anti-microbial principles of selected remedial plants from Southern India. Asian Pac J Trop Biomed 2011; 1(4): 298–305. doi: 10.1016/s2221-1691(11)60047-6.
17. Kujawska M, Ewertowska M, Adamska T, Ignatowicz E, Flaczyk E, Przeor M, et al. Protective effect of Morus alba leaf extract on N-Nitrosodiethylamine-induced Hepatocarcinogenesis in rats. In vivo 2016; 30(6): 807–12.
18. Yang Y, Zhang T, Xiao L, Yang L, Chen R. Two new chalcones from leaves of Morus alba L. Fitoterapia. 2010; 81(6): 614–16. doi: 10.1016/j.fitote.2010.03.005.
19. Vick SJ, Bovet D, Anderson JR. How do African grey parrots (*Psittacus erithacus*) perform on a delay of gratification task? Anim Cogn 2010; 13(2): 351–8. doi: 10.1007/s10071-009-0284-2.
20. Lee YJ, Choi DH, Kim EJ, Kim HY, Kwon TO, Kang DG, et al. Hypotensive, hypolipidemic, and vascular protective effects of Morus alba L. in rats fed an atherogenic diet. Am J Chin Med 2011; 39(1): 39–52. doi: 10.1142/s0192415x11008634.
21. Jung JW, Ko WM, Park JH, Seo KH, Oh EJ, Lee DY, et al. Isoprenylated flavonoids from the root bark of Morus alba and their hepatoprotective and neuroprotective activities. Arch Pharm Res 2015; 38(11): 2066–75. doi: 10.1007/s12272-015-0613-8.
22. Seo KH, Lee DY, Jeong RH, Lee DS, Kim YE, Hong EK, et al. Neuroprotective effect of prenylated arylbenzofuran and flavonoids from morus alba fruits on glutamate-induced oxidative injury in HT22 hippocampal cells. J Med Food 2015; 18(4): 403–8. doi: 10.1089/jmf.2014.3196.
23. Jiao Y, Wang X, Jiang X, Kong F, Wang S, Yan C. Antidiabetic effects of Morus alba fruit polysaccharides on high-fat diet- and streptozotocin-induced type 2 diabetes in rats. J Ethnopharmacol 2017; 199: 119–27. doi: 10.1016/j.jep.2017.
24. Ye M, Ke Y, Liu B, Yuan Y, Wang F, Bu S, et al. Root bark of Morus alba ameliorates the depressive-like behaviors in diabetic rats. Neurosci Lett 2017; 637: 136–41. doi: 10.1016/j.neulet.2016.11.036.
25. Chang BY, Kim SB, Lee MK, Park H, Kim SY. Nonclinical safety assessment of Morus alba L. fruits: study of 90-D toxicity in Sprague Dawley Rats and genotoxicity in *Salmonella*. J Food Sci 2016; 81(5): T1328–35. doi: 10.1111/1750-3841.13285.
26. Kim SB, Chang BY, Hwang BY, Kim SY, Lee MK. Pyrrole alkaloids from the fruits of Morus alba. Bioorg Med Chem Lett 2014; 24(24): 5656–9. doi: 10.1016/j.bmcl.2014.10.073.
27. Hurley D, McCusker MP, Fanning S, Martins M. *Salmonella*-host interactions – modulation of the host innate immune system. Front Immunol 2014; 5: 481. doi: 10.3389/fimmu.2014.00481.
28. Zhou D, Yang K, Chen L, Zhang W, Xu Z, Zuo J, et al. Promising landscape for regulating macrophage polarization: epigenetic viewpoint. Oncotarget. 2017; 8(34): 57693–706. doi: 10.18632/oncotarget.17027.
29. Chu HB, Zhang TG, Zhao JH, Jian FG, Xu YB, Wang T, Wang M, Tang JY, Sun HJ, Li K, Guo WJ, Zhu XJ. Assessment of immune cells and function of the residual spleen after subtotal splenectomy due to splenomegaly in cirrhotic patients. BMC immunology 2014; 15: 42. doi:10.1186/s12865-014-0042-3

30. Kalupahana RS, Mastroeni P, Maskell D, Blacklaws BA. Activation of murine dendritic cells and macrophages induced by *Salmonella* enterica serovar Typhimurium. Immunology 2005; 115(4): 462–72. doi: 10.1111/j.1365-2567.2005.02180.x.
31. Perkins DJ, Rajaiah R, Tennant SM, Ramachandran G, Higginson EE, Dyson TN, et al. *Salmonella* typhimurium co-opts the host type I IFN system to restrict macrophage innate immune transcriptional responses selectively. J Immunol. 2015; 195(5): 2461–71. doi: 10.4049/jimmunol.1500105.
32. Fernandez-Cabezudo MJ, Mechkarska M, Azimullah S, al-Ramadi BK. Modulation of macrophage proinflammatory functions by cytokine-expressing *Salmonella* vectors. Clin Immunol 2009; 130(1): 51–60. doi: 10.1016/j.clim.2008.08.017.
33. Hamidzadeh K, Mosser DM. Purinergic signaling to terminate TLR responses in macrophages. Front Immunol 2016; 7: 74. doi: 10.3389/fimmu.2016.00074.

***SungYeon Kim**

Institute of Pharmaceutical Research and Development College of Pharmacy Wonkwang University Iksan, Jeonbuk 54538 South Korea
Email: sungykim@wonkwang.ac.kr

15

# Nutrition education, farm production diversity and commercialization on household and individual dietary diversity in Zimbabwe

Conrad Murendo[1]*, Brighton Nhau[2], Kizito Mazvimavi[1], Thamsanqa Khanye[3] and Simon Gwara[1]

[1]International Crops Research Institute for the Semi-Arid Tropics, Bulawayo, Zimbabwe; [2]United Nations, Food and Agriculture Organization, Harare, Zimbabwe; [3]Community Technology Development Organization, Harare, Zimbabwe

*Abstract*

***Background:*** Nutrition education is crucial for improved nutrition outcomes. However, there are no studies to the best of our knowledge that have jointly analysed the roles of nutrition education, farm production diversity and commercialization on household, women and child dietary diversity.
***Objective:*** This article jointly analyses the role of nutrition education, farm production diversity and commercialization on household, women and children dietary diversity in Zimbabwe. In addition, we analyze separately the roles of crop and livestock diversity and individual agricultural practices on dietary diversity.
***Design:*** Data were collected from 2,815 households randomly selected in eight districts. Negative binomial regression was used for model estimations.
***Results:*** Nutrition education increased household, women, and child dietary diversity by 3, 9 and 24%, respectively. Farm production diversity had a strong and positive association with household and women dietary diversity. Crop diversification led to a 4 and 5% increase in household and women dietary diversity, respectively. Furthermore, livestock diversification and market participation were positively associated with household, women, and children dietary diversity. The cultivation of pulses and fruits increased household, women, and children dietary diversity. Vegetable production and goat rearing increased household and women dietary diversity.
***Conclusion:*** Nutrition education and improving access to markets are promising strategies to improve dietary diversity at both household and individual level. Results demonstrate the value of promoting nutrition education; farm production diversity; small livestock; pulses, vegetables and fruits; crop-livestock integration; and market access for improved nutrition.

Keywords: *nutrition education*; *production diversity*; *commercialization*; *dietary diversity*; *Zimbabwe*

The topics on behavior change communication (BCC), farm production diversity, and commercialization within the nutrition debate are gathering enormous interest among researchers, policy makers, and development practitioners. BCC interventions (e.g. promoting consumption of iron-rich foods, hygiene, preservation, and nutrition gardens) seek to improve household and individual nutrition knowledge and encourage behavior change adoption as well as improve decision-making on nutrition and child care as they encourage active participation of both men and women (1–4). Nutrition education increases awareness of malnutrition, benefits of consuming healthy diets, and healthy implications of consuming various foods. In Ethiopia, Hirvonen, Hoddinott, Minten and Stifel (1) found that enhanced nutrition knowledge improved children's dietary diversity only in areas with relatively good market access. Ensuring that caregivers understand what foods are appropriate for young children and women is seen as an integral component of efforts to improve maternal and children's nutritional status. Hence, BCC interventions that seek to improve caregivers' nutrition knowledge have gained popularity among policymakers in developing countries (1, 5, 6). According to Dewey and Adu-Afarwuah (6), BCC has been found to be effective at improving child-feeding practices in a number of randomized control trials in different countries. In Zimbabwe, there is poor dietary diversity as the majority of smallholder farmers heavily rely on maize, the main staple crop, which is not very nutritious. National assessments have shown that only 54% of the population consume acceptable diets and there is lack of protein-rich foods in the diets (7). This provides scope for promoting BCC and nutrition interventions to increase iron-rich foods and protein consumption (7).

Agriculture has a direct impact on household food security and nutrition through three pathways, which are own production, agricultural income, and women empowerment (8–10). In developing countries, agriculture through own production is the main source of diverse and nutritious foods and increased agricultural production through diversified farming can positively result in food availability, diet, and nutrition improvement (11). Agricultural income is another key pathway that can improve household food and nutrition security. Income generated from commercialization – crop and livestock sales and or income earned through farm labor supply increases household income (12). In addition, higher agricultural productivity from own production can result in improved household income through increases in marketable surplus. The improved household income might enable households to better spend their money on food and non-food items, for example, healthcare expenditure which subsequently improves nutrition, health, and welfare (9, 13–16).

Women empowerment is another important pathway to improved household nutrition. Women empowerment influences nutrition through several ways, including time use or caring capacity, workload in agriculture, maternal energy use, and women's control of income and resource allocation (9, 14). Empowered women can efficiently allocate their time for child feeding and caring, agricultural work, and household chores so as to improve household and child nutrition. It is believed that empowering women by giving them access to productive resources to the same level as men would increase yields by 20–30% and reduce the malnourished population by 100–150 million people (17). Furthermore, studies have shown that women's control of income and resources as well as greater access to markets have positive effects on household food and nutrition security as well as child education. According to literature, empowered women are better able to allocate resources for food and health care which can improve household, maternal, and child nutrition (9, 14).

There is a growing body of contrasting literature analyzing the effect of farm production diversity (8, 14, 15, 18–21), commercialization (13, 21), and nutrition knowledge (1) on household, maternal, and child nutrition. Malapit, Kadiyala, Quisumbing, Cunningham and Tyagi (14) found that production diversity positively influenced maternal and child dietary diversity in Nepal. In their study, Koppmair, Kassie and Qaim (21) conclude that farm production diversity and commercialization have a positive association with household, maternal, and child dietary diversity in Malawi. Snapp and Fisher (20) found that although crop diversity was positively associated with dietary diversity, education, income, market access, and availability of improved storage technologies had higher influence on dietary diversity. Carrleto, Corral and Guelfi (13) found little evidence of a positive relationship between commercialization and nutritional status in three countries, namely, Malawi, Tanzania, and Uganda.

The literature on agriculture–nutrition linkages has narrowly focused on farm production diversity and commercialization and only few studies have analyzed the role of nutrition education on household and individual-level nutrition (1). Furthermore, there are no studies to the best of our knowledge that have jointly analyzed the roles of nutrition education, farm production diversity, and commercialization on household, women, and child dietary diversity, especially in Zimbabwe. This is crucial given that there are context-specific factors that facilitate the functioning of impact pathways for improving nutrition (2). Furthermore, we disaggregate farm production diversity into crop and livestock diversity and analyze their separate associations together with nutrition education and commercialization on household, women, and child dietary diversity. Most studies in literature focus on nutrition outcomes at household level and fail to capture the effects at individual level (21). In addition, we investigate the association between specific crop and livestock practices on dietary diversity of household, women, and children. These areas have received little research attention. This paper attempts to fill these gaps by using cross-sectional survey data from 2,815 smallholder farm households randomly selected from eight districts in Zimbabwe.

## Methodology

### *Data collection*

The data used in this article were drawn from Crop and Livestock Production Survey conducted by Food and Agriculture Organization in 2016 as part of the annual assessment of the Livelihoods and Food Security Programme (LFSP). The programme is working to improve food security and nutrition of smallholder farmers and rural communities in eight districts of Zimbabwe (3). A total of 2,815 rural households were surveyed across eight districts (Table 1). In each district, 10 wards were purposively selected to include diversity of agricultural value chains,

*Table 1.* Sample

| District | Household interviewed |
|---|---|
| Gokwe South | 274 |
| Guruve | 391 |
| Kwekwe | 392 |
| Makoni | 306 |
| Mt Darwin | 397 |
| Mutare | 352 |
| Mutasa | 308 |
| Shurugwi | 395 |
| Total | 2,815 |

areas with biofortified crop production, and community -based micro-finance groups. Systematic random sampling was used to select households in each ward. About 36 households were selected per ward using beneficiary lists where the sampling interval was calculated by dividing the total number of beneficiaries by 36. The enumerators visited individual households selected through this process with an allowance of not more than two house recalls after which a replacement household was found. If someone was not present at the time of the visit, the next household on the same list was chosen and not the next-door neighbor. The survey collected information on household characteristics, agricultural practices, household nutrition, maternal and child nutrition, and food security. The total number of women and children (6–23 months of age) in the 2,815 households is 2,285 and 506, respectively.

### *Measurements*

#### Household dietary diversity

A modified Household Dietary Diversity Score (HDDS) (22) was calculated for each household using recall data on consumption of foods over the previous 24 h. In general, shorter recall period improves the accuracy of estimates compared with longer recall periods of 7 days (23). The food items were categorized into 12 different food groups with each food group counting toward the household score if a food item from the group was consumed by anyone in the household in the previous 24 h. The modified HDDS, then, is a count variable from 0 to 12. The food groups used to calculate the modified HDDS included cereals, roots and tubers, vegetables, fruits, meat, eggs, fish and seafood, pulses and nuts, milk and milk products, oils and fats, sugar, and condiments.

#### Women dietary diversity

Women dietary diversity score (WDDS) is measured using the individual dietary diversity score (22) of women aged 15–49 years. We compute individual dietary diversity scores using 24-h dietary recall data of women's own consumption from 11 food groups, namely, starchy staples; pulses; dark green leafy vegetables; vitamin A-rich fruits and vegetables; roots and tubers; other fruits and vegetables; milk and milk products; egg; fish; meat; and sugar and condiments (11, 22).

#### Children's dietary diversity

The child dietary diversity scores (CDDS) were used to determine the quality of the individual child's diet (14, 24). Dietary diversity of infants aged 6–23 months is measured by the number of food groups consumed in the last 24 h out of 16 food groups, namely, cereal-based foods; tubers; orange vegetables; green vegetables; orange fruits; other vegetables and fruits; juice; organ meat; meat; eggs; fish; pulses and nuts; dairy; oils; sugar; and liquids (14).

#### Nutrition education

Households' nutrition education is captured in the data through two questions about whether household received information on nutrition and child feeding and care. These were captured as dummy variables. Recognizing the multidimensional determinants of malnutrition in society, the LFSP project uses pluralistic extension approaches for wider dissemination of nutrition education. Various nutrition messages, for example, healthy eating, four-star diets, dietary diversification, and importance of biofortified crops are disseminated to farmers through various training platforms such as community health clubs, information and communication technology platforms (podcasts, videos, WhatsApp), and field days. These messages are disseminated by public and private extension officers, health officers, project nutritionists, trained community-based volunteers, and lead farmers (25, 26).

#### Farm production diversity

The number of crop and livestock species produced on a farm was used as the measure of farm production diversity (8, 18, 21). This is a simple, unweighted count measure. Second, we split and used the simple, unweighted count of only crop species produced on a farm (crop diversity) and livestock species (livestock diversity) separately. For robustness checks, we reran the model for crop and livestock diversity with a stepwise exclusion of relevant control variables in the model specifications to examine whether this influences the results significantly (27).

#### Commercialization

There are various definitions of commercialization (13). For the purposes of this article, we limit our definition of commercialization to two definitions: (a) household's market participation measured by the incidence of household selling crop and or livestock to the market and (b) the intensity of market participation measured by the share of crop output that the household sells to the market (13). The limitation of the first definition is its inability to measure the intensity of market participation.

### Estimation strategy

To investigate the relationship between nutrition education, farm production diversification, and commercialization on dietary diversity, we estimate the following regression models:

$$DD = b_0 + b_1\text{Nutrition education} + b_2\text{Farm production diversity} + b_3\text{Commercialization} + b_4 I + b_5 H + \varepsilon \quad (1)$$

where, *DD* is the nutrition outcome (i.e. dietary diversity); *I* and *H* are the vectors of individual and household characteristics, respectively; $b_i$ is the parameter to be estimated; and ε is an error term. The parameters $b_1$, $b_2$, and $b_3$ capture how nutrition education, farm production diversity, and commercialization are correlated with dietary diversity, controlling for a set of observable individual and household characteristics. In the extended model specifications, we split farm production diversity into crop and livestock diversity and assess their separate roles on dietary diversity as follows:

$$DD = b_0 + b_1\text{Nutrition education} + b_2\text{Crop diversity} + b_3\text{Livestock diversity} + b_4\text{Commercialization} + b_5 I + b_6 H + \varepsilon \quad (2)$$

In Equation 2, our key parameters of interest are $b_1$, $b_2$, $b_3$ and $b_4$ which capture how nutrition education, crop and livestock diversification and commercialization are correlated with dietary diversity. A positive and significant estimate for $b_1$, $b_2$, $b_3$ and $b_4$ implies that nutrition education, crop, livestock diversity, and commercialization are associated with higher dietary diversity. The dietary diversity is a count variable that can take values between 1 and 12 (or between 1 and 9 when only including the healthier food groups) and is not normally distributed. The goodness-of-fit chi-squared tests for household (1,439, $p > 0.05$) and women dietary diversity (1,308, $p > 0.05$) were not statistically significant revealing that poisson models fit reasonably well (28). For the children dietary diversity, the goodness-of-fit chi-squared test (1,010, $p < 0.001$) is statistically significant, indicating that the data do not fit the poisson model well. Given this, the negative binomial regression which is suitable for over-dispersed data is used for estimating all the three models (28–30). Robust variance estimator is used to obtain correct standard errors for model coefficient estimates in both models (31). For both models, we compute the incident rate ratios (IRRs) and their 95% confidence intervals. The IRRs are interpreted as percent change in the expected count, thus by what percentage the dietary diversity score change when the explanatory variable changes by one unit (30, 32).

## Results

### *Descriptive results*

Table 2 describes household characteristics. The upper part of Table 2 shows dietary diversity at the household level, and individually for women and children. At the household level, mean dietary diversity is 7; that is, the average household has consumed seven food groups during the reference day. Individual-level dietary diversity is lower than those at household level. This is expected because at household level the consumption of all household members is covered, including children above the age of 5 years, adolescents, and male adults (21). About 80% of the sampled households reported to have received information on nutrition, child feeding, and care practices. BCC strategies, for example, healthy eating messages disseminated to households, women, and men through various training platforms are crucial as they increase awareness of eating balanced diets.

The average farm household produces 3.0 and 2.4 different crop and livestock species, respectively. All households grew vegetables and 67% grew pulses. In terms of market participation, 50% of the sample households were engaged in crop and/or livestock sales. About 23.3% were involved in crop sales. On the contrary, about 10% of the harvest from crops is sold. These results reveal that only a small proportion of crop produce is sold to the market. Farm households prioritize food self-sufficiency and only sell surplus to the market. The El-Nino drought of 2015/16 season resulted in poor harvest and thus reduced marketable surplus.

The bottom part of Table 2 shows the variables that we use as covariates in the different specifications of the regression models. Our sample was dominated by male-headed households (72%) with a mean age of 50.7 years. Regarding education, 53% of the household heads had secondary education and above. The household size varied from 1 to 19 members with a mean size of 5.7. Also, mean arable land size holding within the sample was found to be three hectares.

### Food group consumption

As presented in Table 3, food groups that were mostly consumed by households included cereals (99%), condiments/spices/beverages (95%), oils/fats (94.3%), and sugar and sweets (84.9%). Milk and dairy products (24.4%) and eggs (22%) were the least consumed. Among households who had consumed foods from the given food groups, households' own production was the main source of vegetables (81.5%), eggs (80.5%), nuts and pulses (77.3%), and cereals (72.6%), whereas, oils and fats, sugars and sweets, condiments and spices, fish and milk products were mainly acquired through purchasing.

Table 4 shows the main food groups that were consumed by the youngest child. The food groups that were mostly consumed by the youngest child in the household included plain water (94.4%), cereals (78.7%), oils (63.9%), and cereal porridge (56.8%). Fortified baby formula (10.9%), infant formula (11.1%), orange fruits (6.5%), and other liquids (4.2%) were the least consumed. Unfortunately, we have no data on the source of foods consumed. However, the food types that young children eat are mostly acquired through purchasing rather than own production. This may suggest that young children dietary diversity is most likely influenced by income rather than farm production diversity. The results also show that approximately half of the sampled children consumed fruits and nuts.

*Table 2.* Household, farm, and institutional sample characteristics

| Variable | Description | |
|---|---|---|
| Household dietary diversity (mean [SD]; median) | Frequency of consumption of food groups | 7.0 (2.0); 7.0 |
| Women dietary diversity (mean [SD]; median) | Number of food groups consumed by women | 4.2 (1.7); 4.0 |
| Child dietary diversity | Number of food groups consumed by child | 5.7 (3.4); 5.0 |
| Nutrition information | Received nutrition information (1 = yes) | 79 |
| Child feeding and care | Received child feeding and care information (1 = yes) | 77 |
| Farm production diversity (mean [SD]; median) | Number of crop and livestock species reared | 5.4 (1.8); 7.0 |
| Crop diversity (mean [SD]; median) | Number of crop species grown | 3.0 (1.8); 3.0 |
| Livestock diversity (mean [SD]; median) | Number of livestock species reared | 2.4 (1.2); 2.0 |
| Beans and pulses | Grew pulses (1 = yes) | 67 |
| Vegetables | Grew vegetables (1 = yes) | 99 |
| Fruits | Grew fruits (1 = yes) | 49 |
| Cattle | Reared cattle (1 = yes) | 61 |
| Sheep | Reared sheep (1 = yes) | 3 |
| Goats | Reared goats (1 = yes) | 67 |
| Chicken | Reared chicken (1 = yes) | 85 |
| Market participation | Sold crop and livestock (1 = yes) | 50 |
| Market intensity (mean [SD]; median) | Total crop sold over total crop production | 0.1 (0.5); 0.0 |
| Age (mean [SD]; median) | Age of household head (years) | 50.7 (14.6); 48 |
| Gender | Gender of household head (1 = male) | 72 |
| Marital | Marital status of head (1 = married) | 75 |
| Education | Secondary education and above (1 = yes) | 53 |
| Household size (mean [SD]; median) | Household size | 5.7 (2.4); 5.0 |
| Orphans (mean [SD]; median) | Number of orphans | 0.5 (0.9); 0.0 |
| Chronically ill (mean [SD]; median) | Number of chronically ill | 0.1 (0.4); 0.0 |
| Land size (mean [SD]; median) | Total land owned (hectares) | 3.0 (2.2); 2.5 |
| Total income (mean [SD]; median) | Total household income (USD) | 185.0 (405.0); 75 |
| Number of observations | | 2,815 |

Notes: Values are % unless specified as (mean [SD]; median). For all continuous variables, the median is reported, especially for age and income which are skewed.

*Table 3.* Proportion of households which had consumed foods from each food group and main sources of these foods consumed

| | Consumption | | Main source | | | | | |
|---|---|---|---|---|---|---|---|---|
| | | | Own production | | Purchased | | Other | |
| Food group | N | Consumed (%) | N | % | n | % | N | % |
| Cereals | 2,805 | 99.0 | 2,010 | 72.6 | 535 | 19.3 | 223 | 8.1 |
| Roots and tubers | 2,799 | 25.3 | 440 | 62.5 | 218 | 31.0 | 46 | 6.5 |
| Nuts and pulses | 2,795 | 43.6 | 940 | 77.3 | 194 | 16.0 | 82 | 6.7 |
| Green leafy vegetables | 2,802 | 72.1 | 1,642 | 81.5 | 303 | 15.0 | 70 | 3.5 |
| Fruits | 2,802 | 37.1 | 598 | 58.4 | 242 | 24.1 | 184 | 17.5 |
| Meats – beef and poultry | 2,805 | 41.3 | 534 | 46.4 | 544 | 47.3 | 73 | 6.3 |
| Fish | 2,789 | 29.6 | 42 | 5.1 | 722 | 87.7 | 59 | 7.2 |
| Eggs | 2,799 | 22.0 | 491 | 80.5 | 105 | 17.2 | 14 | 2.3 |
| Milk and dairy products | 2,799 | 24.4 | 268 | 39.4 | 379 | 55.7 | 33 | 4.9 |
| Sugar and sweets | 2,792 | 84.9 | 52 | 2.2 | 2,256 | 94.5 | 55 | 3.3 |
| Oils and fats | 2,782 | 94.3 | 184 | 7.0 | 2,369 | 90.7 | 59 | 2.3 |
| Condiments, spices, and beverages | 2,767 | 95.0 | 52 | 2.0 | 2,519 | 96.2 | 48 | 1.8 |

*Table 4.* Proportion of youngest child who had consumed foods from each food group

| Food group | N | Consumed (%) |
|---|---|---|
| Infant formula | 506 | 11.07 |
| Cereal porridge | 506 | 56.76 |
| Fortified baby formula | 505 | 10.89 |
| Cereals | 506 | 78.74 |
| Orange vegetables | 506 | 23.87 |
| Tubers | 506 | 20.12 |
| Green vegetables | 506 | 40.72 |
| Orange fruits | 505 | 6.53 |
| Other vegetables and fruits | 504 | 48.61 |
| Organ meat | 503 | 10.74 |
| Red meat | 505 | 24.55 |
| Poultry | 501 | 20.16 |
| Eggs | 504 | 25.0 |
| Fish | 503 | 14.51 |
| Pulses | 502 | 23.11 |
| Nuts | 502 | 50.40 |
| Milk products | 502 | 21.91 |
| Oils | 498 | 63.86 |
| Sugary foods | 501 | 27.15 |
| Other solids | 493 | 13.18 |
| Plain water | 501 | 94.41 |
| Milk | 498 | 26.71 |
| Fizzy drinks | 502 | 16.14 |
| Maheu | 503 | 43.17 |
| Fruit juice | 492 | 7.52 |
| Tea | 502 | 53.78 |
| Other liquids | 481 | 4.16 |

#### Household dietary diversity and characteristics of HDDS tertiles

In this section, we categorized household into three levels to understand the proportions of household dietary diversity. Since there are no universal cut-offs for categorizing households according to their HDDS, the sample distribution was divided into HDDS tertiles which were characterized as low (0–5), moderate (6–7), and high (8–12) dietary diversity (23, 33). Figure 1 shows that Mt Darwin, Mutare and Makoni had a higher proportion of households with low dietary diversity relative to other districts. On the contrary, Mutasa, Kwekwe and Gokwe South had higher proportion of households with high dietary diversity. About 56 and 52% of the households were categorized as having high diversity in Mutasa and Kwekwe districts, respectively. Higher dietary diversity was confined to districts located in relatively high rainfall regions.

### *Econometric results*

#### Nutrition education, farm production diversity, and commercialization

Table 5 shows estimates of the association between nutrition education and dietary diversity. Results from the negative binomial regression show that nutrition education and in particular access to child feeding and care information has a positive and significant association with household, women, and children dietary diversity. Nutrition education on child feeding and care practices increases household, women, and child nutrition by 3, 9 and 24%, respectively.

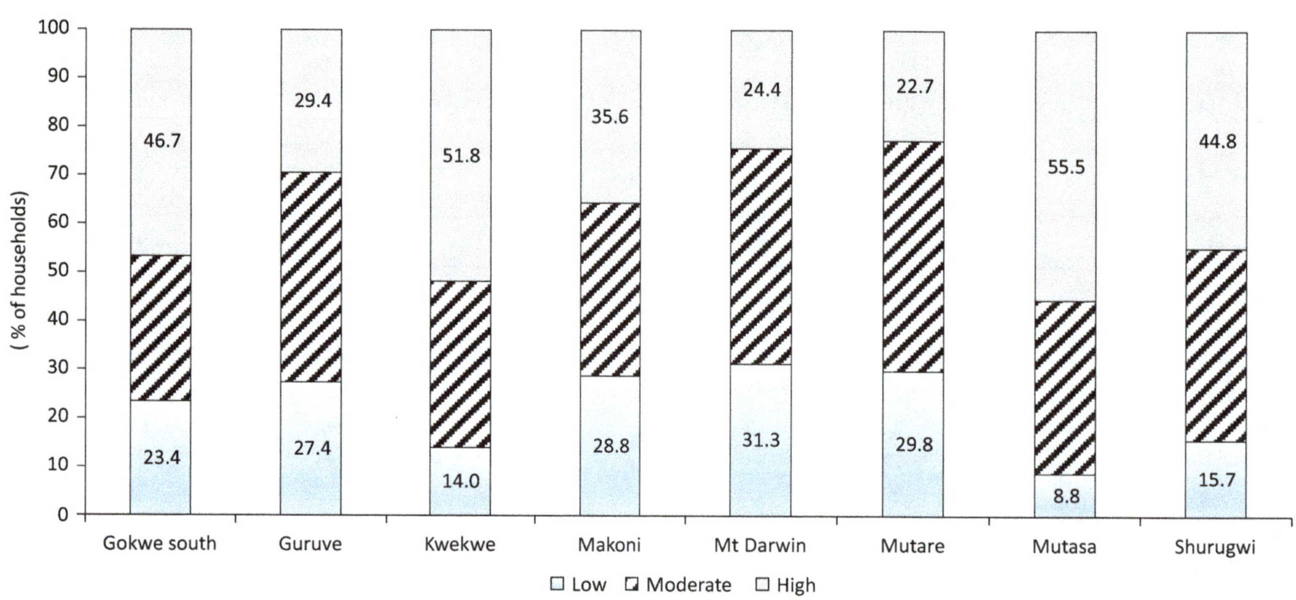


*Fig. 1.* Proportion of households by dietary diversity tertile.

*Table 5.* Nutrition education, farm production diversity, and commercialization on household, women, and child dietary diversity

| | HDDS | WDDS | CDDS |
|---|---|---|---|
| | IRR | IRR | IRR |
| Nutrition information | 1.00 (0.97–1.03) | 0.98 (0.94–1.03) | 1.03 (0.89–1.20) |
| Child feeding and care | 1.03** (1.00–1.06) | 1.09*** (1.04–1.14) | 1.24** (1.04–1.50) |
| Farm production diversity | 1.03*** (1.03–1.04) | 1.04*** (1.03–1.05) | 1.01 (0.98–1.05) |
| Market participation | 1.06*** (1.04–1.09) | 1.13*** (1.09–1.16) | 1.15*** (1.04–1.28) |
| Age | 1.00 (1.00–1.00) | 1.00** (1.00–1.00) | 1.00** (1.00–1.01) |
| Gender | 0.99 (0.95–1.02) | 1.01 (0.95–1.07) | 0.96 (0.83–1.12) |
| Marital | 1.02 (0.98–1.06) | 1.00 (0.94–1.07) | 1.11 (0.92–1.33) |
| Education | 1.06*** (1.03–1.08) | 1.07*** (1.03–1.11) | 1.14** (1.01–1.28) |
| Household size | 1.00 (1.00–1.00) | 0.99** (0.98–1.00) | 0.99 (0.97–1.02) |
| Orphans | 1.00 (0.99–1.01) | 1.01* (0.99–1.03) | 1.04 (0.98–1.10) |
| Chronically ill | 0.99 (0.96–1.01) | 1.00 (0.96–1.04) | 0.93 (0.77–1.14) |
| Land size | 1.00 (1.00–1.01) | 1.01*** (1.00–1.02) | 0.98 (0.96–1.01) |
| Total income | 1.00*** (1.00–1.00) | 1.00*** (1.00–1.00) | 1.00 (1.00–1.00) |
| Gender of child (male) | – | – | 1.03 (0.93–1.14) |
| District dummies | Yes | Yes | Yes |
| Constant | 5.27*** (4.92–5.65) | 2.80*** (2.51–3.12) | 3.32*** (2.32–4.75) |
| No. of observations | 2,801 | 2,272 | 499 |

HDDS, household dietary diversity score; WDDS, women dietary diversity score; CDDS, child dietary diversity score; IRR, incidence rate ratios; CI, confidence interval.

The dependent variables are household, women, and CDDS. Models were estimated with negative binomial estimator. IRRs are shown with 95% CI in parentheses. *, **, and *** Statistically significant at the 10, 5, and 1% level, respectively.

Farm diversification has a positive and significant association with household and women dietary diversity. The sample consists of subsistence-oriented households, who consume the large part of what is produced on the farm and these results are expected. Producing one additional crop or livestock species leads to a 3 and 4% increase in household and women dietary diversity, respectively. Yet, the effects are relatively small. Commercialization is associated with positive nutritional outcomes for household, women, and children. Market participation results in 6, 13, and 15% increase in household, women, and child dietary diversity, respectively. This also confirms the result that children relied on purchased foods.

### Nutrition education, crop and livestock diversification, and commercialization

In Table 6, results from the same type of regression models are shown, but using the crop and livestock species counts as separate independent variables instead of farm production diversity. Nutrition education increases household, women, and children dietary diversity by 3, 9 and 25%, respectively. Increasing crop diversity by one crop species is associated with only a 4 and 5% increase in the number of food groups consumed by the household and women, respectively. Livestock diversity is positively associated with both household and individual dietary diversity. Market participation is associated with 6, 13, and 16% increase in household, women, and children dietary diversity, respectively. Furthermore, education of household head positively influenced household, women, and child nutrition.

#### *Association between individual agricultural practices and nutrition*

In this section, we assessed which agricultural practices might play a greater role in shaping household and women nutrition patterns in the sample (27). With regard to access to information on child feeding and care practices, our results are still robust and suggest that nutrition education is positively and significantly associated with women and child nutrition (Table 7). Nutrition education improves women and child nutrition by 8 and 24%, respectively. We decomposed the crop and livestock diversity to explore the association between individual farming practices and nutrition indicators. Results indicated that the cultivation of pulses and fruits were associated with a significant increase in household, women, and children dietary diversity. The cultivation of pulses increased household, women, and children dietary diversity by 19, 22, and 12%, respectively. Vegetables increased household and

*Table 6.* Nutrition education, crop and livestock diversity, and commercialization on household, women, and child dietary diversity

| | HDDS | WDDS | CDDS |
|---|---|---|---|
| | IRR | IRR | IRR |
| Nutrition information | 1.00 (0.97–1.03) | 0.98 (0.93–1.03) | 1.03 (0.89–1.19) |
| Child feeding and care | 1.03** (1.00–1.06) | 1.09*** (1.04–1.14) | 1.25** (1.05–1.50) |
| Crop diversity | 1.04*** (1.02–1.05) | 1.05*** (1.03–1.07) | 0.98 (0.93–1.04) |
| Livestock diversity | 1.03*** (1.02–1.04) | 1.03*** (1.02–1.05) | 1.04* (1.00–1.09) |
| Market participation | 1.06*** (1.04–1.08) | 1.13*** (1.09–1.16) | 1.16*** (1.04–1.30) |
| Age | 1.00 (1.00–1.00) | 1.00** (1.00–1.00) | 1.00** (1.00–1.01) |
| Gender | 0.99 (0.95–1.02) | 1.01 (0.95–1.07) | 0.96 (0.83–1.12) |
| Marital | 1.02 (0.98–1.06) | 1.00 (0.94–1.07) | 1.11 (0.92–1.33) |
| Education | 1.06*** (1.03–1.08) | 1.07*** (1.03–1.11) | 1.15** (1.02–1.29) |
| Household size | 1.00 (0.99–1.00) | 0.99** (0.98–1.00) | 0.99 (0.97–1.02) |
| Orphans | 1.00 (0.99–1.01) | 1.01* (1.00–1.03) | 1.04 (0.98–1.11) |
| Chronically ill | 0.99 (0.96–1.01) | 1.00 (0.96–1.04) | 0.93 (0.77–1.13) |
| Land size | 1.00 (1.00–1.01) | 1.01*** (1.00–1.02) | 0.99 (0.96–1.02) |
| Total income | 1.00*** (1.00–1.00) | 1.00*** (1.00–1.00) | 1.00 (1.00–1.00) |
| Gender of child (male) | – | – | 1.03 (0.93–1.14) |
| District dummies | Yes | Yes | Yes |
| Constant | 5.25*** (4.90–5.64) | 2.77*** (2.49–3.10) | 3.28*** (2.24–4.79) |
| No. of observations | 2,801 | 2,272 | 499 |

HDDS, household dietary diversity score; WDDS, women dietary diversity score; CDDS, child dietary diversity score; IRR, incidence rate ratios; CI, confidence interval.

The dependent variables are household, women, and CDDS. Models were estimated with negative binomial estimator. IRRs are shown with 95% CI in parentheses. *, **, and ***Statistically significant at the 10, 5, and 1% level, respectively.

*Table 7.* Regression analysis of nutrition education, individual crop and livestock production practices, and commercialization on household and individual-level dietary diversity

| Production system | Individual practice | HDDS | WDDS | CDDS |
|---|---|---|---|---|
| | | IRR | IRR | IRR |
| Nutrition education | Nutrition information | 1.00 (0.97–1.02) | 0.97 (0.93–1.02) | 1.00 (0.87–1.16) |
| | Child feeding and care | 1.02 (1.00–1.05) | 1.08*** (1.04–1.13) | 1.24** (1.05–1.48) |
| Crop | Pulses | 1.19*** (1.17–1.21) | 1.22*** (1.18–1.26) | 1.12** (1.00–1.26) |
| | Vegetables | 1.25*** (1.11–1.42) | 1.27*** (1.11–1.45) | 1.31 (0.89–1.94) |
| | Fruits | 1.24*** (1.21–1.26) | 1.23*** (1.19–1.27) | 1.18*** (1.06–1.31) |
| Livestock | Cattle | 1.03*** (1.01–1.06) | 1.04** (1.00–1.08) | 1.07 (0.95–1.21) |
| | Goats | 1.05*** (1.03–1.07) | 1.07*** (1.03–1.10) | 1.09 (0.97–1.22) |
| | Chickens | 1.02 (0.99–1.04) | 0.99 (0.95–1.04) | 0.88* (0.76–1.01) |
| Market | Market participation | 1.04*** (1.03–1.06) | 1.11*** (1.07–1.14) | 1.15*** (1.04–1.28) |
| | Constant | 3.81*** (3.33–4.36) | 2.08*** (1.77–2.45) | 2.48*** (1.46–4.20) |
| | No. of observations | 2,801 | 2,272 | 499 |

HDDS, household dietary diversity score; WDDS, women dietary diversity score; CDDS, child dietary diversity score; IRR, incidence rate ratios; CI, confidence interval.

The dependent variables are household, women, and CDDS. Models were estimated with negative binomial estimator. IRRs are shown with 95% CI in parentheses. *, **, and ***Statistically significant at the 10, 5, and 1% level, respectively. Model estimated with same covariates as in Table 6.

women dietary diversity by 25 and 27%, respectively. Fruit production is associated with an increase in household, women, and children dietary diversity. Goat rearing was women dietary diversity. Goat rearing increased household and women dietary diversity by 5 and 7%, respectively. Commercialization is positively and significantly associated with household, women, and child nutrition.

*Robustness checks*

We ran a series of robustness checks. First, we re-estimated Equation 2 with commercialization measured as market intensity instead of participation (Table 8). Results confirm that market intensity is positive and significantly associated with household and women nutrition. Study findings do not seem to be driven by the way commercialization is measured. Furthermore, access to child nutrition information positively influences women and children dietary diversity. In addition, results display similar findings and confirm that pulses and fruits are positively associated with household, women, and child dietary diversity. Our results are therefore quite robust.

Second, we reran the model for crop and livestock diversity and market participation as presented earlier in Table 6 with a stepwise exclusion of relevant control variables in the model specification (27, 34). With these variables removed from the model (Table 9), we found that

*Table 8.* Regression analysis of nutrition education, individual crop and livestock production practices, and commercialization on household and individual-level dietary diversity

| | Individual practice | HDDS | WDDS | CDDS |
|---|---|---|---|---|
| | | IRR | IRR | IRR |
| Nutrition education | Nutrition information | 1.00 (0.98–1.03) | 0.99 (0.94–1.03) | 1.02 (0.89–1.18) |
| | Child feeding and care | 1.02 (0.99–1.05) | 1.08*** (1.03–1.13) | 1.23** (1.03–1.47) |
| Crop | Pulses | 1.19*** (1.17–1.21) | 1.22*** (1.18–1.26) | 1.13** (1.01–1.27) |
| | Vegetables | 1.26*** (1.12–1.43) | 1.29*** (1.13–1.47) | 1.30 (0.88–1.94) |
| | Fruits | 1.24*** (1.21–1.26) | 1.23*** (1.19–1.27) | 1.20*** (1.08–1.33) |
| Livestock | Cattle | 1.03*** (1.01–1.05) | 1.04** (1.00–1.07) | 1.06 (0.94–1.19) |
| | Goats | 1.05*** (1.03–1.07) | 1.07*** (1.04–1.11) | 1.09 (0.97–1.22) |
| | Chickens | 1.02 (0.99–1.05) | 1.00 (0.95–1.04) | 0.89 (0.77–1.03) |
| Market | Market intensity | 1.10*** (1.05–1.16) | 1.16*** (1.06–1.26) | 0.98 (0.74–1.30) |
| | Constant | 3.84*** (3.36–4.39) | 2.11*** (1.80–2.48) | 2.61*** (1.54–4.43) |
| | No. of observations | 2,801 | 2,272 | 499 |

HDDS, household dietary diversity score; WDDS, women dietary diversity score; CDDS, child dietary diversity score; IRR, incidence rate ratios; CI, confidence interval.

The dependent variables are household, women, and CDDS. Models were estimated with negative binomial estimator. IRRs are shown with 95% CI in parentheses. *, **, and ***Statistically significant at the 10, 5, and 1% level, respectively. Model estimated with same covariates as in Table 6.

*Table 9.* Robustness checks: nutrition education, crop and livestock diversity, and commercialization on household and women dietary diversity

| | Panel A: Head characteristics (age, sex, marital, and education) excluded | | | Panel B: Wealth (land, income) excluded | | |
|---|---|---|---|---|---|---|
| | HDDS | WDDS | CDDS | HDDS | WDDS | CDDS |
| | IRR | IRR | IRR | IRR | IRR | IRR |
| Nutrition information | 1.00 (0.97–1.03) | 0.98 (0.94–1.03) | 1.03 (0.89–1.20) | 1.00 (0.97–1.03) | 0.98 (0.94–1.03) | 1.02 (0.88–1.18) |
| Child feeding and care | 1.03** (1.00–1.06) | 1.09*** (1.04–1.14) | 1.24** (1.04–1.48) | 1.03** (1.00–1.07) | 1.09*** (1.04–1.14) | 1.26** (1.06–1.50) |
| Crop diversity | 1.04*** (1.03–1.05) | 1.05*** (1.04–1.07) | 0.99 (0.94–1.04) | 1.04*** (1.03–1.05) | 1.06*** (1.04–1.07) | 0.98 (0.93–1.03) |
| Livestock diversity | 1.03*** (1.02–1.04) | 1.04*** (1.02–1.05) | 1.04* (1.00–1.09) | 1.03*** (1.02–1.04) | 1.04*** (1.02–1.05) | 1.05** (1.00–1.09) |
| Market participation | 1.06*** (1.04–1.09) | 1.13*** (1.09–1.16) | 1.16*** (1.05–1.30) | 1.07*** (1.05–1.09) | 1.14*** (1.10–1.17) | 1.18*** (1.06–1.31) |
| Constant | 5.59*** (5.32–5.87) | 3.10*** (2.86–3.36) | 4.48*** (3.29–6.09) | 5.24 (4.89–5.62) | 2.75*** (2.47–3.08) | 3.26*** (2.23–4.76) |
| Observations | 2,801 | 2,272 | 499 | 2,814 | 2,282 | 501 |

HDDS, household dietary diversity score; WDDS, women dietary diversity score; CDDS, child dietary diversity score; IRR, incidence rate ratios; CI, confidence interval.

The dependent variables are household, women, and CDDS. Models were estimated with negative binomial estimator. IRRs are shown with 95% CI in parentheses. *, **, and ***Statistically significant at the 10, 5, and 1% level, respectively. Model estimated with same covariates as in Table 6.

the influence of nutrition education, crop and livestock diversity, and commercialization on household, women, and child nutrition remained significant and positive, thereby providing evidence for the overall robustness of the model. We interpret this as evidence that the main results do not suffer from omitted variable bias (18).

## Discussion

Most households consumed starchy staples, whereas few consumed eggs and animal-based foods. Similar results on consumption of eggs were found in Haiti (33), while Galbete et al. (35) found that diets were concentrated on starchy foods and animal-based products in rural and urban Ghana, respectively. Households' own agricultural production was the main source of foods consumed the day before the survey.

To our knowledge, only few studies have analyzed the role of nutrition education on household and individual-level nutrition. In addition, this is a unique study that jointly examines the effects of nutrition education, farm production diversity, and commercialization on household, women, and children dietary diversity in a developing country context. The results of this study clearly support the role of nutrition education for enhancing household and individual nutrition in Zimbabwe. These findings resonate with Hirvonen, Hoddinott, Minten and Stifel (1) who found that nutrition knowledge leads to considerable improvements in children's dietary diversity in Ethiopia. BCC and nutrition-specific approaches that target women and children are needed to accelerate progress toward improved nutrition (4). The positive association of farm production diversity on dietary diversity confirms the findings of Koppmair, Kassie and Qaim (21) and Malapit, Kadiyala, Quisumbing, Cunningham and Tyagi (14), highlighting the crucial role of farm production diversity on improving household and women dietary diversity. Similarly, Sibhatu, Krishna and Qaim (18) found the positive association between farm production diversity and dietary diversity. We found no association between farm production diversity and child dietary diversity. These results contradict other study findings (4, 21, 34). Our study measured dietary diversity in relatively younger children (6–23 months) compared to other studies, for example, by Koppmair, Kassie and Qaim (21) and Saaka, Osman and Hoeschle-Zeledon (4) that included children up to 5 years. Our results are partly explained by the fact that younger children tend to rely on purchased foods and less on foods from own production.

Crop diversity was significantly and positively associated with household and women dietary diversity and not children dietary diversity. In rural Malawi, Koppmair, Kassie and Qaim (21) and Jones, Shrinivas and Bezner-Kerr (8) found similar results that crop diversification improves dietary diversity. Livestock diversity is positively associated with both household and individual dietary diversity. However, the effects are relatively smaller, suggesting that substantial improvement in dietary diversity would require very high levels of crop and livestock diversity if these were the only strategies available. Other studies found similar results that livestock improves nutrition (36, 37). Kabunga, Ghosh and Webb (36) found that ownership of improved dairy cows enhanced household welfare and child nutrition in Uganda. In Northern Rwanda, Rawlins, Pimkina, Barrett, Pedersen and Wydick (37) highlight the positive association between household ownership of dairy cows and child linear growth.

Results indicated that the cultivation of pulses and fruits were associated with a significant increase in household, women, and children dietary diversity. The important contribution of pulses for nutrition is also highlighted in Kenya (27). Goat rearing was significant and positively correlated with household and women dietary diversity. These results suggest that crop–livestock integration is crucial for improved nutrition. The preservation and storage of fodder for livestock feeding in dry season is one crop–livestock integration activity that needs to be promoted to enhance livestock nutrition. Access to markets for buying food and for selling farm produce increased household, women, and children dietary diversity. Various scholars found similar results for Malawi (21) and Ethiopia (1, 38). Hence, improving access to markets through better infrastructure and institutions is a promising strategy to improve nutrition.

## Conclusion and policy implications

This study investigated the role of nutrition education, farm production diversity, and commercialization on household, women, and child dietary diversity. We used data collected in 2016 in eight LFSP districts in Zimbabwe. There is renewed attention on the factors that directly affect household and individual-level nutritional status, and efforts are being made to ensure that caregivers and individuals understand which diets are appropriate for which age groups. In turn, this has led to the use of BCC interventions that seek to improve household and individual nutrition knowledge and encourage behavior change adoption. BCC interventions are also expected to improve decision-making on nutrition and child care since they encourage active participation of both men and women. In this study, we find that nutrition knowledge leads to improvements in household, women, and children's dietary diversity. Overall, results demonstrate the potential value of promoting nutrition education via BCC interventions to enhance household and individual-level nutrition. BCC strategies, for example, messages on healthy eating and balanced diets should be disseminated to households, women, children, and men through various platforms, for example, print and electronic media, food fairs, field days, and school curriculums and dramas to enhance improved nutrition.

The results show that farm production diversity had a strong and positive association with household and women dietary diversity. These results suggest that farm production diversification has the potential to improve household and women nutrition, highlighting the importance of individual-level analysis. Furthermore, when farm production is disaggregated, our results show that crop diversity is positively associated with household and women dietary diversity. The association between individual farming practices and nutrition shows interesting results. The cultivation of pulses and fruits is positively associated with household, women, and child dietary diversity, while vegetables and goats had significant relationship with household and women dietary diversity only. This suggests that interventions that promote pulses, vegetables, fruits, and small stock production maximize nutritional content of diets and are beneficial for household, women, and child nutrition.

Market participation is positively associated with household, women, and child dietary diversity. Smallholder farmers have limited access to markets to sell their products. They often live in remote locations where infrastructure is poor and buyers do not travel. In addition, they have poor skills to negotiate with buyers and also lack access to credit. Therefore, improving access to markets through better infrastructure and institutions and promoting programs that link farmers to the market are promising strategies to improve nutrition.

These findings demonstrate the importance of household and individual-level analysis. Furthermore, results demonstrate the significant role of women crops: pulses and vegetables on women and child nutrition. Interventions that minimize trade-offs between women child care and agricultural production should be promoted, for example, the adoption and use of labor-saving technologies such as fuel-efficient stoves, shellers, and ridgers. Taken together, the results show the need to promote nutrition education, farm production diversification, and commercialization as complementary interventions for improving household and individual nutrition.

## Limitations

This article is based on cross-sectional data which were collected at a single point in time. This study has limitations in that we cannot account for seasonality in diets. We have data on whether the household, women, and child consumed different foods, but we do not have information on the quantities consumed. In addition to this, as the study considered only the 24-h recall method, it might not accurately reflect participants past feeding dietary habit. Moreover, there might be a recall bias, and being a self-reported study might not give the exact figure of the minimum dietary diversity practice. Furthermore, establishing causality with cross-section data is a challenge. Even if we are able to find a good instruments, the instrumental variable regression results will only be as good as the underlying instruments. Future research might need to consider use of panel data to address these shortcomings. Finally, the study findings are based on a LFSP targeting the poor and vulnerable households and as such our results are not nationally representative.

## Acknowledgements

The authors are grateful to the farmers and extension staff in the survey districts for their enthusiasm and collaboration in providing information during fieldwork. We are grateful to the UK Department for International Development through Food and Agriculture Organization for funding the research. We acknowledge the research assistants for providing constructive and very useful comments that improved the survey tool as well as collecting the data.

## Conflicts of interest and funding

The authors declare that they have no conflicts of interest. The article is original work and has not been submitted for publication elsewhere.

## References

1. Hirvonen K, Hoddinott J, Minten B, Stifel D. Children's diets, nutrition knowledge, and access to markets. World Dev 2017; 95: 303–15.
2. Jones AD. Critical review of the emerging research evidence on agricultural biodiversity, diet diversity, and nutritional status in low- and middle-income countries. Nutr Rev 2017; 75(10): 769–82.
3. LFSP. Livelihoods and Food Security Programme Zimbabwe. Available from: https://lfspzim.com/what-is-lfsp/background/projects/ [cited 3 March 2018].
4. Saaka M, Osman SM, Hoeschle-Zeledon I. Relationship between agricultural biodiversity and dietary diversity of children aged 6–36 months in rural areas of Northern Ghana. Food Nutr Res 2017; 61: 1391668.
5. Pelto GH, Martin SL, van Liere MJ, Fabrizio CS. Perspectives and reflections on the practice of behaviour change communication for infant and young child feeding. Matern Child Nutr 2016; 12: 245–61.
6. Dewey KG, Adu-Afarwuah S. Systematic review of the efficacy and effectiveness of complementary feeding interventions in developing countries. Matern Child Nutr 2008; 4(Suppl 1): 24–85.
7. Zimbabwe Vulnerability Assessment Committee. Zimbabwe Vulnerability Assessment Committee (ZimVAC) rural livelihoods assessment. Harare, Zimbabwe; 2016. Available from: http://www.fnc.org.zw/downloads/Bulletins/2016%20Bulletins/ZimVAC%202016%20Rural%20Livelihoods%20Assessment.pdf [cited 4 July 2017].
8. Jones AD, Shrinivas A, Bezner-Kerr R. Farm production diversity is associated with greater household dietary diversity in Malawi: findings from nationally representative data. Food Policy 2014; 46: 1–12.
9. Carletto G, Ruel M, Winters P, Zezza A. Farm-level pathways to improved nutritional status: introduction to the special issue. J Dev Stud 2015; 51: 945–57.
10. Ruel MT, Alderman H. Nutrition-sensitive interventions and programmes: how can they help to accelerate progress in improving maternal and child nutrition? Lancet 2013; 382: 536–51.

11. Arimond M, Wiesmann D, Becquey E, Carriquiry A, Daniels MC, Deitchler M, et al. Simple food group diversity indicators predict micronutrient adequacy of women's diets in 5 diverse, resource-poor settings. J Nutr 2010; 140: 2059S–69S.
12. Akaakohol MA, Aye GC. Diversification and farm household welfare in Makurdi, Benue State, Nigeria. Dev Stud Res. 2014; 1: 168–75.
13. Carletto C, Corral P, Guelfi A. Agricultural commercialization and nutrition revisited: empirical evidence from three African countries. Food Policy 2017; 67: 106–18.
14. Malapit HJL, Kadiyala S, Quisumbing AR, Cunningham K, Tyagi P. Women's empowerment mitigates the negative effects of low production diversity on maternal and child nutrition in Nepal. J Dev Stud. 2015; 51: 1097–123.
15. Pellegrini L, Tasciotti L. Crop diversification, dietary diversity and agricultural income: empirical evidence from eight developing countries. Can J Dev Stud 2014; 35: 211–27.
16. Seng K. The effects of nonfarm activities on farm households' food consumption in rural Cambodia. Dev Stud Res 2015; 2: 77–89.
17. Quisumbing AR, Meinzen-Dick R, Raney TL, Croppenstedt A, Behrman JA, Peterman A. Gender in agriculture. Dordrecht: Springer Netherlands; 2014.
18. Sibhatu KT, Krishna VV, Qaim M. Production diversity and dietary diversity in smallholder farm households. Proc Natl Acad Sci U S A 2015; 112: 10657–62.
19. Shively G, Sununtnasuk C. Agricultural diversity and child stunting in Nepal. J Dev Stud 2015; 51: 1078–96.
20. Snapp SS, Fisher M. 'Filling the maize basket' supports crop diversity and quality of household diet in Malawi. Food Security 2015; 7: 83–96.
21. Koppmair S, Kassie M, Qaim M. Farm production, market access and dietary diversity in Malawi. Public Health Nutr 2017; 20(2): 325–35.
22. Swindale A, Bilinsky P. Household dietary diversity score (HDDS) for measurement of household food access: indicator guide: indicator guide (v. 2): food and nutrition technical assistance project. FHI360/FANTA: Washington, DC; 2006.
23. Swindale A, Ohri-Vachaspati P. Measuring household food consumption: a technical guide: food and nutrition technical assistance project. FHI360/FANTA: Washington, DC; 2004.
24. Muhoozi GKM, Atukunda P, Mwadime R, Iversen PO, Westerberg AC. Nutritional and developmental status among 6- to 8-month-old children in southwestern Uganda: a cross-sectional study. Food Nutr Res 2016; 60: 30270.
25. Kansiime MK, Watiti J, Mchana A, Jumah R, Musebe R, Rware H. Achieving scale of farmer reach with improved common bean technologies: the role of village-based advisors. J Agric Educ Extension 2018; 1071: 1–18.
26. Kiptot E, Franzel S. Voluntarism as an investment in human, social and financial capital: evidence from a farmer-to-farmer extension program in Kenya. Agric Hum Values 2014; 31: 231–43.
27. Romeo A, Meerman J, Demeke M, Scognamillo A, Asfaw S. Linking farm diversification to household diet diversification: evidence from a sample of Kenyan ultra-poor farmers. Food Security 2016; 8: 1069–85.
28. Cameron AC, Trivedi PK. Microeconometrics using Stata. College Station, TX: Stata Press; 2010.
29. Greene WH. Econometric analysis. 7th ed. Boston, MA: Prentice Hall; 2012.
30. Hilbe JM. Negative binomial regression. 2nd ed. Cambridge: Cambridge University Press; 2011.
31. Wilber ST, Fu R. Risk ratios and odds ratios for common events in cross-sectional and cohort studies. Acad Emerg Med 2010; 17: 649–51.
32. Long JS, Freese J. Regression models for categorical dependent variables using Stata. [place unknown]: [publisher unknown]; 2014.
33. Pauzé E, Batal M, Philizaire Y, Blanchet R, Sanou D. Determinants of diet quality among rural households in an intervention zone of Grande Anse, Haiti. Food Security 2016; 8: 1123–34.
34. Galbete C, Nicolaou M, Meeks KA, de-Graft Aikins A, Addo J, Amoah SK, et al. Food consumption, nutrient intake, and dietary patterns in Ghanaian migrants in Europe and their compatriots in Ghana. Food Nutr Res 2017; 61: 1341809.
35. Kabunga NS, Ghosh S, Webb P. Does ownership of improved dairy cow breeds improve child nutrition? A pathway analysis for Uganda. PLoS One 2017; 12: e0187816.
36. Hirvonen K, Hoddinott J. Agricultural production and children's diets: evidence from rural Ethiopia. Agric Econ 2017; 48: 469–80.
37. Rawlins R, Pimkina S, Barrett CB, Pedersen S, Wydick B. Got milk?: the impact of Heifer International's livestock donation programs in Rwanda on nutritional outcomes. Food Policy 2014; 44: 202–13.
38. Sibhatu KT, Qaim M. Rural food security, subsistence agriculture, and seasonality. PLoS One 2017; 12: e0186406.

***Conrad Murendo**
International Crops Research Institute for the Semi-Arid Tropics
P. O. Box 776
Bulawayo, Zimbabwe
Email: cmurendo@hotmail.com

# 16

# Pre-pregnancy and early pregnancy dietary behavior in relation to maternal and newborn health in the Norwegian Fit for Delivery study – a post hoc observational analysis

Elisabet R. Hillesund[1*], Elling Bere[1], Linda R. Sagedal[2,3], Ingvild Vistad[2,3], Hilde L. Seiler[1], Monica K. Torstveit[1] and Nina C. Øverby[1]

[1]Department of Public Health, Sports and Nutrition, University of Agder, Kristiansand, Norway; [2]Department of Obstetrics and Gynecology, Sørlandet Hospital HF, Kristiansand, Norway; [3]Department of Research, Sørlandet Hospital HF, Kristiansand, Norway

*Abstract*

***Background:*** Randomized controlled trials targeting maternal dietary and physical activity behaviors during pregnancy have generally failed to accomplish reductions in the prevalence of adverse maternal and neonatal outcomes. Interventions carried out during pregnancy could thus be missing the mark in maximizing intervention health benefit.

***Objective:*** To investigate whether *pre-pregnancy* and *early pregnancy* dietary behavior as reported at inclusion into the Norwegian Fit for Delivery (NFFD) trial was associated with maternal and neonatal outcomes irrespective of subsequent randomization assignment.

***Design:*** The study is a post-hoc observational analysis of data from a randomized controlled lifestyle intervention. We constructed two diet scores from participant responses to a 43-item questionnaire that addressed dietary behavior in retrospect (*pre-pregnancy* diet score) and dietary behavior at inclusion (*early pregnancy* diet score), respectively. The diet scores ranged from 0 to 10, with higher score reflecting healthier dietary behavior. Associations between diet scores and maternal and neonatal health outcomes were estimated in multivariate logistic regression models.

***Results:*** A total of 591 women were eligible for analysis. A one-point increase in *pre-pregnancy* diet score was associated with lower odds of excessive gestational weight gain (GWG) (odds ratio $[OR]_{adj}$: 0.92; 95% confidence interval [CI]: 0.84–1.00, $p = 0.050$), preterm delivery ($OR_{adj}$: 0.81; 95% CI: 0.68–0.97, $p = 0.019$), and birthweight ≥ 4,000 g ($OR_{adj}$: 0.88; 95% CI: 0.78–0.99, $p = 0.038$). A one-point increase in *early pregnancy* diet score was associated with lower odds of excessive GWG ($OR_{adj}$: 0.88; 95% CI: 0.79–0.97, $p = 0.009$), preterm delivery ($OR_{adj}$: 0.82; 95% CI: 0.67–0.99, $p = 0.038$), and preeclampsia ($OR_{adj}$: 0.78; 95% CI: 0.62–0.99, $p = 0.038$).

***Discussion:*** Higher diet score either pre-pregnancy or in early pregnancy was protectively associated with excessive GWG and preterm delivery, whereas the protective association with high birthweight was confined to *pre-pregnancy* diet and with preeclampsia to *early pregnancy* diet.

***Conclusions:*** Both pre-pregnancy and early pregnancy dietary behavior was associated with important maternal and neonatal health outcomes in the NFFD dataset.

Keywords: *diet; neonatal outcome; diet score; preconception; preconception diet; pregnancy complications; pregnancy health; preeclampsia; preterm birth; gestational weight gain*

Excessive gestational weight gain (GWG) has been identified as a potentially modifiable risk factor for adverse pregnancy outcomes based on consistent findings from several observational studies (1). In the randomized controlled Norwegian Fit for Delivery (NFFD) study, we targeted maternal weight gain through a lifestyle intervention during pregnancy and demonstrated that dietary advice and supervised exercise groups during pregnancy improved dietary behavior and physical activity level, and resulted in lower GWG compared to the control group who received standard care (2). There was, however, no accompanying reduction in common pregnancy complications such as gestational diabetes mellitus (GDM), preeclampsia, or preterm delivery, and no significant between-group differences in birthweight or other neonatal outcomes following the intervention. Other large and well-designed randomized controlled trials (RCTs) have reported similar findings, namely, a modest effect of pregnancy interventions on diet quality, physical activity level, and reduced GWG, but little or no effect on other measurable aspects of maternal and neonatal health (3–5). An individual patient data meta-analysis compiling data from several RCTs targeting lifestyle during pregnancy recently confirmed the lack of intervention effect on pregnancy complications and neonatal health outcomes despite self-reported improvement in diet and physical activity (6). Findings from large prospective observational studies have, on the other contrary, repeatedly indicated protective associations between healthier maternal diet and pregnancy complications such as preeclampsia (7, 8), preterm delivery (8–12), and GDM (13).

These seemingly contradictory findings from observational versus experimental studies could possibly be reconciled by taking into account the time window represented by the dietary data. The abovementioned observational studies information on maternal diet was collected during pregnancy. High correlations have previously been demonstrated between presently reported diet and diet reported several years ahead in the general population (14). Dietary data collected during pregnancy may thus simultaneously represent longer-term diet and complicate the interpretation of whether observed associations between diet and pregnancy outcomes relate to diet during pregnancy per se or rather to maternal pre-pregnancy diet and nutritional status before conception. This distinction could be of considerable public health interest, because pregnancy complications such as GDM, preterm birth, and preeclampsia are relatively common and may hamper maternal and newborn immediate and long-term health with associated large individual and socioeconomic life course costs (15). Effective prevention strategies and relevant stages for prevention are therefore being searched for (16).

In the NFFD study, participants responded to questions about diet and dietary behavior both at the time of inclusion around week 15 of pregnancy and, in retrospect, to identical questions covering the period before getting pregnant. This left us with the opportunity to investigate both pre-pregnancy and early pregnancy dietary behavior in relation to subsequent maternal and neonatal outcomes and compare the respective effect sizes. The aim of this observational post-hoc analysis was thus to investigate whether NFFD participants' dietary behavior *before* inclusion, assessed both pre-pregnancy and in early pregnancy, was associated with aspects of maternal and neonatal health irrespective of subsequent randomization assignment.

## Methods

The present paper is a post-hoc analysis carried out among pregnant women participating in the NFFD study (17). We treated the study population as a cohort for investigating pre-intervention diet–outcome associations independently of randomization assignment but took potential randomization-related effects into account by adjusting for randomization status in the analyses and by carrying out sensitivity analyses confined to the control group. Although the main study and effects of the lifestyle intervention have been thoroughly described elsewhere (2), they have been briefly described below.

### *The Norwegian Fit for Delivery trial*

The NFFD study is a population-based lifestyle RCT carried out among nulliparous pregnant women in Southern Norway between 2009 and 2013 (ClinicalTrials.gov ID NCT01001689). The main aim of the study was to facilitate optimal GWG through dietary advice and twice-weekly supervised exercise lessons, and thereby reducing the number of infants with high birthweight. The study protocol and the effectiveness of the intervention on various outcomes have been published previously (17–21).

### *Participants*

Women were eligible for participation if they were 18 years or older, nulliparous, had pre-pregnancy body mass index (BMI) ≥19 kg/m$^2$, were 20 weeks pregnant or less at inclusion, carrying a single fetus, literate in Norwegian or English, and had provided written consent (2). Exclusion criteria comprised pre-existing diabetes mellitus, disabilities precluding participation in a physical fitness program, ongoing substance abuse, or planned relocation outside the study area before delivery. Out of 1,610 potentially eligible women, a total of 606 nulliparous women agreed to participate and were consecutively enrolled from eight health care clinics between September 2009 and February 2013. Mean gestational age at inclusion was 15 weeks. Participants were randomly assigned to the control ($n$ = 303) or intervention group ($n$ = 303), respectively. Twelve women were later withdrawn from the study because of miscarriage ($n$ = 6), twin pregnancy ($n$ = 2), and relocation outside study area ($n$ = 4). One woman was excluded from participation in the trial due to very low BMI after being mistakenly included, and two women withdrew from the trial without giving permission to use data. A total of 591 participants were thus included in intention-to-treat analyses in the main study and were also eligible for the observational analyses in the present study.

### *The 10 dietary behaviors that were targeted in the diet intervention*

The diet intervention aimed at facilitating optimal GWG and otherwise promoting a healthy pregnancy through simple diet rules aimed at heightening participant reflection on dietary behavior (see below). We based the intervention components on 10 dietary recommendations developed specifically for the study. The rationale for the 10 recommendations has been published previously (22).

The 10 dietary recommendations in the NFFD trial are the following (19):

1. Eat regular meals
2. Drink water when thirsty
3. Eat vegetables with dinner every day
4. In-between meals – choose fruits and vegetables
5. Eat sweets and snacks only when you really appreciate it
6. Choose small portion sizes of unhealthy foods
7. Limit your intake of added sugar
8. Limit your intake of salt
9. Do not eat beyond satiety
10. Read nutritional labels

Women randomized to the intervention group received an illustrated booklet describing the dietary recommendations and their simplified rationale shortly after randomization. The recommendations were reinforced and tailored to the individual in two telephone sessions with a trained advisor, scheduled approximately 4–6 weeks apart. The intervention also comprised access to supervised exercise classes twice weekly, including strength training and cardiovascular exercise at moderate intensity. Women in the control group received routine pregnancy care but answered the same questionnaires and received the same medical follow-up as intervention participants, including extra ultrasound investigations and blood tests. The present paper addresses pre-intervention dietary behavior in relation to maternal and neonatal health outcomes.

### *The Norwegian Fit for Delivery diet score*

We operationalized pre-intervention dietary behavior as a *pre-pregnancy* and an *early pregnancy* diet score, respectively. The scores were designed to reflect participant degree of compliance with the 10 dietary recommendations prior to inclusion into the study. Both diet scores were built from 10 subscales, each subscale referring to a corresponding dietary behavior. The subscales were built from participants' responses to the baseline questionnaire that included a 43-item questionnaire with food frequency questions (FFQ) and questions about aspects of dietary behavior. All 43 questions addressed pre-pregnancy diet in retrospect, and present diet at the time of inclusion (e.g. 'how often did you drink water before you became pregnant?' and 'how often do you drink water now?'). The questionnaire only covered selected aspects of diet and dietary behavior, mainly the dietary aspects that were targeted in the NFFD intervention (22). The subscales could be single variables or sum scores constructed from relevant questionnaire responses. Each subscale was dichotomized with the sample median as cutoff, and participants with the healthier behavior were assigned '1' in each subscale, whereas the other half of the sample was assigned '0'. Individual diet scoring thus ranged from 0 to 10, with higher score indicating healthier behavior. For some of the analyses, participants were categorized as having low [0–3], medium [4–5], or high [6–10] diet score. Supplementary Table 1 provides an overview of the variables that were included in each subscale including cutoffs for scoring in each individual subscale. In brief, the behaviors that yielded scoring in the pre-pregnancy and early pregnancy subscales were as follows:

1. having ≥24 main meals/week (≥25 in the early pregnancy subscale)
2. 44% or more of drinking events being water (≥46% in the early pregnancy subscale)
3. having vegetables with dinner ≥5 times/week
4. choosing fruits or vegetables for in-between meal snacks ≥3 times/week (≥5 times/week in the early pregnancy subscale)
5. never eating sweets and snacks without appreciation
6. buying small portion size of one or more unhealthy food items (soda, salty crisps, or chocolate)
7. consuming sugar-rich food items once a day or less
8. consuming fast-foods, snacks, or other salty food less than daily
9. eating beyond satiety less than once a week
10. reading nutrition labels on foods sometimes or often.

A detailed description of the construction of the diet score and its test–retest reliability has been published previously (22).

### *Maternal and child outcomes*

Outcomes in the present study were excessive and inadequate GWG, preeclampsia, preterm delivery, GDM, and various measures of birthweight. Birth records and hospital charts were reviewed in retrospect to validate information on maternal and neonatal outcomes (2)

All participants were weighed at their healthcare clinic at inclusion, and at Sorlandet Hospital at 30 gestational-weeks (Tanita BC 418, Tokyo, Japan). Height was measured with a stadiometer (Seca Leicester, Hamburg, Germany). Pre-pregnancy BMI ($kg/m^2$) was calculated based on self-reported pre-pregnancy weight (kg) and measured height (m). Participants were also weighed on admission to the delivery ward. If admission weight was not available, the last weight in the prenatal record was recorded with its corresponding date. Total weight gain

*Table 1.* Maternal characteristics and correlation with pre-pregnancy and early pregnancy diet scores in the Norwegian Fit for Delivery study ($n$ = 591)

| Maternal characteristics | Number included | Percentage | Pre-pregnancy diet score Mean (SD) | Early pregnancy diet score Mean (SD) |
|---|---|---|---|---|
| **Age at inclusion (years)** | 591 | | | |
| **<25** | 149 | 25.2 | 4.3 (2.1) | 4.7 (1.9) |
| **25–29** | 273 | 46.2 | 4.5 (2.2) | 4.9 (2.1) |
| **30–34** | 129 | 21.8 | 4.8 (2.1) | 5.2 (2.1) |
| **35+** | 40 | 6.8 | 4.7 (2.4) | 5.4 (1.9) |
| **Education (years)** | 588 | | | |
| **≤12** | 187 | 31.8 | 4.0 (2.1) | 4.6 (2.0) |
| **13–15** | 192 | 32.7 | 4.6 (2.2) | 4.9 (2.1) |
| **≥16** | 209 | 35.5 | 5.1 (2.1) | 5.4 (2.0) |
| **Missing** | 3 | | | |
| **BMI category pre-pregnancy** | 590 | | | |
| **<25.0** | 426 | 71.5 | 5.4 (1.9) | 5.0 (1.6) |
| **25.0–29.9** | 119 | 20.8 | 4.4 (2.1) | 4.8 (2.0) |
| **≥30.0** | 45 | 7.6 | 4.4 (2.4) | 5.1 (1.9) |
| **Missing** | 1 | | | |
| **Current smoking** | | | | |
| **No smoking** | 589 | 96.1 | 4.6 (2.2) | 5.0 (2.1) |
| **Current smoking** | 23 | 3.9 | 3.1 (1.8) | 4.1 (1.9) |
| **Missing** | 2 | | | |
| **Marital status** | 589 | | | |
| **Married/boyfriend/partner** | 567 | 96.3 | 4.6 (2.2) | 5.0 (2.1) |
| **Other** | 22 | 3.7 | 4.2 (2.1) | 4.5 (1.7) |
| **Missing** | 2 | | | |
| **Occupation** | | | | |
| **Work outside home** | 496 | 84.2 | 4.6 (2.2) | 4.9 (2.0) |
| **Student** | 51 | 8.7 | 5.1 (2.2) | 5.5 (2.2) |
| **Unemployed** | 23 | 3.9 | 4.2 (1.6) | 4.8 (2.0) |
| **Sick leave/disabled** | 11 | 1.9 | 3.5 (2.0) | 4.9 (1.9) |
| **Homemaker** | 8 | 1.4 | 3.6 (1.7) | 4.1 (1.4) |
| **Missing** | 2 | | | |
| **Income (NOK)** | | | | |
| **≤400,000** | 183 | 31.2 | 4.3 (2.2) | 4.7 (2.0) |
| **400,001–700,000** | 163 | 27.8 | 4.5 (2.1) | 5.1 (2.1) |
| **>700,000** | 202 | 34.4 | 4.9 (2.2) | 5.1 (2.0) |
| **Refrain from response** | 39 | 6.6 | 4.2 (2.4) | 4.9 (2.1) |
| **Missing** | 4 | | | |
| **Physical activity level in early pregnancy**[a] | 481 | | | |
| **Low activity** | 127 | 26.4 | 4.2 (1.9) | 4.7 (1.8) |
| **Medium activity** | 280 | 58.2 | 4.8 (2.3) | 5.3 (2.2) |
| **High activity** | 74 | 15.4 | 5.0 (2.3) | 5.0 (2.0) |
| **Missing** | 110 | | | |
| **Randomization status** | 591 | | | |
| **Control** | 295 | 49.9 | 4.6 (2.2) | 5.0 (2.1) |
| **Intervention** | 296 | 50.1 | 4.5 (2.1) | 5.0 (2.1) |

BMI, Body Mass Index; NOK, Norwegian currency (1 US Dollar).

[a]Based on responses to the International Physical Activity Questionnaire short form (IPAQ-SF) and scored and categorized according to IPAQ analysis algorithms into physical activity categories (27)

was calculated for women who delivered at ≥37 gestational-weeks with measured weight available within 2 weeks of admission (2). Excessive GWG was defined as pregnancy weight gain measured at term exceeding the optimal range proposed by the 2009 Institute of Medicine (IOM) guidelines, that is, >16.0 kg if normal weight, >11.5 kg if overweight, and >9.0 kg if obese pre-pregnancy (1). Inadequate GWG was defined as weight gain below the BMI-specific optimal range, that is, <11.5 kg if normal weight, <7.0 kg if overweight, and <5.0 kg if obese pre-pregnancy (1). Inadequate and excessive GWG were treated as dichotomous variables in the analyses (excessive GWG yes/no and inadequate GWG yes/no).

Participants underwent a glucose tolerance test in gestational week 30, with measurement of fasting serum glucose after overnight fasting, and postprandial level 2 h after intake of 75 g of glucose. Glucose levels ≥7.8 mmol/l at 2 h were classified as elevated, based on 2006 WHO criteria (23). The diagnosis of GDM was subsequently ascertained from hospital charts.

Preeclampsia was diagnosed based on guidelines adopted by the Norwegian Federation of Obstetricians and Gynecologists; an increase in blood pressure to at least ≥140 systolic or 90 mm Hg diastolic after 20th gestational week combined with proteinuria (protein excretion of at least 0.3 g/24 h or ≥1+ on dip-stick), both measured at least twice (2, 24). Severe preeclampsia was defined as preeclampsia before 34 weeks of pregnancy and/or severity of symptoms, as documented in hospital charts. Cases of eclampsia and HELLP-syndrome (preeclampsia affecting hemolysis, liver function, and platelet counts) were included as severe preeclampsia cases.

Preterm delivery was defined as delivery before 37 completed weeks of gestation. Estimated date of confinement was determined as part of routine prenatal care for all participants, based on ultrasound examinations supplemented with date of the last menstrual cycle.

We assessed birthweight according to widely used cutoffs for macrosomia (≥4,000 g and ≥4,500 g) and low birthweight (<2,500 g) (25), and relative to national reference values for gestational age and gender. Being small for gestational age (SGA) was defined as birthweight below the 10th percentile and being large for gestational age (LGA) was equivalent to birthweight ≥90th percentile, both calculated according to sex and gestational age-specific references from the Medical Birth Registry of Norway (MBRN) (26).

*Sociodemographic variables and potential confounders*

Information on maternal age, education, marital status, occupation, income, smoking, pre-pregnancy weight and early pregnancy physical activity level was collected from the baseline questionnaire completed upon inclusion. BMI was calculated from self-reported pre-pregnancy weight and height measured with a stadiometer at inclusion (Secca Leicester, Hamburg, Germany). Physical activity level was assessed with the International Physical Activity Questionnaire short form (IPAQ-SF) (27, 28) that quantifies frequency and duration of physical activity in the intensity categories: vigorous, moderate, walking and sitting during the last 7 days (27). In addition to intensity, frequency and duration of physical activity are assessed. Responses were scored according to IPAQ-SF analysis algorithms into three categories denoting low, medium or high physical activity level.

*Statistics*

Statistical analyses were performed with SPSS for IBM statistical software package version 24.0 (IBM Corporation, Armonk, NY, USA). A two-sided $p$-value of ≤ 0.05 was considered significant. Maternal age, weight, height, and BMI are presented with mean and standard deviation (SD). Sociodemographic variables are presented with number and proportions (%). We calculated mean diet score for each category of the sociodemographic variables to visualize covariance between *pre-pregnancy* and *early pregnancy* diet scores and potential confounders.

We compared dietary intake across diet score categories and presented this information with median and interquartile range (IQR) as Supplementary Table 2. Prevalence of maternal and neonatal outcomes were similarly compared across low, medium and high diet score categories and tested for trend across categories with the Mantel-Haenszel statistics (29).

We estimated crude and adjusted odds ratios (OR) and 95% confidence intervals (CI) for all outcomes with the continuous *pre-pregnancy* and *early pregnancy* diet scores as main exposure in separate tables. In the multivariate models, we included the following potential confounders: maternal age at inclusion (continuous), marital status (husband/boyfriend/partner or living alone), pre-pregnancy BMI (continuous), educational attainment (≤12, 13–15, and ≥16 years), household income (≤400,000, 401,000–700,000, and >700,000 NOK/year, equivalent to <52,000, 52,000–91,000, and <91,000 dollars/year, assessed from exchange rate on 18 September 2017), and randomization assignment (control/intervention). In the *early pregnancy* analyses, we additionally included current smoking (yes/no). A total of 110 participants had missing information on early pregnancy physical activity level. We therefore fit a third *early pregnancy* model that included early pregnancy physical activity level (low, medium, or high) along with the other potential confounders.

Given the randomized controlled design, and the fact that the intervention group improved diet and physical activity behaviors compared to the control group between randomization and delivery (19), we performed sensitivity analyses by rerunning all pre-pregnancy and early pregnancy models confined to the control group who received no intervention.

*Table 2.* Difference in prevalence of maternal and neonatal outcomes across *pre-pregnancy* and *early pregnancy* diet score categories ($n = 591$)

| Obstetrical outcomes | Included in the analysis | Number of cases | Pre-pregnancy diet score categories | | | | Early pregnancy diet score categories | | | |
|---|---|---|---|---|---|---|---|---|---|---|
| | | | Low N = 195 (33.0%) | Medium N = 204 (34.5%) | High N = 192 (32.5%) | *p*-trend* | Low N = 151 (25.5%) | Medium N = 204 (34.5%) | High N = 236 (*n* = 39.9%) | *p*-trend* |
| **Adequacy of pregnancy weight gain (term)**[a] | | | % | % | % | | % | % | % | |
| **Excessive** | 531 | 258 | 52.7 | 49.2 | 42.8 | **0.033** | 49.7 | 51.3 | 44.8 | 0.197 |
| **Inadequate** | 527 | 110 | 19.4 | 22.8 | 20.8 | 0.546 | 19.6 | 22.3 | 20.7 | 0.604 |
| **Gestational diabetes**[b] | | | | | | | | | | |
| **Elevated 2-h glucose tolerance test (WHO criteria)** | 582 | 53 | 6.3 | 13.9 | 6.9 | 0.808 | 5.4 | 12.5 | 8.6 | 0.432 |
| **Preeclampsia**[c] | | | | | | | | | | |
| **All cases combined** | 582 | 25 | 4.7 | 3.5 | 4.8 | 0.965 | 7.4 | 2.5 | 3.9 | 0.151 |
| **Severe preeclampsia/HELLP/ eclampsia**[d] | 582 | 15 | 3.1 | 2.0 | 2.7 | 0.772 | 5.4 | 1.0 | 2.1 | 0.090 |
| **Preterm delivery** | | | | | | | | | | |
| **Prior to 37 weeks (all)** | 591 | 34 | 8.7 | 5.9 | 2.6 | **0.010** | 12.6 | 3.4 | 3.4 | **<0.001** |
| **Prior to 37 weeks (preeclampsia excluded)** | 557 | 24 | 7.1 | 4.6 | 1.1 | **0.005** | 9.4 | 3.1 | 2.2 | **0.002** |
| **Neonatal outcomes** | | | | | | | | | | |
| **Birthweight > 4,000 g (term)** | 557 | 75 | 18.0 | 12.5 | 10.2 | **0.029** | 17.4 | 14.7 | 10.5 | **0.041** |
| **Birthweight > 4,500 g (term)** | 557 | 7 | 1.1 | 1.0 | 1.6 | 0.677 | 3.0 | 1.0 | 0.4 | **0.042** |
| **LGA > 90th centile**[e] | 591 | 18 | 3.1 | 4.4 | 2.6 | 0.390 | 4.0 | 3.9 | 1.7 | 0.168 |
| **Birthweight <2.5 kg (term)** | 557 | 7 | 1.1 | 1.6 | 1.1 | 0.958 | 0.0 | 2.0 | 1.3 | 0.385 |
| **SGA < 10th centile**[e] | 591 | 58 | 8.2 | 6.9 | 14.6 | **0.036** | 6.6 | 8.8 | 12.7 | **0.043** |
| **Newborn birthweight, mean (SD)** | 591 | | 3,440 (524) | 3,452 (523) | 3,397 (490) | 0.528[f] | 3,412 (585) | 3,476 (501) | 3,403 (470) | 0.291[f] |

LGA, large for gestational age; SGA, small for gestational age.
*P-trend across diet score categories (Mantel-Haenszel statistics).
[a]Weight gain outside Institute of Medicine (IOM) 2009 BMI-specific recommendations, calculated for term pregnancies only (1).
[b]WHO 1999 criteria at gestational week 30: Elevated 2-h glucose ≥7.8 mmol/l (23).
[c]Based on guidelines adopted by the Norwegian Federation of Obstetricians and Gynecologists; an increase in blood pressure to at least ≥140 systolic or 90 mm Hg diastolic after 20th gestational week combined with proteinuria (protein excretion of at least 0.3 g/24 h or ≥1+ on dip-stick), both measured at least twice (24). Nine participants did not have information on preeclampsia recorded.
[d]Defined as preeclampsia diagnosed before 34 weeks of pregnancy and/or severity of symptoms, as documented in hospital charts. Cases of eclampsia and HELLP-syndrome were included.
[e]Birth weight centiles calculated according to offspring sex and gestational age, based on data from the Medical Birth Registry of Norway (MBRN) (26).
[f]One-way ANOVA.

*Ethics*

Written informed consent was obtained from all participants before inclusion into the study. The study was approved by the Norwegian Regional Committee for Medical Research Ethics South East C (REK reference 2009/429). The authors assert that all procedures contributing to this work comply with the ethical standards of the Norwegian Regional Committee for Medical Research Ethics and with the Helsinki Declaration of 1975, as revised in 2008. The NFFD trial has the Clinical Trials registration: clinicaltrial.gov NCT0100168.

*Results*

Descriptive information about the 591 participants is presented in Table 1. Mean age at inclusion was 28.0 years (SD 4.4, range18–44). Included women were 168.7 cm tall (SD 6.2) and weighed 67.5 kg (SD12.2). Mean pre-pregnancy BMI was 23.7 kg/m$^2$ (SD 3.9). Mean *pre-pregnancy* and *early pregnancy* diet score across categories of the sociodemographic variables are presented in Table 1. There was a positive correlation with educational attainment for both diet scores ($p < 0.001$) and a negative correlation with smoking status ($p < 0.05$). Pre-pregnancy diet score was positively correlated with early pregnancy physical activity level ($p = 0.029$). Neither age, pre-pregnancy BMI, marital status, income nor occupation was significantly associated with the diet scores. A comparison of the dietary characteristics associated with low, medium, and high diet scores in both *pre-pregnancy* and in *early pregnancy* are presented in Supplementary Table 2. Higher diet score implied more frequent consumption of main meals, fruits, vegetables, and water, and less frequent consumption of sweetened beverages, sweets, and snacks. There was considerable correlation between the continuous *pre-pregnancy* and *early pregnancy* diet scores ($r_{Pearson} = 0.59$, $p < 0.001$).

*Maternal and newborn outcomes*

Differences in prevalence of maternal and child outcomes with low, medium, and high *pre-pregnancy* and *early pregnancy* diet scores, respectively, are presented in Table 2. There were significant trends toward lower prevalence of excessive GWG, preterm delivery, and macrosomia, across *pre-pregnancy* diet score categories, but concurrent higher prevalence of SGA with higher diet scores. For the *early pregnancy* diet score, we observed significant trends toward lower prevalence of preterm delivery and macrosomia with higher diet score, and a concurrent higher prevalence of SGA.

Mean GWG was 15.0 kg (SD 6.0). The overall prevalence of excessive and inadequate GWG was 48.6 and 20.9%, respectively, leaving 30.5% with optimal GWG. There were significant inverse associations between a one-point increase in *pre-pregnancy* and *early pregnancy* diet scores and odds of excessive GWG in crude and adjusted models (Tables 3 and 4) but no association between the diet scores and inadequate GWG.

A total of 53/582 (9.1%) NFFD participants were diagnosed with GDM. The highest prevalence of GDM was observed among women in the medium diet score category, whether assessed *pre-pregnancy* (13.9%) or in *early pregnancy* (12.5%) (Table 2). There was, however, no association between *pre-pregnancy* and *early pregnancy* diet scores and GDM in multivariate analyses (Tables 3 and 4).

A total of 25/582 participants (4.3%) developed preeclampsia, with 15/582 (2.6%) classified as severe cases. Early pregnancy diet score was protectively associated with preeclampsia risk in model 3 when adjusted for pre-pregnancy physical activity level in addition to other potential confounders (Table 4). The same trend was observed for severe preeclampsia, although not significant.

A total of 34/591 women (5.8%) delivered preterm. Women with low *early pregnancy* diet score had the highest prevalence of preterm delivery (12.5%), while women with high diet score *pre-pregnancy* had the lowest prevalence (2.6%) (Table 2). There were significant inverse associations between the diet scores and preterm delivery, whether assessed pre-pregnancy or in early pregnancy (Tables 3 and 4). The same pattern was observed when pregnancies complicated by preeclampsia were excluded from the analysis.

A total of 75/557 (13.5%) newborns had birthweight ≥4,000 g at term, and 7/557 (1.3%) had birthweight ≥4,500 g. A total of 18/591 (3.0%) were classified as LGA. Both the *pre-pregnancy* and *early pregnancy* diet score were inversely associated with birthweight above 4 kg in crude models, but the association was attenuated and no longer significant in the adjusted models (Tables 3 and 4). The *early pregnancy* diet score was associated with lower risk of birthweight above 4.5 kg, but the association was attenuated after adjustment for *early pregnancy* physical activity level (Table 4). There were no significant associations between the diet scores and other measures of fetal growth.

*Sensitivity analyses*

There was no formal interaction between randomization assignment and the diet scores. We nevertheless reran all *pre-pregnancy* and *early pregnancy* models confined to the control group to assess the associations in a non-intervention setting. This made no substantial difference in the direction or magnitude of the estimates although some of the associations were no longer significant because of the smaller sample (Supplementary Tables 3a and 3b).

*Discussion*

In this study, we investigated whether and how degree of maternal compliance with a set of predefined dietary

*Table 3.* Associations between *pre-pregnancy* NFFD diet score and maternal and newborn outcomes ($n = 591$)

| Obstetrical outcomes | No. included in the analysis | No. of cases | Pre-pregnancy model 1 Crude | | | Pre-pregnancy model 2 Adjusted[a] | | |
|---|---|---|---|---|---|---|---|---|
| | | | OR | 95% CI | *p*-value | OR[a] | 95% CI | *p*-value |
| **Adequacy of weight gain (at term)**[b] | | | | | | | | |
| **Excessive** | 528 | 256 | **0.91** | **0.84–0.98** | **0.019** | **0.92** | **0.84–1.00** | **0.050** |
| **Inadequate** | 524 | 110 | 1.03 | 0.93–1.13 | 0.576 | 1.02 | 0.92–1.12 | 0.766 |
| **Gestational diabetes**[c] | | | | | | | | |
| **Elevated 2-h glucose tolerance test (WHO criteria)** | 578 | 53 | 1.06 | 0.93–1.20 | 0.403 | 1.07 | 0.94–1.23 | 0.314 |
| **Preeclampsia**[d] | | | | | | | | |
| **Preeclampsia total** | 578 | 25 | 0.99 | 0.82–1.19 | 0.900 | 0.97 | 0.81–1.18 | 0.784 |
| **Severe preeclampsia/HELLP/ eclampsia**[e] | 578 | 15 | 0.93 | 0.73–1.18 | 0.564 | 0.93 | 0.73–1.19 | 0.573 |
| **Preterm delivery** | | | | | | | | |
| **Prior to 37 weeks** | 586 | 34 | **0.81** | **0.68–0.96** | **0.014** | **0.81** | **0.68–0.97** | **0.019** |
| **Prior to 37 weeks (preeclampsia cases excluded)** | 553 | 24 | **0.76** | **0.62–0.93** | **0.008** | **0.77** | **0.62–0.95** | **0.013** |
| **Neonatal outcomes** | | | | | | | | |
| **Birthweight > 4,000 g (term)** | 552 | 75 | **0.87** | **0.77–0.98** | **0.016** | **0.88** | **0.78–0.99** | **0.038** |
| **Birthweight > 4,500 g (term)** | 552 | 7 | 0.82 | 0.57–1.17 | 0.275 | 0.76 | 0.52–1.14 | 0.183 |
| **LGA >90th centile**[f] | 591 | 18 | 0.80 | 0.63–1.00 | 0.049 | 0.91 | 0.64–1.02 | 0.071 |
| **Birthweight < 2.5 kg (term)** | 552 | 7 | 0.90 | 0.64–1.28 | 0.567 | 0.92 | 0.63–1.33 | 0.646 |
| **SGA < 10th centile**[f] | 586 | 57 | 1.08 | 0.95–1.22 | 0.242 | 1.09 | 0.95–1.24 | 0.217 |

LGA, large for gestational age; SGA, small for gestational age.
[a]Multivariable associations between pre-pregnancy diet score and outcomes are expressed as odds ratios (OR) with 95% confidence intervals (95% CI) and corresponding *p*-values, adjusted for maternal age (continuous), educational attainment (≤12, 13–15, ≥6 years), marital status (cohabiting yes/no), family income (4 categories), pre-pregnancy BMI (continuous), and randomization assignment (control/intervention).
[b]Weight gain outside Institute of Medicine (IOM) 2009 recommendations, calculated for term pregnancies only (1).
[c]WHO 1999 criteria at gestational week 30: Elevated 2-h glucose ≥7.8 mmol/l (23).
[d]Based on guidelines adopted by the Norwegian Federation of Obstetricians and Gynecologists; an increase in blood pressure to at least ≥140 systolic or 90 mm Hg diastolic after 20th gestational week combined with proteinuria (protein excretion of at least 0.3 g/24 h or ≥1+ on dip-stick), both measured at least twice (24).
[e]Defined as preeclampsia diagnosed before 34 weeks of pregnancy and/or severity of symptoms, as documented in hospital charts. Cases of eclampsia and HELLP-syndrome were included.
[f]Birth weight centile calculated according to offspring sex and gestational age, based on data from the Medical Birth Registry of Norway (MBRN) (26).

behaviors assessed both pre-pregnancy and in early pregnancy was associated with maternal and neonatal outcomes in the NFFD dataset. For the outcomes excessive GWG and preterm delivery, respectively, we found protective associations of similar magnitude with *pre-pregnancy* and *early pregnancy* dietary behavior. Lower odds of high birthweight were only observed with increasing *pre-pregnancy* diet score, whereas lower odds of preeclampsia were only observed with increasing *early pregnancy* diet score. No association between the two diet scores and GDM was observed in this sample.

To our knowledge, no other study has investigated both pre-pregnancy and early pregnancy dietary behavior in the same individuals in relation to subsequent maternal and neonatal outcomes. Having done so, allows for speculation regarding sensitive periods for the role of diet and dietary behaviors in the prevention of adverse pregnancy outcomes. Our findings suggest a protective influence of healthier pre-pregnancy dietary behavior on GWG, preterm delivery, and newborn macrosomia, but possibly also an independent protective influence of early pregnancy dietary behavior on preeclampsia risk. Although aspects of dietary behavior changed from pre-pregnancy to early pregnancy among NFFD participants (30, 31), the correlation between the two diet scores in the present study was high.

### *Gestational weight gain*

The protective associations observed between pre-pregnancy and early pregnancy dietary behavior and excessive GWG support the relevance of targeting the chosen dietary behaviors for optimizing GWG. A recent observational study from Greece reported that higher adherence to the Mediterranean diet prior to pregnancy was

*Table 4.* Associations between *early pregnancy* NFFD diet score and maternal and newborn outcomes ($n$ = 591)

| Obstetrical outcomes | No. included in the analysis | No. of cases | Early pregnancy model 1 Crude | | | Early pregnancy model 2 Adjusted[a] | | | Early pregnancy model 3 Adjusted[b] | | |
|---|---|---|---|---|---|---|---|---|---|---|---|
| | | | OR | 95% CI | *p*-value | OR[a] | 95% CI | *p*-value | OR[b] | 95% CI | *p*-value |
| **Adequacy of weight gain (term)**[c] | | | | | | | | | | | |
| **Excessive** | 528 | 256 | **0.90** | **0.83–0.98** | **0.019** | **0.90** | **0.83–0.99** | **0.024** | **0.88** | **0.79–0.97** | **0.009** |
| **Inadequate** | 524 | 110 | 1.05 | 0.95–1.17 | 0.331 | 1.05 | 0.94–1.17 | 0.381 | 1.02 | 0.95–1.19 | 0.374 |
| **Gestational diabetes**[d] | | | | | | | | | | | |
| **Elevated 2-h glucose tolerance test (WHO criteria)** | 578 | 53 | 1.02 | 0.88–1.17 | 0.815 | 1.00 | 0.86–1.15 | 0.949 | 0.98 | 0.83–1.16 | 0.810 |
| **Preeclampsia**[e] | | | | | | | | | | | |
| **Preeclampsia total** | 578 | 25 | 0.93 | 0.76–1.13 | 0.461 | 0.90 | 0.73–1.10 | 0.325 | **0.78** | **0.62–0.99** | **0.038** |
| **Severe preeclampsia/HELLP/ eclampsia**[f] | 582 | 15 | 0.91 | 0.71–1.17 | 0.457 | 0.90 | 0.67–1.17 | 0.429 | 0.74 | 0.54–1.01 | 0.060 |
| **Preterm delivery** | | | | | | | | | | | |
| **Prior to 37 weeks** | 587 | 34 | **0.77** | **0.65–0.92** | **0.004** | **0.77** | **0.64–0.92** | **0.005** | **0.82** | **0.67–0.99** | **0.038** |
| **Prior to 37 weeks (preeclampsia cases excluded)** | 555 | 24 | **0.77** | **0.62–0.95** | **0.014** | **0.77** | **0.62–0.96** | **0.018** | 0.81 | 0.64–1.02 | 0.068 |
| **Neonatal outcomes** | | | | | | | | | | | |
| **Birthweight > 4,000 g (term)** | 552 | 75 | **0.86** | **0.76–0.98** | **0.018** | 0.89 | 0.78–1.01 | 0.061 | 0.91 | 0.79–1.05 | 0.185 |
| **Birthweight > 4,500 g (term)** | 552 | 7 | **0.58** | **0.39–0.89** | **0.011** | **0.54** | **0.35–0.84** | **0.006** | 0.60 | 0.33–1.10 | 0.097 |
| **LGA >90th centile**[g] | 586 | 18 | 0.80 | 0.63–1.01 | 0.060 | 0.79 | 0.62–1.01 | 0.062 | 0.80 | 0.60–1.09 | 0.166 |
| **Birthweight < 2.5 kg (term)** | 552 | 7 | 1.18 | 0.82–1.71 | 0.368 | 1.25 | 0.84–1.86 | 0.267 | 1.20 | 0.79–1.83 | 0.387 |
| **SGA < 10th centile**[g] | 586 | 57 | 1.12 | 0.98–1.28 | 0.107 | 1.13 | 0.98–1.29 | 0.089 | 1.10 | 0.94–1.28 | 0.225 |

LGA, large for gestational age; SGA, small for gestational age.

[a]Multivariable associations between early pregnancy diet score and the outcomes are expressed as odds ratios (OR) with 95% confidence intervals (95% CI) and corresponding *p*-values. A *p*-value of ≤ 0.05 is considered significant. Early pregnancy model 2 is adjusted for maternal age (continuous), educational attainment (≤12, 13–15, ≥6 years), marital status (married/cohabiting yes/no), family income (4 categories), pre-pregnancy BMI (continuous), current smoking (yes/no), and randomization assignment (control/intervention).

[b]Model 3 is adjusted for all variables in model 2 and in addition early pregnancy physical activity level (3 categories). There was a large number of missing values in model 3 due to missing information on early pregnancy physical activity level ($n$ = 110).

[c]Weight gain outside Institute of Medicine (IOM) 2009 recommendations (1)

[d]WHO 1999 criteria at gestational week 30: Elevated 2-h glucose ≥7.8 mmol/l (23).

[e]Based on guidelines adopted by the Norwegian Federation of Obstetricians and Gynecologists; an increase in blood pressure to at least ≥140 systolic or 90 mm Hg diastolic after 20th gestational week combined with proteinuria (protein excretion of at least 0.3 g/24 h or ≥1+ on dip-stick), both measured at least twice (24).

[f]Defined as preeclampsia diagnosed before 34 weeks of pregnancy and/or severity of symptoms, as documented in hospital charts. Cases of eclampsia and HELLP-syndrome were included.

[g]Birth weight percentile calculated according to offspring sex and gestational age, based on data from the Medical Birth Registry of Norway (MBRN) (26).

associated with decreased risk for deviation from the maternal recommended GWG (32).

NFFD women with high diet score *pre-pregnancy* had similar prevalence of excessive GWG as women in the intervention group (41.6% vs. 42.8%) (2) and almost one in two participants in the NFFD cohort exceeded BMI-specific recommendations for GWG which compares well with findings from the MoBa cohort (33). Given the high prevalence of excessive GWG in all diet score categories, more research is needed to identify successful interventions for optimizing GWG.

#### *Preterm delivery*

Preterm birth is strongly associated with perinatal and infant mortality (34), and even late preterm birth may have negative consequences for long-term health and development (35). Rates of preterm birth vary widely among and within countries, and modifiable determinants are searched for (16). We observed inverse associations of similar strength between *pre-pregnancy* and *early* pregnancy diet scores and subsequent preterm delivery. Our findings are in agreement with previous observations of protective associations between healthy dietary patterns during pregnancy and subsequent preterm delivery (8, 9, 11, 12), and higher risk with unhealthy dietary patterns (12, 36). In the National Danish Birth Cohort (DNBC), a consistent dose–response association between Western diet score and risk of preterm delivery was observed (OR: 1.30, 95% CI: 1.13, 1.49 for highest vs. lowest quintile). Grieger et al. derived dietary patterns from retrospectively reported *pre-pregnancy* diet in 309 women and found that higher pre-pregnancy score on a high-protein/fruit pattern was associated with lower odds of subsequent preterm delivery (OR: 0.31; 95% CI: 0.50, 0.91 for each SD higher score) (37). The NFFD diet score reflect constellations of maternal dietary behaviors with potential favorable impact on maternal hormones, metabolism, immunologic factors, inflammation, antioxidant defense, and energy balance, all of which might influence the risk of preterm delivery (34). Given the magnitude and strength of the associations between *pre-pregnancy* and *early pregnancy* diet score and preterm delivery, it was somewhat surprising that there was no reduction in preterm delivery in the NFFD intervention group. If a true relationship exists between pregnancy dietary behavior and risk of preterm delivery, this lack of intervention effect on preterm delivery could imply a time-dependent association, that is, that interventions need to be implemented earlier in pregnancy or even before pregnancy to be effective. Other possibilities are insufficient intensity of the NFFD intervention to impact on preterm delivery risk, insufficient dietary difference between control and intervention group, or that other aspects of the lifestyle intervention negated potential protective effects of diet.

#### *Preeclampsia*

Preeclampsia is another serious complication of pregnancy that may threaten maternal survival and severely affect fetal growth and development (38). There was no association between *pre-pregnancy* diet score and preeclampsia in the present study. A significant protective association was, however, observed between *early pregnancy* dietary behavior when the model was adjusted for physical activity level (Table 4), indicating that the protective association with early pregnancy diet was negatively confounded by physical activity level. Fewer preeclampsia cases occurred in the intervention group, but the difference was not significant (OR: 0.65; 95% CI: 0.29–1.47) (2). Importantly, the NFFD trial was not powered to detect between-group differences for this outcome. A meta-analysis of lifestyle interventions during pregnancy by Allen et al. found that dietary interventions resulted in an estimated 33% reduction in preeclampsia prevalence (39), supporting an independent influence of dietary factors during pregnancy. We only found one other study that prospectively investigated associations between *pre-pregnancy* diet and subsequent hypertensive disorders of pregnancy. This study reported a protective dose–response association between *pre-pregnancy* consumption of a Mediterranean-style dietary pattern and subsequent risk of hypertensive disorders of pregnancy (quartile 4 vs. quartile 1: RR, 0.58; 95% CI, 0.42, 0.81) (40).

#### *Newborn birthweight*

Only seven children had birthweight ≥4,500 g, so associations between the diet scores and this outcome should be interpreted with caution. The observation that higher diet score was associated with lower odds of high birthweight might point to pre-pregnancy and the first trimester as a window of opportunity regarding healthy fetal growth. Given that excessive GWG is strongly associated with macrosomia (41, 42), efforts to avoid excessive GWG are likely to simultaneously influence fetal fuel availability and birthweight in addition to potential direct influences of diet and dietary behavior on fetal tissue accretion (43). The higher prevalence of newborn SGA among women with high *pre-pregnancy* and *early pregnancy* diet score highlights that there is also a risky side of presumably healthy dietary behaviors, and that energy balance–related behaviors might compromise fetal fuel availability if taken too far. There was however no significant association between the diet scores and odds of SGA in multivariate analyses, indicating that other maternal characteristics associated with the diet scores might explain the increased prevalence of SGA in the unadjusted analysis in Table 2. Fortunately, the NFFD intervention did not result in increased prevalence of SGA in the intervention group compared to the control group (OR: 1.16, 95% CI: 0.68–2.00, $p = 0.679$) (2).

*Gestational diabetes mellitus*

Surprisingly, the prevalence of GDM was substantially higher in the medium diet score category, whether assessed pre-pregnancy or in early pregnancy. This finding is difficult to explain and should be a target for further investigations in the NFFD dataset. The dietary differences between the diet score categories in Supplementary Table 2 give no clue as to why the medium diet score group should perform worse than the others. There may, however, be dietary characteristics specific to the medium diet score category that was not captured by the NFFD questionnaire. There could also be unmeasured confounding related to maternal risk status, for example, that women susceptible to overweight or obesity (and therefore at a higher risk of GDM) could be more conscious about their diet than women with lower risk, and therefore more likely to be categorized in the medium (or high) diet score category. A pre-pregnancy 'Meats, snacks, and sweets' pattern was associated with higher GDM risk, and a 'Mediterranean-style' pattern with lower risk after adjustment for socioeconomic, reproductive, and lifestyle factors in the Australian Longitudinal Study on Women's Health (44). Large population-based RCTs as well as RCTs targeting overweight and obese gravidas have demonstrated no effect of lifestyle interventions on GDM prevalence despite dietary improvement, increased physical activity, and in some of the studies, even reduced GWG (4, 5, 45). A recent systematic review on primary prevention studies of GDM through nutritional factors summarized that no conclusions can be drawn with regard to the best dietary interventions and that there is a strong need for additional research on this topic (46).

*Strengths and limitations*

There are several strengths to the present study. The participation rate in the trial was high. All women provided dietary data upon inclusion in early pregnancy, and in retrospect, the same dietary data pertaining to the period before getting pregnant. Birth records and hospital charts were reviewed for all participants to confirm data on maternal weight gain and maternal and neonatal outcomes.

Only nulliparous women were included in the study. Nulliparity is associated with higher risk of pregnancy complications compared to multiparous pregnancies (16). Thus, heterogeneity and bias introduced by differential absolute risk of pregnancy complications between nulliparous and multiparous gravidas was avoided, as well as bias related to the high repeatability risk of preterm delivery and preeclampsia in subsequent pregnancies (16).

Sufficient variation in diet is necessary to detect true diet–disease associations in epidemiological studies (14). Randomized controlled diet interventions normally result in rather small mean improvements in diet or dietary behavior and are therefore not suited to assess dose–response relationships in diet–outcome associations (14). The NFFD diet score captured a continuum of combinations of healthy and less healthy dietary behaviors and thus much larger dietary variation than could be obtained in a RCT. Even though the numbers of preterm delivery, preeclampsia, and macrosomia cases were small in this study, we identified significant inverse associations even with these outcomes.

There are, however, also limitations that warrant discussion. Causality cannot be inferred from observational data. We adjusted for randomization assignment in all models and reran all models confined to the control group to avoid bias introduced by the intervention. There could, however, still be residual or unmeasured confounding from participating in a lifestyle intervention trial. The diet scores are likely to capture level of health consciousness in general, which could imply that variation in personal traits not captured by the sociodemographic variables could positively or negatively confound the associations.

The NFFD diet score and subscales have shown acceptable test–retest reproducibility (22) but have not been validated against other methods of operationalizing dietary behavior. Completing questionnaires about diet and frequency of intake challenges participants with complex tasks that increase the risk of misreporting (47). In addition, single-item questions about complex dietary behaviors may not fully capture a specific behavior. Recalling dietary behavior from before getting pregnant adds to the risk of misreporting and could lead to incorrect assignment of diet score values and a less reliable *pre-pregnancy* diet score in general. If random, misreporting would tend to bias the estimates toward null association. Misreporting or measurement error in the other covariates could not only lead to biased estimates but would also tend to bias estimates toward null association. We therefore assume that our estimates are conservative.

The NFFD diet score represents a crude operationalization of dietary behavior and equal weight is given to each dietary behavior regardless of their potential individual impact on the various outcomes. We did not investigate individual dietary behaviors in relation to the outcomes as our aim was to evaluate this constellation of dietary behaviors. It has previously been documented that single behaviors have less power as predictors of complex outcomes such as preterm delivery (48).

The NFFD diet score was primarily constructed to evaluate post-intervention effect of the diet intervention and reflected degree of adherence to the 10 dietary recommendations that were forwarded to the intervention group in the trial (22). It could be argued that it would be better to apply other criteria for scoring in each subscale rather than the statistically driven method of using the median in each subscale as cutoff. Similar methods have, however, been extensively used in evaluating associations between adherence to the Mediterranean diet and subsequent health outcomes (49).

The women participating in the NFFD study were predominantly white, European, highly educated, and nulliparous, and therefore not fully representative of the pregnant background population. This self-selection may have affected outcome prevalence but is less likely to have influenced diet-outcome associations (50).

## Concluding remarks

There are numerous reasons why pregnant women should be encouraged to achieve and maintain a healthy and nutritious diet during pregnancy. The relevance of pre-pregnancy diet for maternal and offspring antenatal and long-term health should, however, be explored as a means to securing maximum benefit of public health interventions. Our findings suggest that NFFD participants' pre-pregnancy compliance with the dietary behaviors targeted in the NFFD trial was beneficially associated with risk of pregnancy and neonatal outcomes such as excessive GWG, preterm delivery, and newborn macrosomia. We did not observe substantial differences between associations with early pregnancy as opposed to pre-pregnancy dietary behavior, except for the lower odds of preeclampsia that was only observed with increasing *early pregnancy* diet score. Based on these findings, we speculate that the previously observed relationship between diet reported during pregnancy and pregnancy complications such as preterm delivery in observational studies could be a representation of a relationship that at least partly exists between maternal pre-pregnancy dietary behavior and the neonatal outcomes in question.

Prospectively collected high-quality dietary data from various time-points before conception and during pregnancy with the possibility of linkage to birth registry data would help identify important windows of opportunity for a healthy pregnancy and a nutritionally sound start to life. RCTs evaluating diet interventions before conception will need to be undertaken to establish causality.

## Acknowledgements

The authors would like to thank the women who participated in the Norwegian Fit for Delivery study. We also thank the health care clinic midwives who recruited participants in early pregnancy and collected inclusion data, and the delivery ward staff who collected data on maternal and newborn study-related outcomes.

## Authors' contributions

LRS, IV, and EB conceived the NFFD trial. NCØ and ERH carried out and supervised the dietary intervention. HLS and MKT developed and supervised the physical activity component of the NFFD trial. ERH, EB, and NCØ designed the present study. ERH analyzed the data and drafted the paper. All authors revised the paper critically.

## Conflict of interest and funding

The authors declare no conflict of interest. The NFFD trial was financed by a grant from South-Eastern Norway Regional Health Authority. Additional funding was provided by the municipalities of southern Norway and by the University of Agder. The funders had no role in design, analysis, or writing of this paper.

## References

1. Rasmussen KM, Yaktine AL, eds. Weight gain during pregnancy: reexamining the guidelines. Washington, DC: The National Academies Press; 2009.
2. Sagedal LR, Overby NC, Bere E, Torstveit MK, Lohne-Seiler H, Smastuen M, et al. Lifestyle intervention to limit gestational weight galn: the Norwegian Fit for Delivery randomised controlled trial. BJOG 2017; 124(1): 97–109.
3. Vinter CA, Jensen DM, Ovesen P, Beck-Nielsen H, Jørgensen JS. The LiP (Lifestyle in Pregnancy) study: a randomized controlled trial of lifestyle intervention in 360 obese pregnant women. Diabetes Care 2011; 34(12): 2502–7.
4. Dodd JM, Turnbull D, McPhee AJ, Deussen AR, Grivell RM, Yelland LN, et al. Antenatal lifestyle advice for women who are overweight or obese: LIMIT randomised trial. BMJ 2014; 348(7948): 11.
5. Poston L, Bell R, Croker H, Flynn AC, Godfrey KM, Goff L, et al. Effect of a behavioural intervention in obese pregnant women (the UPBEAT study): a multicentre, randomised controlled trial. Lancet Diabetes Endocrinol 2015; 3(10): 767–77.
6. Rogozinska E, Marlin N, Jackson L, Rayanagoudar G, Ruifrok AE, Dodds J, et al. Effects of antenatal diet and physical activity on maternal and fetal outcomes: individual patient data meta-analysis and health economic evaluation. Health Technol Assess 2017; 21(41): 1–158.
7. Brantsaeter AL, Haugen M, Samuelsen SO, Torjusen H, Trogstad L, Alexander J, et al. A dietary pattern characterized by high intake of vegetables, fruits, and vegetable oils is associated with reduced risk of preeclampsia in nulliparous pregnant Norwegian women. J Nutr 2009; 139(6): 1162–8.
8. Hillesund ER, Øverby NC, Engel SM, Klungsøyr K, Harmon QE, Haugen M, et al. Associations of adherence to the New Nordic Diet with risk of preeclampsia and preterm delivery in the Norwegian Mother and Child Cohort Study (MoBa). Eur J Epidemiol 2014; 29(10): 753–65.
9. Englund-Ogge L, Brantsaeter AL, Sengpiel V, Haugen M, Birgisdottir BE, Myhre R, et al. Maternal dietary patterns and preterm delivery: results from large prospective cohort study. BMJ 2014; 348: g1446.
10. Englund-Ogge L, Birgisdottir BE, Sengpiel V, Brantsaeter AL, Haugen M, Myhre R, et al. Meal frequency patterns and glycemic properties of maternal diet in relation to preterm delivery: results from a large prospective cohort study. PLoS One 2017; 12(3): e0172896.
11. Chia A-R, de Seymour JV, Colega M, Chen L-W, Chan Y-H, Aris IM, et al. A vegetable, fruit, and white rice dietary pattern during pregnancy is associated with a lower risk of preterm birth and larger birth size in a multiethnic Asian cohort: the Growing

Up in Singapore Towards healthy Outcomes (GUSTO) cohort study. Am J Clin Nutr 2016; 104(5): 1416–23.
12. Martin CL, Sotres-Alvarez D, Siega-Riz AM. Maternal dietary patterns during the second trimester are associated with preterm birth. J Nutr 2015; 145(8): 1857–64.
13. Meinila J, Valkama A, Koivusalo SB, Stach-Lempinen B, Rono K, Lindstrom J, et al. Is improvement in the Healthy Food Intake Index (HFII) related to a lower risk for gestational diabetes? Br J Nutr 2017; 117(8): 1103–9.
14. Willett WC. Nutritional epidemiology. 3rd edn. New York, NY, USA: Oxford University Press; 2013.
15. Hanson MA, Gluckman PD. Early developmental conditioning of later health and disease: physiology or pathophysiology? Physiol Rev 2014; 94(4): 1027–76.
16. Ferrero DM, Larson J, Jacobsson B, Di Renzo GC, Norman JE, Martin JN, Jr., et al. Cross-country individual participant analysis of 4.1 million singleton births in 5 countries with very high human development index confirms known associations but provides no biologic explanation for 2/3 of all preterm births. PLoS One 2016; 11(9):e0162506.
17. Sagedal LR, Overby NC, Lohne-Seiler H, Bere E, Torstveit MK, Henriksen T, et al. Study protocol: fit for delivery – can a lifestyle intervention in pregnancy result in measurable health benefits for mothers and newborns? A randomized controlled trial. BMC Public Health 2013; 13: 132.
18. Sagedal LR, Sanda B, Overby NC, Bere E, Torstveit MK, Lohne-Seiler H, et al. The effect of prenatal lifestyle intervention on weight retention 12 months postpartum: results of the Norwegian Fit for Delivery randomised controlled trial. BJOG 2017; 124(1): 111–21.
19. Hillesund ER, Bere E, Sagedal LR, Vistad I, Øverby NC. Effect of a diet intervention during pregnancy on dietary behavior in the randomized controlled Norwegian fit for delivery study. J Dev Orig Health Dis 2016; 7(5): 538–47.
20. Sagedal LR, Vistad I, Overby NC, Bere E, Torstveit MK, Lohne-Seiler H, et al. The effect of a prenatal lifestyle intervention on glucose metabolism: results of the Norwegian fit for delivery randomized controlled trial. BMC Pregnancy Childbirth 2017; 17(1): 167.
21. Haakstad LA, Sanda B, Vistad I, Sagedal LR, Seiler HL, Torstveit MK. Evaluation of implementing a community-based exercise intervention during pregnancy. Midwifery 2017; 46: 45–51.
22. Øverby NC, Hillesund ER, Sagedal LR, Vistad I, Bere E. The fit for delivery study: rationale for the recommendations and test-retest reliability of a dietary score measuring adherence to 10 specific recommendations for prevention of excessive weight gain during pregnancy. Matern Child Nutr 2015; 11(1): 20–32.
23. World Health Organization. Definition and diagnosis of diabetes mellitus and intermediate hyperglycaemia: report of a WHO/IDF consultation. Geneva, Switzerland: World Health Organization; 2006.
24. Klungsøyr K, Morken NH, Irgens L, Vollset SE, Skjærven R. Secular trends in the epidemiology of pre-eclampsia throughout 40 years in Norway: prevalence, risk factors and perinatal survival. Paediatr Perinat Epidemiol 2012; 26(3): 190–8.
25. Boulet SL, Alexander GR, Salihu HM, Pass M. Macrosomic births in the united states: determinants, outcomes, and proposed grades of risk. Am J Obstet Gynecol 2003; 188(5): 1372–8.
26. Skjaerven R, Gjessing HK, Bakketeig LS. Birthweight by gestational age in Norway. Acta Obstet Gynecol Scand 2000; 79(6): 440–9.
27. Craig CL, Marshall AL, Sjostrom M, Bauman AE, Booth ML, Ainsworth BE, et al. International physical activity questionnaire: 12-country reliability and validity. Med Sci Sports Exerc 2003; 35(8): 1381–95.
28. Sanda B, Vistad I, Haakstad LAH, Berntsen S, Sagedal LR, Lohne-Seiler H, et al. Reliability and concurrent validity of the International Physical Activity Questionnaire short form among pregnant women. BMC Sports Sci Med Rehabil 2017; 9: 7.
29. Veierød M, Lydersen S, Laake P, eds. Logistic regression. In: Hosmer DW, Lemeshow S. Medical statistics in clinical and epidemiological research. Oslo, Norway: Gyldendal Akademisk; 2012, pp. 90–126.
30. Skreden M, Bere E, Sagedal LR, Vistad I, Overby NC. Changes in beverage consumption from pre-pregnancy to early pregnancy in the Norwegian Fit for Delivery study. Public Health Nutr 2015; 18(7): 1187–96.
31. Skreden M, Bere E, Sagedal LR, Vistad I, Overby NC. Changes in fruit and vegetable consumption habits from pre-pregnancy to early pregnancy among Norwegian women. BMC Pregnancy Childbirth 2017; 17(1): 107.
32. Koutelidakis AE, Alexatou O, Kousaiti S, Gkretsi E, Vasios G, Sampani A, et al. Higher adherence to Mediterranean diet prior to pregnancy is associated with decreased risk for deviation from the maternal recommended gestational weight gain. Int J Food Sci Nutr 2018; 69(1): 84–92.
33. Hillesund ER, Bere E, Haugen M, Øverby NC. Development of a New Nordic Diet score and its association with gestational weight gain and fetal growth – a study performed in the Norwegian Mother and Child Cohort Study (MoBa). Public Health Nutr 2014; 17(9): 1909–18.
34. Goldenberg RL, Culhane JF, Iams JD, Romero R. Epidemiology and causes of preterm birth. Lancet 2008; 371(9606): 75–84.
35. Hibbard JU, Wilkins I, Sun L, Gregory K, Haberman S, Hoffman M, et al. Respiratory morbidity in late preterm births. JAMA 2010; 304(4): 419–25.
36. Rasmussen MA, Maslova E, Halldorsson TI, Olsen SF. Characterization of dietary patterns in the Danish national birth cohort in relation to preterm birth. PLoS One 2014; 9(4): e93644.
37. Grieger JA, Grzeskowiak LE, Clifton VL. Preconception dietary patterns in human pregnancies are associated with preterm delivery. J Nutr 2014; 144(7): 1075–80.
38. Sibai B, Dekker G, Kupferminc M. Pre-eclampsia. Lancet 2005; 365(9461): 785–99.
39. Allen R, Rogozinska E, Sivarajasingam P, Khan KS, Thangaratinam S. Effect of diet- and lifestyle-based metabolic risk-modifying interventions on preeclampsia: a meta-analysis. Acta Obstet Gynecol Scand 2014; 93(10): 973–85.
40. Schoenaker DAJM, Soedamah-Muthu SS, Callaway LK, Mishra GD. Prepregnancy dietary patterns and risk of developing hypertensive disorders of pregnancy: results from the Australian Longitudinal Study on Women's Health. Am J Clin Nutr 2015; 102(1): 94–101.
41. Haugen M, Brantsæter AL, Winkvist A, Lissner L, Alexander J, Oftedal B, et al. Associations of pre-pregnancy body mass index and gestational weight gain with pregnancy outcome and postpartum weight retention: a prospective observational cohort study. BMC Pregnancy Childbirth 2014; 14: 201.
42. Kim SY, Sharma AJ, Sappenfield W, Wilson HG, Salihu HM. Association of maternal body mass index, excessive weight gain, and gestational diabetes mellitus with large-for-gestational-age births. Obstet Gynecol 2014; 123(4): 737–44.
43. Brantsaeter AL, Haugen M, Myhre R, Sengpiel V, Englund-Øgge L, Nilsen RM, et al. Diet matters, particularly in pregnancy – results

from MoBA studies of maternal diet and pregnancy outcomes. Norwegian J Epidemiol 2014; 24(1–2): 63–78.
44. Schoenaker DAJM, Soedamah-Muthu SS, Callaway LK, Mishra GD. Pre-pregnancy dietary patterns and risk of gestational diabetes mellitus: results from an Australian population-based prospective cohort study. Diabetologia 2015; 58(12): 2726–35.
45. Sagedal LR, Øverby NC, Bere E, Torstveit MK, Lohne-Seiler H, Småstuen M, et al. Lifestyle intervention to limit gestational weight gaIn: the Norwegian Fit for Delivery randomised controlled trial. BJOG 2017; 124(1): 97–109.
46. Donazar-Ezcurra M, López-del Burgo C, Bes-Rastrollo M. Primary prevention of gestational diabetes mellitus through nutritional factors: a systematic review. BMC Pregnancy Childbirth 2017; 17: 1–5.
47. Westerterp KR, Goris AH. Validity of the assessment of dietary intake: problems of misreporting. Curr Opin Clin Nutr Metab Care 2002; 5(5): 489–93.
48. Savitz DA, Harmon Q, Siega-Riz AM, Herring AH, Dole N, Thorp JM, Jr. Behavioral influences on preterm birth: integrated analysis of the pregnancy, infection, and nutrition study. Matern Child Health J 2012; 16(6): 1151–63.
49. Bach A, Serra-Majem L, Carrasco JL, Roman B, Ngo J, Bertomeu I, et al. The use of indexes evaluating the adherence to the Mediterranean diet in epidemiological studies: a review. Public Health Nutr 2006; 9(1A): 132–46.
50. Nilsen RM, Vollset SE, Gjessing HK, Skjaerven R, Melve KK, Schreuder P, et al. Self-selection and bias in a large prospective pregnancy cohort in Norway. Paediatr Perinat Epidemiol 2009; 23(6): 597–608.

***Elisabet R. Hillesund**
Department of Public Health, Sports and Nutrition
University of Agder
Serviceboks 422
NO-4604 Kristiansand, Norway
Email: elisabet.r.hillesund@uia.no

17

# The impact of worksite interventions promoting healthier food and/or physical activity habits among employees working 'around the clock' hours

Anne Dahl Lassen[1]*, Sisse Fagt[1], Maria Lennernäs[2], Maria Nyberg[3], Irja Haapalar[4,5], Anne V. Thorsen[1], Anna C. M. Møbjerg[6], and Anne M. Beck[6,7]

[1]Division for Risk Assessment and Nutrition, Technical University of Denmark, Kemitorvet, Lyngby, Denmark; [2]Department of Occupational and Public Health Science, University of Gävle, Gävle, Sweden; [3]Department of Food and Meal Science, Kristianstad University, Kristianstad, Sweden; [4]School of Social and Political Sciences, The University of Melbourne, Melbourne, Victoria, Australia; [5]School of Applied Educational Sciences and Teacher Education, Savonlinna, Finland; [6]Institute for Nursing and Nutrition, University College Copenhagen, Copenhagen N, Denmark; [7]Clinical Nutrition Research Unit, Copenhagen University Hospital Herlev-Gentofte, Gentofte, Denmark.

*Abstract*

We conducted a systematic review of randomised studies on the impact of worksite interventions to promote healthier food and/or physical activity among people who work irregular hours 'around the clock', that is, outside of ordinary daytime working hours. The population–intervention–comparator–outcomes–study (PICOS) design format was used. Data sources were PubMed and CINAHL. An updated search was conducted on October 2017 using Google Scholar and the related articles function in PubMed on initially included studies to identify additional studies. Risk of bias was used to assess study quality. A total of seven studies (reports published in 14 papers) were included in the systematic review: Two interventions with a broader lifestyle approach, three focusing on physical exercise and two on providing healthier food or meal options. The studies had sample sizes from 30 to 1,000 and targeted a mixture of occupations, including both male- and female-dominated occupational groups. The interventions lasted from 2 to 12 months. Only one had an extended follow-up. In general, the studies showed small-to-moderate effect sizes on several measures, including dietary and/or physical activity measures, suggesting acceptable effectiveness for interventions involving community-level behaviour change. Our findings highlight a need to further develop and implement well-designed health promotion interventions with comparable outcome measures and effect size reports. A mixture of health promotion strategies is recommended for future practice in this target population, including individually tailored programmes, improving the food and physical activity environment and using broader lifestyle approaches including the use of participatory and empowerment strategies. While more research is needed in this field, the existing knowledge base on effective approaches awaits translation into practice.

*Keywords: public health; health promotion; occupational health; shift work nutrition; participatory and empowerment strategies*

The workplace has been identified as an important setting in which behavioural patterns, including healthy eating, physical activity as well as sleep hygiene, can be promoted (1, 2). Worksites provide a natural social context and could potentially reach a large number of people, including many who would otherwise be unlikely to engage in preventive health behaviour (3, 4). Workers' good health and well-being is vital for workplace competitiveness and productivity, a long life and a high quality of life (5). This is also emphasised in the EU Public Health Programme for 2014–2020 (6), but there appears to be a gap between political intentions and implementation (4, 7–9).

The political agenda is taking place in a context that has been created by major changes in working life. The modern society has become a '24-h society' in which people can buy goods, including food, and go to restaurants 'around the clock'. An increasing amount of people are employed in shift work or working outside the ordinary daytime working period and therefore required to work and eat their meals at unconventional hours (10, 11). As the shift work pattern may vary depending on the time of day, the rotation cycle and the direction of rotation of shifts, and may also involve a mobile working place, it creates additional challenges to the food situation at work (12). While there is no consensus definition of the term 'shift work' in the published scientific literature, it is often referred to as work conducted primarily outside of ordinary daytime working hours and a pattern of shifts that may be permanent or rotating (13).

Approximately 21% of the workforce in Europe participate in shift work (10) which in this review is referred to as working irregular hours or extended hours 'around the clock'. Occupations that would fall into this category can be found within the health care sector, manufacturing sector, retail and service sectors. Previous research has linked shift work and working irregular hours to reduced well-being, increased health risks, metabolic syndrome and obesity (13–15), and to poorer eating habits, including a higher energy intake among shift workers compared with day workers (16). However, it has been suggested that it is the timing of meals and eating occasions, rather than the dietary composition that differs between day and shift workers (17–19). Circadian stress due to eating and sleeping in the wrong phase of inherent circadian rhythms is believed to be a main contributor to metabolic disorders in shift workers (20, 21).

Factors that may negatively affect workers' ability to make healthy food and physical activity choices during working hours include a lack of workers' influence on work organisation and hours worked, lack of social support and feelings of lack of personal agency and control over the job situation. In addition to the negative effects caused by circadian stress, health risks may be increased by the fact that employees working irregular hours often have limited access to healthy meals and snacks at work (22, 23) and that they are not included in workplace health-promoting activities and initiatives to the same extent as workers in day jobs (24).

In line with the adoption of ecological and socio-ecological models in health promotion, a change has been seen towards moving nutrition from a primarily individual issue to an environmental concern addressing both the physical and psychosocial work environment (3, 14, 25). Accordingly, the use of participatory and empowerment strategies has become important in assuring programme responsiveness to employees' needs and priorities (3, 26). Research evidence on the effectiveness of different health promotion strategies, including educational, environmental and/or multi-component strategies, in worksites during ordinary daytime working hours suggests that these may be effective in improving dietary habits (27, 28), increasing physical activity (29), reducing body weight (30–32) and increasing work productivity (33). However, uncertainty exists especially regarding the effectiveness and feasibility of health promotion interventions among the working population working 'around the clock'.

The aim of this study was to conduct a systematic review of randomised studies on the impact of worksite interventions to promote healthier food and/or physical activity among people who work 'around the clock'.

## Material and methods

A systematic review was undertaken and reported according to the guidelines of the PRISMA statement (34). The protocol was registered with Prospero (registration number CRD42016045216).

### *Eligibility criteria*

Criteria for study inclusion were developed using the population–intervention–comparator–outcomes–study (PICOS) design format. The resulting PICOS can be found in Table 1, where 'population' included people working irregular hours (e.g. shift workers in permanent 2-shift work, permanent night work or 3-shift including night work) or extended working hours (e.g. 12- or 24-h shifts) and 'intervention' included studies that focused on developing a healthy working environment defined as interventions to improve dietary habits and/or increase physical activity for a month or more.

The following studies were excluded: interventions conducted among non-shift workers (i.e. workers working ordinary office hours); interventions conducted among workers with extreme work schedules or workers who cross time zones (e.g. astronauts and air crew); interventions conducted in simulated work environments and conditions; literature reviews, commentaries, editorials, opinion pieces, policy documents, consensus statements, study protocols; lacking both pre- and post-intervention critical outcome measures; interventions that were designed to improve profit or turnover; and interventions that were reported in a language other than English.

Critical outcome measures focused on dietary and physical activity. Important outcomes were measures for general well-being, quality of life, sleep circadian rhythm, cognitive performance, mood, psychological stress, blood measurements, body composition, muscle strength, influence on work (e.g. productivity, absenteeism, use of medication, work injuries and medical costs), adverse events and dropouts. Outcomes at both pre- and post-interventions were included, as well as outcomes at follow-up, if reported.

### *Search strategy*

Relevant studies were identified by searching two different electronic databases: PubMed and CINAHL. There were no time restrictions. Date of search was 14 June 2016. A full example of the search terms used in PubMed is outlined in Appendix A. An updated search was conducted

*Table 1.* Study eligibility criteria according to PICOS

| Author/year | N | Sample | Shift system | Intervention | Length | Design | Critical/important outcome measures (Tool) Significant effects highlighted in bold | Risk of bias †) |
|---|---|---|---|---|---|---|---|---|
| Leedo et al. 2017 (51) | 60 M/F | Hospital nurses/nursing-aides/physicians (Denmark)<br>Mean age: 45.1 ± 9.3 years<br>Mean BMI: 24.1 ± 3.5 | Day time workers and shift workers | **Change of meal offer:**<br>Water, healthy snacks and healthy cold meals during each shift versus own lunch | 8 weeks | Cross-over | Anthropometrics (BMI, weight)<br>Reaction time (Go/No-Go test)<br>**Profile of Mood States (POMS) (shift workers)**<br>**Dietary intake (dietary record)** | Low within the larger study. High within the shift workers subsample |
| Matsugaki et al. 2017 (52) | 30 F | Hospital nurses (Japan)<br>Age: 20–40 years<br>BMI: app. 20 | Shift work, full time | **Physical exercise:**<br>Supervised versus non-supervised resistance and aerobic training two sessions/week | 12 weeks | RCT | **$VO_2$ max (cycle)**<br>Muscle strength (knee extension)<br>Anthropometrics (BMI)<br>Body composition (body fat, muscle mass)<br>Blood pressure<br>Pulse rate<br>Blood measurements (**cholesterol**, glucose, oxidative stress)<br>Depression (BDI-II)<br>Profile of Mood States (POMS) | Unclear |
| Härmä et al. 1988 1988 (39, 40) | 75 F | Hospital nurses/Nursing-aides, (Finland)<br>Age: 2<br>0–49 years; BMI? | 38 h/week, irregular rotation of 8–10 h day, evening and night shifts | **Physical exercise**:<br>Training program targeting circulatory and muscular systems (jogging, running, swimming, skiing, walking and gymnastics); 2–6 ×/week, 60–70% maximum heart rate versus usual activity | 4 months | 2-arm RCT (2:1) | **$VO_2$ max (cycle)**<br>**Strength (sit-ups/30s)**<br>**Resting heart rate**<br>WeightBody composition (skinfolds mm)<br>Subjective Sleep (Diary)<br>**Fatigue (questionnaire)**<br>**Sleep Length (h)**<br>Sleep Quality (questionnaire)<br>Body temperature<br>**Alertness (VAS)**<br>Short term memory (SAM-test)<br>**Muscular, GI** and nervous symptoms | High |
| Morgan et al. 2011 and Morgan et al. 2012 (POWER) (41, 42) | 110 M | Overweight/obese aluminium plant workers (Australia)<br>Mean age: 44.4 ± 8.6 years; BMI 30.5 ± 3.6 (45.5% obese) | Four shifts (schedule not reported) | **Lifestyle intervention**:<br>Group-based intervention for weight loss based on Social Cognitive Theory; one-on-one information session, study website, resource booklet, pedometer and financial incentive versus usual activity | 14 weeks | Cluster randomised | **Weight (loss)**<br>**Waist circumference**<br>BMI<br>Blood pressure (**systolic)Resting heart rate**<br>**Physical habits, dietary habits, healthy eating practices, dietary stage of change, self-efficacy *)** (questionnaire)<br>Sleepiness during day (Epworth scale)<br>**Quality of life *) (SF-12)**<br>**Workplace productivity (WLQ)**<br>**Injuries at work**<br>**Absenteeism** | Low |

*Table 1.* Continued

| Author/year | N | Sample | Shift system | Intervention | Length | Design | Critical/important outcome measures (Tool)<br>Significant effects highlighted in bold | Risk of bias †) |
|---|---|---|---|---|---|---|---|---|
| Guillermard et al. 2010 (43) | 1,000 M/F | Worker in factory, nurses, firefighters, police officer, other (France)<br>Age: app. 32 years<br>BMI: app. 24 | 2-shift work or 3-shift work (83%) | **Change of meal offer:**<br>Fermented dairy product containing lactobacillus casei versus placebo to drink (100 g) 2 times per day | 3 months (1 month follow-up) | 2-arm RCT | **Common infectious diseases** (CID) (upper tract, lower tract, GI) (diary + medical examination + pathogens)<br>**Immune parameters**<br>Duration,<br>**Days with fever**<br>Sick leave<br>Medication (prescribed/self-medication)<br>Quality of life (SF-36)<br>Adverse events (BP, heart rate, weight) | Low |
| Lim et al. 2015 (44) | 30 M | Type of work? (South Korea)<br>Age: app. 57 years<br>BMI: app. 23 | Night shift | **Physical exercise:**<br>3 days walking exercise per week (60–79% $VO_2$ max) 3 × 10 min/day versus usual activity | 10 weeks | 2-arm RCT §) | **Weight,** BMI **§)**<br>Body composition (LBM, **% fat**)<br>Blood pressure<br>**Biomarkers** (cathepsins) | High |
| Elliot et al. 2004 (PHLAME pilot) (50) | 33 M? | Fire fighters (USA)<br>Age: app. 44 years<br>BMI: app. 28 | 24 h works followed by 48 h off duty | **Lifestyle intervention:**<br>Team-based curriculum (model 1), individual counsellor meetings (model 2) versus usual care<br>Goals: Increase physical activity, servings of fruit and vegetables, reduce fat, improve energy balance versus information | 6 months | Cluster randomised §) | **Cholesterol** (blood)<br>BMI, Weight.<br>Body composition (skinfold, % fat)<br>**Dietary habits, exercise habits, mediating aspects** (questionnaire)<br>Peak oxygen uptake (treadmill) | High |
| Kuehl et al. 2005 (46)<br>Elliot et al. 2007 (45)<br>Ranby et al. 2011 (48)<br>MacKinnon et al. 2010 (PHLAME) (47) | 599 (397)<br>97%<br>M | Fire fighters (USA)<br>Age: 41 ± 9 years<br>BMI: app. 27 | 24 h works followed by 48 h off duty | **Lifestyle intervention:**<br>Team-based curriculum (model 1), individual counsellor meetings (model 2) versus usual care<br>Goals: Increase physical activity, servings of fruit and vegetables, reduce fat, improve energy balance versus information | 12 months and 4 years follow-up | Cluster randomised | 12 months<br>**BMI, Weight**<br>Body composition (skinfold, mm)<br>**Dietary habits*)**, exercise habits, **well-being** (questionnaire)<br>Peak oxygen uptake (treadmill)<br>Strength (**sit-ups** and sit and reach)<br>**Work injuries**<br>**Days of**<br>**Injury claims**<br>4 years' follow-up<br>Weight<br>Dietary habits, exercise habits, well-being (questionnaire)<br>Peak oxygen uptake (treadmill) | High |
| Kuehl et al. 2013 (PHLAME) (49) | 1,369<br>93%<br>M | Fire fighters (USA)<br>No data about age or BMI | 24 h works followed by 48 h off duty | **Lifestyle intervention**<br>Team-based curriculum (model 1), individual counsellor meetings (model 2) versus usual care<br>Goals: Increase physical activity, servings of fruit and vegetables, reduce fat, improve energy balance versus information | 7 year period | Retrospective data before after intervention comparison | **Compensation claims**<br>**Medical costs** | High ‡) |

M = male, F = female, BMI = body mass index, LBM = lean body mass.
* Some of the parameters are significant; † see text for explanation; † since data are based on the PHLAME study with a high risk of bias; § data different at baseline.

on 18 October 2017 by performing a search on Google Scholar. We also used the related articles function in PubMed on initially included studies to identify additional studies. In addition, a PubMed citation search was conducted on all studies included in the final review.

*Identification of studies*

The titles of the studies generated from the searches were reviewed for inclusion by one author alone. Abstracts from potentially relevant titles were then reviewed against the inclusion and exclusion criteria by two authors. The full texts of articles were obtained for all abstracts deemed to be potentially relevant and were reviewed by three authors. Systematic reviews identified by the search were scrutinised by one author for additional studies. Any disagreements were resolved by discussion and consensus reached before final inclusion. The study selection process from identification to exclusion was documented using the PRISMA flow chart.

*Quality assessment of evidence*

The Cochrane Collaboration's recommended tool for assessing risk of bias was used to assess the risk of bias (35). The potential sources of bias assessed were random sequence generation (selection bias), allocation concealment, blinding of participants and personnel (assessment was made for each) and outcome assessment (detection bias due to knowledge of the allocated interventions), incomplete outcome data, selective outcome reporting and other sources of bias. The studies were classified as containing high, low or unclear risk of bias for each of the criteria for judging risk of bias, and a conclusion regarding the overall risk of bias was made. Classification was based on the judgement of three authors following the guidelines outlined in the Cochrane Handbook.

*Data extraction and description*

Outcome measures sought in the publications were defined as either 'critical' or 'important' according to GRADE (36) (see Table 1). Data were described in the text. Since it was not expected that the included studies would be judged to be clinically homogeneous, no meta-analysis was performed. In cases where statistically significant effects were demonstrated, effect sizes (Cohen's d) of the study interventions were either obtained from the publications when provided or calculated for this review. Cohen proposed interpreting $d = 0.2$ as a small effect size, $d = 0.5$ as a moderate effect size and $d = 0.8$ as a large effect size (37, 38).

## Results

*Articles selected for review*

The initial searches resulted in 1,196 titles. Screening of titles identified 128 abstracts for further assessment. A total of 30 full-text articles were reviewed. Seven studies (reports published in 14 papers) fulfilled the inclusion criteria for the present review (see flow diagram in Fig. 1): Härmä et al. (39, 40), the POWER study (41, 42), Guillermard et al. (43), Lim et al. (44) and the PHLAME study (45–49), including a pilot study (50). Two additional relevant studies were identified in the updated search: Leedo et al. (51) and Matsugaki et al. (52). A list of the excluded full-text articles is available from the last author.

*Details of the studies*

The studies had been performed in different parts of the world, including East Asia, Europe, the United States and Australia (Table 2). The majority of studies were performed in the health care and manufacturing sector among shift workers including nurses and other health care workers (39, 40, 51, 52), plant workers (41, 42), fire fighters (45–50) and different shift workers, including police officers and nurses (43). One study did not report the occupation of the night shift workers (44).

The number of participants within each study was generally small with four studies having between 30 and 75 participants (39, 40, 44, 50–52), while three studies had a larger sample size of between 110 and 1,000 participants (41–43, 45). In all, the participants were young or middle-aged adults. In three studies, the target population included only men or consisted predominantly of male employees (41, 42, 44, 45, 50), two included only women (39, 40, 52) and two studies included both male and female employees (43, 51). The length of the interventions varied from 2 to 12 months.

*Interventions*

*A broader lifestyle intervention approach* was reported in two studies; the POWER (41, 42) and the PHLAME study (45–50). The POWER study (41, 42) involved a 3-month cluster randomised controlled trial among 110 male overweight/obese aluminium plant workers in Australia and focused on weight loss. It included an information session during work, a handbook with provision of information regarding the programme, a study website including a tutorial and a user guide, seven individualised dietary feedback sheets, group-based financial incentives and a pedometer as part of a group-based, cognitive theory-guided weight-loss programme versus usual activity (41). In the PHLAME cluster randomised controlled trial (45–48, 50), two types of intervention among firefighters during duty hours were compared with a control group in a 6-month pilot study with 33 participating firefighters and in a 12-month main study (followed by a scaled-down booster programme the following year and a 4-year follow-up period) with 397 participating firefighters. The first type of intervention involved a *team-centred curriculum* with a group-designated team leader, team leaders'

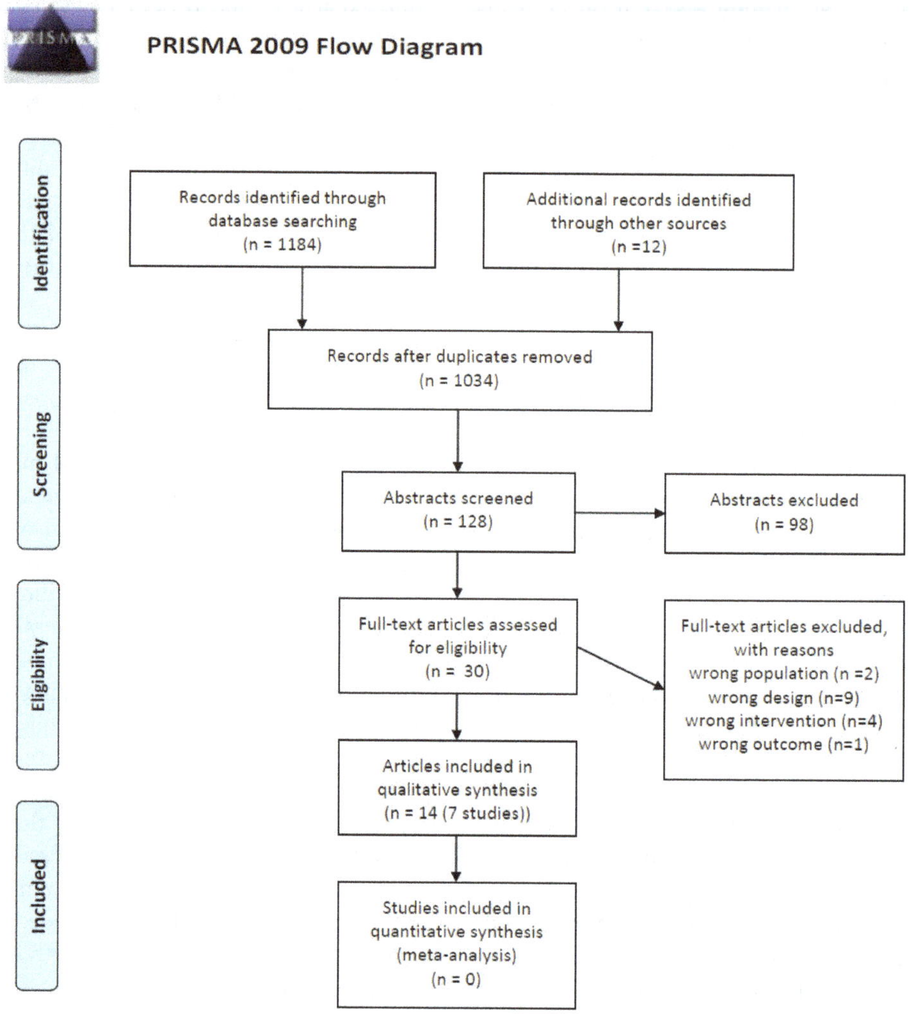


*Fig. 1.* Search strategy, study selection and process of identification of suitable studies.

*Table 2.* Description of the included studies

*Population (P):* People working irregular hours, meaning 'around the clock'

*Intervention (I):* Healthy working environment

*Comparison (C):* Usual care

*Outcomes (O):* Critical: Dietary and physical activity habits
Important: General well-being, quality of life, sleep circadian rhythm, cognitive performance, psychological stress, blood measurements, body composition, muscle strength, influence on work performance, adverse events, dropouts

*Study design:* Randomised controlled trials, cluster-randomised controlled trials and randomised crossover studies

manual, workbooks, lesson plans and team leaders' orientation focusing on healthy nutrition, physical activity and energy balance plus additional core topics, such as stress or sleep. The second type utilised *individual-centred motivational interviewing* with a counsellor to discuss and review the goals, values and priorities for change in firefighters' personal lifestyle behaviours, plus a short follow-up option in person or via phone (45). Further, a retrospective follow-up study over a 6-year period was conducted among the firefighters in the PHLAME study to evaluate medical costs among the fire departments participating in the health promotion intervention department compared with other fire departments (49).

*Physical activity* was the focus of the intervention in three studies (39, 40, 44, 52). In the randomised controlled trial by Härmä et al. (39, 40), a 4-month physical training programme was individually tailored for 75 female nurses in Finland according to their submaximal ergometer test, age and sports habits. In the exercise programme, both circulatory and musculoskeletal systems were activated by jogging, running, swimming, skiing, walking and gymnastics in 2–6 training sessions per week, according to the physical condition of the subject. In a 10-week randomised controlled trial by Lim et al. (44), 30 male night shift workers in South Korea were instructed to include three 10-min walking exercise sessions on 3 days per week into their night routines while at work. Based on the highest heart rate recorded during the $VO_2$ max test, a target zone of the maximal heart rate was established for each subject. The exercise programme was self-monitored, and participants were encouraged to schedule their walking time into their night routines while at work. In a randomised controlled trial by Matsugaki et al. (52), the 12-week exercise programme intervention among 30 female nurses conducting shift work consisted of either exercise under the individual supervision of a physical therapist or voluntary exercise without supervision at the hospital.

*Offering healthier food or meal options* was the focus of the intervention in two studies. Guillermard et al. (43) tested in a randomised controlled trial the effect of offering a fermented dairy product containing *Lactobacillus casei* twice a day as a breakfast and dinner supplement in a placebo-controlled study of 1,000 male and female shift workers in France. This was a 3-month study with 1-month follow-up aiming at reducing the risk of common infections. Leedo et al. (51) tested in a randomised crossover controlled study the effect of 8 weeks of increased availability of healthy meals at work, including a daily cold lunch meal, bottled water and a snack among a total of 59 hospital health care employees, including 16 employees working in shifts.

Additional information about the included studies, that is, the outcomes assessed and significant effects, can be found in Table 2.

### *Study quality*

Three of the studies, Guillermard et al. (43), the POWER study (41, 42) and Leedo et al. (51), were assessed as having a low risk of bias (see Table 2). This includes also the risk of carry-over effect in the crossover study by Leedo et al. (51), based upon the report that the researchers had examined the possible existence of a carry-over effect of treatment sequence on all outcomes. However, the study by Leedo et al. (51) was assessed as having an unclear to high level of bias in the group of shift workers as a subsample within the larger study sample due to small number of subjects. Four studies were assessed as having unclear or high risk of bias, which was mainly due to lack of blinding of participants, personnel or outcome assessment. In these studies, the outcomes may have become influenced by lack of blinding of the allocated interventions and the use of subjective and self-reported outcomes (39, 44, 45, 50, 52), other sources of bias, for example, an imbalance in baseline characteristics (44, 45, 50), a high dropout rate (39, 40) or in situations where the influence of clusters (in the analysis) had not been considered (45, 50).

### *Critical outcomes*

*Dietary habits* were evaluated in the PHLAME study (45, 50), the POWER study (41) and the study by Leedo et al. (51) among firefighters, aluminium plant workers and health care staff, respectively. All three found some significant improvement in dietary behaviour, for example, an increased intake of fruit and vegetables in the PHLAME main study (effect sizes: 0.2 and 0.4 in the individual and team-based groups, respectively) (45), a decreased intake of sweetened beverages in the POWER study (effect size: 0.5 to 0.6) (41) and an increased intake of water among the shift-work subgroup in the study by Leedo et al. when comparing intervention versus control group (not possible to calculate effect size) (51). On the contrary, no intervention effect on fruit and vegetable intake was found in the POWER study (41). PHLAME and POWER studies both used a questionnaire to assess dietary habits, whereas in the study by Leedo et al. (51) participants completed a 4-day self-reported dietary record. In the PHLAME study, mediating factors for the improvement in fruit and vegetable intake included an increased knowledge of the benefits of fruit and vegetable intake (significant for fruit intake) and an improved level of social support (dietary norms) experienced from co-workers (significant for vegetable intake) (45, 47).

*Physical activity* measures included changes in physical activity habits and maximum oxygen uptake and were assessed in four studies (39, 41, 45, 50, 52). All four, expect for the PHLAME main study, found a significant impact on either maximal oxygen uptake ($VO_2$ max) (39, 52) or physical activity habits assessed via questionnaire (41, 50). In the study by Härmä et al., the physical exercise intervention resulted in an improved $VO_2$ max among nurses (effect size: 0.4) (39). Similarly, in the study reported by Matsugaki et al. (52), $VO_2$ max increased significantly in the group receiving exercise supervision (effect size: 0.6) compared with the voluntary exercise group. Contrary to these, the PHLAME lifestyle interventions among firefighters resulted in non-significant impact on $VO_2$ max in the pilot study (46) and in the main study (41). However, the level of physical activity, assessed via questionnaire, was reported to have significantly improved in the team-based group in the PHLAME pilot study (effect size: 1.1) (46).

*Physical strength* was assessed in three studies (39, 45, 52), and a significant impact was reported in all on either number of sit-ups or on muscle strength measured by strength of the knee extensor muscle. Number of sit-ups from baseline to post-intervention increased significantly both in the PHLAME main lifestyle intervention (not possible to calculate effect size) (45) and in the nurses' physical activity study by Härmä et al. (39) (effect size: 0.9). Also, the Matsugaki et al. study (52) reported significant improvement in muscle strength (180 deg/sec KET) among nurses in the supervised exercise group over time (effect size: 1.3).

*Long-term change in diet and physical activity habits* were assessed in the PHLAME study, which included a 4-year follow-up of their participants. The authors concluded that 1-year effects of the programme did not remain over time compared to the control group, but the long-term pattern of behaviours in both groups suggested that the worksites, as a whole, had continued to improve in outcome measures for several years following the programme (47).

#### *Important outcomes*

*General well-being including quality of life* was assessed in three studies via questionnaires (42, 43, 45). Two of the interventions showed significant improvements in either overall well-being or quality of life using different scales. In the PHLAME study, the index of general well-being improved significantly in both types of lifestyle intervention (individual- and team-based) among firefighters (45). The POWER trial used the SF-12 questionnaire and found a significant positive effect of the broader lifestyle intervention on mental health (effect size: 0.7) but not on physical health among aluminium plant workers (42). However, no difference was found by Guillermard et al., who used the original larger SF-36 scale in their study on offering a fermented dairy product as a supplement to reduce the risk of common infections among shift workers (43).

*Sleep circadian rhythm* was examined in two studies. Härmä et al. found a significant positive effect of physical exercise on sleep length and reduction of fatigue among nurses (not possible to calculate effect size) (39), while the POWER study (42) did not observe any significant benefits in sleepiness score of a broader lifestyle intervention for weight loss among aluminium plant workers.

*Psychological stress* was measured in several ways: via blood pressure, heart rate, testosterone level and body temperature in a total of four studies (39–41, 43, 44). Two of them found a significant positive effect on blood pressure and/or heart rate (39, 41), while two did not (43, 44). Morgan et al. (41) found a positive effect of the POWER lifestyle intervention on systolic blood pressure among aluminium plant workers in their group-based weight loss programme compared to control (effect size: 0.5). Psychological stress was assessed via heart rate in three studies. Two of these found a significant positive effect: Härmä et al. (39) offering physical exercise to female nurses (effect size: −0.4) and Morgan et al. (41) offering a lifestyle intervention to aluminium plant workers (effect size: −0.8). In contrast, no difference between intervention and control groups was reported in the study by Guillermard et al. offering two daily fermented dairy products to male and female shift workers (43). Härmä et al. (40) also measured psychological stress by means of body temperature (40) and did not observe any benefit of the intervention in nurses' physical exercise intervention.

*Cognitive performance* was evaluated in three studies using different measures. In two, positive effects were found in cognitive performance measures (40, 51). The study by Härmä et al. found a significant positive effect of physical exercise on alertness in nurses during the night shift (not possible to calculate effect size) (40), and the study by Leedo et al. (51) found a significant positive effect on total mood-related score among the subgroup of shift workers (effect size: 0.3). In the latter study, however, no effect on reaction time was found. Contrary to Leedo et al.'s study (48), Matsugaki et al.'s study did not find any significant effect in total mood-related score among nurses (52).

*Blood measures*, for example, cholesterol and the biomarker cathepsin, were evaluated in three studies (44, 50, 52). All three found significant positive effects: decreased level of LDL-cholesterol in the PHLAME pilot study in both the team- and individual-based groups (effect sizes: −0.2 and −0.4, respectively) (50), increased level of HDL cholesterol among nurses in the supervision exercise group in the study by Matsugaki et al. (effect size: 0.2) (52) and a decrease in cathepsin S and L in the Lim et al.'s study on night shift workers in the exercise intervention group compared to control (effect size: −0.4) (44).

*Body composition* was assessed in all studies except the Leedo et al.'s study (51). Two studies assessing change in lean body mass (LBM) in a physical exercise intervention among night shift workers did not find any effect (44, 52). However, one of these studies found a small but significant positive effect on percentage of body fat (effect size: −0.03) (44), while no difference was observed in the others (39, 45, 52). Finally, Morgan et al. (42) assessed waist circumference and found a positive effect of the intervention among the aluminium plant workers (effect size: −0.6).

*Weight and body mass index (BMI)* were measured in all studies except the one by Guillemard et al. (43). They reported either significant difference in weight loss between intervention and control groups (41, 44), no significant weight changes compared to control group or control period (39, 51, 52), or less weight gain in the intervention group than the control group (45). The POWER study resulted in both significant weight loss and improved BMI among overweight plant workers in the intervention group compared to control (effect sizes: −0.3 and −0.4, respectively) (41). The goal of the PHLAME study was, among others, to improve energy balance among firefighters. This was succeeded during the 1-year intervention, where both the team- and individual-based groups gained less weight than the control group (45). The three studies testing the effect of physical exercise (39, 40, 44, 52) measured weight, and in two, the normal weight participants in the intervention group had a small loss of weight which was more than in the control group, but this type of unintentional weight loss was reported as significant only in the study among night shift workers in the study by Lim et al. (effect size: −0.1) (44). In the study by Leedo et al., the participants kept a stable weight throughout the intervention offering foods and beverages to improve overall dietary intake (51).

*Influence on work performance* was assessed in three studies (41, 43, 46, 49), all with positive outcomes. The POWER study among plant workers (42) assessed work place productivity, injuries at work and absenteeism and found a positive effect on all these outcomes (effect sizes: 0.5 to 0.7). In the retrospective PHLAME follow-up study, a reduction in compensation claims and medical costs was seen (49). Guillermard et al. (43) found a positive significant effect from offering fermented dairy products among shift workers' cumulated days with fever (effect sizes: −1.2) compared to control (only for the whole study phase) but not on the primary outcome, that is, cumulated time with chronic infectious diseases.

*Adverse effects* were only assessed in two studies. Guillermard et al. (43) assessed blood pressure, heart rate and weight, and Matsugaki et al. assessed muscle pain and physical fatigue (52). They did not find any difference between study groups.

## Discussion

The present review carried out a systematic identification, analysis and quality assessment of the evidence on the impact of workplace interventions to promote healthy food and/or physical activity on dietary and physical activity outcome measures among people working 'around the clock' compared with controls receiving usual care. A total of seven studies (reported in 14 papers) were included in the final analysis: two having a broader lifestyle approach, three based on physical exercise and two based on offering healthy meals as a replacement of ordinary meals and offering food supplements to existing workplace meals. In general, a positive effect was seen on several of the outcomes assessed irrespective of the intervention approach.

Taken together, the studies showed small-to-moderate effect sizes on several measures, including dietary and/or physical activity measures, suggesting acceptable effectiveness for interventions involving community-level behaviour change. This review showed moderate positive effects on several critical and important outcomes in the two larger studies with a broader lifestyle approach focusing on dietary habits among aluminium plant workers (the POWER study) (41, 42) and on physical activity among firefighters (the PHLAME study) (45–50). These outcomes included improvements in intake of fruit and vegetables, intake of sweetened drinks, weight status, physical activity, strength and work performance. Moderate positive effects were seen also in the two smaller 'high-intensity' studies using individually tailored or supervised exercise programmes among nurses (39, 40, 52). Here, the outcomes included improvements in physical activity, strength and LDL-cholesterol levels. Small-to-moderate positive effects were seen in the intervention in which a 'one type fits all' exercise programme was added to the routines of night shift workers by Lim et al. (44). Also, in general, limited effects were reported in the study in which a food supplement was offered (43). The outcomes in these studies included improvements in weight status and the biomarker cathepsin in the former, and improvements in incidence of respiratory and gastrointestinal common infectious diseases and work performance in the latter study. Small effects were also shown in the study by Leedo et al. (51), providing health workers with healthy foods and beverages during working hours. This study reported some positive results, including an increase in water intake but did not reach its targets in increasing overall dietary intake, for example, an increase in fruit and vegetable intake. The Leedo et al.'s (51) study outcomes might have shown more effect, had the sample size been larger in terms of the number of shift workers. In light of our literature review, it may be prudent to say that the limited outcomes in these three studies (43, 44, 51) may at least partly be attributable to a lack of use of participatory and empowerment strategies to assure that the intervention content is responsive to the employees' needs and priorities. The unique challenges encountered by shift workers in adhering to a healthy diet are important and should be acknowledged in successful intervention design (41).

In a similar vein, a review by Verweij et al. of worksite interventions, not limited to shift workers, to promote physical activity and dietary behaviour, showed greater effect, for example, success in weight loss, in interventions which contained environment components besides personal components (32). On the contrary, the review by Allan et al. (27) showed that significant change in primary outcome measures of eating behaviours, for example, increased fruit and vegetable consumption, was reported only by about half of the identified worksite interventions that had used solely environmental strategies to alter eating behaviours. Implementing environmental interventions can, according to Tam et al. (31) in their review of long-term effectiveness of work-based lifestyle interventions to tackle overweight and obesity, prove problematic due to the multiple layers of commitment needed at different levels of the organization, for example, support at the management level and on behalf of the participants to ensure sufficient individual participation. Our review concurs with the conclusion of Tam et al. (31) that the most effective interventions may be the ones that are of high intensity or include a specific motivational component besides interventions with multiple lifestyle components.

To conclude, the findings from our review have highlighted a lack of evidence from workplace interventions to promote healthy food and physical activity during working hours among people who work during unorthodox hours, 'around the clock'.

*Quality of the studies reviewed*

Several of the studies were assessed as having an overall high risk of bias with regard to the outcomes (see Table 2). It is important to note that it has probably not been feasible to conduct blinding in terms of participants and staff in the type of interventions studied, that is, focusing on diet or physical activity in real-life settings. Achieving a high-quality rating was especially problematic because of the subjective outcomes (e.g. quality of life) and self-reported measures (via questionnaires) used in many of the reviewed studies in assessing their effect. In future studies in this field, it is, therefore, important to consider more objective outcome parameters. Further, offering an active control condition, as opposed to no treatment control, may facilitate blinding (53). Another major issue possibly contributing to bias in the assessment of outcomes common in the now reviewed studies was an imbalance in baseline characteristics. This may, in turn, have contributed to the lack of effect on some of the outcomes. In addition, only three studies identified primary outcome and presented a power calculation, which reduces their comparability and contribution to evidence base in this field.

*Limitations and strengths of the systematic review*

With our search terms, we identified only seven studies that could be included in the analysis. This is an indication of a lack of studies on the promotion of physical activity and dietary lifestyle changes among employees working 'around the clock'. Due to the small number of studies, a wide mixture of approaches (from broader lifestyle intervention to food supplements), the generally small sample sizes, the variation in intervention duration and the different kind of shift work occupations and settings, we were only able to perform a qualitative extract of main patterns in the effectiveness of the different types of intervention. A higher number of larger well-focused studies are needed to compare different approaches in different types of shift work under irregular working hours and among different occupational groups. For example, the two studies focusing specifically on male shift workers were the ones that employed a broader lifestyle approach and showed evidence of effectiveness. It would be of interest to replicate such an approach among both female and male shift workers and different occupational groups. Women have been frequently reported to engage in far more health-promoting behaviours than men and to obtain healthier lifestyle patterns (54). On the contrary, from a behavioural standpoint, some evidence suggests that men may engage better with a lifestyle programme once committed, although getting them to initially commit might be more challenging (55). A further limitation is the clinical inhomogeneity in the included studies which did not warrant a meta-analysis but would have rendered it meaningless. Finally, a limitation of the search strategy was that articles not published in English were not included and moreover that the updated search in October 2017 was restricted to Google Scholar and PubMed, which may mean that some relevant studies were missed.

The main strengths of this review were that it employed a comprehensive search strategy and brought together research findings on the impact of worksite interventions to promote healthier food and/or physical activity among an understudied but critical group of employees who work 'around the clock'. Despite the fact that the interventions were focused on healthy food and/or physical activities, other beneficial outcomes were measured such as work performance. Of course, a causal relation between diet/physical activity and the important outcomes can be questioned. According to our knowledge, no other systematic review has considered employees working 'around the clock'. Neil-Sztramko et al. (56) has critically reviewed the literature of worksite health-related interventions to prevent negative health effects among shift workers but limited their target group to night shift workers and only two of the 38 studies reviewed had a focus on healthy food or physical activity. These two studies (39–42) have been included in the present review.

*Implications for health promotion programming and practice*

Our review highlights the need for further testing of the broader lifestyle interventions as well as the individualised and high-intensity approaches in the target population. This arises from the two interventions carried out among male participants in the PHLAME study (45–50) and the POWER study (41, 42), and the two physical exercise studies among nurses (39, 40, 52). These studies included some degree of participatory and empowerment strategies, approaches that have been shown to be important in assuring programme responsiveness to employees' needs and priorities (3, 26). The long-term follow-up of the PHLAME study suggested that the participating worksites, as a whole, including the control participants, continued to improve in their outcome measures for several years following the programme (47). This provides further encouragement for knowledge translation into practice. The review also provides some support for improving the food and physical activity environmental strategies within organisations, including the provision of healthy meals and beverages, as in the Leedo et al.'s study (51). However, the study population (51) was too small to make firm conclusions.

In future studies, it is necessary to tailor intervention studies with respect to work schedules, meal breaks and mobile or mixed work places. The special challenges with respect to working irregular hours and circadian stress need to be addressed, that is, to recommend a healthy timing of eating with respect to circadian rhythm factors. Although there are still unsolved issues regarding the association between shift work and disease, we have enough knowledge to prompt preventative action (57).

*Future perspectives*

This review highlights the need for more evidence on the effectiveness of workplace interventions to promote healthy food and physical activity among people working irregular or extended hours 'around the clock'. Future research could focus on the nutritional and social aspects regarding eating behaviour in this target population, for example, to describe the effect of work schedule on dietary intake and meal timing, and the strategies people use in relation to their food and eating during irregular or extended working hours.

In particular, more knowledge is needed on the coping strategies and interventions to support shift workers employed in the retail and service sector in our modern '24-hour society'. This was a sector from which no studies were identified in this review. More research is also needed on effective approaches to promote health and well-being at any age by adopting a life-course approach and including older workers in the studies (58).

## Acknowledgements

Nordic Council of Ministers, Metropolitan University College, Technical University of Denmark, Gävle University and Kristianstad University, Sweden, and the University of Melbourne funded the study but had no influence on the study results reported.

## Conflict of interest and funding

None of the authors have any conflicts of interest to declare. Nordic Council of Ministers, Metropolitan University College, Danish Technical University, Gävle University, Kristianstad University and the University of Melbourne.

## References

1. Smith SA, Lake AA, Summerbell C, Raujo-Soares V, Hillier-Brown F. The effectiveness of workplace dietary interventions: protocol for a systematic review and meta-analysis. Syst Rev 2016; 5(1): 20.
2. Lassen AD, Thorsen AV, Haapala I, Wiklund ML, Nyberg M, Beck AM, et al. Food at work around the clock – the Nordic Model. Report from a Nordic Workshop, November 4, 2016, Copenhagen, Denmark. Copenhagen: National Food Institute, Technical University of Denmark; 2017.
3. Lassen AD, Thorsen AV, Sommer HM, Fagt S, Trolle E, Biltoft-Jensen A, et al. Improving the diet of employees at blue-collar worksites: results from the 'food at work' intervention study. Public Health Nutr 2011; 14(6): 965–74.
4. Guazzi M, Faggiano P, Mureddu GF, Faden G, Niebauer J, Temporelli PL. Worksite health and wellness in the European Union. Prog Cardiovasc Dis 2014; 56(5): 508–14.
5. The World Economic Forum. Working towards wellness: the business rationale. Geneva; World Economic Forum 2008.
6. European Commission. EU Health Programme 2014–2020. 2014. Available from: http://ec.europa.eu/health/programme/policy/2014-2020/index_en.htm [cited April 2018].
7. European Agency for Safety and Health at Work. Motivation for employees to participate in workplace health promotion. A literature review. Luxembourg: Publications Office of the European Union, 2012.
8. European Agency for Safety and Health at Work. Well-being at work creating a positive work environment. A literature review. Luxembourg: Publications Office of the European Union, 2013.
9. Toker S, Heaney CA, Ein-Gar D. Why won't they participate? Barriers to participation in worksite health promotion programmes. Eur J Work Organ Psychol 2015; 24(6): 866–81.
10. Eurofound. Sixth European Working Conditions Survey. Luxembourg: Publications Office of the European Union; 2017.
11. National Research Centre for the Working Environment. Working hours measured as 'other than regular daytime work' 2012 to 2016 Arbejdstid målt med 'andet end fast dagarbejde' 2012 til 2016. 2018. Available from: www.arbejdsmiljodata.nfa.dk [cited 15 April 2018].
12. Lindén AL, Lagnevik M, Sjöberg K, Svederberg E, Jönsson H, Nyberg M. Mat hälsa och oregelbundna arbetstider [English translation: Food, health and irregular working hours]. Research Reports in Sociology, 2005: 1. Department of Sociology, Lund, Lund University; 2005.
13. Esquirol Y, Perret B, Ruidavets JB, Marquie JC, Dienne E, Niezborala M, et al. Shift work and cardiovascular risk factors: new knowledge from the past decade. Arch Cardiovasc Dis 2011; 104(12): 636–68.
14. Antunes LC, Levandovski R, Dantas G, Caumo W, Hidalgo MP, Obesity and shift work: chronobiological aspects. Nutr Rev Rev 2010; 23(1): 155–68.
15. Nea FM, Kearney J, Livingstone MB, Pourshahidi LK, Corish CA. Dietary and lifestyle habits and the associated health risks in shift workers. Nutr Rev Rev 2015; 28(2): 143–66.
16. Hulsegge G, Boer JM, van der Beek AJ, Verschuren WM, Sluijs I, Vermeulen R, et al. Shift workers have a similar diet quality but higher energy intake than day workers. Scand J Work Environ Health 2016; 42(6): 459–68.
17. Holmback U, Forslund A, Lowden A, Forslund J, Akerstedt T, Lennernas M, et al. Endocrine responses to nocturnal eating – possible implications for night work. Eur J Nutr 2003; 42(2): 75–83.
18. Lennernas M, Hambraeus L, Akerstedt T. Shift related dietary-intake in day and shift workers. Appetite 1995; 25(3): 253–65.
19. Lowden A, Moreno C, Holmback U, Lennernas M, Tucker P, Eating and shift work – effects on habits, metabolism and performance. Scand J Work Environ Health 2010; 36(2): 150–62.
20. Asher G, Sassone-Corsi P. Time for food: the intimate interplay between nutrition, metabolism, and the circadian clock. Cell 2015; 161(1): 84–92.
21. Froy O. The relationship between nutrition and circadian rhythms in mammals. Front Neuroendocrinol 2007; 28(2–3): 61–71.
22. Hemio K, Puttonen S, Viitasalo K, Harma M, Peltonen M, Lindstrom J. Food and nutrient intake among workers with different shift systems. Occop Environ Med 2015; 72(7): 513–20.
23. Lemaire JB, Wallace JE, Dinsmore K, Lewin AM, Ghali WA, Roberts D. Physician nutrition and cognition during work hours: effect of a nutrition based intervention. BMC Health Serv Res 2010; 10: 241.

24. Nabe-Nielsen K, Jorgensen MB, Garde AH, Clausen T. Do working environment interventions reach shift workers? Int Arch Occup Environ Health 2016; 89(1): 163–70.
25. Dorfman L, Wallack L. Moving nutrition upstream: the case for reframing obesity. J Nutr Educ Behav 2007; 39(2 Suppl): S45–50.
26. Brandstetter S, Rueter J, Curbach J, Loss J. A systematic review on empowerment for healthy nutrition in health promotion. Public Health Nutr 2015; 18(17): 3146–54.
27. Allan J, Querstret D, Banas K, de Bruin M. Environmental interventions for altering eating behaviours of employees in the workplace: a systematic review. Obes Rev 2017; 18(2): 214–26.
28. Maes L, Van Cauwenberghe E, Van Lippevelde W, Spittaels H, De Pauw E, Oppert JM, et al. Effectiveness of workplace interventions in Europe promoting healthy eating: a systematic review. Eur J Public Health 2012; 22(5): 677–83.
29. Malik SH, Blake H, Suggs LS. A systematic review of workplace health promotion interventions for increasing physical activity. Br J Health Psychol 2014; 19(1): 149–80.
30. Schroer S, Haupt J, Pieper C. Evidence-based lifestyle interventions in the workplace-an overview. Occup Med (Lond) 2014; 64(1): 8–12.
31. Tam G, Yeung MPS. A systematic review of the long-term effectiveness of work-based lifestyle interventions to tackle overweight and obesity. Prevent Med 2018; 107: 54–60.
32. Verweij LM, Coffeng J, van Mechelen W, Proper KI. Meta-analyses of workplace physical activity and dietary behaviour interventions on weight outcomes. Obes Rev 2011; 12(6): 406–29.
33. Jensen JD. Can worksite nutritional interventions improve productivity and firm profitability? A literature review. Perspect Public Health 2011; 131(4): 184–92.
34. Liberati A, Altman DG, Tetzlaff J, Mulrow C, Gotzsche PC, Ioannidis JPA, et al. The PRISMA statement for reporting systematic reviews and meta-analyses of studies that evaluate healthcare interventions: explanation and elaboration. BMJ 2009; 339: b2700.
35. Higgins JPT, Green S. Cochrane handbook for systematic reviews of interventions version 5.1.0. The Cochrane Collaboration; 2011. Available from http://handbook.cochrane.org [cited April 2018].
36. Guyatt G, Oxman AD, Akl EA, Kunz R, Vist G, Brozek J, et al. GRADE guidelines: 1. Introduction-GRADE evidence profiles and summary of findings tables. J Clin Epidemiol 2011; 64(4): 383–94.
37. Cohen J. Statistical power analysis for the behavioural sciences. Hillsdale, NJ: Erlbaum; 1988.
38. Social Science Statistics. Effect size calculators. 2018. Available from: http://www.socscistatistics.com/effectsize/Default3.aspx [cited April 2018].
39. Härma MI, Ikmarinen J, Knauth P, Rydell SA, Hannnenin O. Physical training intervention in female shift workers I. The effekcts of intervention on fitness fatique sleep and psychosomatic symptoms. Ergonomics 1988; 31(1): 39–50.
40. Härma MI, Ilmarinen J, Knauth P, Rutenfranz J, Hannnenin O. Physical training intervention in female shift workers II. The effects of intervention on the circadian rhythms of alertness short-term memory and body temperature. Ergonomics 1988; 31(1): 51–63.
41. Morgan PJ, Collins CE, Plotnikoff RC, Cook AT, Berthon B, Mitchell S, et al. Efficacy of a workplace-based weight loss program for overweight male shift workers: the workplace POWER (Preventing Obesity Without Eating like a Rabbit) randomized controlled trial. Prev Med 2011; 52(5): 317–25.
42. Morgan PJ, Collins CE, Plotnikoff RC, Cook AT, Berthon B, Mitchell S, et al. The Impact of a workplace-based weight loss program on work-related outcomes in overweight male shift workers. J Occup Environ Med 2012; 54(2): 122–7.
43. Guillemard E, Tanguy J, Flavigny A, de la Motte S, Schrezenmeir J. Effects of consumption of a fermented dairy product containing the probiotic Lactobacillus casei DN-114 001 on common respiratory and gastrointestinal infections in shift workers in a randomized controlled trial. J Am Coll Nutr 2010; 29(5): 455–68.
44. Lim ST, Min SK, Kwon YC, Park SK, Park H. Effects of intermittent exercise on biomarkers of cardiovascular risk in night shift workers. Atherosclerosis 2015; 242(1): 186–90.
45. Elliot DL, Goldberg L, Kuehl KS, Moe EL, Breger RK, Pickering MA. The PHLAME (Promoting Healthy Lifestyles: Alternative Models' Effects) firefighter study: outcomes of two models of behavior change. J Am Diet Assoc 2007; 49(2): 204–13.
46. Kuehl KS, Elliot DL, Goldberg L, Moe E. The PHLAME study: short-term economic impact of health promotion. J Investig Med 2005; 53(1): S127.
47. MacKinnon DP, Elliot DL, Thoemmes F, Kuehl KS, Moe EL, Goldberg L, et al. Long-term effects of a worksite health promotion program for firefighters. Am J Health Behav 2010; 34(6): 695–706.
48. Ranby KW, MacKinnon DP, Fairchild AJ, Elliot DL, Kuehl KS, Goldberg L. The PHLAME (Promoting Healthy Lifestyles: Alternative Models' Effects) firefighter study: testing mediating mechanisms. J Occup Health Psychol 2011; 16(4): 501–13.
49. Kuehl KS, Elliot DL, Goldberg L, Moe EL, Perrier E, Smith J. Economic benefit of the PHLAME wellness programme on firefighter injury. Occup Med (Lond) 2013; 63(3): 203–9.
50. Elliot DL, Goldberg L, Duncan TE, Kuehl KS, Moe EL, Breger RKR, et al. The PHLAME firefighters' study: feasibility and findings. Am J Health Behav 2004; 28(1): 13–23.
51. Leedo E, Beck AM, Astrup A, Lassen AD. The effectiveness of healthy meals at work on reaction time, mood and dietary intake: a randomised cross-over study in daytime and shift workers at a university hospital. Br J Nutr 2017; 118(2): 121–9.
52. Matsugaki R, Kuhara S, Saeki S, Jiang Y, Michishita R, Ohta M, et al. Effectiveness of workplace exercise supervised by a physical therapist among nurses conducting shift work: a randomized controlled trial. J Occup Health 2017; 59(4): 327–35.
53. Byrd-Bredbenner C, Wu F, Spaccarotella K, Quick V, Martin-Biggers J, Zhang Y. Systematic review of control groups in nutrition education intervention research. Int J Behav Nutr Phys Act 2017; 14(1): 91.
54. Lassen AD, Lehmann C, Andersen EW, Werther MN, Thorsen AV, Trolle E, et al. Gender differences in purchase intentions and reasons for meal selection among fast food customers. Opportunities for healthier and more sustainable fast food. Food Qual Prefer 2016; 47: 123–9.
55. Kent LM, Morton DP, Rankin PM, Gobble JE, Diehl HA. Gender differences in effectiveness of the Complete Health Improvement Program (CHIP). J Nutr Educ Behav 2015; 47(1): 44–52.
56. Neil-Sztramko SE, Pahwa M, Demers PA, Gotay CC. Health-related interventions among night shift workers: a critical review of the literature. Scand J Work Environ Health 2014; 40(6): 543–56.
57. Knutsson A. Mortality of shift workers. Scand J Work Environ Health 2017; 43(2): 97–8.
58. European Agency for Safety and Health at Work. Safer and healthier work at any age: analysis report of workplace good practices and support needs of enterprises. A report. Luxembourg: Publications Office of the European Union, 2016.

***Anne Dahl Lassen**
National Food Institute
Danish Technical University
Email: adla@food.dtu.dk

# 18

# Efficacy and safety of *Eurycoma longifolia* (Physta®) water extract plus multivitamins on quality of life, mood and stress

Annie George[1,2], Jay Udani[3], Nurhayati Zainal Abidin[1] and Ashril Yusof[4]*

[1]Institute of Biological Sciences, Faculty of Science, University of Malaya, Kuala Lumpur, Malaysia; [2]Biotropics Malaysia Berhad, Lot 21, Jalan U1/19, Section U1, Hicom-Glenmarie Industrial Park, 40150 Shah Alam, Malaysia; [3]Agoura Hills, CA, USA; [4]Exercise Science, Sports Centre, University of Malaya, 50603 Kuala Lumpur, Malaysia

*Abstract*

***Background:*** The use of alternative and complementary medicines to alleviate stress has increased to avoid the negative effects of pharmaceutical drugs.

***Objective:*** This study investigated the safety and efficacy of *Eurycoma longifolia* in combination with multivitamins (EL+MV) versus placebo on improving quality of life (QoL), mood and stress in moderately stressed healthy participants.

***Methods:*** This randomised, double-blind, placebo-controlled 24-week study enrolled 93 participants aged 25–65 years, with a body mass index of 18–30 kg/m$^2$, scoring ≤18 in tension and ≤14 in fatigue subscale of Profiles of Mood Scores (POMS) questionnaire and supplemented with EL+MV or placebo. The primary endpoints were QoL measured by 12-Item Short Form Health Survey (SF-12) questionnaire and mood measured by POMS. The secondary endpoint was stress measured by Multi-Modal Stress Questionnaire (MMSQ). The safety of the intervention product was measured by complete metabolic panel, lipid and renal analysis including several immune parameters.

***Results:*** While there were no significant between-group differences, within-group improvements were observed in the SF-12 QoL, POMS and MMSQ domains. In the SF-12 domain, improvements were seen in role limitation due to emotional health ($P = 0.05$), mental component domain ($P < 0.001$), emotional well-being ($P < 0.001$), social functioning ($P = 0.002$) as well as vitality ($P = 0.001$) at week 12. An increasing trend in POMS-vigour domain was also observed in the EL+MV group at week 12. A 15% decrease in physical stress domain ($P < 0.05$) compared with 0.7% in the placebo group was also observed in MMSQ. When the subjects were subgrouped according to age, 25–45 and 46–65 years of age, for primary outcomes, between-group significance was observed in the 25–45 year group in the social functioning domain of SF-12 ($P = 0.021$) and POMS-vigour ($P = 0.036$) in the 46–65 year group. No significant changes were observed in vital signs and complete metabolic panel. Regarding immune parameters, the lymphocytes increased significantly in the active group ($P \leq 0.05$). In total, 13 adverse events were reported: six on placebo and seven on EL+MV.

***Conclusion:*** EL+MV may support the QoL, mood, stress and immune parameters in healthy participants.

Key words: *Eurycoma longifolia; multivitamins; quality of life; mood; stress*

Unresolved stress greatly increases the risk of developing depression, consequently becoming a topic of public health awareness and therapeutic interventions. Depression afflicts approximately 20–25% of women and 10–17% of men during their lifetime (1). While certain drugs like fluoxetine (Prozac) and sertraline (Zoloft) have been used to treat stress and anxiety disorders and, in recent years, the anti-depressant setraline, there is a concern that one can be addicted to and dependent on drug usage (2). Alternative and complementary medicines, such as herbal supplements, have emerged as substitutes to conventional therapeutics for ameliorating depression and maintaining mental well-being (3–5).

In South East Asia, where traditional/herbal medicine is popular, supplementation with *Eurycoma longifolia* Jack, Simaroubaceae (*Tongkat Ali* or Malaysian ginseng), has been shown to be efficacious for alleviating stress (6), as well as many other ailments including fever, arthritis, high blood pressure, diabetes, low energy or libido, bacterial infections and cancer (7–9). *Eurycoma longifolia* (EL) is a slender evergreen tree mainly found in Malaysia, Indonesia and the Philippines. Derivatives of this plant have been used to restore and enhance energy levels, to improve physical and mental performance, endurance and stamina (9) and quality of life (QoL), as evidenced by a decrease in aging males symptoms score and an increase in serum testosterone levels (10). Another related study showed improvement in QoL and sexual well-being in men, specifically in the domains of 'physical function' and 'vitality' (11). The roots of EL are largely responsible for its biological activity due to the presence of alkaloids, quassinoids, quassinoid diterpenoids, eurycomacoside, eurycolactone, laurylcolactone or eurycomalactone and pasakbumin-B (7) and peptides (12). It has been demonstrated to reduce stress through the reduction of cortisol (6) with a concurrent increase in lymphocytes and natural killer cells (13). These active ingredients in EL and in other plants, such as mountain ginseng (*Panax ginseng*), may be responsible for improving QoL, as well as combating stress without adverse effects (11, 14–16). A recent 4-week, randomised clinical study on moderately stressed participants consuming water extract from EL reported significant improvements in mood, tension, anger and confusion (6). This was accompanied by a reduction in cortisol and increased testosterone levels. Another study investigated the effect of EL on the immune status of moderately stressed subjects (13), whereby a 1-month supplementation of 200 mg EL extract per day nearly significantly improved vigour measured by Profile of Mood States (POMS) while scores for immunological vigour also improved.

Micronutrient deficiencies contribute to stress and depression (5). Indeed, low levels of folic acid may be correlated with depressive symptomatology (16) that can be ameliorated by mineral supplementation (17). Multinutrient formulations have a significantly greater effect in reducing stress and anxiety in subjects than single interventions alone (18). In addition, a recent study demonstrated that a formulation consisting of multivitamins, minerals and herbal extracts was more effective than placebo in significantly reducing the overall score on a depression, anxiety and stress scale, as well as improving alertness and general daily functioning in healthy older men (19). Furthermore, a high dose of vitamin B complex with vitamin C and minerals led to significant improvements in ratings on Perceived Stress Scales, General Health Questionnaire and the 'vigour' subscale of POMS in healthy males (20).

While preclinical and clinical studies lend credence to the ability of EL to improve mood which was possibly linked to hormonal balance favouring elevated mood (21), efficacy studies of EL in combination with micronutrients and conducted in accordance with established standards are currently lacking. The objective of this study was to investigate the safety and efficacy of a multivitamin mix in combination with EL water extract on QoL, mood and stress of moderately stressed but healthy participants.

## Materials and methods

This study was conducted in accordance with the Guidelines for Good Clinical Practice (ICH-6) and the Declaration of Helsinki. Institutional Review Board (IRB) approval was obtained from IntegReview Ethical Review Board, an independent IRB located in Austin, TX, USA, comprising scientific and non-scientific members of mostly medical doctors, on 17 January 2014 prior to initiation of any study-related activities. The IRB reviewed the protocol, medical ethics, informed consent, advertisement, stipend and compliance to protocol. The study was conducted at Medicus Research LLC, a clinical research site located at Agoura Hills, CA, USA. Written informed consent was obtained from volunteers prior to all study procedures. The recruitment and follow-up took place from 7 February 2014 to 13 March 2015.

### *Study design*

This was a randomised, double-blind, placebo-controlled parallel study with a 12-week efficacy and a 24-week safety period. The allocation *ratio* of participants in each of the comparison groups was 1:1. Efficacy was measured at 6 and 12 weeks, with safety and adverse events at 6, 12 and 24 weeks. The participants were required to make a total of four visits to the clinical trial site at Medicus Research LLC, Agoura Hills, CA.

At screening/baseline (week 0), inclusion/exclusion criteria, medical history and concomitant therapies were reviewed; baseline demographic data were collected; heart rate, respiratory rate, blood pressure and oral temperature were measured; and body mass index (BMI) was calculated. Fasting blood samples were obtained for assessment of complete blood count (CBC), comprehensive metabolic panel (CMP) including kidney function (estimated glomerular filtration rate, blood urine nitrogen [BUN], creatinine and bilirubin), liver function (aspartate aminotransferase, alanine transaminase), lipid panel (total cholesterol [TC], high-density lipoprotein-cholesterol [HDL-C], low-density lipoprotein-cholesterol [LDL-C], and triglycerides), testosterone (free and total) and urinalysis (leukocyte esterase, amorphous and calcium oxalate crystals). A urine pregnancy test was conducted on females with child-bearing potential. Electrocardiogram (EKG) was performed and POMS (22), SF-12 QoL (23), and Multi-Modal Stress Questionnaire (MMSQ) (24) were administered. Participants were dispensed a 6-week supply of the investigational product, a daily dosing diary and a 3-day food recall. Subjects who met all the study inclusion criteria and none of the exclusion criteria were enrolled in the study. After eligibility was confirmed, all volunteers received a randomisation number.

Participants returned to the clinic at weeks 6, 12 and 24 after having fasted for 10 h for assessment of medical and concomitant medication history. Vital signs and anthropometric measures, compliance and adverse events, and current medical history were reviewed. Fasting blood was collected for CBC, CMP, lipid panel, testosterone (free and total) measurements and urinalysis was performed. EKG was performed at baseline and at week 24.

POMS, SF-12 and MMSQ questionnaires were administered and a daily dosing diary and a 3-day food recall were dispensed at baseline, week 6 and week 12 only. At week 6, participants were dispensed a 6-week supply of the investigational product and at week 12, a 12-week supply of the investigational product. Participants maintained their daily diary for the duration of the study period and were required to record concomitant therapies and adverse events.

*Participants*

Study participants were recruited from the general population by online advertising, recruiting and available clinical trial databases. Inclusion criteria were as follows: healthy volunteers between 25 and 65 years of age, BMI 18–30 kg/m$^2$ and having self-reported moderate stress. Moderate stress was defined as a measure of both the tension and fatigue subscale of the POMS questionnaire. Participants who scored ≤18 in the tension subscale and ≤14 in the fatigue subscale were considered as having moderate stress. The tension subscale items are tense, on edge, uneasy, restless, nervous and helpless. A highest score (4 = extremely) for each of these items will give a total subscale score of ≤24 in tension and ≤20 in fatigue. An upper cut-off limit was determined, that is, a scoring of ≤18 in the tension subscale and ≤14 in the fatigue subscale, to exclude subjects who might fall within extremely stressed and possibly depressed category that will require medication and possibly cannot be addressed with health supplementation of multinutrients. The subjects were furthermore required to answer a Yes/No questionnaire in the inclusion/exclusion criteria as to whether they perceived themselves to having mid-level stress at work as a result of employment and life balance.

Exclusion criteria: participants were excluded if they were pregnant, lactating, planning to become pregnant or unwilling to use adequate contraception during the duration of the study, or had a history of immune system disorders, neurological disorders, temporal arthritis, ulcerative colitis, history of cancer within 2 years prior to enrolment, any active infection, or infection requiring antibiotics within 30 days of enrolment, significant gastrointestinal conditions including, but not limited to, inflammatory bowel disease, eating disorders, untreated hypothyroidism and use of herbal products containing androgenic/anxiolytic activity within 30 days prior to enrolment.

*Investigational product*

The investigational product (50 mg per tablet) was a proprietary water extract of EL root (Physta® also known as LJ100 in the USA). The multivitamin mix consisted of ascorbic acid (50 mg), retinyl acetate (4,000 IU), cholecalciferol (200 IU), Dl-alpha tocopherol acetate (15 IU), thiamine mononitrate (1.5 mg), riboflavin (1.7 mg), pyridoxine hydrochloride (2 mg), cyanocobalamin (0.001 mg), folic acid (0.2 mg), niacinamide (20 mg), D-biotin (0.15 mg), copper (2 mg), iron (10 mg), magnesium (10 mg), manganese (2.5 mg), selenium (0.005 mg), zinc (5 mg) and calcium (100 mg). The placebo contained microcrystalline cellulose, polyvinylpyrrolidone, sodium starch glycolate, colloidal silicon dioxide and magnesium stearate. The investigational product was produced under good manufacturing practices (GMP) requirements by Unison Nutraceutical Sdn Bhd and stored in a dry place at room temperature. Participants were instructed to consume either EL+MV or the placebo starting the day following the baseline visit, one tablet daily in the morning with water for 24 weeks.

*Outcome measures*

The primary and secondary outcomes measures were assessed by questionnaires at week 0 (Visit 0), week 6 (Visit 1) and 12 (Visit 2). The primary outcome measure for this study was the assessment of the efficacy of EL+MV versus placebo on mood and QoL. Mood state was assessed using the POMS questionnaire, which consisted of the following: total mood disturbance and its subscales, tension, depression, anger, fatigue, confusion and vigour. The POMS rated emotional and physical aspects of mood as ranging from 'not at all (1 point)' to 'extremely (5 points)'. A lower score, except for vigour, indicates better mood.

The POMS Iceberg profile, designed for assessing active/healthy individuals (25), was also analysed. QoL was assessed by the SF-12 questionnaire which measured the following domains: physical component summary, mental component summary, physical functioning, role limitations due to physical health, role limitations due to emotional health, energy/fatigue ratio (vitality), emotional well-being, social functioning, pain and general health. Scores on the SF-12 scales ranged from 0 to 100, with higher scores indicating better health.

The secondary objective was to assess stress using MMSQ, which measured the following subscales: total, behavioural, cognitive and physical. The MMSQ rated emotional and physical aspects of stress as ranging from 'never (1 point)' to 'constantly (5 points)'.

Safety and tolerability of the investigational product were assessed through changes in CBC, CMP, lipid panel, total and free testosterone, urinalysis and vital signs at all visits. The study would be temporarily stopped for any of the following: if WHO Grade 3 toxicity is experienced by four or more patients or WHO Grade 4 toxicity is experienced by two or more patient(s).

#### *Compliance*

The dispensed study product compliance diaries were returned to the clinic and participants who were non-compliant with their diaries were reminded of their obligations regarding appropriate study compliance.

#### *Sample size*

The sample size was calculated using the G*Power 3.0.10 software based on a reference value proposed by Perazzo et al. (26), which assessed QoL (SF-12) following treatment of Gerovital (a multivitamin and mineral combined with Panax ginseng extract) and placebo. In addition, a between-factor repeated-measure analysis of variance (ANOVA) with a level of significance ($\alpha$) of 0.05 (two sided) and power of 80% was considered, while the ratio between trial and control group was set at 1, resulting in 36 subjects per group. A 20% loss to follow-up was considered relevant, thus resulting in 45 subjects per group.

#### *Randomisation*

Stratified randomisation sequences were created with computer-generated random numbers, which allocated subjects based on sex (male/female) into two groups. Demographic stratifications based on gender were set and crossed. Patients were randomly assigned to order of treatment (placebo or active) using simple randomisation based on the atmospheric noise method and sequential assignment was used to determine group allocation (GraphPad Prism 6). A computer-generated list of random numbers was used in order to allocate participants. The results of these two randomisations were combined and assigned as the final randomisation sequence for this trial. Allocation, enrolment and assignment of participants to products were performed by the staff of Medicus Research LLC who did not perform any analyses or clinical procedures. The allocation information was disclosed to the investigator, subjects and a statistician after all measurements were completed. The investigational product was stored in a sequentially numbered Study Product Container in a locked cabinet with limited access.

#### *Statistical analysis*

The modified per-protocol analysis included subjects with at least one post-dose completed visit and participants who completed all visits of the 24-week study and consumed the product. Subgroup analysis was performed based on gender for testosterone measurements, domains within questionnaires and age groups. The safety analysis was based on all randomised participants known to have taken at least one dose of the investigational or placebo products. Subgroup analysis of primary endpoints was performed for the age groups, 25–45 and 46–65 years, due to perceived stress from increased responsibilities in the older age group and potential hormonal variances which affect QoL in these subgroups.

All evaluations were performed using the software package R 3.2.2 (R Core Team, 2015). Descriptive statistics were calculated for each group and statistical comparisons were performed using the analysis of covariance (ANCOVA) adjusting for baseline values. Numerical endpoints that are intractably non-normal were assessed by the Mann-Whitney U test; in these instances, only the comparisons of the changes from baseline were considered in the formal testing between groups. Statistical comparisons for baseline characteristics, lipid and testosterone levels, and measures of safety (haematology, blood chemistry, anthropometrics and vital signs) were performed using ANOVA. For categorical endpoints, the differences in proportions between groups were formally tested by the Fisher's exact test. The Shapiro–Wilk normality test was carried out to determine data normality when $P > 0.05$. Within-group comparisons on numeric endpoints were made using Student's paired $t$-test or, in the case of intractable non-normality, the Wilcoxon signed rank test. Differences were considered significant at $P \leq 0.05$. Subgroup analysis based on gender differences was conducted for testosterone measurements only.

### Results

#### *Participant baseline characteristics*

A total of 120 participants were screened and a total of 93 subjects were enrolled, of which 7 were lost to follow-up due to the long enrolment period of 6 months (Fig.1). There were 28 females and 19 males in the EL + multivitamins group (EL+MV), and 20 females and 19 males in the placebo group. The demographic characteristics of participants were not significantly different in terms of age, BMI, employment and relationship status between groups at baseline (Table 1).

More than 94% of participants in both groups were employed and were predominantly Caucasian in ethnicity. There were no significant differences in CBC, CMP and urinalysis, anthropometric measures and vital signs between groups at baseline (Table 2). Analysis of POMS-Tension-Anxiety mood state subscale showed participants to be moderately stressed.

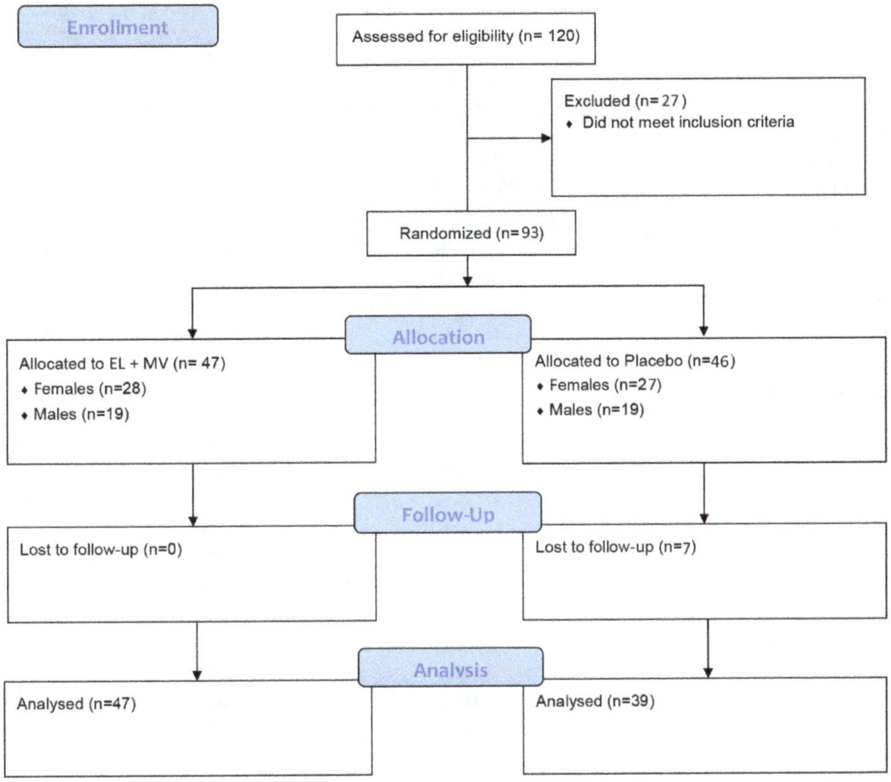


*Fig. 1.* Study flowchart. A total of 120 participants were screened, of which 93 were randomised in the study, with 47 in the EL+MV group and 39 in the placebo group enrolledas the modified per-protocol population in the final analysis. EL+MV, *E. longifolia* + multivitamin.

### *Primary endpoints*

#### SF-12 questionnaire on QoL

POMS, SF-12 and MMSQ scores obtained by all participants in the study before and after supplementation with EL+MV group or placebo are presented in Table 3. There were no significant between-group differences reported in physical component, mental component, physical functioning, role limitations due to physical health, role limitations due to emotional health, vitality, emotional well-being, social functioning, pain and general health domains as assessed by the SF-12 questionnaire, but several within-group significant findings were observed (Table 3).

Participants supplemented with EL+MV reported significant improvements from baseline, with 9.7% improvement in role limitation due to emotional health at week 6 ($P = 0.003$) and 9.2% at week 12 ($P = 0.05$) (Fig. 2a) and a further 11.3% improvement in vitality (energy/fatigue ratio) at week 12 ($P = 0.001$) (Fig. 2b). Similar improvements from baseline were not reported by participants in the placebo group.

Participants supplemented with EL+MV reported a significant increase in the mental component domain at weeks 6 ($P = 0.001$) and 12 ($P < 0.001$), with an increase of 24.6% in the EL+MV compared to 12.7% in the placebo group at week 12. The placebo group only had significant improvements at week 6 ($P = 0.007$). In the emotional well-being domain, significant improvements were observed in both groups, with a 23% ($P < 0.001$) and 6.9% ($P < 0.01$) improvement observed at week 12, respectively, in the EL+MV and placebo groups. The social functioning domain for participants supplemented with EL+MV significantly improved by 11.3% at week 12 ($P = 0.002$) but only by 7.5% at week 6 ($P = 0.01$) in the placebo group.

A subgroup analysis of subjects based on age group 25–45 years had $n = 29$ on treatment and $n = 24$ on placebo, while age subgroup 46–65 years had $n = 18$ on treatment and $n = 12$ on placebo. Primary and secondary outcome measures of POMS, SF-12 and MMSQ revealed a 14.4% increase in the social functioning score within the SF-12 questionnaire in the 25–45-year subgroup of the EL+MV group, achieving a between-group significance ($P = 0.021$). Changes in other domains remained non-significant.

#### Profile of mood states questionnaire on mood

There were no significant between-group differences reported in total mood disturbance, tension, depression, anger, fatigue, confusion and vigour assessed by POMS

*Table 1.* Demographics and anthropometric measures of all 86 participants enrolled in the study.

| | EL+MV (n = 47) | Placebo (n = 36) | P-value[§] |
|---|---|---|---|
| Age (years) | | | |
| Mean ± SD | 40.6 ± 12.3 | 41.0 ± 9.9 | 0.744[σ] |
| Median (min – max) | 36 (25 – 62) | 39.5 (25 – 62) | |
| Gender (n[%]) | | | |
| Female | 28 (60%) | 18 (50%) | 0.504 |
| Male | 19 (40%) | 18 (50%) | |
| BMI (kg/m$^2$) | | | |
| Mean ± SD (n) | 23.9 ± 3.20 | 25.0 ± 3.24 | 0.124 |
| Median (min – max) | 23.4 (18.1 – 35) | 24.8 (18.3 – 31.8) | |
| Tobacco use (n[%]) | | | |
| Current smoker | 7 (16%) | 4 (11%) | 0.505 |
| Non-smoker | 31 (69%) | 29 (81%) | |
| Past smoker | 7 (16%) | 3 (8%) | |
| Alcohol use (n[%]) | | | |
| Current consumer | 31 (67%) | 22 (61%) | 0.739 |
| Non-drinker | 11 (24%) | 12 (33%) | |
| Past drinker | 4 (9%) | 2 (6%) | |
| Ethnicity (n[%]) | | | |
| African-American | 5 (11%) | 4 (11%) | 0.384 |
| Asian | 3 (6%) | 2 (6%) | |
| Caucasian | 32 (68%) | 18 (51%) | |
| Latino/Hispanic | 3 (6%) | 7 (20%) | |
| Other | 4 (9%) | 4 (11%) | |
| Current employment (n[%]) | | | |
| Employed | 44 (96%) | 33 (94%) | 1.000 |
| Not employed | 2 (4%) | 2 (6%) | |
| Relationship status (n[%]) | | | |
| Divorced | 4 (9%) | 3 (8%) | 0.318 |
| Domestic partnership | 1 (2%) | 1 (3%) | |
| Married | 12 (26%) | 8 (22%) | |
| Separated | 0 (0%) | 4 (11%) | |
| Single | 28 (60%) | 19 (53%) | |
| Widowed | 2 (4%) | 1 (3%) | |
| Have children (n[%]) | | | |
| No | 32 (71%) | 18 (50%) | 0.067 |
| Yes | 13 (29%) | 18 (50%) | |
| Systolic blood pressure (mmHg) | | | |
| Mean ± SD (n) | 117.7 ± 14.3 | 118.4 ± 13.5 | 0.819 |
| Median (min – max) | 117 (91 – 154) | 119 (91 – 150) | |
| Diastolic blood pressure (mmHg) | | | |
| Mean ± SD (n) | 74.5 ± 10.6 | 77.0 ± 10.9 | 0.296 |
| Median (min – max) | 73 (50 – 105) | 75 (60 – 99) | |
| Heart Rate (beats per minute) | | | |
| Mean ± SD (n) | 66.2 ± 10.7 | 64.5 ± 9.5 | 0.468 |
| Median (min – max) | 66 (42 – 94) | 65 (41 – 84) | |
| Body temperature (°F) | | | |
| Mean ± SD (n) | 98.14 ± 0.44 | 98.16 ± 0.64 | 0.868 |
| Median (min – max) | 98.2 (97.2 – 99.8) | 98.1 (96.4 – 99.6) | |
| Respiratory rate (per minute) | | | |
| Mean ± SD (n) | 14.57 ± 1.96 | 14.95 ± 1.60 | 0.354 |
| Median (min – max) | 15 (12 – 20) | 15 (12 – 18) | |

[σ]Between-group comparison was made using the independent Student's *t*-test.

[§]Between-group comparisons were performed using Fisher's exact test. The variable *n* indicates the number of subjects analysed. Demographics data were not available for three participants.

*Table 2.* CBC and CMP safety parameters assessed in participants at all visits.

| Item | Reference value | Group | Screening (Week 0) | Week 6 | Week 12 | Week 24 |
|---|---|---|---|---|---|---|
| AST | 7 –≤70 U/L | EL + MV | 24.8 ± 10.1 | 23.9 ± 7.8 | 29.3 ± 27.1 | 21.5 ± 7.9 |
| | | Placebo | 25.2 ± 9.0 | 23.7 ± 10.2 | 24.3 ± 11.1 | 29.1 ± 36.1 |
| ALT | 12 – <90 U/L | EL + MV | 21.5 ± 13.4 | 21.5 ± 9.4 | 22.9 ± 14.5 | 21.2 ± 16.7* |
| | | Placebo | 23.5 ± 14.9 | 21.1 ± 12.4*# | 22.0 ± 13.5** | 22.3 ± 16.2 |
| ALP | 39–117 IU/L | EL + MV | 64.5 ± 19.2 | 63.7 ± 19.8 | 63.8 ± 19.1 | 59.2 ± 20.3 |
| | | Placebo | 66.9 ± 18.9 | 67.1 ± 18.4 | 67.5 ± 17.1 | 66.1 ± 19.7 |
| Total bilirubin | ≤25 μmol/L | EL + MV | 0.62 ± 0.36 | 0.53 ± 0.32 | 0.454 ± 0.284 | 0.463 ± 0.213 |
| | | Placebo | 0.62 ± 0.36 | 0.53 ± 0.33 | 0.450 ± 0.244 | 0.474 ± 0.350 |
| Sodium | 133–148 mmol/L | EL + MV | 141.18 ± 1.85 | 141.30 ± 2.47 | 140.8 ± 4.7 | 138.9 ± 6.5 |
| | | Placebo | 141.17 ± 2.50 | 141.08 ± 2.20 | 140.8 ± 4.9 | 141.0 ± 2.8 |
| Potassium | 3.3–5.7 mmol/L | EL + MV | 4.21 ± 0.35 | 4.39 ± 1.25 | 4.24 ± 0.37 | 4.20 ± 0.37 |
| | | Placebo | 4.17 ± 0.27 | 4.24 ± 0.32 | 4.61 ± 1.74* | 4.36 ± 0.39* |
| Chloride | 98–115 mmol/L | EL + MV | 102.48 ± 1.97 | 102.42 ± 2.29 | 101.5 ± 3.9 | 99.2 ± 5.7*** |
| | | Placebo | 103.17 ± 2.66 | 102.73 ± 1.79 | 101.9 ± 4.1* | 100.9 ± 2.8*** |
| Carbon dioxide | 18–29 mmol/L | EL + MV | 26.98 ± 1.99 | 28.6 ± 11.3 | 25.4 ± 3.4* | 23.43 ± 2.93*** |
| | | Placebo | 26.64 ± 2.26 | 24.9 ± 3.9* | 24.8 ± 2.8* | 23.97 ± 2.65*** |
| Anion gap | 3–11 mEq/L | EL + MV | 12.3 ± 3.5 | 13.3 ± 5.0 | 16.6 ± 5.6*** | 20.0 ± 3.3*** |
| | | Placebo | 11.7 ± 3.2 | 14.8 ± 5.7* | 17.0 ± 5.3*** | 19.8 ± 4.2*** |
| Calcium | 8.4–10.4 mg/dL | EL + MV | 9.61 ± 0.40 | 9.60 ± 0.40 | 9.26 ± 1.58 | 9.04 ± 0.67*** |
| | | Placebo | 9.56 ± 0.41 | 9.51 ± 0.41 | 9.47 ± 0.59 | 9.19 ± 0.45** |
| Glucose | 70–109 mg/dL | EL + MV | 94.9 ± 8.6 | 93.5 ± 9.6 | 95.2 ± 11.4 | 89.0 ± 11.6** |
| | | Placebo | 92.2 ± 10.2 | 93.3 ± 6.4 | 91.6 ± 10.5 | 88.5 ± 16.3 |
| Blood urea nitrogen | 8.0–20.0 mg/dL | EL + MV | 13.2 ± 3.1 | 13.4 ± 4.4 | 12.8 ± 3.1 | 14.7 ± 11.3 |
| | | Placebo | 13.4 ± 3.7 | 12.9 ± 4.0 | 12.9 ± 5.2 | 13.1 ± 4.1 |
| Creatinine | 0.47–0.79 mg/dL | EL + MV | 0.795 ± 0.152 | 0.782 ± 0.147 | 0.777 ± 0.172 | 0.770 ± 0.204 |
| | | Placebo | 0.794 ± 0.200 | 0.768 ± 0.220 | 0.812 ± 0.247 | 0.774 ± 0.192 |
| Blood urea nitrogen: creatinine ratio | 10:1 –20:1 | EL + MV | 17.1 ± 4.7 | 17.8 ± 5.3 | 17.1 ± 4.2 | 17.8 ± 4.8 |
| | | Placebo | 17.6 ± 5.3 | 17.6 ± 5.9 | 16.3 ± 5.0 | 17.4 ± 4.9 |
| Estimated glomerular filtration rate | 50–≥120 mL/min/1.73 $m^2$ | EL + MV | 64.6 ± 13.1 | 69.2 ± 19.5 | 78.2 ± 23.2*** | 92.1 ± 28.2*** |
| | | Placebo | 62.6 ± 9.5 | 74.9 ± 32.4**# | 83.5 ± 30.9** | 93.1 ± 23.6*** |
| Total serum protein | 6.7–8.3 g/dL | EL + MV | 7.13 ± 0.37 | 7.09 ± 0.41 | 8.0 ± 6.2 | 6.72 ± 0.56***# |
| | | Placebo | 7.13 ± 0.47 | 7.02 ± 0.45 | 7.0 ± 0.6 | 7.09 ± 0.48 |
| Serum albumin | 3.5 to 5.5 g/dL | EL + MV | 4.63 ± 0.29 | 4.60 ± 0.30 | 4.59 ± 0.43 | 4.42 ± 0.48**# |
| | | Placebo | 4.54 ± 0.34 | 4.56 ± 0.33 | 4.56 ± 0.38 | 4.55 ± 0.31 |
| Globulin | 2.6–4.6 g/dL | EL + MV | 2.493 ± 0.277 | 2.49 ± 0.30 | 2.36 ± 0.29* | 2.31 ± 0.51***# |
| | | Placebo | 2.586 ± 0.304 | 2.46 ± 0.35* | 2.45 ± 0.33 | 2.53 ± 0.32 |
| Albumin : globulin ratio | 0.8–2.0 | EL + MV | 1.877 ± 0.251 | 1.875 ± 0.260 | 1.958 ± 0.205 | 1.99 ± 0.35* |
| | | Placebo | 1.778 ± 0.251 | 1.897 ± 0.320*# | 1.894 ± 0.269* | 1.83 ± 0.30 |
| Total cholesterol | 120–219 mg/dL | EL + MV | 195 ± 46 | 194 ± 43 | 192 ± 43 | 180 ± 36* |
| | | Placebo | 184 ± 34 | 184 ± 41 | 184 ± 40 | 177 ± 40 |
| Triglycerides | 30–149 mg/dL | EL + MV | 89 ± 52 | 104 ± 99 | 111 ± 90 | 91 ± 54 |
| | | Placebo | 98 ± 75 | 111 ± 171 | 118 ± 110 | 97 ± 53 |
| HDL cholesterol | 40–95 mg/dL | EL + MV | 74.8 ± 22.6 | 73.7 ± 23.2 | 72.7 ± 24.9 | 61.5 ± 17.9*** |
| | | Placebo | 69.3 ± 20.5 | 67.5 ± 24.3 | 63.0 ± 20.9** | 61.3 ± 18.7&** |
| LDL cholesterol | 65–139 mg/dL | EL + MV | 102 ± 38 | 100 ± 41 | 99 ± 34 | 103 ± 33 |
| | | Placebo | 95 ± 28 | 95 ± 29 | 97 ± 31 | 99 ± 28 |
| Coronary risk factor (cholesterol : HDL) | <3.3 | EL + MV | 2.79 ± 0.99 | 2.87 ± 1.07 | 4.3 ± 8.6* | 3.26 ± 1.18*** |
| | | Placebo | 2.87 ± 1.03 | 3.07 ± 1.71 | 3.1 ± 1.1** | 3.15 ± 1.06** |

*Table 2.* Continued

| Item | Reference value | Group | Screening (Week 0) | Week 6 | Week 12 | Week 24 |
|---|---|---|---|---|---|---|
| VLDL cholesterol | 2 to 30 mg/dL | EL + MV | 17.9 ± 10.4 | 20.9 ± 19.7 | 22.1 ± 18.1 | 18.2 ± 10.9 |
| | | Placebo | 19.5 ± 14.9 | 22.3 ± 34.3 | 23.6 ± 22.0 | 19.4 ± 10.6 |
| White blood cell | 3,300–9,000/μL | EL + MV | 6.06 ± 1.65 | 5.60 ± 1.55* | 5.57 ± 1.47* | 5.88 ± 1.41 |
| | | Placebo | 5.93 ± 1.86 | 6.10 ± 2.07 | 5.86 ± 1.58 | 5.43 ± 1.34 |
| Red blood cell | 430–570 10^4/mL | EL + MV | 4.71 ± 0.44 | 4.69 ± 0.49 | 4.64 ± 0.42* | 4.63 ± 0.45* |
| | | Placebo | 4.79 ± 0.47 | 4.70 ± 0.46 | 4.70 ± 0.42 | 4.60 ± 0.40*** |
| Haemoglobin | M: 13.5–17.5 g/dL | EL + MV | 14.69 ± 1.29 | 14.58 ± 1.44 | 14.38 ± 1.32** | 14.30 ± 1.42** |
| | F: 11.5–15.0 g/dL | Placebo | 14.61 ± 1.45 | 14.40 ± 1.49 | 14.44 ± 1.53 | 13.98 ± 1.36*** |
| Haematocrit | M: 39.7–52.4% | EL + MV | 43.2 ± 3.5 | 43.3 ± 3.7 | 43.1 ± 3.4 | 43.0 ± 3.7 |
| | F: 34.8–45.0% | Placebo | 43.3 ± 3.6 | 42.8 ± 3.3 | 43.4 ± 3.8 | 42.3 ± 3.4* |
| Blood platelet | 14.0–34.0 ×10^3/mm$^3$ | EL + MV | 248 ± 57 | 255 ± 61# | 256 ± 80 | 277 ± 76** |
| | | Placebo | 227 ± 57 | 223 ± 50 | 239 ± 49* | 245 ± 81* |
| Mean corpuscular volume | 85–102 fl | EL + MV | 92.1 ± 3.9 | 92.6 ± 4.4 | 92.9 ± 4.3* | 93.0 ± 4.1* |
| | | Placebo | 90.7 ± 5.4 | 91.4 ± 5.2 | 92.3 ± 4.9* | 90.7 ± 11.6 |
| Mean corpuscular haemoglobin | 28.0–34.0 pg | EL + MV | 31.22 ± 1.38 | 31.11 ± 1.47 | 31.00 ± 1.50 | 30.91 ± 1.14* |
| | | Placebo | 30.57 ± 2.13 | 30.67 ± 2.13 | 30.72 ± 2.10 | 30.42 ± 2.02* |
| Mean corpuscular haemoglobin concentration | 30.2–35.1% | EL + MV | 33.95 ± 0.92 | 33.61 ± 1.12 | 33.39 ± 1.22* | 33.24 ± 0.99*** |
| | | Placebo | 33.74 ± 1.15 | 33.57 ± 1.43 | 33.26 ± 1.24* | 33.01 ± 1.19*** |
| Neutrophil count | 1.6–8.0 ×10^9/L | EL + MV | 55.5 ± 10.8 | 53.5 ± 10.9# | 52.2 ± 10.6* | 54.9 ± 9.5 |
| | | Placebo | 56.1 ± 10.1 | 57.3 ± 9.8 | 55.8 ± 9.0 | 56.8 ± 7.7 |
| Lymphocyte count | 0.8–3.0 ×10^9/L | EL + MV | 32.5 ± 9.2 | 34.6 ± 9.8 | 35.4 ± 9.1*# | 33.2 ± 8.4 |
| | | Placebo | 32.6 ± 8.6 | 32.4 ± 9.5 | 32.4 ± 6.9 | 32.9 ± 6.6 |
| Monocyte count | 0.1–1.5 × 10^9/L | EL + MV | 7.33 ± 2.01 | 8.00 ± 2.32 | 7.93 ± 1.94 | 8.09 ± 2.47 |
| | | Placebo | 7.42 ± 1.67 | 7.27 ± 1.90 | 8.19 ± 2.72 | 7.65 ± 1.91 |
| Eosinophil count | 0.0–0.7× 10^9/L | EL + MV | 3.2 ± 4.0 | 3.08 ± 2.20 | 3.28 ± 2.47 | 3.22 ± 2.35 |
| | | Placebo | 2.8 ± 3.3 | 2.40 ± 1.93 | 2.45 ± 1.97 | 2.25 ± 1.20 |
| Basophil count | 0.0–0.2× 10^9/L | EL + MV | 1.56 ± 0.89 | 1.42 ± 1.32 | 1.23 ± 1.76** | 0.60 ± 0.54*** |
| | | Placebo | 1.29 ± 0.56 | 1.08 ± 0.59 | 1.17 ± 2.30** | 0.48 ± 0.46*** |

*$P < 0.05$, **$P < 0.01$, ***$P < 0.001$, significant within-group differences and #significant between-group differences in *E. longifolia* + multivitamins (EL+MV) group ($n$ = 44–47) and the placebo group ($n$ = 34–36).

questionnaire. Within group, participants supplemented with EL+MV and placebo reported significant improvements in several of the POMS domains. An increasing trend was observed in the vigour domain of the EL+MV group at week 12.

The POMS Iceberg profile was applied to the POMS raw scores of healthy, moderately stressed population of participants in this study. Average baseline profiles showed that participants in both groups had the expected normal profiles. A normal profile consists of a peak in vigour with tension, depression, anger, fatigue and confusion making up the trough of the profile (Fig. 3). In the subgroup analysis of the POMS scores, participants between the ages of 46 and 65 years showed significant between-group improvement in vigour ($P = 0.036$) by 14.1% in the EL+MV group, observed by the mean change from weeks 0 to 12.

### *Secondary outcomes*

#### Multi-modal stress questionnaire on stress

There were no significant between-group differences in self-reported total, behavioural, cognitive and physical stress by participants, as assessed by the MMSQ questionnaire (Table 3).

Significant within-group effects were observed in several domains in both groups, but only for the EL+MV group, significant reduction in physical stress was observed at week 12 ($P < 0.05$), as evidenced by a reduction of 15% compared to 0.7% in the placebo group only at week 6 ($P < 0.05$). The decrease in cognitive stress and total stress in the EL+MV group was significant ($P < 0.001$) compared to the placebo group ($P < 0.01$) at week 12.

*Table 3.* POMS and SF-12 MMSQ scores in all participants in the study.

| | Before supplementation | | *P*-value | After supplementation–week 6 | | *P*-value | After supplementation – week 12 | | *P*-value |
|---|---|---|---|---|---|---|---|---|---|
| | EL+MV | Placebo | | EL+MV | Placebo | | EL+MV | Placebo | |
| **POMS†** | | | | | | | | | |
| Tension-anxiety | 8.3 ± 4.4 | 9.8 ± 5.7 | 0.289 | 6.6 ± 4.0** | 6.8 ± 4.2*** | 0.909 | 5.4 ± 2.9 *** | 6.4 ± 4.0*** | 0.489 |
| Depression-dejection | 8.7 ± 9.5 | 10.6 ± 11.5 | 0.892 | 5.7 ± 9.1** | 5.6 ± 8.0** | 0.821 | 3.5 ± 5.4*** | 5.2 ± 7.7* | 0.427 |
| Anger-hostility | 5.1 ± 5.1 | 7.2 ± 8.5 | 0.682 | 3.9 ± 6.3 | 4.5 ± 6.3* | 0.976 | 2.4 ± 3.5** | 4.2 ± 5.8 | 0.162 |
| Vigour-activity | 15.0 ± 6.1 | 16.6 ± 6.1 | 0.237 | 15.1 ± 6.6 | 16.4 ± 6.1 | 0.453 | 16.3 ± 5.4 | 16.5 ± 5.8 | 0.974 |
| Fatigue-inertia | 6.2 ± 5.7 | 6.7 ± 5.5 | 0.673 | 5.2 ± 5.4 | 5.5 ± 4.7 | 0.634 | 4.2 ± 4.6* | 3.2 ± 3.9*** | 0.268 |
| Confusion-bewilderment | 6.0 ± 4.0 | 7.9 ± 4.9 | 0.108 | 4.96 ± 2.88 | 5.19 ± 2.72** | 0.521 | 4.63 ± 2.03 | 5.31 ± 3.01* | 0.576 |
| Overall mood | 19 ± 27 | 25 ± 36 | 0.651 | 11.2 ± 27.3* | 11.1 ± 25.3** | 0.962 | 3.8 ± 18.6*** | 7.9 ± 23.8** | 0.485 |
| **SF-12†** | | | | | | | | | |
| Physical component | 56.2 ± 5.5 | 54.9 ± 4.8 | 0.294 | 54.1 ± 5.8* | 55.1 ± 3.2 | 0.332 | 53.8 ± 4.6** | 53.7 ± 5.3 | 0.930 |
| Mental component | 28.4 ± 11.2 | 32.0 ± 10.8 | 0.148 | 33.4 ± 9.9** | 35.8 ± 8.6** | 0.266 | 35.4 ± 9.4*** | 36.0 ± 8.9 | 0.749 |
| Physical functioning | 53.4 ± 7.6 | 52.5 ± 9.4 | 0.781 | 52.7 ± 9.3 | 54.7 ± 5.4 | 0.413 | 53.7 ± 6.3 | 54.0 ± 7.7 | 0.391 |
| Role limitations-physical | 28.43 ± 2.60 | 28.88 ± 1.98 | 0.444 | 28.84 ± 1.93 | 29.14 ± 1.31 | 0.517 | 28.74 ± 2.01 | 28.62 ± 2.18 | 0.817 |
| Role limitations-emotional | 18.5 ± 4.7 | 20.5 ± 3.9 | 0.044 | 20.3 ± 3.6** | 20.9 ± 3.5 | 0.341 | 20.2 ± 4.2* | 21.6 ± 2.9 | 0.101 |
| Energy/fatigue | 44.7 ± 11.6 | 48.3 ± 11.7 | 0.158 | 47.3 ± 10.6 | 51.2 ± 10.0 | 0.081 | 49.7 ± 10.1** | 51.2 ± 10.6 | 0.465 |
| Emotional well-being | 34.6 ± 13.0 | 40.7 ± 11.6 | 0.274 | 37.5 ± 12.7** | 42.8 ± 11.7* | 0.429 | 42.7 ± 10.8*** | 43.5 ± 11.6** | 0.797 |
| Social functioning | 46.7 ± 9.9 | 49.1 ± 8.9 | 0.284 | 49.5 ± 8.5 | 52.8 ± 6.5* | 0.066 | 52.0 ± 6.3** | 50.2 ± 8.2 | 0.446 |
| Pain | 54.3 ± 5.2 | 54.2 ± 5.4 | 0.966 | 53.2 ± 7.6 | 55.4 ± 4.8 | 0.207 | 53.0 ± 7.0 | 54.5 ± 5.3 | 0.404 |
| General health | 56.6 ± 5.6 | 56.1 ± 5.1 | 0.487 | 56.5 ± 5.5 | 56.1 ± 6.0 | 0.843 | 55.9 ± 5.2 | 54.7 ± 7.9 | 0.888 |
| **MMSQ†** | | | | | | | | | |
| Physical stress | 47.6 ± 13.6 | 43.8 ± 13.0 | 0.198 | 45.2 ± 13.1 | 43.5 ± 11.2* | 0.071 | 40.4 ± 9.1* | 40.3 ± 9.5 | 0.277 |
| Behavioural stress | 22.1 ± 5.5 | 21.6 ± 5.0 | 0.700 | 20.6 ± 5.2* | 19.6 ± 3.4** | 0.323 | 19.6 ± 4.7*** | 19.2 ± 4.5*** | 0.673 |
| Cognitive stress | 16.5 ± 6.0 | 14.2 ± 5.8 | 0.094 | 14.0 ± 5.4*** | 12.2 ± 3.9** | 0.091 | 12.4 ± 3.7*** | 11.8 ± 4.2** | 0.520 |
| Overall stress | 86.1 ± 23.0 | 79.7 ± 21.3 | 0.209 | 79.8 ± 21.4* | 72.2 ± 14.6** | 0.064 | 75.5 ± 18.0*** | 71.3 ± 15.7** | 0.181 |

POMS, SF-12 and MMSQ scores are depicted as mean ± SD.
*$P \le 0.05$, **$P \le 0.01$, ***$P \le 0.001$, significant within-group difference in *E. longifolia* + multivitamins (EL+MV) ($n$ = 47) and placebo group ($n$ = 36).
†Between-group comparisons were made using ANCOVA.

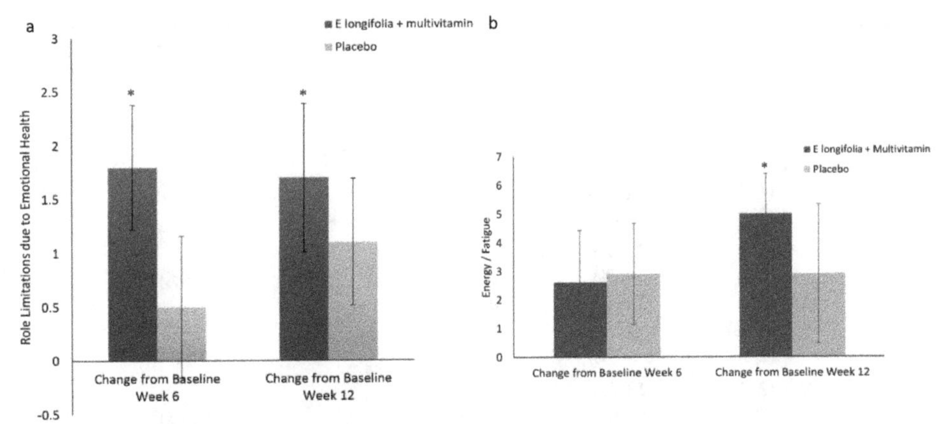


*Fig. 2.* (a) Changes in role limitation due to emotional health in EL+MV ($n$ = 46) and placebo ($n$ = 35) groups. Participants consuming *E. longifolia* + multivitamins displayed a significant improvement in role limitation due to emotional health at week 6 (9.7%; $P$ = 0.003) and week 12 (9.2%; $P$ = 0.05) when compared to baseline. Axes represent change in scores that numerically capture domains in the SF-12 questionnaire. Within-group comparisons were made using the paired $t$-test. Mean ± SE values. *$P \le 0.05$. (b) Energy/fatigue ratio in EL+MV ($n$ = 46) and placebo ($n$ = 35) groups. Only participants consuming *E. longifolia* + multivitamins showed a significant increase (11.2%, $P$ = 0.001) in their energy/fatigue ratio at week 12 when compared to baseline. Axes represent change in scores that numerically capture domains in the SF-12 questionnaire. Within-group comparisons were made using the paired $t$-test. Mean ± SE values. *$P \le 0.05$.

### Compliance

Compliance, which was assessed by counting the returned unused test product at each visit, was calculated by determining the number of dosage units taken divided by the number of dosages expected to have been taken multiplied by 100. The overall mean compliance was greater than 99% in both EL+MV and placebo groups.

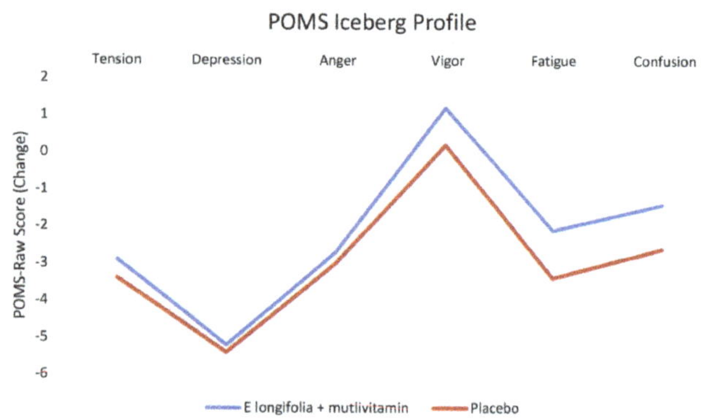


*Fig. 3.* Changes in POMS Iceberg profiles in EL+MV ($n = 46$) and placebo ($n = 36$) groups. Changes in POMS Iceberg profiles based on the raw POMS mood state subscales were consistent with that of healthy and active individuals in tension, depression, anger, vigour, fatigue and confusion in *E. longifolia* + multivitamins and placebo groups. Vigour activity in placebo group was reduced compared to an increase in the supplemented group. Axes represent change in scores that numerically capture domains in POMS Iceberg profile.

No participants were removed from the study due to low compliance (less than 80%).

### Safety parameters

Anthropometric measures and vital signs (systolic and diastolic blood pressure, body temperature, respiratory rate and heart rate) were similar between EL+MV and placebo groups after 24 weeks of supplementation. Participants consuming EL+MV showed incidental differences in their respiratory rate at week 12 ($P = 0.03$) and mean diastolic blood pressure at week 6 ($P = 0.02$) compared to the placebo, but not at other time points (Table 1). However, all excursions were within a normal clinical reference range for the duration of the study.

Reduction in neutrophil count at week 6 ($P = 0.03$) and an increase in lymphocyte count at week 12 ($P = 0.01$) versus placebo were observed (Table 2). Mean platelet volume increased in the EL+MV at weeks 12 ($P < 0.001$) and 24 ($P < 0.001$) and in the placebo group at weeks 6 ($P = 0.03$), 12 ($P < 0.001$) and 24 ($P < 0.001$) compared to baseline, but all values remained within their normal laboratory range (Table 2).

Participants in the EL+MV group showed a decrease in glucose concentration ($P = 0.005$) and TC($P = 0.03$) at 24 weeks compared to baseline (Table 2). Urinalysis revealed a difference in the presence of leukocyte esterase at week 6 ($P = 0.008$), with 25% of participants in the EL+MV group testing negative (Table 4). Nine per cent more participants in the placebo group tested positive

*Table 4.* Urinalysis of all participants in the study based on the number of subjects ($n$).

| | | Presence of leukocyte esterase (n) | | | | Presence of calcium oxalate crystals (n) | | |
|---|---|---|---|---|---|---|---|---|
| | | EL+MV | Placebo | *P*-value§ | | EL+MV | Placebo | *P*-value§ |
| Week 0 (screening) | 1+ | 5 (11%) | 1 (3%) | | | | | |
| | 2+ | 2 (4%) | 0 (0%) | | Few | 0 (0%) | 3 (9%) | |
| | 3+ | 1 (2%) | 1 (3%) | 0.121 | None | 44 (100%) | 31 (91%) | 0.079 |
| | Negative | 34 (74%) | 32 (94%) | | | | | |
| | Trace | 4 (9%) | 0 (0%) | | | | | |
| Week 6 | 1+ | 2 (5%) | 0 (0%) | | | | | |
| | 2+ | 0 (0%) | 2 (6%) | | Few | 3 (9%) | 7 (27%) | |
| | 3+ | 2 (5%) | 0 (0%) | 0.008 | None | 31 (91%) | 19 (73%) | 0.085 |
| | Negative | 38 (88%) | 25 (76%) | | | | | |
| | Trace | 1 (2%) | 6 (18%) | | | | | |
| Week 12 | 1+ | 3 (7%) | 2 (6%) | | | | | |
| | 2+ | 1 (2%) | 1 (3%) | | Few | 1 (6%) | 2 (17%) | |
| | 3+ | 1 (2%) | 1 (3%) | 0.108 | None | 17 (94%) | 10 (83%) | 0.548 |
| | Negative | 35 (85%) | 21 (66%) | | | | | |
| | Trace | 1 (2%) | 7 (22%) | | | | | |
| Week 24 | 1+ | 2 (5%) | 0 (0%) | | | | | |
| | 2+ | 3 (7%) | 2 (6%) | | Few | 2 (25%) | 2 (50%) | |
| | 3+ | 0 (0%) | 0 (0%) | 0.744 | None | 6 (75%) | 2 (50%) | 0.547 |
| | Negative | 35 (80%) | 28 (88%) | | | | | |
| | Trace | 4 (9%) | 2 (6%) | | | | | |

§Between-group analysis was made using the Fisher's exact test. $P \leq 0.05$ is statistically significant.

for the presence of calcium oxalate crystals in the urine compared to EL+MV group (Table 4).

### Testosterone levels

There was no between-group significance; however, a significant time effect within group changes in testosterone levels was observed. Serum total testosterone decreased in the placebo group at week 6 compared to during screening ($P = 0.009$) (Fig. 4a). This decrease continued till weeks 12 and 24, but was not observed in the EL+MV group. In contrast, free serum testosterone levels increased in both groups ($P < 0.001$) (Fig.4b).

However, there was an increase in free testosterone levels in males supplemented with EL+MV from 1.67 ± 2.35 ng/dL at baseline to 11.4 ± 24.9 ng/dL, double the increase seen in the placebo group, from 1.4 ± 12.7 ng/dL to 6.4 ± 2.9 ng/dL (Table 5). An increase in free testosterone levels from 0.15 ± 0.3 ng/dL in the EL+MV and 0.12 ± 0.4 ng/dL in the placebo group at baseline to 1.05 ± 0.9 ng/dL and 1.3 ± 1.3 ng/dL, respectively, at week 24 was observed in female participants. There were no significant between-group differences in free testosterone levels in both genders.

### Adverse events

In this clinical study, there were a total of 13 adverse events reported by 13 participants: six (urinary tract infection, blood in urine, nasal congestion, nasopharyngitis [$n = 2$] and migraine) of which were in the placebo group and 7 (food poisoning, kidney infection, fracture, influenza, vomiting, nausea and urinary tract infection) were in the EL+MV group.

## Discussion

This study evaluated the efficacy and safety of EL+MV in healthy males and females with moderate stress. The demographics of the population studied were middle class and lower middle class individuals who worked hard to sustain their families and maintain their lifestyles while juggling work-related requirements. The participants were employed and experienced self-reported job-related stress due to work responsibilities, particularly when responsibility and authority were mismatched (27).

Participants on EL+MV reported a significant improvement in their mental component domain, suggesting they felt 'calm and peaceful', emotional well-being and improvement in energy/fatigue profile after the 12-week supplementation. This supports the results of the POMS analysis with regard to the vigour activity domain, which reported an increasing trend in the EL+MV group. These results were further supported by the POMS Iceberg profiles that showed optimal peaks of vigour activity and a decrease in the negative mood clusters, contributing to the trough values of the profile in both EL+MV and placebo groups. This concept has previously been applied to assess physical activity and mood among healthy individuals (28, 29). After the 12-week supplementation, the POMS Iceberg profiles favoured an improvement in vigour among participants in the EL+MV group. Previous studies with nutritionally enriched coffee (28) and adaptation to competitive sports (30) have reported a similar shift to healthy POMS Iceberg profiles, akin to positive mood states associated with the use of multivitamins and protein supplements in other stressed populations (31). In another study, a significant improvement in mood by a reduction in tension and anxiety domain of the POMS was found ($P = 0.054$) in stressed subjects with EL supplementation (13).

Participants on EL+MV reported significant improvement in role limitation due to emotional health and in social functioning domains, suggesting an enhancement in their QoL, social interactions and related activities.

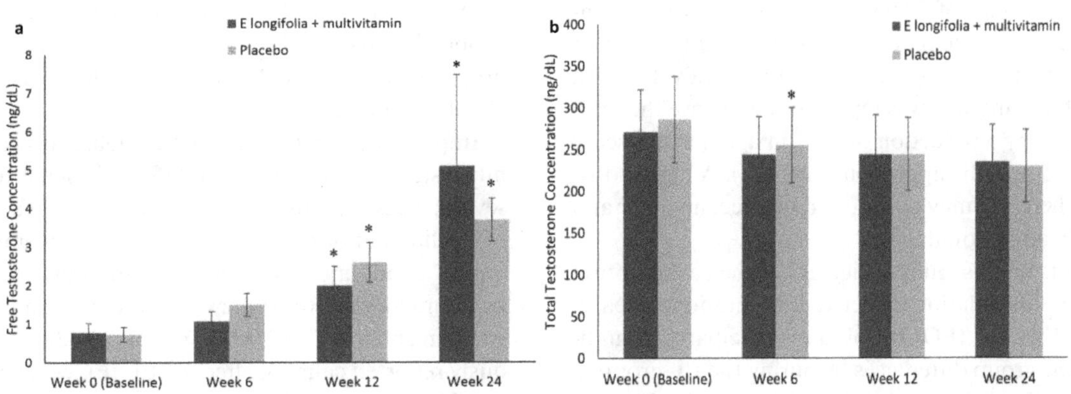


*Fig. 4.* (a) Serum total testosterone levels in EL+MV ($n = 44$) and placebo groups ($n = 36$). Serum total testosterone decreased significantly ($P = 0.009$) in the placebo group at week 6 compared to baseline. Within-group comparisons were made using the paired $t$-test. Mean ± SE values.*$P \leq 0.05$. (b) Serum free testosterone levels in EL+MV ($n = 44$) and placebo ($n = 36$) groups. Serum free testosterone increased significantly in both groups ($P < 0.001$). Larger percentage increases were observed in the *E. longifolia* + multivitamins group. Within-group comparisons were made using the paired $t$-test. Mean ± SE values.*$P \leq 0.05$.

*Table 5.* Mean concentrations of testosterone in female and male participants.

| | Female | | | Male | | |
|---|---|---|---|---|---|---|
| | EL+MV | Placebo | *P*-value (*t*-test)† | EL+MV | Placebo | *P*-value (*t*-test)† |
| | Mean ± SD (*n*) Within Group *P*-value | Mean ± SD (*n*) Within Group *P*-value | | Mean ±SD (*n*) Within Group *P*-value | Mean ± SD (*n*) Within Group *P*-value | |
| **Total testosterone concentration (ng/dL)** | | | | | | |
| Week 0 (baseline) | 15.9 ± 12.7 (26) | 20.5 ± 12.6 (19) | 0.270 | 641 ± 198 (18) | 582 ± 177 (17) | 0.269 |
| Week 6 | 18.3 ± 14.2 (26) | 17.8 ± 9.6 (20) | 0.723 | 570 ± 193 (18) | 468 ± 230 (17) | 0.184 |
| | 21.6 ± 22.0 (23) | 29.4 ± 28.6 (17) | 0.155 | 563 ± 189 (16) | 458 ± 188 (17) | 0.118 |
| Week 24 | 18.6 ± 13.2 (28) | 20.0 ± 13.1 (19) | 0.737 | 573 ± 208 (18) | 434 ± 154 (16) | 0.070 |
| Change from weeks 0 to 6 | 1.9 ± 6.5 (24) *P* = 0.223‡ | −2.9 ± 10.2 (19) *P* = 0.556‡ | 0.271 | −64 ± 125 (17) *P* = 0.058‡ | −124 ± 156 (15) *P* = 0.003‡ | 0.246 |
| Change from weeks 0 to 12 | 5.3 ± 14.0 (21) *P* = 0.203‡ | 8.6 ± 33.3 (16) *P* = 0.660‡ | 0.530 | −74 ± 153 (16) *P* = 0.094‡ | −130 ± 152 (15) *P* = 0.005‡ | 0.401 |
| Change from weeks 0 to 24 | 1.9 ± 8.1 (26) *P* = 0.115‡ | ± 8.5 (18) *P* = 0.433‡ | 0.839 | −79 ± 155 (17) *P* = 0.049‡ | −127 ± 185 (14) *P* = 0.017‡ | 0.710 |
| **Free testosterone concentration (ng/dL)** | | | | | | |
| Week-0 (baseline) | 0.15 ± 0.30 (26) | 0.12 ± 0.44 (19) | 0.239 | 1.67 ± 2.35 (18) | 1.40 ± 1.27 (17) | 0.298 |
| Week-6 | 0.39 ± 0.62 (26) | 0.27 ± 0.50 (20) | 0.456 | 2.04 ± 2.19 (18) | 2.95 ± 2.53 (17) | 0.276 |
| Week-12 | 0.85 ± 0.78 (23) | 0.68 ± 1.04 (17) | 0.175 | 3.7 ± 4.2 (16) | 4.6 ± 3.1 (17) | 0.231 |
| Week-24 | 1.05 ± 0.89 (28) | 1.36 ± 1.37 (19) | 0.931 | 11.4 ± 24.9 (18) | 6.4 ± 2.9 (16) | 0.506 |
| Change from week-0 to -6 | 0.16 ± 0.43 (24) *P* = 0.132‡ | 0.09 ± 0.31 (19) *P* = 0.888‡ | 0.304 | −0.04 ± 1.72 (17) *P* = 0.678‡ | 1.72 ± 2.51 (15) *P* = 0.030‡ | 0.086 |
| Change from week-0 to 12 | 0.62 ± 0.76 (21) *P* < 0.001‡ | 0.53 ± 0.99 (16) *P* = 0.025‡ | 0.249 | 2.0 ± 4.4 (16) *P* = 0.130‡ | 3.4 ± 3.0 (15) *P* = 0.002‡ | 0.151 |
| Change from week-0 to-24 | 0.86 ± 0.93 (26) *P* < 0.001‡ | 1.26 ± 1.34 (18) *P* < 0.001‡ | 0.519 | 9.7 ± 25.9 (17) *P* = 0.005‡ | 5.3 ± 2.9 (14) *P* < 0.001‡ | 0.218 |

‡Within-group analysis was made using the Wilcoxon signed rank test. Significant within-group difference in *E. longifolia* + multivitamins (EL+MV) and placebo groups;

†Between-group analysis was made using the *t*-test. Probability values $P \leq 0.05$ are statistically significant; $n$ = number of subjects.

A significant between-group improvement in the 25–45 years subgroup in the social functioning domain could be explained by the higher occurrence of mood and anxiety disorder generally increasing with age (30), hence the extract at a low dosage of 50 mg EL/day, not showing an intervention effect in the older subgroup, instead having an effect in the younger subgroup. In another study, EL with a dosage of 200 mg/day was reported to improve the QoL demonstrated by a reduction of 38% in aging males score (QoL) after 1-month supplementation (10). A higher dosage of EL therefore may be required to affect an older and otherwise healthy population.

The results of this study indicate that the consumption of EL+MV formulation affected the emotional health (SF-12) and vigour (POMS) of the participants. Significant between-group differences favouring the EL group in the vigour activity domain of POMS for the 46–65 years age group could be due to the physical fitness since the reduction in muscle strength in the upper and lower limbs, changes in body fat percentages and endurance increase with age and poor nutrition (31). Hence, an intervention effect may have probably arisen from muscle and strength improvement (32, 33), anti-ageing and enhancement of vigour (13) properties of EL. In addition, participants consuming EL+MV showed a significant decrease in glucose concentrations from baseline to the end of the study, supporting its previously reported anti-hyperglycaemic properties *in vivo* (34, 35) which overall may contribute to well-being of subjects.

Improvement in mood with the highest decrease in cognitive stress subscale in the MMSQ – which is made up of several questions that include a participant's perception of 'feeling out of control', 'inability to concentrate', 'feeling no good' and a general sense of things being 'really bad' and a desire to 'run away and hide' – in participants supplemented with EL+MV is possibly due to the previously reported calming effect of EL (6), which is corroborated by animal studies demonstrating the anti-anxiolytic effects of EL (22). It was observed that there were more parents with children in the placebo group. It is surprising however that the mean for MMSQ (stress) at baseline was lower in all four domains in the placebo group in spite of them having more children. The POMS, however, had higher baseline means in individual domains. The SF-12 had mixed baseline values where either placebo or treatment group had higher baseline values. There were no between-group differences in all domains at baseline. There were also more women in the treatment group, which may have contributed to higher mean at baseline in MMSQ compared to placebo since stress was more prevalent among women (36).

A large placebo effect as well as large standard deviations in POMS total mood disturbance and its subscales, however, perhaps contributed to the absence of between-group significance in the questionnaires tested. Furthermore, it is also plausible that the lower dose of EL (50 mg/day) used in the current formulation may not have provided the clinical benefits achieved with the higher dose (200 mg/day) used in previous studies which showed improvements in tension, anger and confusion with EL supplementation (6). A reduction in negative mood states mediated by phytochemicals has been demonstrated in numerous studies, with placebo effects ranging from 1 to 50% (37–41); therefore, the 10–12% placebo effect seen with SF-12 and MMSQ and nearly 70% in POMS in the current study is not surprising. Thus, the lower dose of EL and a substantial placebo effect exacerbated by the large statistical deviations observed in the current study may have obscured the efficacy of EL+MV. This is a challenge in clinical trials conducted on a healthy population as the effects of nutrition interventions are subtle, whereas drug trials compare exposure with no exposure, and nutrition trials compare higher and lower exposures. Everyone consumes nutrients in their diet; therefore, subtle differences may be difficult to detect and have long latency periods. Taken together, these limitations and considerations mean that it is difficult to demonstrate statistically significant benefit between groups (42). In addition, due to the lack of significant difference between groups in primary and secondary outcomes, a comparison was made in both outcomes across groups and within groups at multiple time points, and also in subgroup analyses by sex and age. This could contribute to type II error, lack of between-group statistical significance and false positives. The problem of multiple comparisons to be counteracted by, for example, Bonferroni analysis, may be considered.

Within the safety parameters, significant increase in lymphocytes similar to earlier reports (15, 43, 44) was observed. Furthermore, micronutrients contribute to the body's natural defences by supporting physical barriers (skin/mucosa), cellular immunity and antibody production. Vitamins A, B6, B12, C, D, E and folic acid and the trace elements iron, zinc, copper and selenium work in synergy to support the protective activities of the immune cells, whereby vitamins A, C, E and zinc assist in enhancing the skin barrier function (45). Combining EL with micronutrients thus is anticipated to provide health benefits through hormonal balance and optimal nutritional requirements.

Participants in this study showed a significant decrease in neutrophils that degranulate to release proteases during pathogenesis and psychological stress (46). Stress also enhances neutrophilia and neutrophil counts (47) without concurrent increase in eosinophils or monocytes (48), which was also noted in this study. Plant extracts are known to reduce leukocyte esterase (49) and calcium oxalate crystals (50) in urine, similar to observations made in this study, which suggests fewer urinary abnormalities associated with EL+MV. It can be speculated that EL is a nutritional adaptogen (51), an agent that rejuvenates the body through restoration, which may regulate neutrophils and leukocyte esterase release. It is plausible that the EL+MV-mediated improvement in emotional health and vitality may be associated with changes in these immune parameters.

Importantly, serum total testosterone levels in the EL+MV group did not alter, while it decreased in the placebo group. The stress hormone cortisol increases under stressed states and as a result, the opposite effect is that the testosterone levels dip. It is possible through the absence of the hormone modulating effect of EL and multinutrients, the cortisol levels as a result of stress may have increased, hence causing the reduction in testosterone levels (52). However, there was an increase in free testosterone levels in males in the EL+MV group. Increase in free testosterone levels is a measure of bioavailable testosterone (53). Our results are in agreement with other studies showing a 10.3% increase in free testosterone with EL in combination of *Polygonum minus* supplementation compared to 4.3% with the placebo (54), and EL-mediated enhancement of free testosterone levels by 46.8% in subjects suffering from hypogonadism (10). A supplementation with testosterone improves mood, energy, friendliness and decreased negative mood (55). Eurypeptides, a bioactive peptide of 4.3 kDa with testosterone-modulating properties identified in EL (10), may restore normal testosterone levels by influencing the release of free testosterone from its binding hormone, sex-hormone-binding globulin, which results in improvement in QoL (10, 55). Eurypeptides enhance metabolism of pregnenolone and progesterone to yield more dehydroepiandrosterone and androstenedione (10, 44, 56) by activating the CYP17 (17α-hydroxylase and 17,20lyase) enzyme (10). In addition, even though levels of free testosterone increased significantly from baseline in females in both groups, the increase was higher in the placebo group compared to EL+MV group, rendering it non-significant between groups. Therefore, EL+MV and the adaptogenic nature of EL may be considered safe in women, preventing an increase in free testosterone, which is related to conditions such as hirsutism and polycystic ovary syndrome (57).

There were no significant and sustained changes from baseline or against placebo in relevant blood, liver and kidney laboratory tests. This product was well-tolerated and safe in the population studied, with no serious adverse events reported, which corroborates findings from previous randomised and controlled clinical trials evaluating EL (11). This study did not measure cortisol levels, which perhaps may have provided valuable information to understand the efficacy of EL+MV on various stress indicators and immunological parameters. This is a limitation of the study and should be considered when conducting future clinical studies.

Observational studies and clinical trials evaluating the efficacy of EL on mood, stress and testosterone levels have consistently shown favourable changes in these parameters, thereby providing a rationale for its incorporation into new formulations of multivitamins. Multivitamin supplementation enhanced mood by 15% and energy levels by 17% (58) and reduced depressive symptoms since inadequacy of key micronutrients has been associated with poor mood states (19). Therefore, it is reasonable to speculate that EL synergises health benefits exerted by multivitamins through improvement in mood states, vigour and a reduction in stress. The effect of intervention on depressed subjects could be evaluated in the future since the subjects used in this study were healthy subjects with only mid-level stress and not in a depressed state. There are differences and similarities in the way drugs affect a depressed mental state compared to the product. For example, fluoxetine (Prozac) and sertraline (Zoloft) are newer medicines that act as selective serotonin reuptake inhibitors (SSRIs). The product in this study appears to affect energy and mood levels most likely via hormonal modulation (testosterone) and nutritional supplementation, for example, vitamins B complex and C, which also affect mood (20). Vitamin B complex is involved in the metabolism of S-adenosylmethionine (SAM), a donator of methyl groups, which plays a decisive role in the functioning of the nervous system and in the formation of neurotransmitters (e.g. serotonin) (59). The target of the vitamins is similar, whereas the target of EL is different for this study. There could be a lack of intervention effect in subjects with chronic stress or depressed state; hence, one needs to be open to a more prescription-based therapy than nutritional supplementation for beyond everyday moderate stress. With unrealistic expectations to treat depression or stress related to suffering from, for example, advanced disease, there is a risk of dropping traditional medication exacerbated with a fear of potential interactions between EL and other medications. It is however noteworthy that recent research on herb–drug interaction of EL was weak and inconclusive due to the dissimilarities between investigated solvent extract and aqueous extract of EL (60).

## Conclusions

This study reports significant within-group improvements in QoL, mood and stress of moderately stressed participants supplemented with EL+MV for 12 weeks. Despite the placebo effects, participants supplemented with EL+MV reported improvements in vigour, mental component, emotional well-being, cognition and testosterone levels possibly through hormonal balance and nutritional supplementation. The stress-related changes in neutrophils and leukocyte esterase suggest the counteracting effect of EL+MV supplementation; hence, further research is warranted. Significant between-group improvements in the social functioning domain of SF-12 observed in the 25–45 years age group and vigour domain of POMS in the 46–65 years age group supplemented with EL+MV indicate the efficacy of the supplement in particular spheres of influence, particularly relating to age. EL+MV was found to be safe and well-tolerated in this 24-week supplementation study on moderately stressed participants.

## Acknowledgements

The authors would like to thank the volunteers for their time and participation in the study; Ms. Sasikala Chinnappan for assisting in the data management and Dr. Joseph Antony for the statistics and editing of the manuscript.

## Conflict of interest and funding

The study was funded by NKEA Research Grant Scheme (NRGS) EPP#1 under the Ministry of Agriculture and Agro Based Industry, Malaysia. Annie George is an employee of Biotropics Malaysia Berhad. The authors have no potential conflict of interest.

## References

1. Liu RT, Alloy LB. Stress generation in depression: a systematic review of the empirical literature and recommendations for future study. Clin Psychol Rev 2010; 30(5): 582–93. doi: 10.1016/j.cpr.2010.04.010
2. Fernandes AC, Chandran D, Khondoker M, Dewey M, Shetty H, Dutta R, et al. Demographic and clinical factors associated with different antidepressant treatments: a retrospective cohort study design in a UK psychiatric healthcare setting. BMJ Open 2018; 8(9): e022170. doi: 10.1136/bmjopen-2018-022170
3. Schrader E. Equivalence of St John's wort extract (Ze 117) and fluoxetine: a randomized, controlled study in mild-moderate depression. Int Clin Psychopharmacol 2000; 15(2): 61–8. doi: 10.1097/00004850-200015020-00001
4. Edwards D, Heufelder A, Zimmermann A. Therapeutic effects and safety of Rhodiolarosea extract WS® 1375 in subjects with life-stress symptoms – results of an open-label study. Phytother Res 2012; 26(8): 1220–5. doi: 10.1002/ptr.3712

5. Kaplan BJ, Crawford SG, Field CJ, Simpson JS. Vitamins, minerals, and mood. Psychol Bull 2007; 133(5): 747–60. doi: 10.1037/0033-2909.133.5.747
6. Talbott SM, Talbott JA, George A, Pugh M. Effect of Tongkat Ali on stress hormones and psychological mood state in moderately stressed subjects. J Int Soc Sports Nutr 2013; 10(1): 28. doi: 10.1186/1550-2783-10-28
7. Wizneh FM, Asmawi MZ. *Eurycoma longifolia* jack (simarubaceae); advances in its medicinal potentials. Pharmacognosy J 2014; 6(4): 1–9. doi: 10.5530/pj.2014.4.1
8. Bhat R, Karim AA. Tongkat Ali (*Eurycoma longifolia* Jack): a review on its ethnobotany and pharmacological importance. Fitoterapia 2010; 81(7): 669–79. doi: 10.1016/j.fitote.2010.04.006
9. Goreja WG. Tongkat Ali: The tree that cures a hundred diseases. Vol. 2. New York: Amazing Herb Press, TNC International Inc.; 2004, pp. 10–11.
10. Tambi MI, Imran MK, Henkel RR. Standardised water-soluble extract of Eurycoma longifolia, Tongkat Ali, as testosterone booster for managing men with late-onset hypogonadism. Andrologia 2012; 44(Suppl 1): 226–30. doi: 10.1111/j.1439-0272.2011.01168.x
11. Ismail SB, Wan Mohammad WM, George A, Nik Hussain NH, Musthapa Kamal ZM, Liske E. Randomized clinical trial on the use of PHYSTA freeze-dried water extract of *Eurycoma longifolia* for the improvement of quality of life and sexual well-being in men. Evid Based Complement Alternat Med 2012; 2012: 429268. doi: 10.1155/2012/429268
12. Sambandan TG, Rha CK, Kadir AA, Aminudim N, Saad J, Mohammed M. Bioactive fraction of *Eurycoma longifolia*. [7132117 B2.]. United States Patent; 2006. https://patents.google.com/patent/US20040087493A1/en.
13. George A, Suzuki N, Abas AB, Mohri K, Utsuyama M, Hirokawa K, et al. Immunomodulation in middle-aged humans via the ingestion of Physta® standardized root water extract of *Eurycoma longifolia* Jack-arandomized, double-blind, placebo-controlled, parallel study. Phytother Res 2016; 30(4): 627–35. doi:10.1002/ptr.5571
14. Coleman CI, Hebert JH, Reddy P. The effects of Panax ginseng on quality of life. J Clin Pharm Ther 2003; 28(1): 5–15. https://doi.org/10.1046/j.1365-2710.2003.00467.x.
15. Kaneko H,Nakanishi K. Proof of the mysterious efficacy of ginseng: basic and clinical trials: clinical effects of medical ginseng, Korean red ginseng: specifically, its anti-stress action for prevention of disease. J Pharmacol Sci 2004; 95(2): 158–62. https://doi.org/10.1254/jphs.FMJ04001X5.
16. Fava M, Abraham M, Clancy-Colecchi K, Pava JA, Matthews J, Rosenbaum JF. Eating disorder symptomatology in major depression. J Nerv Ment Dis 1997; 185: 140–4.
17. Benton D, Cook R. The impact of selenium supplementation on mood. Biol Psychiatry 1991; 29(11): 1092–8. http://dx.doi.org/10.1016/0006-3223(91)90251-G.
18. Kaplan BJ, Rucklidge JJ, Romijn AR, Dolph M. A randomised trial of nutrient supplements to minimise psychological stress after a natural disaster. Psychiatry Res 2015; 228: 373–9. doi: 10.1016/j.psychres.2015.05.080
19. Harris E, Kirk J, Rowsell R, Vitetta L, Sali A, Scholey AB, et al. The effect of multivitamin supplementation on mood and stress in healthy older men. Hum Psychopharmacol 2011; 26(8): 560–7. doi: 10.1002/hup.1245
20. Kennedy DO, Veasey R, Watson A, Dodd F, Jones E, Maggini S, et al. Effects of high-dose B vitamin complex with vitamin C and minerals on subjective mood and performance in healthy males. Psychopharmacology (Berl) 2010; 211(1): 55–68. doi: 10.1007/s00213-010-1870-3
21. Ang HH, Cheang HS. Studies on the anxiolytic activity of *Eurycoma longifolia* Jack roots in mice. Jpn J Pharmacol 1999; 79(4): 497–500.
22. McNair D, Lorr M, Droppleman L. Profile of Mood States (POMS). San Diego, California: Multi-Health Systems Inc.; 1992.
23. Jenkinson C, Layte R, Jenkinson D, Lawrence K, Petersen S, Paice C, et al. A shorter form health survey: can the SF-12, replicate results from the SF-36 in longitudinal studies? J Public Health Med 1997; 19(2): 179–86.
24. Lefebvre RC, Sandford SL. A multi-modal questionnaire for stress, J Hum Stress 1985; 11(2): 69–75.
25. Morgan WP, Brown DR, Raglin JS, O'Connor PJ, Ellickson KA. Psychological monitoring of overtraining and staleness. Br J Sports Med 1987; 21(3): 107–14.
26. Perazzo FF, Fonseca FLA, Souza GHB, Maistro EL, Rodrigues M, Jose CT. Carvalho. Double-blind clinical study of a multivitamin and polymineral complex associated with Panax ginseng extract (Gerovital®). Open Complement Med J 2010; 2: 100–4. doi: 10.2174/1876391X01002010100
27. Dewe PJ, O'Driscoll MP, Cooper CL. Theories of psychological stress at work. In: Gatchel RJ, Schultz IZ eds. Handbook of occupational health and wellness. New York: Springer Science; 2012, pp. 23–38.
28. Hoffman JR, Kang J, Ratamess NA, Jennings PF, Mangine G, Faigenbaum AD. Thermogenic effect from nutritionally enriched coffee consumption. J Int Soc Sports Nutr 2006; 3: 35–41. doi: 10.1186/1550-2783-3-1-35
29. Casanova N, Palmeira-de-Oliveira A, Pereira A, Crisostomo LD, Travassos B, Costa AM. Cortisol, testosterone and mood state variation during an official female football competition. J Sports Med Phys Fitness 2016; 56(6): 775–81.
30. Byers AL, Yaffe K, Covinsky KE, Friedman MB, Bruce ML. High occurrence of mood and anxiety disorders among older adults: The National Comorbidity Survey Replication. Arch Gen Psychiatry 2010; 67(5): 489–96. doi: 10.1001/archgenpsychiatry.2010.35
31. Milanović Z, Pantelić S, Trajković N, Sporiš G, Kostić R, James N. Age-related decrease in physical activity and functional fitness among elderly men and women. Clin Interv Aging 2013; 8: 549–56. doi:10.2147/CIA.S44112
32. Henkel RR, Wang R, Bassett SH, Chen T, Liu N, Zhu Y, et al. Tongkat Ali as a potential herbal supplement for physically active male and female seniors – a pilot study. Phytother Res 2014; 28(4): 544–50. doi: 10.1002/ptr.5017
33. Hamzah S, Yusof A. The ergogenic effects of *Eurycoma longifolia* Jack: a pilot study. Br J Sports Med 2003; 37: 465–6.
34. Husen R, Pihie AH, Nallappan M. Screening for antihyperglycaemic activity in several local herbs of Malaysia. J Ethnopharmacol 2004; 95(2–3): 205–8. doi: 10.1016/j.jep.2004.07.004
35. Li CH, Liao JW, Liao PL, Huang WK, Tse LS, Lin CH, et al. Evaluation of acute 13-week subchronic toxicity and genotoxicity of the powdered root of Tongkat Ali (*Eurycoma longifolia* Jack). Evid Based Complement Alternat Med 2013; 2013: 102987. doi: 10.1155/2013/102987

36. Chaplin TM, Hong K, Bergquist K, Sinha R. Gender differences in response to emotional stress: an assessment across subjective, behavioral, and physiological domains and relations to alcohol craving. Alcohol Clin Exp Res 2008; 32(7): 1242–50. doi:10.1111/j.1530-0277.2008.00679
37. Bradwejn J, Zhou Y, Koszycki D, Shlik J. A double-blind, placebo-controlled study on the effects of Gotu Kola (*Centella asiatica*) on acoustic startle response in healthy subjects. J Clin Psychopharmacol 2000; 20(6): 680–4.
38. Jana U, Sur TK, Maity LN, Debnath PK, Bhattacharyya D. A clinical study on the management of generalized anxiety disorder with *Centella asiatica*. Nepal Med Coll J 2010; 12(1): 8–11.
39. Lopresti AL, Maes M, Maker GL, Hood SD, Drummond PD. Curcumin for the treatment of major depression: a randomised, double-blind, placebo controlled study. J Affect Disord 2014; 167: 368–75. doi: 10.1016/j.jad.2014.06.001
40. Stojanovska L, Law C, Lai B, Chung T, Nelson K, Day S, et al. Maca reduces blood pressure and depression, in a pilot study in postmenopausal women. Climacteric 2015; 18(1): 69–78. doi: 10.3109/13697137.2014.929649
41. Terauchi M, Horiguchi N, Kajiyama A, Akiyoshi M, Owa Y, Kato K, et al. Effects of grape seed proanthocyanidin extract on menopausal symptoms, body composition, and cardiovascular parameters in middle-aged women: a randomized, double-blind, placebo-controlled pilot study. Menopause 2014; 21(9): 990–6. doi: 10.1097/GME.0000000000000200
42. Moyer MW. Nutrition: vitamins on trial. Nature 2014; 510(7506): 462–4. doi: 10.1038/510462a
43. Muhamad AS, Ooi FK, Chen CK. Effects of *Eurycoma longifolia* on natural killer cells and endurance running performance. Int J Sports Sci Coach 2015; 5(3): 93–8. doi: 10.5923/j.sports.20150503.01
44. Tambi MI. Standardized water soluble extract of *Eurycoma longifolia* maintains healthy aging in man. Aging Male 2007; 10: 77–87. doi: 10.1111/j.1439-0272.2011.01168.x
45. Maggini S, Wintergerst ES, Beveridge S, Hornig DH. Selected vitamins and trace elements support immune function by strengthening epithelial barriers and cellular and humoral immune responses. Br J Nutr 2007; 98(1): S29–35. doi: 10.1017/S0007114507832971
46. Hwang TI, Juang GD, Yeh CH, Chang YH, Chou KY, Chen HE. Hormone levels in middle-aged and elderly men with and without erectile dysfunction in Taiwan. Int J Impot Res 2006; 18(2): 160–3. doi: 10.1038/sj.ijir.3901382.
47. Nishitani N, Sakakibara H. Association of psychological stress response of fatigue with white blood cell count in male daytime workers. Ind Health 2014; 52(6): 531–4. doi: 10.2486/indhealth.2013-0045
48. Darko DF, Rose J, Gillin JC, Golshan S, Baird SM. Neutrophilia and lymphopenia in major mood disorders. Psychiatry Res 1988; 25(3): 243–51.
49. Vicariotto F. Effectiveness of an association of a cranberry dry extract, D-mannose, and the two microorganisms Lactobacillus plantarum LP01 and Lactobacillus paracasei LPC09 in women affected by cystitis: a pilot study. J Clin Gastroenterol 2014; 48(Suppl 1): S96–101. doi: 10.1097/MCG.0000000000000224
50. Bashir S, Gilani AH. Antiurolithic effect of Bergenia ligulata rhizome: an explanation of the underlying mechanisms. J Ethnopharmacol 2009; 122(1): 106–16. doi: 10.1016/j.jep.2008.12.004
51. Thu HE, Mohamed IN, Hussain Z, Jayusman PA, Shuid AN. *Eurycoma longifolia* as a potential adoptogen of male sexual health: a systematic review on clinical studies. Chin J Nat Med 2017; 15(1): 0071–80. doi: 10.1016/S1875-5364(17)30010-9
52. Sherman GD, Lerner JS, Josephs RA, Renshon J, Gross JJ. The interaction of testosterone and cortisol is associated with attained status in male executives. J Pers Soc Psychol 2016; 110(6): 921–9. doi: 10.1037/pspp0000063
53. Speroff L, Glass RH, Kase NG. Clinical gynecologic endocrinology and infertility. 5th edn. Baltimore, MD: Lippincott, Williams and Wilkins; 1994.
54. Udani JK, George AA, Musthapa M, Pakdaman MN, Abas A. Effects of a proprietary freeze-dried water extract of *Eurycoma longifolia* (Physta) and Polygonum minus on sexual performance and well-being in men: arandomized, double-blind, placebo-controlled study. Evid Based Complement Alternat Med 2014; 2014: 179529. doi: 10.1155/2014/179529
55. Bain J. The many faces of testosterone. Clin Interv Aging 2007; 2(4): 567–76.
56. Tambi MI, Imran MK. *Eurycoma longifolia* Jack in managing idiopathic male infertility. Asian J Androl 2010; 12(3): 376–80. doi: 10.1038/aja.2010.7
57. Manni A, Pardridge WM, Cefalu W, Nisula BC, Bardin CW, Santner SJ, et al. Bioavailability of albumin-bound testosterone. J Clin Endocrinol Metab 1985; 61(4): 705–10. doi: 10.1210/jcem-61-4-705
58. Sarris J, Cox KH, Camfield DA, Scholey A, Stough C, Fogg E, et al. Participant experiences from chronic administration of a multivitamin versus placebo on subjective health and wellbeing: a double-blind qualitative analysis of a randomised controlled trial. Nutr J 2012; 11: 110. doi: 10.1186/1475-2891-11-110
59. Karakuła H, Opolska A, Kowal A, Domański M, Płotka A, Perzyński J. [Does diet affect our mood? The significance of folic acid and homocysteine]. Pol Merkur Lekarski 2009; 26(152): 136–41.
60. Young MH, In SK, Rehman SU, Choe K, Yoo HH. *In vitro* evaluation of the effects of *Eurycoma longifolia* extract on CYP-mediated drug metabolism. Evid Based Complement Alternat Med 2015; 2015: 631329. doi: 10.1155/2015/631329


***Dr. Ashril Yusof**
Exercise Science, Sports Centre, University of Malaya,
50603 Kuala Lumpur, Malaysia.
Email: ashril@um.edu.my

# 19

# Sufficient iodine status among Norwegian toddlers 18 months of age – cross-sectional data from the Little in Norway study

Inger Aakre[1]*, Maria Wik Markhus[1], Marian Kjellevold[1], Vibeke Moe[2], Lars Smith[2] and Lisbeth Dahl[1]

[1]Food Security and Nutrition, Institute of Marine Research, Bergen, Norway; [2]Department of Psychology, University of Oslo, Oslo, Norway

*Abstract*

***Background***: Inadequate iodine intake has been identified in several population groups in the Nordic countries over the past years; however, studies of iodine status in infants and toddlers are scarce.
***Objective***: The aim of this study is to evaluate the iodine status and dietary iodine sources among 18-month-old toddlers from Norway.
***Methods***: Cross-sectional and country representative data from the Little in Norway study were used. All children who had given a spot urine sample at 18 months age were included ($n$ = 416). Urinary iodine concentration (UIC) was determined by inductively coupled plasma mass-spectrometry. Dietary habits and supplement use were measured by a food frequency questionnaire.
***Results***: Median (25th–75th percentiles [p25–p75]) UIC was 129 (81–190) μg/L while estimated median (p25–p75) habitual iodine intake was 109 (101–117) μg/day. None of the children were below the estimated average requirement (EAR) of 65 μg/day or above the upper intake level of 180 μg/day. There were no differences in either UIC or estimated habitual iodine intake between different geographic areas in Norway. Milk was the most important iodine source, contributing an estimated 70% to the total iodine intake, while other foods rich in iodine such as seafood and enriched baby porridge contributed about 30%.
***Conclusions***: The iodine status among 18-month-old toddlers from different geographic areas in Norway was sufficient, indicated by a median UIC above the WHO cutoff of 100 μg/L. This was further supported by the estimated habitual iodine intake, where none of the participants were below the EAR. Milk was an important iodine source in this age group; thus children with a low intake might be at risk of insufficient iodine intake.

Keywords: *Iodine; Urinary iodine concentration; Iodine intake; Dietary iodine intake; Toddlers*

Infants and toddlers are particularly vulnerable to inadequate iodine nutrition, as iodine is crucial for optimal child growth and development (1, 2) through the many functions of the thyroid hormones (3, 4). Thus, iodine deficiency has been pointed out as one of the main factors that prevent children from achieving their developmental potential (5). Even though the global work towards eliminating iodine deficiency disorders has been successful (6, 7), iodine deficiency has been reemerging in Europe (8); and inadequate iodine status has been reported in several European countries during recent years (9–12).

Iodine is present in relatively few food groups, and iodized salt is the most important source globally (13). In Norway, the permitted iodine level of 5 μg/g in table salt is too low to be considered a significant iodine source in the population (9). However, animal feed is enriched with iodine in Norway; therefore milk, dairy products, and eggs have significant levels of iodine. Marine fish, especially lean fish such as cod, haddock, and saithe, and fish products also have high levels of iodine (14, 15). Industry-manufactured baby food is enriched with iodine; thus among toddlers this is an important iodine source as well as breast milk or formula (16). Dietary surveys among Norwegian toddlers revealed that only 35% and 4% were still breastfed at 12 (17) and 24 months of age (18), respectively. Young children in the weaning period are therefore dependent on iodine-rich complementary foods in order to reach an intake of 50–70 μg/day as recommended in the Nordic countries (19).

As the consumption of milk, yoghurt, and lean fish has been declining in Norway, recent studies have reported insufficient iodine status among pregnant and lactating women (20–23). An association between insufficient iodine intake in pregnant Norwegian women and poorer developmental status in children at 3 years of age has also been found (24). Infants and young children have therefore been identified as a vulnerable group regarding insufficient iodine intake. Recently published data among 5-year-old preschool children ($n$ = 220) and 3–9-year-old children ($n$ = 47) showed iodine sufficiency in these groups, with a median urinary iodine concentration (UIC) of 132 and 148 µg/L, respectively (25, 26). Studies among infants and toddlers remain scarce; however, iodine status was measured in a study of Norwegian toddlers under the age of 2 with cow's milk protein allergy. This study found a median UIC of 159 ug/L, indicating sufficient iodine status (27). The main objective of this paper is to assess iodine status in toddlers 18 months of age participating in the Little in Norway study (LiN). To our knowledge, this is the first paper from Norway to present data on iodine status and its relation to dietary habits among healthy children less than 2 years of age.

## Subjects and methods

### *Study design and subjects*

This paper is based on data from the LiN project (ISRCTN registry number 66710572), a prospective population-based cohort study conducted between September 2011 and November 2014. The study was established to investigate pre- and postnatal risk factors influencing child development from pregnancy to 18 months of age. Pregnant women at nine primary health clinics across all four Norwegian health regions were recruited. The data collection included questionnaires completed by the mothers and biological samples of mother and child. In total, 1,036 pregnant women consented to participate in the LiN cohort. In this paper, cross-sectional data from toddlers 18 months of age were used, as well as background characteristics of their mothers at study enrollment. Of the 1,036 participating pregnant women, 777 children were still participating at 18 months age. Not all toddlers were able to give a urine sample at the time of data collection and some failed due to technical issues. Thus, the final sample size consisted of 416 toddlers 18 months of age, along with their mothers. Further details regarding study attrition for the participants have been described elsewhere (28).

### *Urinary iodine concentration*

UIC was assessed in spot urine samples from the children using Uricol collection pack (Sterisets International B.V., SteriSets GP Supplies, Newcastle Urine Collection Pack, UK). The urine was extracted from the pad with a syringe and transferred to CryoTubes (CryoTubes™ Vials, Nunc A/S, Roskilde, Denmark) for storage at −18°C pending analysis. Content of iodine in urine was determined by inductively coupled plasma mass-spectrometry at the Institute of Marine Research in Norway. Further description of the analytic method and accuracy has been published elsewhere (23).

### *Estimated habitual iodine intake*

The children's habitual food intake was mapped by the mothers of the children answering questions about average intake of selected food items and dishes through an online questionnaire. There were 13 questions concerning the general diet, of which nine questions concerned iodine-containing food items, where intake of yoghurt, porridge, fish, and fish products was assessed. Frequency responses were recorded as never/rarely to seven times per week or more. There was one question assessing intake of eggs, where the frequency responses ranged from less than one egg per week to eight or more per week. There were nine questions assessing intake of fats and oils, of which questions regarding margarine and butter were relevant for iodine intake. The frequency responses ranged from never to daily. There was one question regarding breast milk intake at 18 months of age, where the frequency responses ranged from once in the last 24 h to 10 times or more. However, there were no data available from Norway regarding the amount of breast milk consumed among 18-month-old children. Nor has data regarding breast milk intake been registered in the national dietary surveys for 1- and 2-year-old children in Norway (17, 18). Therefore, children still breastfed at 18 months were excluded from the iodine intake estimations. The intake frequencies related to yoghurt, porridge, fish/fish products, eggs, and butter/margarine were converted to daily amounts using data from a national nutrition survey among children 2 years of age (18) and multiplied with the iodine concentration for each food item or dish. In all calculations, iodine content reported in the Norwegian Food Composition Table (29) was used. The questionnaire did not contain intake of milk and cheese, which are important dietary iodine sources in Norway. Mean intake of milk, white cheese/cheese spread and brown cheese/whey cheese spread among Norwegian 2-year-olds, both users and non-users of the food, was used to calculate the iodine contribution from these foods. In total, milk and cheese were estimated to contribute 79 µg/day, which was applied in the estimation of daily iodine intake among all non-breastfed children.

The frequency responses of the major iodine-contributing foods – fish, yoghurt, and porridge – were divided into low/medium consumption and high consumption using the following criteria: high consumption of fish: lean fish or fish products for dinner at least two to three times per week and fish (fatty and lean) as bread topping at least four to six times per week; high consumption of yoghurt: at least four to six times per week; high consumption of fish and yoghurt: both intake of fish and yoghurt was high; high consumption of porridge: (homemade or industry manufactured) at least four to six times per week.

*Definitions of iodine status and iodine intake*

The epidemiological criteria for assessing iodine nutrition based on median UIC for children were used in this study (13). For children less than 2 years of age a median UIC <100 μg/L indicates insufficient iodine status, while a median UIC ≥100 indicates adequate iodine status. In the Nordic Nutrition Recommendations, an iodine intake of 50–70 μg/day is estimated to be sufficient for infants and children <2 years of age (19). However, as the Nordic Nutrition Recommendations does not have an average requirement for young children, the estimated average requirement (EAR) from the US Institute of Medicine of 65 μg/day was used for evaluating the habitual iodine intake from food (30). To assess excessive iodine intakes, the World Health Organization's (WHO) upper intake level (UL) of 180 μg/day for children under 2 years was used (31).

*Background characteristics and anthropometry*

The mothers answered a precoded questionnaire concerning background variables for themselves and their children. The WHO body mass index (BMI) (kg/m$^2$) was used to classify underweight, normal weight, overweight, and obesity, defined by BMI < 18.5 kg/m$^2$, BMI = 18.5–24.9 kg/m$^2$, BMI = 25.0–29.9 kg/m$^2$, and BMI ≥ 30 kg/m$^2$, respectively (32). The children's height and weight were registered at the primary health clinic by trained health personnel. The gender-specific $z$-scores height-for-age, weight-for-age, weight-for-height (WHZ), and BMI-for-age (BMIz) were calculated using the WHO macro for SPSS (33, 34). A child was categorized as undernourished if WHZ or BMIz, was <−2, and overweight if WHZ or BMIz was above 2.

*Ethics*

Ethics approval for the survey was given by the Regional Committees for Medical Research Ethics (2011/560 REK Sør-Øst). Written informed consent was provided by the mothers on behalf of themselves and their children. All aspects of the study agreed with the latest version of the Helsinki Declaration.

*Statistics*

Normally distributed data were presented as mean ± SD. Non-normally distributed data were presented as median and 25th–75th percentiles (p25–p75). Due to the skewed distribution, non-parametric tests were used for two-sided tests of differences between groups (Mann–Whitney U test). The UIC among children was used as dependent variable in linear regression analyses. Because of skewed distribution, UIC was log2-transformed. Background characteristics (from Table 1) and dietary variables (from Table 4) were assessed for associations in simple linear models. All variables with an association ($p < 0.20$) were selected for the preliminary multiple model, which included the following: iodine supplements during pregnancy, high consumption of fish, high consumption of fish and yoghurt, high consumption of porridge. By backwards stepwise selection conducted manually, variables with a significant association at $p \leq 0.05$ were included in the final model. Analysis of the residuals was performed to examine the fit of the model.

**Results**

Background characteristics of mothers and toddlers are presented in Table 1. The distribution of participants between different geographic regions in Norway was quite even. Mean age among the mothers was 30 years, and 82% had higher education at university level. The gender distribution among the toddlers was even, with 52% boys and 48% girls. Almost 10% of the toddlers were still breastfed, 67% had received breast milk previously, while 4.6% had never been breastfed. Only 0.7 and 5.3% were wasted and overweight, respectively, according to weight-for-length $z$-scores. In total, 60.8% of the toddlers received dietary supplements, and cod liver oil was the most commonly used supplement.

Table 2 presents the UIC among the toddlers in different geographical regions of Norway and across all areas. The median UIC (p25–p75) was 129 (81–190) μg/L. As indicated by Fig. 1, 34% had UIC below 100 μg/L, 59% had UIC between 100 and 200 μg/L and 7% had UIC above 300 μg/L. There were no significant or substantial differences in UIC between different geographical regions or genders. The children who had never been breastfed had higher median UIC (149 μg/L) than children who were no longer breastfed. The children who were still breastfed had a median UIC of 117 μg/L; however the differences in UIC between breastfeeding statuses were not statistically significant. Children who were attending kindergarten had similar median UIC as children who were not attending kindergarten.

Intake frequencies of iodine-rich foods are shown in Table 3. Yoghurt was commonly consumed among the toddlers; however, 22% were given yoghurt ≤1 time/week. About two-thirds of the children were given porridge, either industry manufactured or homemade ≤1 time/week. About 80, 70, and 80% of the children were given fatty fish, lean fish, or fish products for dinner ≤1 time/week, respectively. Baby food with fish was not commonly consumed, with 95% in the category of less than or equal to

*Table 1.* Characteristics of Norwegian mothers and toddlers 18 months of age

| Characteristics of mothers | (*n* = 416) | Characteristics of toddlers | (*n* = 416) |
|---|---|---|---|
| Age, years | 30.3 ± 4.7 | Boy | 217 (52.2) |
| BMI, kg/m²[a] | 23.8 ± 4.5 | Girl | 198 (47.6) |
| <18.5 | 15 (3.6) | Never been breastfed | 19 (4.6) |
| 18.5–24.9 | 233 (56.9) | Stopped breastfeeding | 279 (67.1) |
| ≥25 | 101 (24.3) | Still breastfed | 41 (9.9) |
| Education level | | Breastfeeding frequency per 24 h[c] | |
| Primary and secondary school | 7 (1.7) | 1 time | 6 (14.6) |
| High school | 67 (16.2) | 2–3 times | 25 (61.0) |
| <4 years of university[b] | 167 (40.1) | ≥4 times | 10 (24.4) |
| ≥4 years of university[b] | 174 (41.8) | Weight-for-length/height, z-score | 0.6 ± 1.0 |
| Work situation | | <−2 (wasted) | 3 (0.7) |
| Work full-time | 319 (76.7) | >2 (overweight) | 22 (5.3) |
| Work part-time | 29 (7.0) | BMI-for-age, *z-score* | 0.5 ±1.01 |
| Student | 58 (13.9) | <−2 (underweight) | 5 (1.2) |
| Unemployed | 9 (2.2) | >2 (overweight) | 21 (5.0) |
| Geographic region | | Supplement use (all types) weekly | 253 (60.8) |
| Mid-Norway | 134 (32.2) | Cod liver oil | 151 (36.3) |
| North Norway | 80 (19.2) | Vitamin D drops | 84 (20.2) |
| Western Norway | 89 (21.4) | Omega-3 | 19 (4.6) |
| Eastern Norway | 112 (26.9) | Multivitamin mixture | 40 (9.6) |
| Use medication for thyroid disorder | 15 (3.6) | Iron | 1 (0.2) |
| Used iodine supplements during pregnancy | 91 (21.9) | Other | 14 (3.4) |

Values are presented as mean ± SD and *n* (%).
[a]Body mass index before pregnancy.
[b]University or university college.
[c]Breastfeeding frequency among children still breastfed (*n* = 41). Missing values: 67 missing from women's BMI; 1 missing from mother's education; 1 missing from geographic area; 1 missing from use of medication for thyroid disorder; 93 missing from iodine supplements during pregnancy; 1 missing from tobacco use in pregnancy; 1 missing from work situation; 1 missing from gender of child; 77 missing from breastfeeding status; 21 missing from anthropometric measures of children; 90 missing from supplement use in children.

*Table 2.* Urinary iodine concentration (UIC) among Norwegian toddlers 18 months of age by different geographical regions and characteristics (*n* = 416)

| | UIC (µg/L) | | | | Min | Max |
|---|---|---|---|---|---|---|
| | Median | p25–p75 | Mean | SD | | |
| Total (*n* = 416) | 129 | 81–190 | 148 | 97 | 8 | 688 |
| Gender | | | | | | |
| Boys (*n* = 217) | 139 | 83–258 | 147 | 95 | 12 | 687 |
| Girls (*n* = 198) | 128 | 75–199 | 150 | 100 | 8 | 688 |
| Geographic region | | | | | | |
| Mid-Norway (*n* = 134) | 125 | 69–186 | 138 | 83 | 8 | 426 |
| North Norway (*n* = 80) | 136 | 94–195 | 149 | 83 | 17 | 349 |
| Western Norway (*n* = 89) | 144 | 88–220 | 170 | 125 | 14 | 688 |
| Eastern Norway (*n* = 112) | 125 | 75–182 | 143 | 95 | 14 | 515 |
| Breastfeeding status | | | | | | |
| Never been breastfed (*n* = 19) | 149 | 76–212 | 169 | 126 | 24 | 515 |
| Stopped breastfeeding (*n* = 279) | 130 | 74–201 | 146 | 91 | 8 | 539 |
| Still breastfed (*n* = 41) | 117 | 85–188 | 144 | 87 | 19 | 422 |
| Kindergarten attendance | | | | | | |
| Yes (*n* = 332) | 131 | 81–190 | 148 | 94 | 8 | 687 |
| No (*n* = 68) | 126 | 73–195 | 148 | 114 | 16 | 688 |

There were no significant differences in UIC between gender ($p = 0.461$), geographic areas ($p = 0.321$), breastfeeding status ($p = 0.854$), or kindergarten attendance ($p = 0,311$) tested by Kruskal–Wallis test/Mann–Whitney U test.

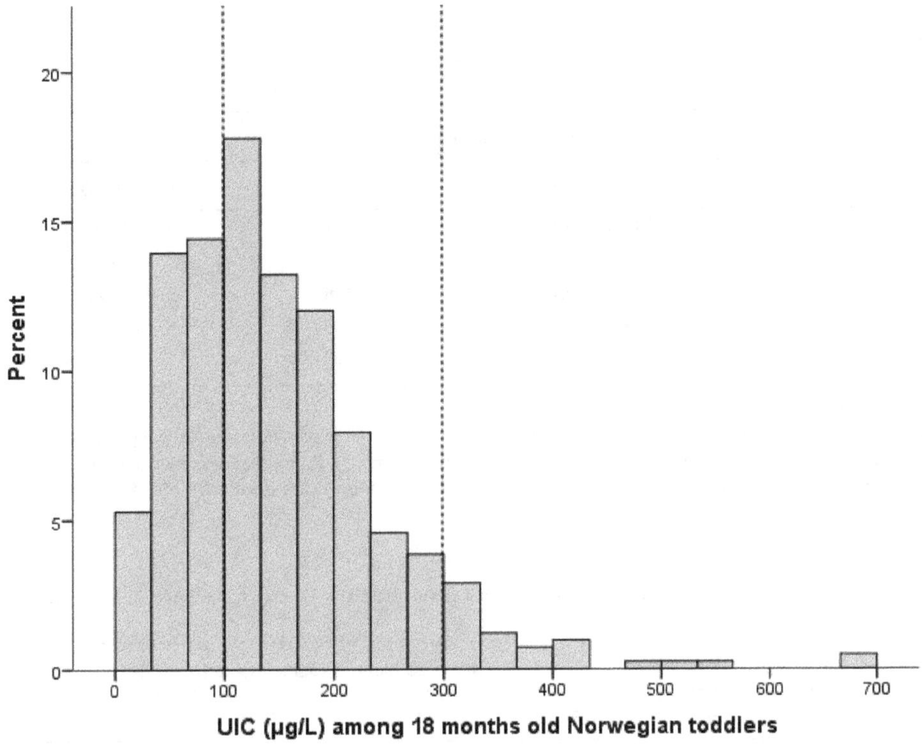


*Fig. 1.* Distribution of urinary iodine concentration (UIC) among Norwegian children 18 months of age: 33% had UIC below 100 µg/L, 59% had UIC between 100 and 299 µg/L, and 7% had UIC above 300 µg/L ($n$ = 416).

*Table 3.* Frequency of intake (times/week) of iodine-rich foods among Norwegian toddlers 18 months of age ($n$ = 340[a])

| Iodine-rich foods | Never/rarely | 1 time per week | 2–3 times per week | ≥4 times per week |
|---|---|---|---|---|
| | *n* (%) | *n* (%) | *n* (%) | *n* (%) |
| Yoghurt | 41 (12) | 35 (10) | 95 (28) | 169 (50) |
| Porridge (industry manufactured) | 193 (57) | 28 (8) | 37 (11) | 82 (24) |
| Porridge (homemade) | 147 (43) | 85 (25) | 62 (18) | 46 (14) |
| Fatty fish, dinner | 69 (20) | 202 (59) | 67 (20) | 2 (1) |
| Lean fish, dinner | 80 (19) | 221 (53) | 39 (12) | 0 |
| Fish products, dinner | 55 (16) | 225 (66) | 55 (16) | 5 (2) |
| Baby food with fish (industry manufactured) | 296 (87) | 28 (8) | 15 (4) | 1 (0.3) |
| Fatty fish, spread | 171 (50) | 64 (19) | 64 (19) | 41 (12) |
| Lean fish, spread | 141 (42) | 78 (23) | 87 (26) | 34 (10) |
| Eggs | 86 (32) | 96 (36) | 63 (24) | 22 (8) |

Values given in *n* (%) within participants with dietary intake category.
[a]*n* = 340 for all foods except eggs where *n* = 267.

once a week. Lean fish products such as caviar and fish-cakes and fatty fish products such as mackerel or salmon were consumed as bread spread among 31 and 36% 2–3 times/week or more frequently, respectively, while the rest consumed fish as bread topping ≤1 time/week. Sixty-eight percent consumed eggs less than or equal to once a week.

UIC according to low/medium and high consumption frequencies of iodine-rich foods is shown in Table 4. There were no substantially or statistically significant differences in UIC between the different consumption categories for any of the foods. There were quite a few children with a high consumption frequency of fish (20%). Yoghurt was more frequently consumed, and 50% had a high intake. Only 12% had a high frequency in intake of both fish and yoghurt. Industry-manufactured porridge is enriched with iodine in Norway; nevertheless, there were no difference in

*Table 4.* Urinary iodine concentration (UIC) among Norwegian toddlers 18 months of age with low/medium consumption frequency and high consumption frequency of iodine-rich foods ($n$ = 340)

| | UIC (µg/L) | | | |
|---|---|---|---|---|
| | Low/medium consumption | | High consumption[a] | |
| | Median (p25–p75) | *n* | Median (p25–p75) | *n* |
| Fish | 134 (83–200) | 271 | 117 (56–200) | 69 |
| Yoghurt | 123 (79–200) | 171 | 132 (75–200) | 169 |
| Fish and yoghurt | 131 (81–200) | 298 | 117 (55–198) | 42 |
| Porridge, industry-manufactured | 129 (81–193) | 258 | 123 (55–208) | 82 |
| Porridge, homemade | 129 (76–205) | 294 | 119 (73–185) | 46 |

Values given as median (p25–p75).
[a]Fish: Lean fish or fish products for dinner at least 2–3 times/week, and lean fish or fatty fish as bread topping at least 4–6 times/week. Yoghurt: at least 4–6 times/week. Fish and yoghurt: both intake of fish and yoghurt was high. Porridge (homemade or industry-manufactured): at least 4–6 times/week. Differences in UIC between consumption frequencies were tested by Mann–Whitney U test for each of the food groups. None were statistically significant.

*Table 5.* Estimated habitual iodine intake among non-breastfed Norwegian toddlers 18 months of age in different geographical regions of Norway ($n$ = 232[a])

| | Estimated habitual iodine intake (µg/day) | | | | | |
|---|---|---|---|---|---|---|
| | Median | p25–p75 | Mean | SD | Min | Max |
| Total (*n* = 232) | 109 | 101–117 | 110 | 13 | 82 | 157 |
| Geographic region | | | | | | |
| Mid-Norway (*n* = 76) | 110 | 101–116 | 109 | 11 | 90 | 157 |
| North Norway (*n* = 44) | 105 | 97–120 | 105 | 12 | 84 | 149 |
| Western Norway (*n* = 51) | 107 | 101–118 | 109 | 13 | 82 | 138 |
| Eastern Norway (*n* = 61) | 113 | 102–124 | 114 | 14 | 88 | 145 |

[a]149 missing from dietary data and 35 excluded as they were still breastfed. Iodine intake from milk and cheese have been estimated based on data from 2-year-old children (18) and were estimated to contribute 79 µg iodine/day.

median UIC between the group who received homemade porridge and those who received industry-manufactured porridge.

All the dietary variables among children included in Table 4, as well as background characteristics of the mothers and children, were tested for associations in linear regression models. None of the food consumption variables or background characteristics for mothers or children had a significant association with the children's UIC. Table 5 shows the estimated habitual iodine intake from the main dietary iodine sources (yoghurt, milk, cheese, fish/fish products, porridge, eggs, butter/margarine) among non-breastfed children 18 months of age in Norway. Estimated median (p25–p75) habitual iodine intake was 109 (101–117) µg/day for all children across geographic regions (where the estimated iodine contribution from milk and cheese is included). There was no substantial difference in estimated habitual iodine intake between the different geographic regions. None of the children were below the EAR (65 µg/day) or above the UL (180 µg/day). Estimated iodine intake from milk and cheese contributed about 72% of the total iodine mean intake, while fish contributed about 12% and other foods about 16%.

## Discussion

The Norwegian toddlers in this study had adequate iodine status, as indicated by a median UIC of 129 µg/L, which is above the WHO cutoff of 100 µg/L. This finding was supported by the estimated habitual iodine intake, which was 109 µg/day. None of the children had an estimated habitual iodine intake below the EAR of 65 µg/day or above the UL of 180 µg/day. There were no substantial differences in either UIC or iodine intake between different geographic areas of Norway. These findings are in line with the local small-scale Norwegian studies among toddlers with cow's milk protein allergy and young children presented in the introduction (25–27).

Infant formula is enriched with iodine in Norway, and the average iodine content of several products of prepared formula intended for consumption from 6 months age, using data from the food composition table, is 15 μg/100 g (29). A recent study among lactating Norwegian women found that the median iodine concentration in breast milk was 68 μg/L (7 μg/100 g) (20), about half of the iodine content found in formula. The children who were never breastfed might still receive formula at 18 months of age, which could explain why the median UIC was highest in this group. A correlation with UIC and use of infant formula has been reported by others (35, 36). Similar results to ours were also found in the mentioned study of 57 infants under the age of 2 with cow's milk protein allergy, where the breastfed children had lower UIC than the children who received formula or were weaned (27).

Intake of milk, formula, and cheese was not recorded in this study, which is a major limitation to the dietary data, as milk is an important component in the diet of young Norwegian children (17, 18). In our study, yoghurt was the most frequently consumed iodine-rich food. Fish and fish products were not as frequently consumed and about 52% consumed fish or fish products (all types) for dinner no more than once a week and 42% as bread spread no more than once a week (data not shown). Similar results were found in a Norwegian study among preschool children (4–6 years of age); however, the consumption of fish as bread spread was higher than in our study (26). Portion sizes were not registered in this study; however data from all the Nordic countries suggest that fish consumption is generally low among preschool children, including Norway (37). This is in line with our findings, where the majority had an intake below the recommendation for 2-year-old children (38). We did not find any substantial difference in UIC between different consumption frequencies of yoghurt, fish, porridge, or eggs, which was in line with the findings from the regression model where none of the dietary intake variables were associated with UIC. This suggests that milk probably made a large contribution to the total iodine intake among the children in this study. Milk as an important contributor to young children's iodine status in Norway has also been found by others (25). Recent studies suggest that pregnant and lactating women in Norway have mild to moderate iodine deficiency (20–23). Others have also found adequate iodine status among children, while mothers from the same population were iodine deficient (39–41). In line with our findings, this has been suggested to be caused by a relatively higher consumption of milk among children (25, 39). On the other hand, as pointed out by Trøan et al., children with a high milk consumption may be at risk of excessive iodine intakes in Norway as the iodine content of milk is relatively high (42).

The median estimated habitual iodine intake was lower than the median UIC. There are several challenges related to dietary assessment, in addition to the mentioned limitation of using extrapolated intake values for milk and cheese. Only the main dietary iodine-containing food items were included in the estimated habitual intake, and missed sources (e.g. vegetables, meat, and bread) cannot be ruled out. Portion sizes from a national survey among 2-year-old children were used. As dietary habits rapidly change in the weaning period (43), the portion sizes may not be accurate for toddlers 18 months of age. Also, most toddlers in this study were attending kindergarten (79.8%, data not shown), which may further complicate dietary assessment as the parents have less control of food consumption. Nevertheless, the estimated habitual iodine intake indicated sufficient iodine status in this age group, which was in line with the WHO epidemiological criteria for assessing iodine nutrition by median UIC. Further, the estimated habitual iodine intake allows one to assess the iodine status at an individual level, as opposed to the UIC, which provides valuable information. None of the children had an estimated iodine intake below the EAR or above the UL.

## Conclusion

Iodine is a crucial nutrient during the first 1,000 days of life (44), and children under 2 years of age have been identified as a particularly vulnerable group for inadequate iodine intake by the WHO (31). Thus, the iodine status among young children should be carefully monitored. This study showed that the iodine status among 18-month-old toddlers was sufficient. Further, milk seemed to be the major iodine-contributing food item among these children, and the intake of fish and enriched porridge was low. Children with low intake of milk could therefore potentially be at risk of insufficient iodine intake in Norway.

## Acknowledgements

We are grateful to all the families that participated in the Little in Norway study and all research assistants at the public health clinics. A special warm thanks to Unni Tranaas Vannebo for her positive and enthusiastic engagement in organizing the project data collection. Thanks to Anne Karin Syversen for taking care of all the collected biological samples and to Tonja Lill Eidsvik and Berit Solli for technical assistance with the laboratory work. The Research Council of Norway (grant number 196156) and the Norwegian Seafood Research Fund, FHF (grant number 900842) supported the work.

## Conflict of interest and funding

The authors declare no conflict of interest. The Research Council of Norway (grant number 196156) and the Norwegian Seafood Research Fund, Fiskeri og Havbruksnæringens Forskningsfond (grant number 900842) supported the work.

## References


1. Zimmermann MB, Jooste PL, Pandav CS. Iodine-deficiency disorders. Lancet 2008; 372(9645): 1251–62. https://doi.org/10.1016/S0140-6736(08)61005-3.
2. Zimmermann BM. The role of iodine in human growth and development. Semin Cell Dev Biol 2011; 22(6): 645–52. https://doi.org/10.1016/j.semcdb.2011.07.009.
3. Brent GA. Mechanisms of thyroid hormone action. J Clin Invest 2012; 122(9): 3035–43. https://doi.org/10.1172/JCI60047
4. Bernal J. Thyroid hormones and brain development. Vitam Horm 2005; 71: 95–122. https://doi.org/10.1016/S0083-6729(05)71004-9.
5. Walker SP, Wachs TD, Grantham-McGregor S, Black MM, Nelson CA, Huffman SL, et al. Inequality in early childhood: risk and protective factors for early child development. Lancet 2011; 378(9799): 1325–38. https://doi.org/10.1016/S0140-6736(11)60555-2.
6. Andersson M, Karumbunathan V, Zimmermann MB. Global iodine status in 2011 and trends over the past decade. J Nutr 2012; 142(4): 744–50. https://doi.org/10.3945/jn.111.149393.
7. IGN. Iodine Global Network, 2016. Annual Report. Zürich, Switzerland: Iodine Global Network; 2016.
8. Lazarus JH. Iodine status in Europe in 2014. Eur Thyroid J 2014; 3(1): 3–6. https://doi.org/10.1159/000358873.
9. Nyström HF, Brantsæter AL, Erlund I, Gunnarsdottir I, Hulthén L, Laurberg P, et al. Iodine status in the Nordic countries – past and present. Food Nutr Res 2016; 60(1): 31969. https://doi.org/10.3402/fnr.v60.31969.
10. Bath SC, Steer CD, Golding J, Emmett P, Rayman MP. Effect of inadequate iodine status in UK pregnant women on cognitive outcomes in their children: results from the Avon Longitudinal Study of Parents and Children (ALSPAC). Lancet 2013; 382(9889): 331–7. https://doi.org/10.1016/S0140-6736(13)60436-5.
11. Manousou S, Dahl L, Heinsbaek Thuesen B, Hulthen L, Nystrom Filipsson H. Iodine deficiency and nutrition in Scandinavia. Minerva Med 2017; 108(2): 147–58. https://doi.org/10.23736/S0026-4806.16.04849-7.
12. Torlinska B, Bath S, Janjua A, Boelaert K, Chan S-Y. Iodine status during pregnancy in a region of mild-to-moderate iodine deficiency is not associated with adverse obstetric outcomes; Results from the Avon Longitudinal Study of Parents and Children (ALSPAC). Nutrients 2018; 10(3): 291. http://dx.doi.org/10.3390/nu10030291.
13. WHO. Assessment of iodine deficiency disorders and monitoring their elimination. A guide for programme managers. Geneva, Switzerland: World Health Organization, International Council for Control of Iodine Deficiency Disorders, United Nations Children's Fund; 2007.
14. Dahl L, Meltzer HM. The iodine content of foods and diets: Norwegian perspectives. In: Preedy VR, Burrow GN, Watson RR, eds. Comprehensive handbook of iodine. Nutritional, biochemical, pathological and therapeutic aspects. London: Academic Press; 2009, pp. 345–52.
15. Nerhus I, Wik Markhus M, Nilsen BM, Øyen J, Maage A, Ødegård ER, et al. Iodine content of six fish species, Norwegian dairy products and hen's egg. 2018; p. 62. Available from: https://dx.doi.org/10.29219/fnr.v62.1291 [cited 25 May 2018].
16. Meltzer HM, Torheim LE, Brandsæter AL, Madar A, Abel MH, Dahl L. Risiko for jodmangel i Norge. Identifisering av et akutt behov for tiltak. Oslo, Norway: Nasjonalt råd for ernæring; 2016.
17. Lande B, Helleve A. Amming og spedbarns kosthold. Landsomfattende undersøkelse 2013. Oslo: The Norwegian Directorate of Health; 2013.
18. Kristiansen AL, Frost AL, Lande B. Diet among 2 year olds. National dietary survey – Småbarnskost. Oslo, Norway: The Norwegian Directorate of Health; 2009.
19. Nordic Council of Ministers. Nordic Nutrition Recommendations 2012: integrating nutrition and physical activity. 5 ed. Copenhagen: Nordisk Ministerråd; 2014, 627 p. http://dx.doi.org/10.6027/Nord2014-002.
20. Henjum S, Lilleengen AM, Aakre I, Dudareva A, Gjengedal ELF, Meltzer HM, et al. Suboptimal iodine concentration in breastmilk and inadequate iodine intake among lactating women in Norway. Nutrients 2017; 9(7): 643. https://doi.org/10.3390/nu9070643.
21. Brantsæter AL, Abel MH, Haugen M, Meltzer HM. Risk of suboptimal iodine intake in pregnant Norwegian women. Nutrients 2013; 5(2): 424–40. http://dx.doi.org/10.3390/nu5020424.
22. Henjum S, Aakre I, Lilleengen A, Garnweidner-Holme L, Borthne S, Pajalic Z, et al. Suboptimal iodine status among pregnant women in the Oslo Area, Norway. Nutrients 2018; 10(3): 280. http://dx.doi.org/10.3390/nu10030280.
23. Dahl L, Wik Markhus M, Sanchez P, Moe V, Smith L, Meltzer H, et al. Iodine Deficiency in a study population of Norwegian pregnant women – results from the little in Norway Study (LiN). Nutrients 2018; 10(4): 513. https://doi.org/10.3390/nu10040513.
24. Abel MH, Caspersen IH, Meltzer HM, Haugen M, Brandlistuen RE, Aase H, et al. Suboptimal maternal iodine intake is associated with impaired child neurodevelopment at 3 years of age in the Norwegian Mother and Child Cohort Study. J Nutr 2017; 147(7): 1314–24.https://doi.org/10.3945/jn.117.250456.
25. Brantsæter A, Knutsen H, Johansen N, Nyheim K, Erlund I, Meltzer H, et al. Inadequate iodine intake in population groups defined by age, life stage and vegetarian dietary practice in a Norwegian convenience sample. Nutrients 2018; 10(2): 230. https://doi.org/10.3390/nu10020230.
26. Nerhus I, Odland M, Kjellevold M, Midtbø LK, Markhus MK, Graff IE, et al. Iodine status in Norwegian preschool children and associations with dietary sources of iodine – FINS-KIDS study. Eur J Nutr 2018: 1–9. https://doi.org/10.1007/s00394-018-1768-0.
27. Thomassen RA, Kvammen JA, Eskerud MB, Júlíusson PB, Henriksen C, Rugtveit J. Iodine status and growth in 0–2-year-old infants with cow's milk protein allergy. J Pediatr Gastroenterol Nutr 2017; 64(5): 806–11. doi: 10.1097/MPG.0000000000001434.
28. Fredriksen E, von Soest T, Smith L, Moe V. Parenting stress plays a mediating role in the prediction of early child development from both parents' perinatal depressive symptoms. J Abnorm Child Psychol 2018: 1–6. https://doi.org/10.1007/s10802-018-0428-4.
29. Norwegian Food Safety Authority, The Norwegian Directorate of Health, University of Oslo. The Norwegian food composition table. Oslo, Norway: Norwegian Food Safety Authority, The Norwegian Directorate of Health, University of Oslo; 2011.
30. IOM. Reference intakes for vitamin A, vitamin k, arsenic, boron, chromium, copper, iodine, iron, manganese, molybdenum, nickel, silicon, vanadium and zinc: a report of the Panel on Micronutrients, Subcommittees on Upper Reference Levels of Nutrients and Interpretation and Uses of Dietary Reference Intakes, and the Standing Committee on the Scientific Evaluation of Dietary Reference Intakes. Washington, DC: Institute of Medicine; 2001.
31. Andersson M, De Benoist B, Delange F, Zupan J, Secretariat W. Prevention and control of iodine deficiency in pregnant

and lactating women and in children less than 2-years-old: conclusions and recommendations of the technical consultation. Public Health Nutr 2007; 10(12): 1606. https://doi.org/10.1017/S1368980007361004.
32. WHO. Global database on body mass index. BMI classification: World Health Organization; 2004. Available from: http://apps.who.int/bmi/index.jsp?introPage=intro_3.html [cited 29 May 2018].
33. WHO. WHO Anthro (version 3.2.2, January 2011) and macros 2011. Available from: http://www.who.int/childgrowth/software/en/ [cited 20 May 2018].
34. WHO. WHO Child Growth Standards. Length/height-for age, weight-for -age, weight-for-length, weight-for-height and body mass index-for-age. Methods and development. Geneva, Switzerland: World Health Organization; 2006.
35. Skeaff SA, Ferguson EL, McKenzie JE, Valeix P, Gibson RS, Thomson CD. Are breast-fed infants and toddlers in New Zealand at risk of iodine deficiency? Nutrition 2005; 21(3): 325–31. https://doi.org/10.1016/j.nut.2004.07.004.
36. Andersson M, Aeberli I, Wüst N, Piacenza AM, Bucher T, Henschen I, et al. The Swiss iodized salt program provides adequate iodine for school children and pregnant women, but weaning infants not receiving iodine-containing complementary foods as well as their mothers are iodine deficient. J Clin Endocrinol Metab 2010; 95(12): 5217–24. https://doi.org/10.1210/jc.2010-0975.
37. Fagt S, Gunnarsdottir I, Hallas-Møller T, Helldán A, Ingi Halldorsson T, Knutsen H, et al. Nordic dietary surveys: study designs, methods, results and use in food-based risk assessments. Copenhagen: Nordic Council of Ministers; 2012.
38. Norwegian Directorate of Health. Norwegian guidelines on diet, nutrition and physical activity. Oslo, Norway: Norwegian Directorate of Health; 2014.
39. Vandevijvere S, Mourri AB, Amsalkhir S, Avni F, Oyen HV, Moreno-Reyes R. Fortification of bread with iodized salt corrected iodine deficiency in school-aged children, but not in their mothers: a national cross-sectional survey in Belgium. Thyroid 2012; 22(10): 1046–53. https://doi.org/10.1089/thy.2012.0016.
40. Andersson M, Berg G, Eggertsen R, Filipsson H, Gramatkovski E, Hansson M, et al. Adequate iodine nutrition in Sweden: a cross-sectional national study of urinary iodine concentration in school-age children. Eur J Clin Nutr 2009; 63(7): 828–34. doi: 10.1038/ejcn.2008.46.
41. Granfors M, Andersson M, Stinca S, Akerud H, Skalkidou A, Poromaa IS, et al. Iodine deficiency in a study population of pregnant women in Sweden. Acta Obstet Gynecol Scand 2015; 94(11): 1168–74. https://doi.org/10.1111/aogs.12713.
42. Trøan G, Dahl L, Margrete Meltzer H, Hope Abel M, Geir Indahl U, Haug A, et al. A model to secure a stable iodine concentration in milk. Food Nutr Res 2015; 59(1): 29829. https://doi.org/10.3402/fnr.v59.29829.
43. WHO. Guiding principles for complementary feeding of the breastfed child. Geneva, Switzerland: World Health Organization; 2003.
44. Velasco I, Bath S, Rayman M. Iodine as essential nutrient during the first 1000 days of life. Nutrients 2018; 10(3): 290. http://dx.doi.org/10.3390/nu10030290.

***Inger Aakre**
Institute of Marine Research
P.O. Box 2029 Nordnes
NO-5817 Bergen, Norway
Email: inger.aakre@hi.no

# Permissions

All chapters in this book were first published in F&NR, by Swedish Nutrition Foundation; hereby published with permission under the Creative Commons Attribution License or equivalent. Every chapter published in this book has been scrutinized by our experts. Their significance has been extensively debated. The topics covered herein carry significant findings which will fuel the growth of the discipline. They may even be implemented as practical applications or may be referred to as a beginning point for another development.

The contributors of this book come from diverse backgrounds, making this book a truly international effort. This book will bring forth new frontiers with its revolutionizing research information and detailed analysis of the nascent developments around the world.

We would like to thank all the contributing authors for lending their expertise to make the book truly unique. They have played a crucial role in the development of this book. Without their invaluable contributions this book wouldn't have been possible. They have made vital efforts to compile up to date information on the varied aspects of this subject to make this book a valuable addition to the collection of many professionals and students.

This book was conceptualized with the vision of imparting up-to-date information and advanced data in this field. To ensure the same, a matchless editorial board was set up. Every individual on the board went through rigorous rounds of assessment to prove their worth. After which they invested a large part of their time researching and compiling the most relevant data for our readers.

The editorial board has been involved in producing this book since its inception. They have spent rigorous hours researching and exploring the diverse topics which have resulted in the successful publishing of this book. They have passed on their knowledge of decades through this book. To expedite this challenging task, the publisher supported the team at every step. A small team of assistant editors was also appointed to further simplify the editing procedure and attain best results for the readers.

Apart from the editorial board, the designing team has also invested a significant amount of their time in understanding the subject and creating the most relevant covers. They scrutinized every image to scout for the most suitable representation of the subject and create an appropriate cover for the book.

The publishing team has been an ardent support to the editorial, designing and production team. Their endless efforts to recruit the best for this project, has resulted in the accomplishment of this book. They are a veteran in the field of academics and their pool of knowledge is as vast as their experience in printing. Their expertise and guidance has proved useful at every step. Their uncompromising quality standards have made this book an exceptional effort. Their encouragement from time to time has been an inspiration for everyone.

The publisher and the editorial board hope that this book will prove to be a valuable piece of knowledge for researchers, students, practitioners and scholars across the globe.

# List of Contributors

**Priscilia Lianto and Huilian Che**
Beijing Advanced Innovation Center for Food Nutrition and Human Health, College of Food Science and Nutritional Engineering, China Agricultural University, Beijing, 100083, P.R. China
College of Food Science and Nutritional Engineering, China Agricultural University, Beijing, 100083, P.R. China

**Yani Zhang and Feng He**
College of Food Science and Nutritional Engineering, China Agricultural University, Beijing, 100083, P.R. China

**Fredrick O. Ogutu**
Food Technology Division of Kenya Industrial Research and Development Institute, South C – Popo Rd., Off Mombasa Rd., PO Box 30650-00100, Nairobi, Kenya

**Wenbo Ye, Liang Liu, Juan Yu, Qiang Yong and Yimin Fan**
Jiangsu Co-Innovation Center of Efficient Processing and Utilization of Forest Resources, Jiangsu Key Lab of Biomass-Based Green Fuel and Chemicals, College of Chemical Engineering, Nanjing Forestry University, Nanjing, China

**Shilin Liu**
College of Food Science and Technology, Huazhong Agricultural University, Wuhan, China

**Yueyue Meng, Bailiang Li, Da Jin, Meng Zhan, Jingjing Lu and Guicheng Huo**
Key Laboratory of Dairy Science, Ministry of Education, Northeast Agricultural University, Harbin, China

**Bodil Ohlsson, Gassan Darwiche and Bodil Roth**
Department of Internal Medicine, Skåne University Hospital, Lund University, Malmö, Sweden

**Peter Höglund**
Department of Clinical Chemistry and Pharmacology, Skåne University Hospital, Lund University, Lund, Sweden

**Elizabeth A. Wood and Katharine McNamara**
Department of Environmental & Global Health, College of Public Health and Health Professions, University of Florida, Gainesville, FL, USA

**Agata Kowalewska**
Department of Food Science & Human Nutrition, College of Agricultural and Life Sciences, University of Florida, Gainesville, FL, USA

**Nargiza Ludgate**
Department of Animal Sciences, College of Agriculture and Life Sciences, University of Florida, Gainesville, FL, USA

**Ruth J. Kamoto, William Kasapila and Tinna A. Ng'ong'ola-Manani**
Department of Food Science and Technology, Lilongwe University of Agriculture and Natural Resources (LUANAR), Lilongwe, Malawi

**Chenyan Lv, Yifei Wang, Cui Zhou, Weiwei Ma, Rong Xiao and Huanling Yu**
School of Public Health, Beijing Key Laboratory of Environmental Toxicology, Capital Medical University, Beijing, China

**Yuexin Yang**
National Institute for Nutrition and Health, Chinese Center for Disease Control and Prevention, Beijing, China

**Holly L. Rippin, Jayne Hutchinson, Charlotte E. L. Evans and Janet E. Cade**
Nutritional Epidemiology Group (NEG), School of Food Science and Nutrition, University of Leeds, Leeds, United Kingdom

**Jo Jewell and Joao J. Breda**
Division of Noncommunicable Diseases and Promoting Health through the Life-Course, World Health Organization Regional Office for Europe, UN City, Marmorvej 51, 21000 Copenhagen, Denmark

**Karianne Svendsen, Hege Berg Henriksen and Monica H. Carlsen**
Department of Nutrition, Institute of Basic Medical Sciences, University of Oslo, Oslo, Norway

**Beate Østengen and Vibeke H. Telle-Hansen**
Faculty of Health Sciences, Oslo Metropolitan University, Oslo, Norway

**David R. Jacobs Jr.**
Division of Epidemiology and Community Health, School of Public Health, University of Minnesota, Minneapolis, USA

**Kjetil Retterstøl**
Department of Nutrition, Institute of Basic Medical Sciences, University of Oslo, Oslo, Norway
The Lipid Clinic, Department of Endocrinology, Morbid Obesity and Preventive Medicine, Oslo University Hospital, Oslo, Norway

**Minxian Rong, Yuesheng Qiu, Yiyuan Wang and Hong Deng**
Department of Nutrition and Food Hygiene, Guangdong Provincial Key Laboratory of Tropical Disease Research, School of Public Health, Southern Medical University, Guangzhou, China

**Pei Wang**
Wuhan Centers for Disease Prevention and Control, Wuhan, China

**Yungang Liu**
Department of Toxicology, Guangdong Provincial Key Laboratory of Tropical Disease Research, School of Public Health, Southern Medical University, Guangzhou, China

**Evelina Höglund, Susanne Ekman and Berit Albinsson**
RISE Research Institutes of Sweden, Agrifood and Bioscience, Göteborg, Sweden

**Gunnel Stuhr-Olsson and Christina Lundgren**
Findus Special Foods, Bjuv, Sweden

**Michael Signäs**
Medirest Compass Group AB, Kista, Sweden

**Christina Karlsson**
ICA Sverige AB, Solna, Sweden

**Elisabet Rothenberg**
Food and Meal Science, Kristianstad University, Kristianstad, Sweden

**Karin Wendin**
Food and Meal Science, Kristianstad University, Kristianstad, Sweden
Department of Food Science, University of Copenhagen, Copenhagen, Denmark

**Asnake Ararsa Irenso and Gudina Egata Atomsa**
School of Public Health, Haramaya University, Harar, Ethiopia

**Jianguo Chen**
Inner Mongolia Mengniu Diary Industry Group Co, Ltd, China

**Xue Shi, Yang Chen and Qiyang He**
Institute of Medicinal Biotechnology, Peking Union Medical College and Chinese Academy of Medical Sciences, Beijing, China

**Hanqiao Liang and Chi Cheng**
China Center of Industrial Culture Collection, China National Research Institute of Food and Fermentation Industries, Beijing, China

**BoYoon Chang and SungYeon Kim**
Institute of Pharmaceutical Research and Development, College of Pharmacy, Wonkwang University, Iksan, Jeonbuk, South Korea

**BongSeong Koo and HyeonCheol Lee**
ForBioKorea Co., Ltd. Seoul, South Korea

**Joa Sub Oh**
College of Pharmacy, Dankook University, Cheonan, South Korea

**Conrad Murendo, Kizito Mazvimavi and Simon Gwara**
International Crops Research Institute for the Semi-Arid Tropics, Bulawayo, Zimbabwe

**Brighton Nhau**
United Nations, Food and Agriculture Organization, Harare, Zimbabwe

**Thamsanqa Khanye**
Community Technology Development Organization, Harare, Zimbabwe
Elisabet R. Hillesund, Elling Bere, Hilde L. Seiler, Monica K. Torstveit and Nina C. Øverby
Department of Public Health, Sports and Nutrition, University of Agder, Kristiansand, Norway

**Linda R. Sagedal and Ingvild Vistad**
Department of Obstetrics and Gynecology, Sørlandet Hospital HF, Kristiansand, Norway
Department of Research, Sørlandet Hospital HF, Kristiansand, Norway

**Anne Dahl Lassen, Sisse Fagt and Anne V. Thorsen**
Division for Risk Assessment and Nutrition, Technical University of Denmark, Kemitorvet, Lyngby, Denmark

**Maria Lennernäs**
Department of Occupational and Public Health Science, University of Gävle, Gävle, Sweden

**Maria Nyberg**
Department of Food and Meal Science, Kristianstad University, Kristianstad, Sweden

**Irja Haapalar**
School of Social and Political Sciences, The University of Melbourne, Melbourne, Victoria, Australia
School of Applied Educational Sciences and Teacher Education, Savonlinna, Finland

**Anna C. M. Møbjerg**
Institute for Nursing and Nutrition, University College Copenhagen, Copenhagen N, Denmark

**Anne M. Beck**
Institute for Nursing and Nutrition, University College Copenhagen, Copenhagen N, Denmark Clinical Nutrition Research Unit, Copenhagen University Hospital Herlev-Gentofte, Gentofte, Denmark

**Annie George**
Institute of Biological Sciences, Faculty of Science, University of Malaya, Kuala Lumpur, Malaysia
Biotropics Malaysia Berhad, Lot 21, Jalan U1/19, Section U1, Hicom-Glenmarie Industrial Park, 40150 Shah Alam, Malaysia

**Jay Udani**
Agoura Hills, CA, USA

**Nurhayati Zainal Abidin**
Institute of Biological Sciences, Faculty of Science, University of Malaya, Kuala Lumpur, Malaysia

**Ashril Yusof**
Exercise Science, Sports Centre, University of Malaya, 50603 Kuala Lumpur, Malaysia

**Xiujing Dou, Junlan Han, Qiuyuan Ma, Baojing Cheng, Anshan Shan, Nan Gao and Yu Yang**
Institute of Animal Nutrition, Northeast Agricultural University, Harbin, China

**Anthony O. Obilana**
Food Technology Department, Cape Peninsula University of Technology, Bellville Campus, Cape Town, South Africa

**Barthi Odhav**
Biotechnology and Food Technology Department, Durban University of Technology, Durban, South Africa

**Victoria A. Jideani**
Food Technology Department, Cape Peninsula University of Technology, Bellville Campus, Cape Town, South Africa

**Inger Aakre**
Food Security and Nutrition, Institute of Marine Research, Bergen, Norway

**Maria Wik Markhus**
Food Security and Nutrition, Institute of Marine Research, Bergen, Norway

# Index

www.ingramcontent.com/pod-product-compliance
Lightning Source LLC
LaVergne TN
LVHW060519210926
848485LV00005B/1106